SARCOMAS

SARCOMAS

Evidence-Based Diagnosis and Management

EDITORS

Jonathan C. Trent, MD, PhD
Professor of Medicine
Director, Sarcoma Program
Associate Director for Clinical Research
Sylvester Comprehensive Cancer Center
University of Miami Health System
Miami, Florida

Andrew E. Rosenberg, MD
Professor and Vice Chair
Director, Bone and Soft Tissue Pathology
Department of Pathology
Miller School of Medicine
University of Miami
Miami, Florida

Raphael Pollock, MD, PhD, FACS
Director
Kathleen Wellenreiter Kotz Chair in Cancer Research
The Ohio State University Comprehensive Cancer Center
Columbus, Ohio

Thomas F. DeLaney, MD
Andres Soriano Professor of Radiation Oncology, Harvard Medical School
Radiation Oncologist, Department of Radiation Oncology
Associate Medical Director, Francis H. Burr Proton Therapy Center
Co-Director, Center for Sarcoma and Connective Tissue Oncology
Massachusetts General Hospital
Boston, Massachusetts

demosMEDICAL
An Imprint of Springer Publishing

Springer Publishing Company, LLC
11 West 42nd Street, New York, NY 10036
www.springerpub.com
connect.springerpub.com/

Acquisitions Editor: David D'Addona
Compositor: Exeter Premedia Services Private Ltd.

ISBN: 978-0-8261-4852-0
ebook ISBN: 978-0-8261-4853-7
DOI: 10.1891/9780826148537

20 21 22 23 24 / 5 4 3 2

The author and the publisher of this Work have made every effort to use sources believed to be reliable to provide information that is accurate and compatible with the standards generally accepted at the time of publication. Because medical science is continually advancing, our knowledge base continues to expand. Therefore, as new information becomes available, changes in procedures become necessary. We recommend that the reader always consult current research and specific institutional policies before performing any clinical procedure or delivering any medication. The author and publisher shall not be liable for any special, consequential, or exemplary damages resulting, in whole or in part, from the readers' use of, or reliance on, the information contained in this book. The publisher has no responsibility for the persistence or accuracy of URLs for external or third-party Internet websites referred to in this publication and does not guarantee that any content on such websites is, or will remain, accurate or appropriate.

Medicine is an ever-changing science. Research and clinical experience are continually expanding our knowledge, in particular our understanding of proper treatment and drug therapy. The authors, editors, and publisher have made every effort to ensure that all information in this book is in accordance with the state of knowledge at the time of production of the book. Nevertheless, the authors, editors, and publisher are not responsible for any errors or omissions or for any consequence from application of the information in this book and make no warranty, expressed or implied, with respect to the content of this publication. Every reader should examine carefully the package inserts accompanying each drug and should carefully check whether the dosage schedules therein or the contraindications stated by the manufacturer differ from the statements made in this book. Such examination is particularly important with drugs that are either rarely used or have been newly released on the market.

Library of Congress Cataloging-in-Publication Data

Names: Trent, Jonathan C., editor. | Rosenberg, Andrew, 1953- editor. | Pollock, Raphael E., editor. | De Laney, Thomas F., editor.
Title: Sarcomas : evidence-based diagnosis and management / editors, Jonathan C. Trent, Andrew E. Rosenberg, Raphael Pollock, Thomas F. DeLaney.
Other titles: Sarcomas (Trent)
Description: New York, NY : Demos Medical Publishing, [2020] | Includes bibliographical references and index.
Identifiers: LCCN 2020011266 (print) | LCCN 2020011267 (ebook) | ISBN 9780826148520 (hardcover) | ISBN 9780826148537 (ebook)
Subjects: MESH: Sarcoma—diagnosis | Sarcoma—therapy
Classification: LCC RC263 (print) | LCC RC263 (ebook) | NLM QZ 345 | DDC 616.99/4—dc23
LC record available at https://lccn.loc.gov/2020011266
LC ebook record available at https://lccn.loc.gov/2020011267

Jonathan C. Trent: https://orcid.org/0000-0001-6169-5238
Andrew E. Rosenberg: https://orcid.org/0000-0002-4536-8824
Raphael Pollock: https://orcid.org/0000-0002-0443-1583
Thomas F. DeLaney: https://orcid.org/0000-0002-0346-3487

Publisher's Note: **New and used products purchased from third-party sellers are not guaranteed for quality, authenticity, or access to any included digital components.**

Printed in the United States.

Contents

Contributors

Pamela Abdayem, MD, Medical Oncologist, Department of Medical Oncology, Gustave Roussy, Villejuif, France

Mark Agulnik, MD, Professor, Division of Hematology/Oncology, Northwestern University, Chicago, Illinois

Catherine M. Albert, MD, Assistant Professor, Seattle Children's Research Institute, Seattle, Washington; Department of Pediatrics, University of Washington, Seattle, Washington

Borislav A. Alexiev, MD, Associate Professor, Division of Pathology, Northwestern University, Chicago, Illinois

Warren Alperstein, MD, Assistant Professor, Department of Pediatrics, Miller School of Medicine, University of Miami, Miami, Florida

Giacomo Giulio Baldi, MD, Medical Oncologist, Mesenchymal Tumor and Rare Cancer Unit, Department of Cancer Medicine, Fondazione IRCCS Istituto Nazionale dei Tumori, Milan, Italy; Medical Oncologist, Department of Medical Oncology, Hospital of Prato, Prato, Italy

Meena Bedi, MD, Associate Professor, Department of Radiation Oncology, Medical College of Wisconsin, Milwaukee, Wisconsin

Robert S. Benjamin, MD, Clinical Professor, Department of Sarcoma Medical Oncology, The University of Texas MD Anderson Cancer Center, Houston, Texas

Jomjit Chantharasamee, MD, Clinical Instructor, Department of Medicine, Faculty of Medicine, Siriraj Hospital, Mahidol University, Bangkok, Thailand

John Charlson, MD, Associate Professor, Division of Hematology–Oncology, Medical College of Wisconsin, Milwaukee, Wisconsin

Edward Y. Cheng, MD, Mairs Family Professor, Department of Orthopaedic Surgery and Cancer Center, University of Minnesota, Minneapolis, Minnesota

Matthew Chin, MD, MS, Orthopaedic Oncology Fellow, Department of Orthopaedic Oncology, The University of Texas MD Anderson Cancer Center, Houston, Texas

Sheila Ann Conway, MD, FAOA, Professor and Chief, Division of Orthopedic Oncology, Program Director, Orthopedic Surgery Residency, Program Director, Musculoskeletal Oncology Fellowship Program, Department of Orthopedics, Miller School of Medicine, University of Miami, Miami, Florida

Angelo Paolo Dei Tos, MD, Professor of Pathology, Department of Medicine, University of Padua School of Medicine, Padua, Italy

Julio A. Diaz-Perez, MD, Fellow in Bone and Soft Tissue Pathology, Department of Pathology, Miller School of Medicine, University of Miami, Miami, Florida

Sarah Dumont, MD, PhD, Medical Oncologist, Department of Medical Oncology, Gustave Roussy, Villejuif, France

Andrea P. Espejo-Freire, MD, Hematology/Oncology Fellow, Division of Hematology/Oncology, Department of Medicine, Sylvester Comprehensive Cancer Center, Miller School of Medicine, University of Miami, Miami, Florida

Chiara Fabbroni, MD, Medical Oncologist in training, Department of Medical Oncology, Fondazione IRCCS Istituto Nazionale dei Tumori, Milan, Italy

Mark Fairweather, MD, Assistant Professor, Department of Surgery, Brigham and Women's Hospital, Center for Sarcoma and Bone Oncology, Dana-Farber Cancer Institute, Boston, Massachusetts

Stéphanie Gaillard, MD, PhD, Assistant Professor, Department of Oncology, Division of Gynecology Oncology, Department of Gynecology and Obstetrics, Johns Hopkins School of Medicine, Baltimore, Maryland

Erika L. Garbrecht, MD, Orthopedic Musculoskeletal Oncology Fellow, Department of Orthopedics, Jackson Memorial Hospital, University of Miami, Miami, Florida

Suzanne George, MD, Clinical Director, Center for Sarcoma and Bone Oncology, Dana-Farber Cancer Institute, Harvard Medical School, Boston, Massachusetts

Valerie P. Grignol, MD, Assistant Professor of Surgery, Division of Surgical Oncology, Department of Surgery, The Ohio State University, Columbus, Ohio

Alessandro Gronchi, MD, Chair of Sarcoma Service, Department of Surgery, Fondazione IRCCS Istituto Nazionale dei Tumori, Milan, Italy

John C. Hardaway, MD PhD, Fellow, Department of Surgical Oncology, Roger Williams Medical Center, Providence, Rhode Island; Department of Surgery, Boston University School of Medicine, Boston, Massachusetts

Sara E. Helmig, MD, Assistant Member, Solid Tumor Division, St. Jude Children's Research Hospital, Memphis, Tennessee

Francis Hornicek, MD, PhD, Chair, Department of Orthopaedic Surgery, UCLA, Los Angeles, California

Chelsea R. Horwood, MD, MPH, PGY4 General Surgery Resident, Wexner Medical Center, The Ohio State University, Columbus, Ohio

Emily E. Jonczak, MD, Division of Hematology/Oncology, Department of Medicine, Sylvester Comprehensive Cancer Center, Miller School of Medicine, University of Miami, Miami, Florida

Steven C. Katz, MD, Associate Professor, Department of Surgical Oncology, Roger Williams Medical Center, Providence, Rhode Island; Department of Surgery, Boston University School of Medicine, Boston, Massachusetts

David M. King, MD, Chairman and Paul A. Jacobs, MD, Professor in Orthopedic Surgery, Medical College of Wisconsin, Milwaukee, Wisconsin

David G. Kirsch, MD, PhD, Barbara Levine University Professor, Vice Chair for Basic and Translational Research, Department of Radiation Oncology, Duke University Medical Center, Durham, North Carolina

Jessica W. Lee, MD, Resident, Department of Radiation Oncology, Duke University Medical Center, Durham, North Carolina

Luyuan Li, MD, PhD, Post-doctoral Fellow, Sylvester Comprehensive Cancer Center, University of Miami Health System, Miami, Florida

David Liebner, MD, Assistant Professor of Medicine, The Ohio State University Comprehensive Cancer Center, Columbus, Ohio

J. Andrew Livingston, MD, MS, Assistant Professor, Department of Sarcoma Medical Oncology, The University of Texas MD Anderson Cancer Center, Houston, Texas

Motasem Al Maaieh, MD, Associate Professor, Director of Spinal Oncology, Department of Orthopedic Surgery, University of Miami, Miami, Florida

A. Craig Mackinnon, MD, PhD, Director, Division of Genomics, Diagnostics, and Bioinformatics; Professor, Department of Pathology, The University of Alabama at Birmingham, Birmingham, Alabama

Kyle Maughan, BA, Medical Student, Department of Interventional Radiology, Miller School of Medicine, University of Miami, Miami, Florida

Prasoon Mohan, MD, Assistant Professor, Department of Clinical Interventional Radiology, Jackson Memorial Hospital, University of Miami, Miami, Florida

Carlo Morosi, MD, Medical Oncologist, Department of Radiology, Fondazione IRCCS Istituto Nazionale dei Tumori, Milan, Italy

Paari Murugan, MBBS, MD, Associate Professor, Department of Laboratory Medicine and Pathology, University of Minnesota, Minneapolis, Minnesota

Christian M. Ogilvie, MD, Associate Professor, Department of Orthopaedic Surgery and Cancer Center, University of Minnesota, Minneapolis, Minnesota

Alberto Pappo, MD, Member, Director, Solid Tumor Division, St. Jude Children's Research Hospital, Memphis, Tennessee

Amanda Parkes, MD, Assistant Professor, Section of Hematology/Oncology, Department of Medicine, Carbone Comprehensive Cancer Center, University of Wisconsin, Madison, Wisconsin

Shreyaskumar R. Patel, MD, RR Herring Distinguished Professor, Department of Sarcoma Medical Oncology, The University of Texas MD Anderson Cancer Center, Houston, Texas

Seth M. Pollack, MD, Associate Member, Clinical Research Division, Fred Hutchinson Cancer Research Center, Seattle, Washington; Associate Professor, Division of Oncology, University of Washington, Seattle, Washington

Juan A. Pretell, MD, Musculoskeletal Oncology Surgeon, Division of Musculoskeletal Oncology, Associate Professor of Orthopedics, Miller School of Medicine, University of Miami, Miami, Florida

Ravin Ratan, MD, Assistant Professor, Department of Sarcoma Medical Oncology, The University of Texas MD Anderson Cancer Center, Houston, Texas

Chandrajit P. Raut, MD, MSc, Professor, Department of Surgery, Brigham and Women's Hospital, Center for Sarcoma and Bone Oncology, Dana-Farber Cancer Institute, Boston, Massachusetts

Steven I. Robinson, MBBS, Assistant Professor of Oncology, Division of Medical Oncology, Mayo Clinic, Rochester, Minnesota

Andrew E. Rosenberg, MD, Professor and Vice Chair, Director, Bone and Soft Tissue Pathology, Department of Pathology, Miller School of Medicine, University of Miami, Miami, Florida

Jagteshwar Sandhu, MD, Clinical Research Assistant, Department of Interventional Radiology, Jackson Memorial Hospital, University of Miami, Miami, Florida

Roberta Giovanna Sanfilippo, MD, Medical Oncologist, Department of Medical Oncology, Fondazione IRCCS Istituto Nazionale dei Tumori, Milan, Italy

Brian Schulte, MD, Fellow, Division of Hematology/Oncology, Northwestern University, Chicago, Illinois

Angeles Alvarez Secord, MD, MHS, Professor, Division of Gynecology Oncology, Department of Obstetrics and Gynecology, Duke Cancer Institute, Duke University Medical Center, Durham, North Carolina

César Serrano, MD, PhD, Head, Sarcoma Translational Research Program, Sarcoma Unit, Oncology Department, Vall d'Hebron Institute of Oncology (VHIO), Vall d'Hebron University, Barcelona, Spain

Jack F. Shern, MD, Lasker Clinical Research Scholar, Pediatric Oncology Branch, Center for Cancer Research, National Cancer Institute, Bethesda, Maryland

Arun S. Singh, MD, Assistant Professor, Sarcoma Service, Division of Hematology–Oncology, UCLA, Los Angeles, California

Neeta Somaiah, MD, Associate Professor, Department of Sarcoma Medical Oncology, The University of Texas MD Anderson Cancer Center, Houston, Texas

Felipe F. de Souza, MD, Musculoskeletal Radiology, Department of Radiology, Jackson Memorial Hospital, University of Miami, Miami, Florida

Silvia Stacchiotti, MD, Medical Oncologist, Mesenchymal Tumor and Rare Cancer Unit, Department of Cancer Medicine, Fondazione IRCCS Istituto Nazionale dei Tumori, Milan, Italy

Ty K. Subhawong, MD, Associate Professor of Clinical Radiology and Orthopaedics, Department of Radiology, Sylvester Comprehensive Cancer Center, University of Miami, Miami, Florida

David Ilan Suster, MD, Fellow in Bone and Soft Tissue Pathology, Department of Pathology, Massachusetts General Hospital, Boston, Massachusetts

Gabriel Tinoco, MD, FACP, Assistant Professor of Medicine, The Ohio State University Comprehensive Cancer Center, Columbus, Ohio

Jonathan C. Trent, MD, PhD, Professor of Medicine, Director for Sarcoma Program, Associate Director for Clinical Research, Sylvester Comprehensive Cancer Center, University of Miami Health System, Miami, Florida

Matteo Trucco, MD, Associate Member, Pediatric Institute, Cleveland Clinic Children's Hospital, Cleveland, Ohio

William W. Tseng, MD, Associate Professor of Surgery, Department of Surgery (Surgical Oncology), University of Southern California, Keck School of Medicine, Los Angeles, California

Shree Venkat, MD, Assistant Professor, Department of Clinical Interventional Radiology, Jackson Memorial Hospital, University of Miami, Miami, Florida

Jennifer Wang, BA, Medical Student, Department of Surgery (Surgical Oncology), University of Southern California, Keck School of Medicine, Los Angeles, California

Brigitte C. Widemann, MD, Chief, Pediatric Oncology Branch, Head, Pharmacology and Experimental Therapeutics Section, Center for Cancer Research, National Cancer Institute, Bethesda, Maryland

Breelyn A. Wilky, MD, Associate Professor, Division of Medical Oncology, Department of Medicine, University of Colorado School of Medicine, Aurora, Colorado

Preface

Bone and soft tissue sarcomas are a heterogeneous collection of over 170 distinct clinical entities. The prevalence of next-generation sequencing has accelerated the molecular classification and discovery of several new sarcoma entities and led to treatment paradigms. Sarcoma clinicians are applying the tools of precision medicine to identify driver mutations and select novel medications or agents in clinical trial. The landscape of sarcoma diagnosis and management is rapidly evolving with the advent of new diagnostic tools, precision medicine, immunotherapy, and cell-based therapies. The current knowledge base with the inclusion of recent advances serves the foundation for which each author has built his or her chapter of this book.

It is impossible to learn all the critical details of each sarcoma subtype during training or even as a junior faculty member. It takes many years as a practicing sarcoma oncologist to gain familiarity with the subtleties of each subtype. We created *Sarcomas: Evidence-Based Diagnosis and Management* in order to provide relevant information to trainees, oncologists who would like to learn more about sarcomas, and even experienced sarcoma oncologists. This book was designed to allow the reader to not only learn the latest information about sarcoma diagnosis and management, but also rapidly access content via the physical book, computer, or their smart device amid a busy clinic. Content was structured by the most common sarcoma histologic subtypes as well as by general concepts. As sarcoma diagnosis and management require an experienced multidisciplinary team, we included overview chapters from each of the medical disciplines involved in the care of sarcoma patients. Importantly, each author was chosen based on his or her expertise specific to the content of the chapter.

Learning the nuances and caveats of sarcoma patient care requires more than didactic lectures or reading text. Each histologic subtype chapter includes a case-based study in which the reader is able to follow the diagnostic and treatment thought processes as the author illustrates his or her management of a complex medical situation. These cases illustrate commonly encountered situations in busy sarcoma clinics and allow the reader to apply the skills learned from the preceding chapter in understanding the authors' diagnostic and therapeutic approach. Significantly, the exceptional and novel digital version of this book allows rapid access to chapters or information through keyword searches at any time by computer, tablet, or smartphone.

We, the editors, designed this book to facilitate management of sarcoma patients in an era of rapidly evolving sarcoma diagnoses and novel therapeutic approaches. Because each chapter was composed by a true expert in the field, the information provided herein is the latest available. We have no doubt this practical book will be a game-changing and incredibly useful tool that will be utilized today and for many years in the future.

Jonathan C. Trent
Andrew E. Rosenberg
Raphael Pollock
Thomas F. DeLaney

Abbreviations

ACT	adoptive cellular transfer
ALL	acute lymphoblastic leukemia
ARMS	alveolar rhabdomyosarcoma
ASPS	alveolar soft part sarcoma
ATRA	all-*trans* retinoic acid
CAR	chimeric antigen receptor
CAR-T	chimeric antigen receptor T cells
CCR	chemokine receptor
CEA	carcinoembryonic antigen
CK	cytokeratins
COG	Children's Oncology Group
CR	complete remission
CRS	cytokine release syndrome
CTA	cancer testis antigens
CTL	cytotoxic T lymphocytes
CTLA-4	cytotoxic T lymphocyte-associated antigen 4
CXCR	chemokine ligand
DD	dedifferentiated
DFS	disease-free survival
EFS	event-free survival
EMA	epithelial membrane antigen
EpSSG	European Soft Tissue Sarcoma Group
ERBB2	human epidermal growth factor receptor 2/neu
ERMS	embryonal rhabdomyosarcoma
ES	epithelioid sarcoma
EWS	Ewing sarcoma
FDG-PET	fluorodeoxyglucose-PET
FISH	fluorescence in situ hybridization
FNCLCC	French Federation of Comprehensive Cancer Centers (*Fédération Nationale des Centres de Lutte Contre le Cancer*)
GD2	disialoganglioside
GIST	gastrointestinal stromal tumor
HAI	hepatic artery infusion
HAIP	hepatic artery infusion pump
HFG	hepatocyte growth factor
HITM	hepatic immunotherapy for metastases
HLA	human leukocyte antigen

HPF	high-powered field
IE	ifosfamide, etoposide
IFP	interstitial fluid pressure
IFS	infantile fibrosarcoma
IgTCR	immunoglobulin T cell receptor
IL	interleukin
IPCTM	Intraperitoneal CAR-T infusion
IRS	Intergroup Rhabdomyosarcoma Study Staging System
LAK	lymphokine-activated killer cells
LDH	lactate dehydrogenase
LSS	limb-sparing/salvage surgery
mAb	monoclonal antibody
MAP	methotrexate, doxorubicin, cisplatin
MDACC	MD Anderson Cancer Center
MDSC	myeloid-derived suppressor cells
MHC	major histocompatibility complex
MITF	microphthalmia transcription factor
MST	median survival time
NCI	National Cancer Institute
NKAE	expanded natural killer cells
NRSTS	non-rhabdomyosarcoma soft tissue sarcoma
ORR	objective response rate
OS	overall survival
PCR	polymerase chain reaction
PD	progressive disease
PD1/PD-L1	programmed death 1/programmed death ligand 1
PEDD	pressure-enabled drug delivery
PFS	progression-free survival
POG	Pediatric Oncology Group
PPTP	Pediatric Preclinical Testing Program
PR	partial response
RECIST	Response Evaluation Criteria in Solid Tumors
RMS	rhabdomyosarcoma
RT	radiation therapy
RT-PCR	reverse transcription polymerase chain reaction
SBRT	stereotactic body radiation therapy
scFv	single-chain variable fragment
SD	stable disease
SEER	Surveillance, Epidemiology, and End Results
SPECT	single-photon emission computed tomography
STIR	short-tau inversion recovery
STS	soft tissue sarcoma
TAA	tumor-associated antigen
TAM	tumor-associated macrophages
TBI	total body irradiation
TCR	T-cell receptor

TFE3	transcription factor E3
Th1	T helper type 1
TIL	tumor-infiltrating lymphocytes
TKI	tyrosine kinase inhibitor
TME	tumor microenvironment
TNF	tumor necrosis factor
TNM	tumor, node, metastases
Treg	T regulatory cell
UPS	undifferentiated pleomorphic sarcoma
VA	vincristine, actinomycin D
VAC	vincristine, actinomycin D, cyclophosphamide
VDC	vincristine, doxorubicin, cyclophosphamide
VEGF	vascular endothelial growth factor
VZV	varicella zoster virus
WD	well differentiated

Acknowledgments

We would like to thank the many sarcoma patients, caregivers, and advocates throughout the world who have supported clinical research and helped shape our understanding of old and new treatments for bone and soft tissue sarcomas. We would also like to thank our colleagues and mentors who instilled the drive to improve patient outcomes and taught us the knowledge not found in typical textbooks, which we have purposefully included in this book. Ultimately, we thank our families and friends who have supported us during the writing of this book.

Introduction

Robert S. Benjamin

The book you are about to read is a compilation of current knowledge of the diagnosis and treatment of several different specific sarcomas of soft tissue and bone, as well as the diagnostic and therapeutic modalities employed. Traditionally, sarcomas have been divided into two groups, those arising in the soft tissue and those arising in bone. Initially, the only diagnostic approaches were physical examination to assess tenderness or presence of a mass; plain radiography, especially for primary bone tumors; and light microscopy of hematoxylin and eosin (H&E)-stained slides. The only therapeutic modality was radical surgery, usually amputation, even for soft tissue tumors of the extremities, because less radical approaches led to local recurrence in 70% of cases.[1]

Radiation was the first nonsurgical therapeutic modality, but its use in the treatment of sarcomas was limited. Only rhabdomyosarcoma[2] and Ewing sarcoma[3] were notably sensitive to radiation, and for this reason, radiation replaced amputation in the treatment of Ewing sarcoma. After all, since all the patients, mostly children and adolescents, were going to die of metastatic disease within a year or two of diagnosis, why use mutilating surgery if the pain of the primary tumor could be controlled with radiation? The other sarcomas were considered to be radioresistant.

Soft tissue sarcomas were treated as a single entity by medical oncologists, whereas the common bone tumors, osteosarcoma, Ewing sarcoma, and chondrosarcoma, were always treated differently. Ewing sarcoma was the first bone tumor for which chemotherapy had an impact.[3] Chondrosarcomas are still not responsive to standard chemotherapy. Osteosarcoma was initially resistant to chemotherapy that worked for Ewing sarcoma as well as other chemotherapeutic agents available in the 1960s. In the early 1970s, Wang et al. reported the responses of osteosarcoma to Adriamycin (before the name doxorubicin was invented),[4] and Jaffe reported the responses of osteosarcoma to high-dose methotrexate.[5] That was the beginning of the modern era of chemotherapy, and you will read more details about current treatment in this book.

For soft tissue sarcomas, the activity of actinomycin D, vincristine, and alkylating agents against rhabdomyosarcoma was discovered early by pediatric oncologists,[6] but other sarcomas were found to be resistant. Only with the development of Adriamcyin was moderate activity noted.[7–10] Gottlieb added dacarbazine to Adriamycin (ADIC) with improvement in response rate and duration,[11] and subsequently added vincristine and then cyclophosphamide (CyVADIC) with little further improvement, but he made several important observations.[10] First, there was a very steep dose–response curve for Adriamycin, such that the response rate for sarcomas doubled between 45 and 75 mg/m^2.[12] Second, although most histologic types of sarcoma had similar response rates, leiomyosarcomas arising from the gastrointestinal (GI) tract had much lower response rates than those arising at other primary sites.[10] We now know that the vast majority of GI leiomyosarcomas diagnosed at that time were actually gastrointestinal stromal tumors (GISTs).

Because most sarcomas responded similarly to Adriamycin, medical oncologists took it for granted that sarcomas were all the same and that histologic type was not important. We should have realized the fallacy of that thinking. After all, rhabdomyosarcoma and Ewing sarcoma responded to actinomycin D, and osteosarcoma responded to high-dose methotrexate and cisplatin, but it was not until ifosfamide, the next drug to show activity against sarcomas, was studied that the difference in response rates between different sarcomas became apparent. Several different studies showed that ifosfamide was more active against synovial sarcomas and less active against leiomyosarcomas than against the other histologic types of sarcomas included in the studies.[13–15] It certainly makes sense that different sarcomas have different sensitivities and behaviors. No oncologist would think of treating adenocarcinoma of the breast, lung, and colon in the same way. Why do so with sarcomas?

Unfortunately, the rarity of sarcomas makes it challenging to perform studies of each interesting new agent in each of the 75 or more individual sarcomas. Unless a specific target can be identified, as was the case with imatinib in GIST, investigators need to pursue hints of activity when they are discovered. The best example is the activity of paclitaxel in angiosarcomas. Casper et al. noted an impressive response during an otherwise negative Phase 2 study,[16] pursued the observation in eight of nine other patients with angiosarcoma,[17] and established paclitaxel as a highly active agent against cutaneous angiosarcomas. Similarly, Grosso et al. observed that two of the responders to trabectedin had myxoid liposarcoma. His group pursued the observation and found that in myxoid liposarcoma, 40% of patients responded by conventional criteria (in contrast to <10% with other histologic types of sarcoma), another 40% responded with decreasing tumor enhancement, and only 10% had progressive disease.[18] Clearly, mining databases of institutional and group experience will be valuable in developing leads for further study. Similarly, pooling multi-institutional data on the behavior of rarer sarcomas may provide the best information into treatment of tumors too rare to study without a good lead. Before concluding that rare sarcoma subsets are resistant to chemotherapy, let us get the data.

Now it is clear that sarcomas are a collection of similar, but not identical, diseases. This book reviews the state of the art in the natural history and treatment of a number, but notably a minority, of these tumors. It also provides an up-to-date review of the modalities employed in the diagnosis and treatment of sarcomas. People frequently refer to liposarcoma as if it were a single entity, but from a clinical point of view, liposarcoma is no more specific than sarcoma. There are separate chapters here on dedifferentiated liposarcoma and myxoid liposarcoma, which are biologically, morphologically, radiologically, clinically, and therapeutically distinct. Well-differentiated liposarcoma has no medical therapy at this time and pleomorphic liposarcoma is too rare and poorly studied to warrant a chapter, but they represent the extremes of benign and aggressive behavior of the sarcomas of adipocytic origin.

The most impressive clinical changes in the management of sarcomas during my career have come from improved diagnostic techniques. Whereas GISTs were clinically different from leiomyosarcomas, even before the name was recognized,[10] they are now not only easily diagnosed with confidence by most pathologists, but can also be subclassified by molecular genotyping of clinical significance.[19–22] Imaging techniques have undergone remarkable improvements, permitting surgeons and radiation oncologists to clearly define the extent and location of sarcomas as well as the anatomic structures involved by or immediately adjacent to the tumors. Whereas in the past amputation was the only approach to an extremity sarcoma and many retroperitoneal sarcomas were considered inoperable, careful resection of the tumors and preservation of function are now the norm. This is all made possible by the advanced imaging techniques used today. Medical oncologists take advantage of modern imaging to define target tumors to assess the effects of treatment, but rarely take advantage of the additional information such as tumor enhancement[23] or fluorodeoxyglucose (FDG) avidity[23,24] in measuring tumor response, relying on the criteria devised when the only diagnostic techniques were physical examination and chest x-ray study.[25]

This book is a compilation of the work of many of the world's experts on the diagnosis and management of sarcomas. As such, it is a critical reference for anyone interested in any aspect of sarcoma diagnosis and treatment and is well worth the read.

REFERENCES

1. Clark RL Jr, Martin RG, White EC, Old JW. Clinical aspects of soft-tissue tumors. *AMA Arch Surg*. 1957;74(6):859–870. doi:10.1001/archsurg.1957.01280120037004.
2. Perry H, Chu FC. Radiation therapy in the palliative management of soft tissue sarcomas. *Cancer*. 1962;15:179–183. doi:10.1002/1097-0142(196201/02)15:1<179::aid-cncr2820150125>3.0.co;2-b.
3. Johnson RE, Senyszyn JJ, Rabson AS, Peterson KA. Treatment of Ewing's sarcoma with local irradiation and systemic chemotherapy. A progress report. *Radiology*. 1970;95(1):195–197. doi:10.1148/95.1.195.
4. Wang JJ, Cortes E, Sinks LF, Holland JF. Therapeutic effect and toxicity of adriamycin in patients with neoplastic disease. *Cancer*. 1971;28(4):837–843. doi:10.1002/1097-0142(1971)28:4<837::aid-cncr2820280406>3.0.co;2-4.
5. Jaffe N. Recent advances in the chemotherapy of metastatic osteogenic sarcoma. *Cancer*. 1972;30(6):1627–1631. doi:10.1002/1097-0142(197212)30:6<1627::aid-cncr2820300631>3.0.co;2-h.
6. Pratt CB. Response of childhood rhabdomyosarcoma to combination chemotherapy. *J Pediatr*. 1969;74(5):791–794. doi:10.1016/s0022-3476(69)80145-9.
7. Bonadonna G, Monfardini S, De Lena M, Fossati-Bellani F. Clinical evaluation of adriamycin, a new antitumour antibiotic. *Br Med J*. 1969;3(5669):503–506. doi:10.1136/bmj.3.5669.503.
8. O'Bryan RM, Luce JK, Talley RW, et al. Phase II evaluation of adriamycin in human neoplasia. *Cancer*. 1973;32(1):1–8. doi:10.1002/1097-0142(197307)32:1<1::aid-cncr2820320101>3.0.co;2-x.

9. Benjamin RS, Wiernik PH, Bachur NR. Adriamycin chemotherapy–efficacy, safety, and pharmacologic basis of an intermittent single high-dosage schedule. *Cancer*. 1974;33(1):19–27. doi:10.1002/1097-0142(197401)33:1<19::aid-cncr2820330107>3.0.co;2-m.
10. Gottlieb J, Baker LH, O'Brien RM, et al. Adriamycin (NSC-123127) used alone and in combination for soft tissue and bony sarcomas. *Cancer Chemother Rep*. 1975;6:271–282.
11. Gottlieb JA, Baker LH, Quagliana JM, et al. Chemotherapy of sarcomas with a combination of adriamycin and dimethyl triazeno imidazole carboxamide. *Cancer*. 1972;30(6):1632–1638. doi:10.1002/1097-0142(197212)30:6<1632::aid-cncr2820300632>3.0.co;2-s.
12. O'Bryan RM, Baker LH, Gottlieb JE, et al. Dose response evaluation of adriamycin in human neoplasia. *Cancer*. 1977;39(5):1940–1948. doi:10.1002/1097-0142(197705)39:5<1940::aid-cncr2820390505>3.0.co;2-0.
13. Antman KH, Montella D, Rosenbaum C, Schwen M. Phase II trial of ifosfamide with mesna in previously treated metastatic sarcoma. *Cancer Treat Rep*. 1985;69(5):499–504. https://www.ncbi.nlm.nih.gov/pubmed/3924401.
14. Le Cesne A, Antoine E, Spielmann M, et al. High-dose ifosfamide: circumvention of resistance to standard-dose ifosfamide in advanced soft tissue sarcomas. *J Clin Oncol*. 1995;13(7):1600–1608. doi:10.1200/JCO.1995.13.7.1600.
15. Benjamin RS, Legha SS, Patel SR, Nicaise C. Single-agent ifosfamide studies in sarcomas of soft tissue and bone: the M.D. Anderson Experience. *Cancer Chemother Pharmacol*. 1993;31(suppl 2):S174–S179.
16. Casper ES, Waltzman RJ, Schwartz GK, et al. Phase II trial of paclitaxel in patients with soft-tissue sarcoma. *Cancer Invest*. 1998;16(7):442–446. doi:10.3109/07357909809011697.
17. Fata F, O'Reilly E, Ilson D, et al. Paclitaxel in the treatment of patients with angiosarcoma of the scalp or face. *Cancer*. 1999;86(10):2034–2037. doi:10.1002/(SICI)1097-0142(19991115)86:10<2034::AID-CNCR21>3.0.CO;2-P.
18. Grosso F, Jones RL, Demetri GD, et al. Efficacy of trabectedin (ecteinascidin-743) in advanced pretreated myxoid liposarcomas: a retrospective study. *Lancet Oncol*. 2007;8(7):595–602. doi:10.1016/S1470-2045(07)70175-4.
19. Rutkowski P, Nowecki ZI, Debiec-Rychter M, et al. Predictive factors for long-term effects of imatinib therapy in patients with inoperable/metastatic CD117(+) gastrointestinal stromal tumors (GISTs). *J Cancer Res Clin Oncol*. 2007;133(9):589–597. doi:10.1007/s00432-007-0202-4.
20. Heinrich MC, Owzar K, Corless CL, et al. Correlation of kinase genotype and clinical outcome in the North American Intergroup Phase III Trial of imatinib mesylate for treatment of advanced gastrointestinal stromal tumor: CALGB 150105 Study by Cancer and Leukemia Group B and Southwest Oncology Group. *J Clin Oncol*. 2008;26(33):5360–5367. doi:10.1200/JCO.2008.17.4284.
21. Gastrointestinal Stromal Tumor Meta-Analysis Group (MetaGIST). Comparison of two doses of imatinib for the treatment of unresectable or metastatic gastrointestinal stromal tumors: a meta-analysis of 1,640 patients. *J Clin Oncol*. 2010;28(7):1247–1253. doi:10.1200/JCO.2009.24.2099.
22. Heinrich MC, Maki RG, Corless CL, et al. Primary and secondary kinase genotypes correlate with the biological and clinical activity of sunitinib in imatinib-resistant gastrointestinal stromal tumor. *J Clin Oncol*. 2008;26(33):5352–5359. doi:10.1200/JCO.2007.15.7461.
23. Choi H, Charnsangavej C, Faria SC, et al. Correlation of computed tomography and positron emission tomography in patients with metastatic gastrointestinal stromal tumor treated at a single institution with imatinib mesylate: proposal of new computed tomography response criteria. *J Clin Oncol*. 2007;25(13):1753–1759. doi:10.1200/JCO.2006.07.3049.
24. Schuetze SM, Rubin BP, Vernon C, et al. Use of positron emission tomography in localized extremity soft tissue sarcoma treated with neoadjuvant chemotherapy. *Cancer*. 2005;103(2):339–348. doi:10.1002/cncr.20769.
25. Moertel CG, Hanley JA. The effect of measuring error on the results of therapeutic trials in advanced cancer. *Cancer*. 1976;38(1):388–394. doi:10.1002/1097-0142(197607)38:1<388::aid-cncr2820380156>3.0.co;2-a.

I

Epidemiology and General Principles

1

Medical Oncology

Ravin Ratan and Shreyaskumar R. Patel

INTRODUCTION

While surgery ± radiation therapy remains the definitive therapy for localized, resectable, low-risk sarcomas, a significant portion of patients will require additional treatment with systemic agents owing to high risk for recurrence or development of metastatic disease. Systemic therapy of sarcoma can be broadly classified to have three separate, but often coincident goals: downstaging of a localized tumor to improve the prospects for local control with better preservation of function, treatment of high-risk localized disease to decrease the risk of distant metastatic recurrence, and treatment of metastatic and unresectable disease with the goal of symptom palliation and life prolongation. Appropriate selection of therapy used in a given scenario will take into account which of these goals are pertinent to the patient being treated, the age and comorbid conditions of that patient, acceptability of the toxicity profile of the agent or combination of agents, previous agents with which the patient may have been treated, and increasingly, specific histologic type of the tumor to be treated.

Interpreting the literature with respect to efficacy of agents also depends on thoughtful consideration of endpoints examined in clinical trials and in the clinic. The gold standard endpoint for patients treated on clinical trials is the median overall survival (OS), commonly defined as the time from initiation of treatment to the death of half the patients treated. While intuitively important, a change in OS by the agent under study can be difficult to prove in clinical trials as every intervention a patient receives before and after an experimental treatment is also going to impact survival. Patients may go on to receive multiple additional lines of systemic therapy, radiation treatments, and surgery, which may be applied to both arms in a comparison study and may make a survival improvement less observable or statistically significant. This issue is particularly pronounced in patients who are treated in a clinical trial with crossover design in which the intervention is made available to both groups, but in a different sequence. Thus, OS is most reliable in patient populations with limited treatment options, without a crossover study design, or in patients who are likely to be cured by the intervention and not require additional therapy.

To get around some of the limitations inherent in proving a better OS associated with a treatment, many trials have also reported median progression-free survival (PFS), defined as the time from initiation of therapy to progression of disease of half the treated patients, with progression defined by specified criteria (in modern studies, this is usually RECIST 1.1). PFS is often viewed as a surrogate endpoint for OS, in that if a patient's cancer is slowed by a certain amount of time, one might assume that the patient's life has been prolonged by the same amount of time. This may not hold true if (a) the treatment causes late toxicity that results in death or (b) the patient receives less subsequent treatment (e.g., high rates of a lethal second cancer, months or years after treatment) or (c) there is organ dysfunction that precludes additional systemic therapy or (d) the treatment somehow modifies future disease biology (making the tumor more or less susceptible to subsequent lines of therapy or more or less likely to metastasize).

Other endpoints are also of interest in specific situations. In a patient who has a tumor that is unresectable or borderline resectable, one may be most likely to use a therapy associated with higher dimensional response rate (RR), defined as the percentage of patients receiving a response based on imaging (usually RECIST 1.1). RR is also likely to be important for patients with highly symptomatic disease for which tumor shrinkage could help achieve palliation.

Measurement of RR and PFS is reliant on accurate criteria by which to determine patients who are responding or progressing on therapy. In earlier eras of treatment, physicians relied on clinical response (e.g., a patient's clinically evident tumor is smaller, softer, or less painful) or dimensions on plain x-rays. With the widespread use of CT and MRI for following disease, most modern studies have employed

World Health Organization (WHO) or, more recently, the RECIST criteria (Response Evaluation Criteria in Solid Tumors), which rely on bidimensional or unidimensional cross-sectional measurements of selected lesions. These criteria are not without their downfalls. It is a well-described phenomenon that a responding tumor may not decrease in size, even though at the time of surgery after treatment, 100% necrosis is observed with acellular matrix being the only remnant of the tumor. This is particularly common in gastrointestinal stromal tumor (GIST), in which lesions will often remain stable in size or even get larger and more cystic as they respond. These responding tumors often demonstrate decreased density and decreased enhancement on cross-sectional imaging. Consequently, in many studies of GIST, RECIST measurements are supplemented by Choi criteria measurements, which examine both size and decrease in attenuation when judging response. Tumors treated with immunotherapy also sometimes demonstrate apparent increase in size related to immune infiltration prior to stabilizing or shrinking. Immune-related response criteria (irRC) have been proposed and are now in common usage in immunotherapy-based clinical trials to identify false progression and capture delayed responses in these patients.

Given the rarity of soft tissue sarcoma in general and even more so for specific subtypes, oncologists are frequently asked to make decisions regarding systemic therapy treatment options in the absence of proven survival benefit and often based on small or underpowered studies. This holds for all scenarios, but is particularly pronounced in the adjuvant and neoadjuvant setting, where clinical trials have, as a rule, been underpowered to demonstrate statistical significance of what would be considered clinically meaningful improvements in OS.

What follows is a discussion of the agents commonly used to treat most soft tissue sarcomas, with a discussion of data surrounding each agent and combination, and situations in which they are commonly used. We also discuss the adjuvant and neoadjuvant treatment of sarcomas, a historically controversial proposition in which we believe improved patient selection tools and supportive therapies are making the approach more appealing for the right patient.

AGENTS IN THE TREATMENT OF METASTATIC DISEASE

Doxorubicin

Most first-line regimens employ doxorubicin as a single agent or in combination. The drug has been used since the 1970s, and early in its history, it became apparent that higher doses result in higher RRs, an effect that was less pronounced in other studied malignancies.[1]

Often discussed is cardiac toxicity related to high lifetime doses of doxorubicin. Given that most modern sarcoma regimens employ doxorubicin at 75 mg/m^2, six doses get patients to 450 mg/m^2, the dose at which the incidence of heart failure seems to increase. Several strategies have been employed to decrease this apparent cardiac risk. The 450 mg/m^2 threshold is based on bolus administration of the drug without dexrazoxane cardioprotection. When the drug is administered over longer periods of time (48–72 hours in our practice), the incidence of cardiac damage declines. This comes at the cost of increased mucositis, which, in some patients, can be severe enough to interfere with oral intake or serve as a source of fever in the setting of neutropenia, which may result in hospitalization. Another strategy to mitigate cardiac toxicity from doxorubicin has been administration of the chelating agent, dexrazoxane. Theoretical concerns with dexrazoxane include theoretical protection of the tumor from the cytotoxic effects of doxorubicin and increased risk of secondary malignancies. Long-term follow-up of survivors of childhood cancers treated with dexrazoxane does not demonstrate worse cancer outcomes, and data regarding secondary malignancies are equivocal. Either of these approaches raises the cumulative dose at which the incidence of cardiomyopathy begins to increase. The cumulative dose of 450 mg/m^2 is not an absolute limit, but may be exceeded in situations in which the potential benefit of doxorubicin outweighs the potential risk of cardiomyopathy.

Dacarbazine

Initially demonstrated to have anticancer effect around the same time as doxorubicin, dacarbazine remains in common use today both as a single agent and in combination for the treatment of soft tissue sarcoma. Contemporary clinical trials have used dacarbazine as a comparator arm in randomized studies for agents being examined in pretreated patients (trabectedin and eribulin) and demonstrated median PFS of 1.5 to 2.6 months and RRs in the range of 5% to 7% using RECIST criteria. Subgroup analysis suggests the drug may be more active in leiomyosarcomas than other treated subtypes (notably, liposarcomas).[2,3] The side effect profile of the drug as a single agent is generally mild, though it is highly emetogenic and does require appropriate nausea prophylaxis.

Cyclophosphamide and Ifosfamide

Cyclophosphamide has a long-standing history of use in the treatment of sarcomas. In modern therapy, it remains a cornerstone of combinations directed at the treatment of pediatric sarcomas like Ewing sarcoma and rhabdomyosarcoma.

In other sarcoma subtypes seen more commonly in adults and in relapsed pediatric sarcomas, ifosfamide came to be of interest because of its clear single-agent activity in the relapsed setting. Similar to doxorubicin, RRs appear to increase as the dose of ifosfamide administered increases. A randomized study comparing ifosfamide 5 g/m^2 (a low to moderate dose in the era of hematopoietic growth factors) to cyclophosphamide 1,200 mg/m^2 (the dose used in most modern regimens) demonstrated a significantly increased RR in the group of patients receiving ifosfamide.[4] Most subsequent soft tissue sarcoma combination regimens have integrated ifosfamide rather than cyclophosphamide. In pediatric tumors, particularly Ewing sarcoma, addition of ifosfamide and etoposide to a cyclophosphamide-containing regimen improved the OS for children with localized disease and is now the standard regimen in the United States.[5] Ifosfamide, however, is more cumbersome to administer and requires experience and expertise, given the possibilities of significant myelosuppression, nephrotoxicity, central neurotoxicity, and an increased risk of hemorrhagic cystitis.

MAID, AIM, and Other Anthracycline-Based Combinations

As such drugs as doxorubicin, cyclophosphamide, ifosfamide, and dacarbazine have come into common use in the treatment of soft tissue sarcomas, there has been interest in combinations of these agents that may be additive or synergistic and provide incremental benefit either in likelihood of response, PFS, and/or OS.

Initially available around the same time period as doxorubicin, dacarbazine was the first agent to be studied as an addition to doxorubicin in the treatment of soft tissue sarcomas. Several studies demonstrated improved RR and PFS, but none were adequately powered to demonstrate OS benefit.[6–8]

Other combinations incorporated cyclophosphamide or ifosfamide, either to doxorubicin alone or to doxorubicin and dacarbazine. In the 1980s, a combination of cyclophosphamide, vincristine, doxorubicin, and dacarbazine was the most active combination available with respect to RR, though without a demonstrated OS benefit.[9] As ifosfamide gradually replaced cyclophosphamide as the more active agent in treatment of soft tissue sarcoma, investigators removed vincristine (with its limited single-agent activity in non-small cell soft tissue sarcoma) and replaced cyclophosphamide with ifosfamide. The resulting mesna, Adriamycin (doxorubicin), ifosfamide, and dacarbazine (MAID) regimen demonstrated a high RR, though again without a statistically significant survival benefit, and became the standard combination therapy through the 1990s.[7] The availability of hematopoietic growth factors allowed for yet another advance, the intensification of dose in agents with a dose–response curve (doxorubicin and ifosfamide). In order to maximize the doses of these agents, dacarbazine was removed from the regimen. The resulting Adriamycin (doxorubicin), ifosfamide, and mesna (AIM) regimen has the highest RRs of any combination reported in soft tissue sarcoma and remains the regimen of choice when inducing a response, which is the primary objective of treatment.[10,11]

The choice of whether to use a doxorubicin-based combination or single-agent doxorubicin in patients with asymptomatic metastatic disease remains controversial. A recent clinical trial attempted to settle this controversy by randomizing 455 patients with advanced soft tissue sarcoma to receive doxorubicin and ifosfamide versus doxorubicin alone. The study demonstrated a longer median PFS for the combination (7.4 vs. 4.6 months, $p = .003$) and overall RR (26% vs. 14%, $p = .0006$). OS also trended toward improvement, but fell short of statistical significance (14.3 vs. 12.8 months, $p = .076$). The results leave room for interpretation, with proponents of combination therapy citing the PFS and RR benefit and nearly statistically improved survival. Opponents of the approach cite the lack of demonstrated OS benefit and clearly increased toxicity with combination therapy.

Gemcitabine and Gemcitabine-Based Combinations

Gemcitabine is a nucleoside analog originally developed as an antiviral agent, but ultimately approved as an antineoplastic drug. It was approved by the U.S. Food and Drug Administration (FDA) in 1996 for the treatment of pancreatic cancer. Several subsequent clinical studies demonstrated the activity of single-agent gemcitabine in soft tissue sarcoma, with RRs ranging from 3% to 18%.[12] The addition of docetaxel to gemcitabine, despite little to no activity of the former as a single agent, also seemed to improve the RRs, with initial nonrandomized studies demonstrating RRs of 14% to 53%.[12] Given the uncontrolled nature of these studies, controversy existed as to whether the higher observed RRs with the combination of gemcitabine and docetaxel were related to synergy between the drugs or that these later combination studies utilized fixed dose rate gemcitabine, administered at 10 mg/m²/min, which has been noted to improve intracellular concentrations of the active metabolite, gemcitabine triphosphate.[13]

To settle this debate, the Sarcoma Alliance for Research through Collaboration (SARC) ran a study using a Bayesian adaptive approach to randomize patients to gemcitabine alone versus gemcitabine and docetaxel. The study demonstrated improved outcomes with the addition of docetaxel to single-agent gemcitabine, including a PFS of 6.2 versus 3.0 months and an OS of 17.9 versus 11.5 months, establishing the combination of gemcitabine and docetaxel as a standard treatment for soft tissue sarcoma in the United States. Of note, the addition of docetaxel was also associated with many more treatment discontinuations related to toxicity.[14] The critique of the study included its small sample size and the statistical design.

Another study performed by the French Sarcoma Group randomized patients with leiomyosarcoma to gemcitabine alone or to the combination of gemcitabine and docetaxel. In contrast to the American study, no improvements in outcomes including RR, PFS, or OS were seen with the addition of docetaxel.[15] These conflicting results have tempered enthusiasm for the gemcitabine and docetaxel combination, especially in light of the added toxicity from docetaxel, and prompted searches for other agents that might be used in combination with gemcitabine. These include drugs such as dacarbazine and vinorelbine.[16,17] Interestingly, the Spanish study randomizing patients to dacarbazine alone versus gemcitabine plus dacarbazine showed improved PFS and OS in favor of the doublet.[16]

Trabectedin

Trabectedin is a novel antineoplastic agent derived from the marine tunicate *Ecteinascidia turbinata*. The mechanism of action is complex; it covalently binds the minor groove of the DNA strand, interfering with DNA replication and the cell cycle, and may also have a myriad of other effects, including disruption of microtubule networks, inhibition of transcription, and other less understood effects on tumor microenvironment.

Early studies demonstrated responses in sarcoma and also established a 24-hour infusion of the agent every 3 weeks as more efficacious than weekly bolus administration. The agent was approved in 2007 by the European regulatory agency for patients with previously treated soft tissue sarcomas. A more recent study conducted in patients with leiomyosarcoma and liposarcoma, in which the efficacy of the drug seemed most pronounced, randomized pretreated patients to receive either single-agent dacarbazine or trabectedin. The study failed to meet its OS endpoint, with a median survival of 12.9 months for trabectedin and 12.4 months for patients receiving dacarbazine. Median PFS, however, was improved at 4.2 versus 1.5 months,[2] which ultimately resulted in approval of trabectedin in the United States for liposarcoma and leiomyosarcoma previously treated with anthracycline.

In several studies conducted prior to the approval of trabectedin and in the subsequent clinical experience with the drug, it has been noted that patients with myxoid/round cell liposarcoma (MRCL) appear to have particularly robust response to trabectedin.[2,18] In a recent study of trabectedin versus doxorubicin-based frontline therapy in translocation-associated sarcomas (approximately a third of which were MRCL), PFS was similar between the two arms. Further interpretation of the data was limited by high attrition rate, related in large part to patients undergoing surgical removal of their tumors, the incidence of this being higher in the trabectedin subgroup.[19] For MRCL, the drug has also been studied in small neoadjuvant studies, in which the overall RR was found to range from 24% to 38%.[20]

Eribulin

Eribulin, a modified analog of halichondrin B, a compound isolated from a marine sponge, was approved for the treatment of breast cancer in 2010 based on data from the EMBRACE study, where it was noted to improve OS in metastatic breast cancer patients. The drug is predominantly felt to be a microtubule dynamics inhibitor, though other mechanisms of action may be important in its clinical effect. Preclinical data demonstrating efficacy in sarcoma subtypes ultimately led to a Phase 2 study conducted by the European Organisation for Research and Treatment of Cancer (EORTC), which demonstrated that leiomyosarcomas and adipocytic tumors (liposarcomas) achieved a 12-week PFS of >30%, which was the prespecified endpoint. These subtypes were subsequently studied in a Phase 3 confirmatory study.[21] This study, enrolling patients with liposarcoma and leiomyosarcoma, randomized patients to treatment with the standard 1.4 mg/m² dose of eribulin or dacarbazine at doses of 850 to 1,200 mg/m². The trial met its primary endpoint of a 2-month improvement in OS with eribulin over dacarbazine (13.5 vs. 11.5 months, $p = .0169$). PFS (X vs. Y months) in the overall study cohort was not improved, suggesting perhaps a mechanism of action other than direct cytotoxicity. Mechanisms including vascular remodeling, improved delivery of subsequent lines of chemotherapy, and modification of metastatic potential have been raised as possibly contributing to the demonstrated survival benefit in the absence of PFS improvement.[22,23]

The subgroup analysis reported in the initial study demonstrated that the OS benefit of eribulin over dacarbazine was limited to patients with liposarcoma, and for this reason, the FDA elected to approve eribulin for liposarcoma only. Subsequent post hoc analysis of only the liposarcoma group from the Phase 3 study demonstrated that among these patients, PFS was improved (2.9 vs. 1.4 months, $p = .0015$) and the magnitude of the OS benefit was larger than in the entire study population (15.6 vs. 8.4 months, $p < .001$).[24]

Of note, despite the lack of improvement seen in clinical endpoints in the study on patients with leiomyosarcoma, an interpretation of the available data may be that eribulin is as efficacious as dacarbazine in patients with leiomyosarcoma, and more effective than dacarbazine in patients with liposarcoma. Despite the lack of FDA approval for this specific histologic diagnosis, eribulin remains an option for treatment of leiomyosarcoma in treatment guidelines.[25,26]

Tyrosine Kinase Inhibitors

Among the so-called targeted agents, the drugs that have had the most impact in the treatment of soft tissue sarcoma are tyrosine kinase inhibitors used in the treatment of GIST. These include FDA approvals for agents such as imatinib, sunitinib, and regorafenib. Their use in the treatment of GIST is discussed elsewhere in this textbook.

For other soft tissue sarcomas, the most commonly used multitargeted tyrosine kinase inhibitor is pazopanib. Based on earlier-phase clinical trials showing promising activity in multiple soft tissue sarcoma subtypes, the drug was studied in the Phase 3 PALLETTE study, which enrolled patients with a wide variety of soft tissue sarcomas and excluded patients with liposarcoma. Compared to placebo, median PFS was improved at 4.6 versus 1.6 months, and there was a trend toward improved OS that was not statistically significant. Dimensional partial responses by RECIST were rare (6% for pazopanib vs. 0% with placebo).[27] Given the paucity of available lines of treatment, its relatively favorable toxicity profile, and its broad approval for most sarcoma subtypes by regulatory agencies, pazopanib continues to be a commonly used agent in pretreated metastatic soft tissue sarcoma, except liposarcomas and GIST.

Immunotherapy

Representing a paradigm shift from traditional cytotoxic therapies and antiangiogenic tyrosine kinase inhibitors, therapies that modulate the endogenous immune system or confer adoptive immunity are of increasing interest across a broad range of tumor types.

The most broadly utilized of these is immune checkpoint blockade. In certain diseases, most notably melanoma, anti-PD1–, anti-PD-L1–, and anti-CTLA-4–directed therapies* have revolutionized treatment and drastically improved outcomes for patients, with long-term responses in patients who previously had few treatment options. PD-1/PD-L1–directed therapies are now approved for a host of malignancies including non-small cell and small cell lung cancers, bladder carcinomas, renal cell carcinoma, squamous cell carcinomas of the head and neck, Hodgkin lymphoma, and cancers with high microsatellite instability. This list continues to grow as additional cancer types are studied. In many of these cases, expression of PD-L1 is used as a biomarker to predict response.

In sarcoma, the largest study reported to date using checkpoint blockade is a study of single-agent pembrolizumab, which examined four cohorts of soft tissue sarcoma patients with leiomyosarcoma, unclassified pleomorphic sarcoma (UPS), synovial sarcoma, and "other" miscellaneous histologic types in addition to three cohorts of patients with bone tumors. Among the soft tissue sarcoma patients, there was an 18% RR and 38% stable disease (SD) rate overall. Responses were primarily seen in the cohorts of patients with UPS and dedifferentiated liposarcoma.[28] Combined checkpoint blockade with nivolumab and ipilimumab has also shown activity, more so than nivolumab alone (RR of 16% vs. 8%) in a study of 85 patients with various sarcoma subtypes, though at the cost of increased toxicity.[29]

Another area of particular interest for immune checkpoint blockade-based therapies has been alveolar soft part sarcoma (ASPS). A Phase 2 study of pembrolizumab and axitinib demonstrated an overall RR of 45.5%.[30] Several other studies have also reported small numbers of patients with this rare sarcoma subtype who responded to therapy with immune checkpoint inhibitors alone or in combination

*PD-1 is programmed cell death protein -1, PDL-1 is programmed cell death protein -1 ligand, and CTLA is cytotoxic t-lymphocyte associated protein.

with other agents.[31,32] In general, these have been small studies that have not resulted in approval of this agent in any sarcoma subtype, but interest remains in pursuing and improving checkpoint blockade-based therapy, particularly in apparently responsive tumors including ASPS, dedifferentiated liposarcoma, and UPS.

Another area of active investigation for immune-based therapies in soft tissue sarcoma is cellular therapies and vaccines directed against the cancer testis antigen NY-ESO-1, which is found with high frequency in patients with myxoid liposarcoma and synovial sarcoma, and with less frequency in other sarcoma subtypes.[33] NY-ESO-1 is not expressed in normal adult tissues outside the testis, making it an ideal target for immune-based approaches.

LV305 is a dendritic cell (DC)-targeted vaccine that aims to induce an endogenous tumor-specific T-cell response. It is an engineered lentiviral particle that selectively targets immature DCs and induces the expression of NY-ESO-1, which is then processed and displayed by major histocompatibility complex (MHC) class I and II molecules that can elicit a T-cell response. In the Phase 1 study, a single partial response (PR) was seen in 24 sarcoma patients treated with the drug; however, over half experienced stable disease and lived longer than might have been expected based on historical comparisons.[34] Subsequent work has focused on combining LV305 with a Toll-like receptor 4 (TLR4) agonist, glucopyranosyl lipid adjuvant (GLA), and recombinant NY-ESO-1, referred to as CMB305. A study of synovial sarcoma and myxoid liposarcoma patients treated with this regimen demonstrated stable disease in 53% of synovial sarcoma patients and 75% of MRCL patients.[34]

While vaccines remain promising, another strategy under active investigation is the use of modified T-cell receptors with affinity for the NY-ESO-1 protein. Small studies utilizing this approach have resulted in meaningful RRs as high as 61% in synovial sarcoma and it remains under active investigation.[35]

Adjuvant and Neoadjuvant Therapy

Given that development and progression of metastatic disease is the largest driver of poor outcomes in soft tissue sarcoma, considerable efforts have been made to examine the utility of chemotherapy in the neoadjuvant or adjuvant setting. These efforts have been hampered by the overall rarity of soft tissue sarcoma in general and specific subtypes of interest in particular, heterogeneous inclusion criteria in studies that do not always reliably identify high-risk patients for treatment, and lack of equipoise at the treating centers, which had made enrollment into randomized studies of adjuvant therapy difficult.

Given the challenges with a small sample size in various studies, perhaps the most compelling evidence of the efficacy of adjuvant chemotherapy comes from two important meta-analyses. The first, published by the Sarcoma Meta-analysis Collaboration (SMAC) in 1997, included 1,568 patients from 14 studies conducted from 1973 to 1990, all having received a doxorubicin-based adjuvant treatment regimen, all at doses lower than those used in modern regimens with growth factor support. This analysis demonstrated an improvement in local recurrence risk, distant (metastatic) recurrence risk, and overall recurrence-free survival. Risk of death also trended lower, but did not achieve statistical significance.[36]

An update to this analysis was reported in 2008. This new report incorporated not only the original 14 doxorubicin-based adjuvant studies discussed in the original SMAC analysis but also four new studies using anthracycline and ifosfamide (though at doses lower than the modern AIM regimen). In addition to again demonstrating improvement in local recurrence rates, distant recurrence rates, and overall recurrence rates, the authors were able to demonstrate an improvement in OS for patients receiving doxorubicin and ifosfamide-based treatments, with an absolute risk reduction of death of 11% in the patients who received doxorubicin and ifosfamide over no treatment.[37]

Since the reporting of this updated meta-analysis, another randomized study was conducted by the EORTC, this time using a more modern regimen of doxorubicin 75 mg/m^2 and ifosfamide 5 g/m^2 (although the dose of ifosfamide was half the dose used in AIM). The study enrolled patients with grade II–III soft tissue sarcomas, with malignant fibrous histiocytoma, liposarcoma, leiomyosarcoma, and synovial sarcoma accounting for 67% of the 176 patients in the control arm and 61% of the 145 patients in the treatment arm. Just under half the patients in each arm had grade III tumors at the central review of pathology. Tumor size ranged from 0.3 to 35 cm in the chemotherapy arm and from 1.2 to 38 cm in the control arm, with the median size being 8.6 and 7.5 cm, respectively. The study failed to show any improvement in relapse-free survival or OS with adjuvant chemotherapy.[38] The major criticism of the study stemmed from the inclusion criteria that allowed patients with lower risk for recurrence (small tumors, intermediate grade, all anatomic sites) to be enrolled in the study and the lower dose of ifosfamide used.

A reanalysis of the data from this EORTC study has recently been reported using a risk stratification tool to better understand the pool of patients enrolled in the study. Using the Sarculator, a recently developed and validated risk assessment nomogram, patients treated on the EORTC adjuvant study with tumors in the extremities and trunk were stratified by their predicted-OS (pr-OS). Patients in the high-risk group had a 10-year pr-OS of ≤51%, the low-risk group had a pr-OS of ≥66%, and the intermediate prognosis patients had a pr-OS from 51% to 66%. This analysis demonstrated half the risk of death (hazard ratio [HR]: 0.46, 95% confidence interval [CI]: 0.23–0.94) in the high-risk group when chemotherapy was given, with the 8-year absolute risk reduction for death being 21.3%, an effect that was not replicated in the intermediate- or low-risk groups.[39]

Similar findings have also been subsequently obtained in the results of ISG-GEIS-FSG-1001, a study of epirubicin and ifosfamide versus subtype-specific neoadjuvant therapy in five sarcoma subtypes (malignant peripheral nerve sheath tumor, myxoid liposarcoma, leiomyosarcoma, synovial sarcoma, and undifferentiated pleomorphic sarcoma). Patients were treated with either three cycles of epirubicin 120 mg/m^2 and ifosfamide 9 g/m^2 or a histology-specific regimen. In this study, the patient's tumors had to be at least 5 cm and deep to investing fascia. Median size of the enrolled tumors was approximately 11 cm in both treatment groups, and the population of tumor types was less heterogeneous than in EORTC 62931, given that it was restricted to only these five tumor types. In this study, patients receiving epirubicin and ifosfamide-based neoadjuvant therapy had a better 46-month disease-free survival rate at 62%, higher than the 36% in the histotype-tailored active chemotherapy group. OS at 46 months was similarly better in the anthracycline plus ifosfamide treatment group. While the study demonstrated that histotype-tailored adjuvant treatment was not better than epirubicin and ifosfamide-based therapy, the most notable finding was the prospectively demonstrated benefit in the epirubicin and ifosfamide arm, the first convincing demonstration of a survival benefit with anthracycline and ifosfamide in a prospective, randomized clinical trial, even when compared to an active control group.[40]

While adjuvant therapy remains in some respects controversial for patients with soft tissue sarcoma, the preponderance of evidence to date does suggest a measurable improvement in disease-free survival and OS. A more pertinent discussion may be how to appropriately risk-stratify patients with localized sarcomas. The Sarculator is a reasonable tool, but remains limited to patients with retroperitoneal, extremity, and trunk sarcomas and only incorporates more common histologic types. Other sites such as the head and neck, the female reproductive tract, intra-abdominal, and intrathoracic locations are not well characterized by the nomogram. In some of these locations, where wide margins may be difficult to obtain, there may be additional benefits to chemotherapy; a consistent finding in adjuvant/neoadjuvant studies has been an improvement in local relapse-free survival.[36]

SUMMARY

Localized approaches such as surgery and radiation therapy are the mainstay for localized, resectable, low-risk sarcoma patients. However, a significant portion of patients requires systemic therapy owing to a high risk for recurrence or the presence of metastatic disease. Systemic therapy for sarcoma patients is generally used to facilitate limb (or organ)-sparing surgery, neoadjuvant/adjuvant treatment of high-risk localized disease to decrease the risk of metastases, and for the treatment of metastatic and locally advanced disease with the objective of symptom palliation and prolongation of life. As discussed previously, many new agents with new mechanisms of action are available to sarcoma patients. A goal in medical oncology is to select the appropriate agent and administer it at the appropriate dose for the appropriate patient. The selection of therapy in a given scenario will consider the overall goals of the patient being treated, the patient's ability to tolerate a treatment, the acceptability of the toxicity profile to the patient, any previous therapies, and, increasingly, the specific histologic subtype of the patient's tumor. In conclusion, we have entered an era with new systemic agents that are offering hope for our patients impacted by sarcoma.

REFERENCES

1. O'Bryan RM, Baker LH, Gottlieb JE, et al. Dose response evaluation of adriamycin in human neoplasia. *Cancer*. 1977;39(5):1940–1948. doi:10.1002/1097-0142(197705)39:5<1940::AID-CNCR2820390505>3.0.CO;2-0
2. Demetri GD, von Mehren M, Jones RL, et al. Efficacy and safety of trabectedin or dacarbazine for metastatic liposarcoma or leiomyosarcoma after failure of conventional chemotherapy: results of a phase III randomized multicenter clinical trial. *J Clin Oncol*. 2015;34(8):786–793. doi:10.1200/jco.2015.62.4734

3. Schoffski P, Maki RG, Italiano A, et al. Randomized, open-label, multicenter, phase III study of eribulin versus dacarbazine in patients with leiomyosarcoma and adipocytic sarcoma. *J Clin Oncol*. 2015;33(suppl):abstr LBA10502. doi:10.1200/jco.2015.33.18_suppl.lba10502
4. Bramwell VH, Mouridsen HT, Santoro A, et al. Cyclophosphamide versus ifosfamide: preliminary report of a randomized phase II trial in adult soft tissue sarcomas. *Cancer Chemother Pharmacol*. 1986;18(suppl 2):S13–S16. doi:10.1007/BF00647440
5. Grier HE, Krailo MD, Tarbell NJ, et al. Addition of ifosfamide and etoposide to standard chemotherapy for Ewing's sarcoma and primitive neuroectodermal tumor of bone. *N Engl J Med*. 2003;348(8):694–701. doi:10.1056/NEJMoa020890
6. Omura GA, Major FJ, Blessing JA, et al. A randomized study of adriamycin with and without dimethyl triazenoimidazole carboxamide in advanced uterine sarcomas. *Cancer*. 1983;52(4):626–632. doi:10.1002/1097-0142(19830815)52:4<626::AID-CNCR2820520409>3.0.CO;2-E
7. Antman K, Crowley J, Balcerzak SP, et al. An intergroup phase III randomized study of doxorubicin and dacarbazine with or without ifosfamide and mesna in advanced soft tissue and bone sarcomas. *J Clin Oncol*. 1993;11(7):1276–1285. doi:10.1200/JCO.1993.11.7.1276
8. Borden EC, Amato DA, Rosenbaum C, et al. Randomized comparison of three adriamycin regimens for metastatic soft tissue sarcomas. *J Clin Oncol*. 1987;5(6):840–850. doi:10.1200/JCO.1987.5.6.840
9. Yap BS, Baker LH, Sinkovics JG, et al. Cyclophosphamide, vincristine, adriamycin, and DTIC (CYVADIC) combination chemotherapy for the treatment of advanced sarcomas. *Cancer Treat Rep*. 1980;64(1):93–98. PMID:7379060.
10. Patel SR, Vadhan-Raj S, Burgess MA, et al. Results of two consecutive trials of dose-intensive chemotherapy with doxorubicin and ifosfamide in patients with sarcomas. *Am J Clin Oncol*. 1998;21(3):317–321. doi:10.1097/00000421-199806000-00025
11. Judson I, Verweij J, Gelderblom H, et al. Doxorubicin alone versus intensified doxorubicin plus ifosfamide for first-line treatment of advanced or metastatic soft-tissue sarcoma: a randomised controlled phase 3 trial. *Lancet Oncol*. 2014;15(4):415–423. doi:10.1016/S1470-2045(14)70063-4
12. Ratan R, Patel SR. Chemotherapy for soft tissue sarcoma. *Cancer*. 2016;122(19):2952–2960. doi:10.1002/cncr.30191.
13. Abbruzzese JL, Grunewald R, Weeks EA, et al. A phase I clinical, plasma, and cellular pharmacology study of gemcitabine. *J Clin Oncol*. 1991;9(3):491–498. doi:10.1200/JCO.1991.9.3.491
14. Maki RG, Wathen JK, Patel SR, et al. Randomized phase II study of gemcitabine and docetaxel compared with gemcitabine alone in patients with metastatic soft tissue sarcomas: results of sarcoma alliance for research through collaboration study 002 [corrected]. *J Clin Oncol*. 2007;25(19):2755–2763. doi:10.1200/JCO.2006.10.4117
15. Pautier P, Floquet A, Penel N, et al. Randomized multicenter and stratified phase II study of gemcitabine alone versus gemcitabine and docetaxel in patients with metastatic or relapsed leiomyosarcomas: a Federation Nationale des Centres de Lutte Contre le Cancer (FNCLCC) French Sarcoma Group Study (TAXOGEM study). *Oncologist*. 2012;17(9):1213–1220. doi:10.1634/theoncologist.2011-0467
16. Garcia-Del-Muro X, Lopez-Pousa A, Maurel J, et al. Randomized phase II study comparing gemcitabine plus dacarbazine versus dacarbazine alone in patients with previously treated soft tissue sarcoma: a Spanish Group for Research on Sarcomas study. *J Clin Oncol*. 2011;29(18):2528–2533. doi:10.1200/JCO.2010.33.6107
17. Dileo P, Morgan JA, Zahrieh D, et al. Gemcitabine and vinorelbine combination chemotherapy for patients with advanced soft tissue sarcomas: results of a phase II trial. *Cancer*. 2007;109(9):1863–1869. doi:10.1002/cncr.22609.
18. Schwartz GK. Trabectedin and the L-sarcomas: a decade-long odyssey. *J Clin Oncol*. 2016;34(8):769–771. doi:10.1200/JCO.2015.63.5938
19. Blay J-Y, Leahy MG, Nguyen BB, et al. Randomised phase III trial of trabectedin versus doxorubicin-based chemotherapy as first-line therapy in translocation-related sarcomas. *Eur J Cancer*. 2014;50(6):1137–1147. doi:10.1016/j.ejca.2014.01.012
20. Assi T, Kattan J, El Rassy E, et al. A comprehensive review of the current evidence for trabectedin in advanced myxoid liposarcoma. *Cancer Treat Rev*. 2019;72:37–44. doi:10.1016/j.ctrv.2018.11.003
21. Schoffski P, Ray-Coquard IL, Cioffi A, et al. Activity of eribulin mesylate in patients with soft-tissue sarcoma: a phase 2 study in four independent histological subtypes. *Lancet Oncol*. 2011;12(11):1045–1052. doi:10.1016/S1470-2045(11)70230-3
22. Young RJ, Woll PJ. Eribulin in soft-tissue sarcoma. *Lancet*. 2016;387(10028):1594–1596. doi:10.1016/S0140-6736(16)00162-8
23. Cortes J, Schoffski P, Littlefield BA. Multiple modes of action of eribulin mesylate: emerging data and clinical implications. *Cancer Treat Rev*. 2018;70:190–198. doi:10.1016/j.ctrv.2018.08.008
24. Demetri GD, Schoffski P, Grignani G, et al. Activity of eribulin in patients with advanced liposarcoma demonstrated in a subgroup analysis from a randomized phase III study of eribulin versus dacarbazine. *J Clin Oncol*. 2017;35(30):3433–3439. doi:10.1200/JCO.2016.71.6605
25. National Comprehensive Cancer Network. *Uterine Neoplasms Version 3.2019*. https://www.nccn.org/professionals/physician_gls/
26. National Comprehensive Cancer Network. *Soft Tissue Sarcoma Version 2.2019*. https://www.nccn.org/professionals/physician_gls/
27. van der Graaf WT, Blay JY, Chawla SP, et al. Pazopanib for metastatic soft-tissue sarcoma (PALETTE): a randomised, double-blind, placebo-controlled phase 3 trial. *Lancet*. 2012;379(9829):1879–1886. doi:10.1016/S0140-6736(12)60651-5

28. Tawbi HA, Burgess M, Bolejack V, et al. Pembrolizumab in advanced soft-tissue sarcoma and bone sarcoma (SARC028): a multicentre, two-cohort, single-arm, open-label, phase 2 trial. *Lancet Oncol*. 2017;18(11):1493–1501. doi:10.1016/S1470-2045(17)30624-1
29. D'Angelo SP, Mahoney MR, Van Tine BA, et al. Nivolumab with or without ipilimumab treatment for metastatic sarcoma (Alliance A091401): two open-label, non-comparative, randomised, phase 2 trials. *Lancet Oncol*. 2018;19(3):416–426. doi:10.1016/S1470-2045(18)30006-8
30. Wilky BA, Trucco MM, Kolonias D, et al. A phase II trial of axitinib plus pembrolizumab for patients with advanced alveolar soft part sarcoma. *J Clin Oncol*. 2018;36(15_suppl):11547. doi:10.1200/JCO.2018.36.15_suppl.11547
31. Groisberg R, Hong DS, Behrang A, et al. Characteristics and outcomes of patients with advanced sarcoma enrolled in early phase immunotherapy trials. *J Immunother Cancer*. 2017;5(1):100. doi:10.1186/s40425-017-0301-y
32. Paoluzzi L, Maki RG. Diagnosis, prognosis, and treatment of alveolar soft-part sarcoma: a review. *JAMA Oncol*. 2019;5(2):254–260. doi:10.1001/jamaoncol.2018.4490
33. Endo M, de Graaff MA, Ingram DR, et al. NY-ESO-1 (CTAG1B) expression in mesenchymal tumors. *Mod Pathol*. 2014;28:587. doi:10.1038/modpathol.2014.155
34. Pollack SM. The potential of the CMB305 vaccine regimen to target NY-ESO-1 and improve outcomes for synovial sarcoma and myxoid/round cell liposarcoma patients. *Expert Rev Vaccines*. 2018;17(2):107–114. doi:10.1080/14760584.2018.1419068
35. Thomas R, Al-Khadairi G, Roelands J, et al. NY-ESO-1 based immunotherapy of cancer: current perspectives. *Front Immunol*. 2018;9:947. doi:10.3389/fimmu.2018.00947
36. Sarcoma Meta-analysis Collaboration. Adjuvant chemotherapy for localised resectable soft-tissue sarcoma of adults: meta-analysis of individual data. *Lancet*. 1997;350(9092):1647–1654. doi:10.1016/S0140-6736(97)08165-8
37. Pervaiz N, Colterjohn N, Farrokhyar F, et al. A systematic meta-analysis of randomized controlled trials of adjuvant chemotherapy for localized resectable soft-tissue sarcoma. *Cancer*. 2008;113(3):573–581. doi:10.1002/cncr.23592
38. Woll PJ, Reichardt P, Le Cesne A, et al. Adjuvant chemotherapy with doxorubicin, ifosfamide, and lenograstim for resected soft-tissue sarcoma (EORTC 62931): a multicentre randomised controlled trial. *Lancet Oncol*. 2012;13(10):1045–1054. doi:10.1016/S1470-2045(12)70346-7
39. Pasquali S, Pizzamiglio S, Touati N, et al. The impact of chemotherapy on survival of patients with extremity and trunk wall soft tissue sarcoma: revisiting the results of the EORTC-STBSG 62931 randomised trial. *Eur J Cancer*. 2019;109:51–60. doi:10.1016/j.ejca.2018.12.009
40. Gronchi A, Ferrari S, Quagliuolo V, et al. Histotype-tailored neoadjuvant chemotherapy versus standard chemotherapy in patients with high-risk soft-tissue sarcomas (ISG-STS 1001): an international, open-label, randomised, controlled, phase 3, multicentre trial. *Lancet Oncol*. 2017;18(6):812–822. doi:10.1016/S1470-2045(17)30334-0

2

Surgical Oncology

Mark Fairweather and Chandrajit P. Raut

INTRODUCTION

Soft tissue sarcomas (STSs) are a rare group of mesenchymal tumors that arise from fat, smooth/skeletal muscle, blood vessels, and connective tissue throughout the body. Gastrointestinal stromal tumors (GISTs) are the most common subtype of sarcoma among a heterogeneous group of over 70 different histologic subtypes.[1] There are approximately 13,000 new diagnoses expected in 2018 in the United States, occurring most commonly in the extremities (60%) followed by the retroperitoneum/abdomen (20%), trunk (10%), and head and neck region (10%).[2,3]

A macroscopically complete resection (R0/R1 resection) is the standard of care for patients with localized STS. There are no data demonstrating a survival benefit for wider pathologic margins. This often requires en bloc resection of the tumor and involved adjacent structures. An R2 resection or resection with gross residual disease should be avoided. Because of the rarity of these tumors, a multidisciplinary evaluation at a high-volume sarcoma center is paramount and has been shown to be associated with improved overall outcomes.[4] After initial radiographic evaluation with either contrast-enhanced CT or MRI, a percutaneous core-needle biopsy (12–16 gauge) is often required to guide the consideration of preoperative chemotherapy and radiation therapy, as well as guide the scope of operation based on histologic subtype and grade.

The primary site of origin of STS is a significant prognostic factor, with patients with retroperitoneal sarcomas (RPSs) generally having a worse prognosis than those with extremity soft tissue sarcomas (ESTSs). Death in patients with RPS is often secondary to local failure, while death in patients with ESTS is often due to distant failure. This difference in outcome is likely influenced not only by variations in distribution of histologic subtypes, but also by anatomic factors associated with the typically large size of tumor at the time of presentation and frequent multivisceral involvement of RPS. Surgical management of STS should be guided not only by the primary site of origin but also by another key prognostic factor, the histologic subtype. Histologic subtype significantly influences patterns of local and distant failure in addition to survival outcomes.[4,5] As a result, instead of a "one-size-fits-all" approach to the surgical management of STS, a histology-specific, site-specific approach is recommended.

This chapter discusses site-specific surgical principles and highlights histology-specific factors that should assist in guiding the operative approach.

EXTREMITY AND TRUNCAL SARCOMA

Extremity and truncal STS often present as a palpable mass and can vary considerably in size at the time of presentation from a small superficial mass to a large, deep compartment thigh mass. After a thorough history and physical examination, radiographic evaluation by MRI (or CT) can be helpful in determining the extent of soft tissue involvement and identify any critical adjacent structures. Imaging alone is very rarely sufficient enough for diagnosis, and percutaneous biopsy is generally recommended. One exception to this is in the case of an atypical lipomatous tumor (ALT)/well-differentiated liposarcoma (WDLPS), which is characterized by a well-encapsulated, homogeneous fat-dense mass, often with thick internal septations (Figure 2.1A and 2.1B). Preoperative biopsy may be deferred in this case with upfront resection of the mass to include a thin rim of normal muscle, fat, or fascia. When biopsy is obtained, a 12- to 16-gauge needle is recommended for a core-needle biopsy, because fine-needle aspiration rarely yields sufficient cellular material for diagnosis and does not maintain enough tissue architecture to distinguish between types of sarcoma, which is critical to optimal treatment planning.

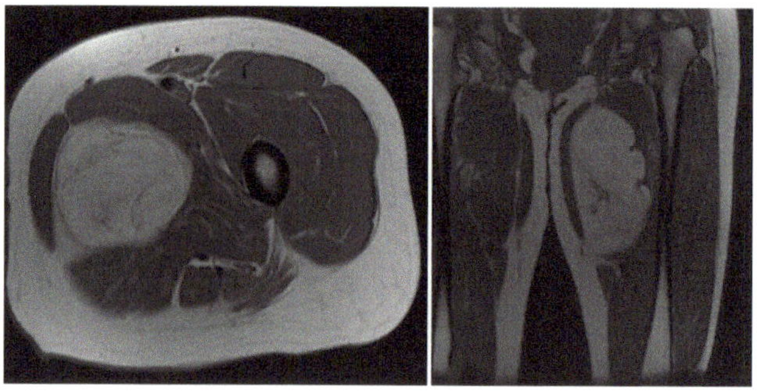

FIGURE 2.1 (A) Axial and (B) coronal images from MRI demonstrating homogeneously T1-hyperintense mass with hypointense internal septations suggestive of an atypical lipomatous tumor.

A core-needle biopsy should be performed using image guidance by an interventional radiologist in order to ensure the solid component of a mass (as opposed to a necrotic or hemorrhagic component) is the target of biopsy when present. While the risk of needle tract seeding is exceedingly rare, the needle tract is typically oriented such that it will be incorporated in either the planned surgical incision or radiation field, though this is not mandatory. An incisional biopsy is rarely indicated; however, when required, the incision should be placed along the long axis of the extremity such that this incision can be incorporated into the incision used for definitive resection.

The landmark randomized controlled trial performed by Rosenberg et al. in 1982 significantly changed the treatment paradigm for ESTS.[6] The results of this trial shifted the historical standard of care from amputation to a limb-sparing approach with no significant difference in overall survival (OS). Optimal outcomes are achieved with multidisciplinary evaluation with utilization of neoadjuvant/adjuvant chemotherapy and/or radiation therapy for tumors with a high risk of local or distant recurrence. The goal of surgery is a function-preserving, limb-conserving resection with negative microscopic margins (R0 resection). Although the data on margin status and survival are conflicting, negative microscopic margins have been shown to significantly improve local control rates.[7–10] Local control and survival may be preserved in the setting of an anticipated positive margin adjacent to a critical underlying structure when combined with preoperative radiation therapy.[11]

The surgical management of ESTS begins with a critical review of preoperative imaging in order to guide placement of incision in relation to the mass and adjacent critical structures. Understanding of functional anatomy is required in order to optimally balance oncologic resection and postoperative functional status. Resection should include the mass with a 1- to 2-cm rim of adjacent subcutaneous fat, muscle, or fascia, although narrower margins suffice when an anatomic barrier (such as fascia) is removed or radiation therapy is also used. Resection of overlying skin may be required and should be anticipated in order to coordinate potential reconstruction with a skin graft, rotational flap, or free flap. If a mass is superficial to the fascia, the fascia can be resected as the deep margin. When the underlying fascia is involved, the fascia should be resected along with the rim of underlying uninvolved muscle. Tumors abutting critical blood vessels, nerves, bone, and other structures require multidisciplinary evaluation as preoperative radiation and chemotherapy may allow these critical structures to be spared from en bloc resection without compromising oncologic outcome.[11,12] When en bloc resection is required, for instance, when a structure is encased by tumor and salvage would require disruption of tumor capsule, vascular reconstruction with an autologous or synthetic graft and nerve reconstruction with an interposition graft can be performed. For periosteal involvement without evidence of bone invasion, the periosteum can be resected as a margin. Prophylactic stabilization of the bone to prevent future fracture can be considered depending on the extent of periosteal stripping as well as the total radiation dose and the degree of circumferential exposure within the radiation field.[13–15] All specimens should be oriented with marking sutures for pathologic examination. Titanium clip placement at the margins of the tumor bed can guide planning of postoperative radiation therapy if indicated.

Atypical Lipomatous Tumor

ALT is the histologic equivalent of WDLPS of the retroperitoneum. ALTs have a homogeneous fat-dense appearance on imaging and may be difficult to distinguish from an intramuscular lipoma. ALTs are low-grade tumors; however, they have a significant local recurrence risk of 20% to 30% with a negligible risk of distant recurrence. While a negative microscopic margin remains the goal, the slow-growing nature of these tumors may allow for a focally positive margin over critical structures in order to preserve limb function. A not uncommon scenario is an incidentally discovered ALT following a marginal excision of a presumed lipoma. Baseline imaging can identify the presence and extent of residual disease. When ALT recurs, the disease-free interval can be long and the growth rate can be slow, so further intervention can be delayed for years and patients can be observed, provided no solid tumor tissue is noted within the area of recurrence on yearly MRI studies. Resection for recurrence may be reserved for those with progressing or symptomatic disease.

Myxofibrosarcoma

Myxofibrosarcomas demonstrate a characteristic growth pattern with a propensity for multiple local recurrences. Commonly arising in the extremities of elderly patients, these tumors have a tendency to infiltrate the surrounding soft tissue with fingerlings often extending beyond the primary appreciable mass of the tumor. When arising intramuscularly, they may be confined by fascial boundaries, but they can frequently demonstrate invasion into adjacent compartments. The microscopic extensions can travel along fascial planes and neurovascular structures and can invade through fascia separating the muscle compartments. Despite local recurrence rates ranging from 18% to 31%, the 5-year OS rates have been reported to be up to 77%.[7,16,17] Multiple local recurrences not only limit limb-salvage approaches but often demonstrate higher histologic grade than the primary lesion and have a greater metastatic propensity.[18] This highlights the need for aggressive upfront local therapy. Resection should aim for wider margins than other sarcomas, typically 2 to 4 cm around the appreciable mass, and is typically combined with either neoadjuvant or adjuvant radiation and/or chemotherapy. Management of the resulting defect often requires complex closure by a reconstructive surgeon. Closure may be delayed by the use of interim dressings, such as a negative pressure wound therapy dressing, to allow pathologic confirmation of negative margin status as well as margin re-excision in the event of positive margins prior to final wound closure.

Myxoid Liposarcoma

Myxoid liposarcoma is the second most common type of liposarcoma after WDLPS. In contrast to most ESTS, which predominately metastasize to the lungs, myxoid liposarcomas demonstrate a unique tumor biology with a predilection for extrapulmonary distant metastases.[19] Distant metastases occur in approximately one-third of patients, with over half of these patients developing bony involvement, with a propensity for the spine.[20] MRI of the spine should be included as part of the staging workup, in addition to CT imaging of the chest, abdomen, and pelvis in these patients. The favorable 5-year local recurrence-free survival (RFS; 97.7%) and metastasis-free survival (89.1%) rates are likely a reflection of their particular sensitivity to chemotherapy and radiation therapy.[21]

Fibromyxoid Sarcoma

Fibromyxoid sarcoma is a low-grade sarcoma that commonly afflicts young male adults, with a propensity for the deep soft tissues of the proximal lower extremities. In contrast to their relatively bland histologic appearance, these tumors demonstrate significant rates of local and distant recurrences, with most recent studies reporting rates of 64% and 45%, respectively.[22] Resection should include a 1- to 2-cm rim of normal adjacent tissue when feasible. Local recurrence and distant metastases have been documented as late as 15 and 45 years, respectively, and emphasize the need for prolonged surveillance in these patients.

Undifferentiated Pleomorphic Sarcoma

Undifferentiated pleomorphic sarcoma (UPS; pleomorphic fibrosarcoma, pleomorphic myxofibrosarcoma) is exclusively an intermediate- or high-grade tumor that was previously categorized under the heading "malignant fibrous histiocytoma." These aggressive tumors are the most common histologic subtype of ESTS and are typically diagnosed in older adults in their sixth and seventh decades of life. UPS has the worst oncologic outcomes of the histologic subtypes arising in the extremity. While these tumors have been reported to demonstrate comparable 5-year local RFS (81.3%) to other common histologic subtypes, 5-year distant metastasis-free survival (DMFS; 56.8%) and disease-specific survival (DSS; 55.6%) are significantly inferior.[23] High rates of unexpected R1 and R2 resections highlight the necessity for multimodality therapy.

RETROPERITONEAL SARCOMA

The retroperitoneum is the primary site in approximately 15% to 20% of patients with STS. The primary site of STS is a known prognostic factor with those arising in the retroperitoneum having a worse prognosis than those arising in the trunk or extremity.[24] Tumors of the retroperitoneum present a unique technical challenge owing to their typically large size at presentation and close proximity to critical structures and often require a multivisceral resection. Patients typically present with a new asymptomatic palpable abdominal mass or as an incidental finding during workup of nonspecific abdominal complaints. Initial radiographic evaluation with contrast-enhanced CT can provide details regarding the extent and involvement of adjacent structures, evaluate for metastatic disease, and potentially provide diagnostic information based on histology-specific imaging characteristics. Percutaneous image-guided biopsy is generally recommended in order to confirm diagnosis and histologic subtype, which will guide multidisciplinary evaluation with medical and radiation oncology. A biopsy may not always be warranted, as in the case of preoperative imaging demonstrating a homogeneous fat-dense mass that is suggestive of a WDLPS (Figure 2.2A and 2.2B). In this case, diagnostic information from a biopsy would likely not change the treatment approach. While there is a theoretical risk of needle track seeding with a biopsy, the reported incidence following biopsy is <2%.[25]

The goal of surgery for RPS is a macroscopically complete (R0/R1) resection of the mass with en bloc resection of directly involved adjacent structures. In contrast to the surgical approach for sarcomas of the extremity where a 2-cm rim of uninvolved surrounding muscle can usually be resected with limited additional morbidity, the close proximity of critical structures in the retroperitoneum requires a balance of oncologic principles and the morbidity associated with resection of these structures. As a result, the appropriate extent of resection and the need to resect adjacent uninvolved structures has been a topic of much debate. Suboptimal 5-year local RFS rates ranging between 42% and 59% despite an R0/R1 resection have prompted the exploration of a more aggressive surgical approach in order to provide improved local control. Some have advocated a compartmental resection approach, which involves a liberal en bloc resection of uninvolved organs in order to obtain a rim of normal tissue surrounding the tumor.[26–28] This more aggressive approach has demonstrated significantly improved local recurrence rates; however, no difference in OS has been observed. While more aggressive surgery may improve R0 resection rates, the prognostic significance of converting an R1 to an R0 resection remains unclear.

While the extent of resection continues to be debated, there are several key surgical principles recognized for RPS. Technical principles and consensus guidelines for the surgical management of RPS have been described.[29–31] A comprehensive knowledge of the retroperitoneum borders and structures is required in order to guide operative planning as well as to respect anatomic distortions due to the typically large size of these tumors. Anatomic considerations such as involvement of end organ vascular supply and organ encasement must be appreciated. Exposure and operative approach are paramount. Multiple incisions can be used based on the size and location of the mass. Choice of incision should be based on surgeon preference, while maximizing exposure in order to allow manipulation of the mass without disruption of the tumor capsule. A midline incision can access the left or right retroperitoneum with mobilization of intra-abdominal structures, though exposure of the subdiaphragmatic regions and the deep aspects of the retroperitoneum can be challenging, particularly in an obese

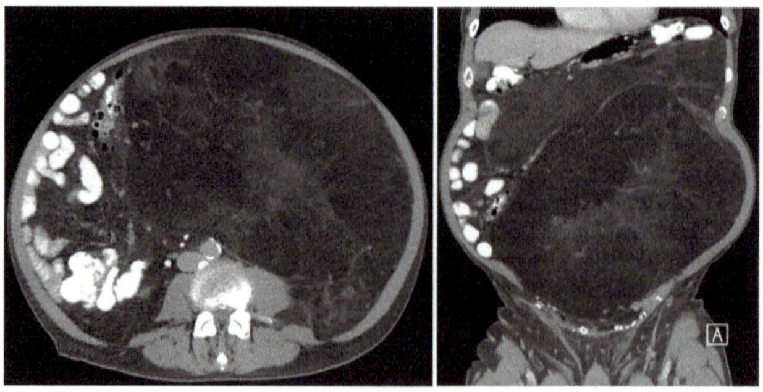

(A) (B)

FIGURE 2.2 (A) Axial and (B) coronal CT images of large homogeneous fat-dense mass with radiographic features consistent with a retroperitoneal WDLPS.

WDLPS, well-differentiated liposarcoma.

TABLE 2.1 Classification System for Rationale for Organ Resection

Category	Criteria
1	Frank organ invasion/tumor origin
2	Tumor involving vascular supply
3	Tumor encasement of organ
4	Tumor adherent to organ
5	Tumor adjacent to organ/required for macroscopic complete resection
6	Other (iatrogenic injury requiring resection, incidental resection for another reason)

patient. Alternatively, with the patient in a lateral decubitus position, a lower midline incision that is extended obliquely across the upper abdomen toward the tip of the ninth or 10th rib can provide optimal exposure for tumors involving the right or left upper quadrants and diaphragm, though this has the downside of cutting across the upper abdominal musculature. This incision can then be extended into the chest as part of a thoracoabdominal incision, if needed. For tumors located in the lower retroperitoneum or lateral side of the pelvis, either a transverse flank or modified Gibson incision can provide extraperitoneal access for smaller, low-grade tumors along the spine, psoas, pelvic sidewall, or sciatic notch.

When considering the need for organ resection, a histology-specific approach should be considered as opposed to a "one-size-fits-all" compartmental resection approach. In contrast to defining the "optimal" extent of resection, a recommended "minimal" extent of anticipated resection can be guided based on histology-specific tumor biology and the likelihood of local invasion. Two recent large studies (>600 patients) have reported histology-specific outcomes for patients undergoing surgery for primary RPS, which have broadened the understanding of the distinct tumor biology associated with individual histologic subtypes.[4,5] Both of these landmark studies demonstrated that local and distant failures are significantly influenced by histologic subtype. Additionally, histologic subtype can also predict the likelihood of histopathologic organ invasion (HOI), and thus necessitate the need for adjacent organ resection.[32] Recently reported data have demonstrated that HOI is present in 26% of resected adjacent organs and is an independent predictor of worse 5-year OS. The likelihood of HOI is influenced by histologic subtype, with patients with dedifferentiated liposarcoma (DDLPS), leiomyosarcoma (LMS), and WDLPS found to have HOI rates of 61%, 56%, and 40%, respectively. Rationale for organ resection may further predict the likelihood of HOI when classified using a six-tier classification system (Table 2.1). HOI has been shown to be present in 65% of organs resected when the surgeon felt the tumor was frankly invading the organ intraoperatively.[33] When a tumor is encasing or adherent to an organ, HOI is present in 19% and 26%, respectively.

Well-Differentiated Liposarcoma

WDLPS is a low-grade malignancy and is the most common subtype of liposarcoma. WDLPS is characterized by a negligible risk of distant failure, but a significant local recurrence risk of approximately 25% at 8 years, which remains constant over time. Surgical management of these tumors and the extent of resection should reflect their less aggressive tumor biology. The lower likelihood of HOI may justify avoiding nephrectomy when possible, as long as the tumor could be removed without violating the tumor capsule. While local failure is the primary cause of disease-specific death, there is typically less of a need for adjacent organ resection, knowing that a local recurrence can often be managed with observation, radiation therapy, or additional surgery.

Dedifferentiated Liposarcoma

DDLPSs are associated with a more aggressive tumor biology characterized by a significant risk of both local and distant failure. These tumors demonstrate a high rate of HOI that necessitates a more aggressive approach to adjacent organ resection. Multimodality therapy should be considered. The results of the recently completed European Organization for Research and Treatment of Cancer (EORTC) Phase 3 trial (STRASS) will better define the role of neoadjuvant radiation therapy in the local control of RPS.[34] Efforts to investigate the utility of systemic chemotherapy in the management of these patients are in development. Review of preoperative imaging is critical in order to appreciate any surrounding well-differentiated homogeneous fat-dense component in addition to the more solid and heterogeneous dedifferentiated component. A common problem noted in sarcoma centers is that patients may undergo surgery for a presumed renal cell carcinoma or ovarian cancer, in which a solid mass is removed, and it then turns out to be DDLPS. The surrounding abnormal fat consistent with WDLPS was not originally recognized, and thus was left behind as a large volume of residual disease.

Leiomyosarcoma

LMS is an aggressive histologic subtype that is thought to originate from a smooth muscle lineage. LMS is characterized by a relatively low risk of local recurrence but a very high risk for distant metastases. An approach to the primary tumor less aggressive than for DDLPS may be justified when the overall outcome in these patients will be ultimately dictated by distant metastases (though an R0/R1 resection, with a margin where possible, is still indicated). These tumors can be technically challenging when arising from the smooth muscle cells of the inferior vena cava or renal vein. The surgical approach for LMS of vascular origin often requires consultation with a vascular surgeon to aid with reconstruction depending on the extent of resection and intraoperative findings.

Solitary Fibrous Tumors

Solitary fibrous tumors (SFTs) are a rare group of sarcomas that are characterized by a more indolent natural history when arising in the retroperitoneum. While malignant and dedifferentiated variants demonstrate more aggressive behavior, the less aggressive classical variant of SFT predominates in the retroperitoneum. These tumors are typically associated with low rates of local recurrence and distant metastasis.[35,36]

Schwannoma

Schwannomas are benign nerve sheath tumors that can occur sporadically or as a manifestation of neurofibromatosis types 1 and 2. Schwannomas are the most common benign tumor arising in the retroperitoneum. These tumors often present as incidental findings on cross-sectional imaging, and percutaneous biopsy is usually warranted in order to rule out more common malignant retroperitoneal tumors. Schwannomas can present a significant technical challenge when arising from a named nerve or from a sacral nerve root at the level of a foramen. The benefit of resection must be carefully weighed against the potential morbidity associated with resection. A subtotal resection can be considered in order to limit morbidity because of the near-negligible risk of local recurrence or malignant transformation.

VISCERAL SARCOMAS

Sarcomas arising from intra-abdominal viscera demonstrate a distinct clinical behavior and require a histology-specific treatment approach. The two most common visceral sarcomas are intra-abdominal visceral LMS and GIST. The discovery that most GISTs express the receptor tyrosine kinase KIT (CD117) by Hirota et al. in 1998 led to more accurate distinction between these two subtypes and, more importantly, transformed the management of GISTs with the development of tyrosine kinase inhibitors.[37]

Gastrointestinal Stromal Tumor

GIST is the most common subtype of sarcoma and accounts for 18% of sarcoma diagnoses. The management of GIST is unique compared to other sarcoma subtypes owing to the presence of the gain-of-function *c-kit* mutation and subsequent efficacy of targeted tyrosine kinase inhibitors in the treatment of these tumors. With *c-kit* mutations present in approximately 85% of GISTs, imatinib mesylate (Gleevec; Novartis, Basel, Switzerland) is considered the standard of care in the neoadjuvant and adjuvant setting in appropriately selected patients.

A macroscopically complete resection is the cornerstone of the management of GIST as it is the only potentially curative therapy. Preoperative workup should include contrast-enhanced CT imaging of the abdomen and pelvis. Routine imaging of the chest for staging is not required because of the rarity of pulmonary metastases. Percutaneous biopsy is typically warranted in order to confirm diagnosis and potentially guide the use of neoadjuvant imatinib therapy. Diagnosis can be confirmed on immunohistochemistry with characteristic expression of markers including *KIT* (CD117, 85%), *CD34* (60%–70%), smooth muscle actin (30%–40%), and S-100 (5%).[38] Additionally, *DOG1* expression is present in >95% of GISTs, is rarely expressed on other tumors, and can identify *KIT*-negative GISTs with/without *PDGFRA* mutations.[39]

Surgery should begin with careful exploration of the abdomen in order to identify any undetected metastatic disease. As is true with RPSs, exposure is critical, so that the tumor can be removed with limited manipulation in order to avoid rupture of the tumor capsule. Wide margins are not required for GIST and due to the low incidence of lymph node metastases, lymphadenectomy is not required. While an R0 resection is optimal, similar rates of RFS have been demonstrated after R1 resection. Typically, localized tumors involving the stomach and small bowel can be approached with a wedge or segmental resection. More extensive resections may be required for tumors involving the proximal stomach/gastroesophageal junction, duodenum, and rectum. For these technically challenging scenarios, the use of neoadjuvant imatinib can be considered to facilitate a less extensive resection. Neoadjuvant imatinib also has utility in potentially downstaging a tumor in order to allow a laparoscopic approach. A laparoscopic approach for gastric GISTs of 2 to 5 cm has been shown to be safe without compromising oncologic outcomes and has subsequently been endorsed by the National Comprehensive Cancer Network (NCCN) guidelines. Outcome data for nongastric sites are sparse and it should only be attempted by oncologic surgeons with an advanced laparoscopic skill set.

GISTs that are 2 cm and smaller require special mention as these are often discovered incidentally and the majority likely do not require surgical resection. Resection of these small GISTs should be considered in the presence of high-risk endoscopic features such as irregular extraluminal border, heterogeneous echo pattern, presence of cystic spaces, and echogenic foci. In the absence of these findings, currently, the NCCN guidelines recommend endoscopic surveillance every 6 to 12 months. Endoscopic removal is generally discouraged because of increased risk of positive margins, tumor spillage, and perforation.

All patients should be evaluated for the need for adjuvant imatinib. Multiple prospective, randomized clinical trials have evaluated the efficacy and duration of adjuvant imatinib.[40–42] The need for adjuvant imatinib is based on the estimation of risk of recurrence, which typically takes into account tumor size, mitotic index, and primary tumor location. Multiple risk calculators have been developed, and in general, at least 36 months of adjuvant imatinib is recommended for patients with intermediate or high risk of recurrence. All patients who undergo neoadjuvant imatinib treatment should be continued on adjuvant imatinib for a total of 36 months of combined treatment owing to the inability to accurately assess recurrence risk from the treated surgical specimen. Treatment therapy and dosing of imatinib can be guided by genotype analysis. While the standard dosing of imatinib is 400 mg/day, extrapolating data from patients with recurrent/metastatic GIST, patients with a *KIT* exon 9 mutation may demonstrate improved results at a higher dose of 800 mg/day.[43] Patients with a succinate dehydrogenase (SDH)-deficient GIST or platelet-derived growth factor receptor-alpha (*PDFGRA*) D842V GIST are insensitive to imatinib treatment and require alternative treatment strategies. Surveillance imaging with CT imaging of the abdomen and pelvis should be obtained every 3 to 6 months for the first 3 to 5 years and then annually thereafter. Routine surveillance imaging of the chest is not indicated because of the rarity of pulmonary metastases.

Visceral LMS

Visceral LMS is the most common non-GIST intra-abdominal visceral sarcoma. Intra-abdominal LMS is much rarer than LMS arising in the retroperitoneum and extremities, and available data are generally limited to case reports and case series. Data reported on visceral LMS before the year 2000 are likely confounded by the inclusion of GISTs that were often misclassified prior to the discovery of their diagnostic molecular marker profile. Visceral LMS lacks *KIT*, *CD34*, and *DOG1* molecular markers, which are present in GISTs, and express smooth muscle markers such as desmin and smooth muscle actin.

Initial workup of visceral LMS is similar to that of GIST with contrast-enhanced CT imaging and endoscopic or percutaneous biopsy. These tumors do differ from GISTs in their propensity to demonstrate a higher rate of local recurrence, whereas GIST rarely recurs locally. The goal of surgery is an R0 resection, with wide margins recommended in order to avoid an R1 resection. Inferred from LMS of the extremity, R1 resection is associated with worse survival. Lymphadenectomy is not indicated for visceral LMS.

The limited data available for visceral LMS suggest they demonstrate similar behavior to their retroperitoneal counterparts. The risk of local and distant failures has been reported to be 21% and 43%, respectively, at 5 years.[44] The lung is the most common site of distant metastases. Notably, distant recurrences have been reported in approximately 10% of patients beyond 5 years from original diagnosis, and this highlights the need for continued surveillance with CT imaging of the chest, abdomen, and pelvis beyond the standard 5 years.

BREAST SARCOMAS

Breast sarcomas are a rare group of tumors that can arise from the breast parenchyma or from the skin of the breast. The two most common histologic types are angiosarcoma and phyllodes tumors. These tumors demonstrate distinctive tumor biologic features that guide their specific treatment approach and overall outcomes.

Primary Angiosarcoma

Primary angiosarcoma arises from the breast parenchyma and is typically seen in young women aged 30 to 50 years. No predisposing risk factors have been identified for primary angiosarcoma. These tumors typically present as a palpable mass and are often diagnosed after a workup including a mammogram, ultrasound, and biopsy. Once diagnosis is confirmed, staging workup should include CT imaging of the chest, abdomen, and pelvis, as well as an MRI study of the breast.

Surgery is the only potentially curative treatment for primary angiosarcomas. Unlike conventional breast cancer that may potentially be amenable to a breast-conserving surgical approach when combined with radiation therapy, the sensitivity of breast angiosarcomas to radiation is unknown (although there is no biologic reason that their sensitivity to radiation would be different from that for sarcomas occurring in other anatomic sites). Therefore, simple mastectomy is the preferred approach. On rare occasions when breast conservation may be an option (small tumor in a woman with breast of an appropriate size that lumpectomy is feasible), surgery short of a mastectomy may be reasonable to consider. However, the utility of radiation therapy, owing to the rarity of reported cases, is uncertain. En bloc resection of skin or pectoralis major may be required in order to obtain an R0 resection if in close proximity. Axillary lymph node dissection is not routinely performed because of the low incidence of reported nodal metastases. While angiosarcomas are often responsive to chemotherapy, the role of chemotherapy in the adjuvant setting is unclear as no definitive benefit has been demonstrated, but could be considered in patients at high risk for recurrence and in the neoadjuvant setting to facilitate breast-sparing surgery. Surveillance usually consists of breast/chest wall MRI and CT of the chest, abdomen, and pelvis.

Secondary Angiosarcoma

Secondary angiosarcomas develop in the setting of prior radiation therapy or chronic lymphedema (Stewart–Treves syndrome). As a result, these patients tend to be older than primary angiosarcoma patients. Radiation-associated breast angiosarcoma often occurs in patients who have undergone breast-conserving surgery followed by radiation for breast carcinoma. This tumor type is distinct from primary angiosarcoma as it arises from the dermis and subcutis in the area of the radiation field.

The surgical approach for radiation-associated breast angiosarcoma reflects its inherent tumor biology and is much more extensive than that for primary angiosarcoma. A radical resection, which involves a mastectomy along with resection of all the skin in the radiation field, is required because of the multifocality of these tumors and the fact that the entire area in the radiation field is at risk for disease. This involves removing all the skin extending from the clavicle superiorly, rectus fascia inferiorly, sternal border medially, and latissimus dorsi laterally. Resection of the pectoralis major muscle may be required if it is directly involved, in order to ensure an R0 resection. Collaboration with a reconstructive team is required to facilitate wound closure with skin grafting and/or rotational flap. This radical approach has been shown to reduce recurrence rates and improve DSS when compared to less extensive resection involving only wide local excision or mastectomy with only partial skin resection.[45] While local recurrences can be appreciated by physical examination, because of a significant risk of distant recurrence, surveillance imaging should include CT imaging of the chest and abdomen.

Phyllodes Tumor

Phyllodes tumors are rare fibroepithelial tumors of the breast that can display varying levels of aggressive behavior. While the majority of these tumors are classified as benign, they can also be categorized as borderline and malignant, depending on the degree of stromal cellular atypia, mitotic activity, presence of infiltrative tumor margins, and presence of stromal overgrowth. Phyllodes tumors often present as a large palpable mass in women in their fifth and sixth decades of life. Core biopsy is typically diagnostic, demonstrating a classic leaf-like architecture on pathologic review.

The surgical approach involves resection with a margin of at least 1 cm. This may be accomplished with a lumpectomy, depending on the size of the tumor; otherwise, a simple mastectomy is required. Axillary lymph node dissection is not required because of the low incidence of regional lymph node involvement. While not indicated for benign phyllodes tumors, adjuvant radiation may be considered in patients with borderline or malignant tumors in order to reduce local recurrence rates.[46] The presence of stromal overgrowth is associated with a high risk of distant recurrence and results in consideration for neoadjuvant/adjuvant chemotherapy. Physical examination is adequate for surveillance of a local recurrence and should be combined with CT imaging of the chest, abdomen, and pelvis for borderline and malignant tumors.

CUTANEOUS SARCOMAS

Sarcomas originating from the dermis and subcutis are a heterogeneous group of tumors that display a wide range of clinical behavior. These tumors may present as a pigmented lesion or subcutaneous nodule that may be difficult to initially distinguish from more common benign and malignant lesions.

Dermatofibrosarcoma Protuberans

Dermatofibrosarcoma protuberans (DFSP) is a rare cutaneous sarcoma that can demonstrate aggressive local behavior. These tumors often present as a slow-growing mass that may manifest as a pigmented skin papule. They commonly arise in the trunk and proximal extremities and often infiltrate the surrounding soft tissue beyond the appreciable mass. Core biopsy can guide the extent of resection; however, often, DFSP may be an incidental finding after initial marginal resection for an unknown superficial mass.

Resection involves wide margins of at least 2 to 4 cm carried down to the level of the underlying fascia. Reconstruction with a skin graft or local flap may be required. Intraoperative margin assessment is challenging as the surrounding fat is not amenable to frozen section analysis. Mohs micrographic surgery is generally not recommended because of lack of long-term results, though it may be considered for tumors in sensitive locations such as the face. Surveillance should include physical examination for detection of a local recurrence. In approximately 5% to 10% of patients, a more aggressive fibrosarcomatous variant will be present. This histologic subtype is associated with a higher rate of local recurrence and propensity for distant metastases. While the surgical approach is similar to that of the classic variant, the behavior of this variant justifies consideration of (neo)adjuvant radiation. Furthermore, surveillance in this subset of patients with the fibrosarcomatous variant may include local imaging with either a chest x-ray or CT imaging of the chest, abdomen, and pelvis.

Atypical Fibroxanthoma

Atypical fibroxanthoma is a cutaneous sarcoma that often arises in sun-exposed skin of the head and neck of older patients. These tumors typically present as a solitary red papule or nodule that may ulcerate and occasionally bleed. Atypical fibroxanthomas demonstrate fairly benign behavior and require resection of the entire tumor with negative margins.

Pleomorphic Dermal Sarcoma

Pleomorphic dermal sarcomas are a group of more aggressive cutaneous sarcomas with a greater propensity for both local and distant recurrence. Pleomorphic dermal sarcomas can be difficult to distinguish from atypical fibroxanthomas; however, the former demonstrates invasion into the subcutaneous fat and may demonstrate a higher mitotic count in addition to lymphovascular and perineural invasion. As a result, resection requires wider margins of at least 2 cm. Adjuvant radiation therapy may be considered. Surveillance should include physical examination of the primary site and CT imaging of the chest.

DESMOID TUMOR

Desmoid tumors are a rare group of tumors that account for <3% of all sarcomas. Also known as desmoid fibromatosis or aggressive fibromatosis, these tumors are histologically benign and lack the ability to metastasize. Desmoid tumors can demonstrate variable clinical behavior and have the ability to be locally aggressive with high local recurrence rates after wide local excision. Desmoid tumors also demonstrate a propensity to occur during pregnancy. Core-needle biopsy can confirm diagnosis and aid in directing management strategy.

While the majority of desmoid tumors occur sporadically, approximately 10% develop in the setting of a germline mutation in the adenomatous polyposis coli (*APC*) gene that is associated with familial adenomatous polyposis (FAP). Desmoids have been reported to develop in 10% to 20% of patients with FAP, with the majority arising within the abdomen and the abdominal wall. Notably, desmoids in patients with FAP also demonstrate a propensity to arise at incision sites from previous surgery. Intra-abdominal desmoids present a technical challenge as they often involve the bowel mesentery and mesenteric vessels, resulting in significant morbidity.

The management of desmoid tumors has evolved with the pendulum swinging away from an aggressive surgical approach to a much more conservative, watchful waiting approach. While some tumors may be locally aggressive, others may demonstrate more indolent behavior and even spontaneously stabilize or regress (approximately 20% spontaneous regression rate). An initial period of observation is recommended for asymptomatic tumors, even when initially resectable. In the setting of progressive or symptomatic disease, multiple options are available, including cytotoxic chemotherapy (doxorubicin ± dacarbazine, liposomal doxorubicin, vinorelbine + methotrexate), tyrosine kinase inhibitors (imatinib, sorafenib), nonsteroidal anti-inflammatory drugs (indomethacin, sulindac), and antihormonal agents (tamoxifen). Surgery is typically reserved for refractory tumors, especially for mesenteric desmoids, where surgery can be associated with significant morbidity. In the case of pregnancy-associated abdominal wall desmoids, surgery can be considered earlier following a period of observation because of favorable outcomes following resection in this cohort of patients.

RECURRENT SARCOMA

While surgery is the mainstay treatment for most STS, despite a successful resection with negative margins, recurrence rates remain significant. Systemic therapies may be the first-line treatment in patients with recurrent disease, particularly those with high-grade tumors. This provides the opportunity to gain control of the disease and allow time to understand the tumor biology and disease trajectory. Surgery in the setting of recurrent disease may be considered in a select group of patients. It is vitally important that these complex patients undergo multidisciplinary evaluation at a sarcoma center in order to optimize outcomes.[4,28,29,47] Site- and histology-specific factors should guide the surgical management in these patients.

Recurrent RPS

The most common cause of death in patients with RPSs is from a local recurrence. The potential survival benefit of surgery must be carefully weighed against the potential morbidity associated with these challenging cases. Resection of a local recurrence or distant metastasis has been shown to significantly improve 5-year OS, compared to those patients who do not undergo resection.[48] Longer time to recurrence is a significant predictor of improved OS.

The surgical management of patients with localized recurrent disease mirrors that of primary disease. The goal of surgery is a macroscopically complete resection with en bloc resection of involved adjacent organs. Surgery in patients with a multifocal recurrence should be considered for palliative purposes weighed against the poor overall outcomes in these patients. The true survival benefit after resection of distant metastases is unclear and should be addressed on a case-by-case basis. The lungs are a common site of metastases and can be considered for resection in the absence of extrathoracic disease, when the primary tumor is treatable/has been treated, and a complete resection can be achieved.[49–51] Surgery is not recommended in patients with a concurrent local recurrence and distant metastasis.

Metastatic GIST

Metastatic disease is present in up to 50% of patients at the time of presentation with GIST.[42] Tyrosine kinase inhibitor therapy is the first-line therapy in patients with metastatic disease. Despite the effectiveness of tyrosine kinase inhibitors in controlling the disease, a complete response is very rare. Additionally, the response to tyrosine kinase inhibitor therapy is not indefinite, with the median time to progression on imatinib being 24 months,[52] on sunitinib malate being 6.8 months[53] (Sutent; Pfizer, New York, NY), and on regorafenib being 4.8 months[54] (Stivarga; Bayer, Leverkusen, Germany). As a result, surgery can play a key role in carefully selected patients, with the aim of prolonging time to progression by removing disease before secondary resistance develops and eliminating resistant clones.

The goal of surgery in patients with metastatic GIST is a macroscopically complete resection and should include en bloc resection of involved adjacent organs. Attempts to conduct a randomized clinical trial to study the outcomes of cytoreductive surgery in patients with metastatic GIST have been unsuccessful because of poor patient accrual. Multiple retrospective studies have demonstrated that cytoreductive surgery may result in prolonged progression-free survival in patients with responsive or stable disease on tyrosine kinase inhibitor therapy at the time of surgery (when compared to surgery in those with progressive disease).[55–59] The morbidity associated with these complex operations must be examined, and prediction of significant postoperative morbidity can be aided by a recently published surgical complexity scoring system.[60] A planned R2 resection may be justified for symptom palliation; however, resection of only tyrosine kinase inhibitor–resistant lesions while leaving lesions that are responsive to treatment likely provides no benefit.

SUMMARY

STSs are composed of a heterogeneous group of tumors that demonstrate distinctive clinical behavior based on their inherent tumor biology. The rarity and complexity of these tumors require multidisciplinary evaluation at a sarcoma center in order to determine optimal therapy and maximize outcomes. Preoperative biopsy and confirmation of accurate diagnosis are paramount in most scenarios and allow a histology-specific approach to treatment. Understanding of the patterns of local and/or distant failure should be one component that helps guide the appropriate extent of resection. Additionally, anatomic considerations and likelihood of adjacent organ involvement should be considered. The optimal extent of resection must be carefully weighed against the associated risks of morbidity and mortality. Close postoperative follow-up and surveillance are required to identify recurrent disease promptly. Surgery can play a significant role in the multimodality treatment of recurrent or metastatic disease in carefully selected patients.

REFERENCES

1. Ducimetiere F, Lurkin A, Ranchere-Vince D, et al. Incidence of sarcoma histotypes and molecular subtypes in a prospective epidemiological study with central pathology review and molecular testing. *PLoS One.* 2011;6(8):e20294. doi:10.1371/journal.pone.0020294
2. American Cancer Society. *Cancer Facts and Figures 2018: Soft Tissue Sarcoma*. Atlanta, GA: American Cancer Society. https://www.cancer.org/cancer/soft-tissue-sarcoma/references.html
3. Clark MA, Fisher C, Judson I, et al. Soft-tissue sarcomas in adults. *N Engl J Med.* 2005;353(7):701–711. doi:10.1056/NEJMra041866
4. Gronchi A, Strauss DC, Miceli R, et al. Variability in patterns of recurrence after resection of primary retroperitoneal sarcoma (RPS): a report on 1007 patients from the Multi-institutional Collaborative RPS Working Group. *Ann Surg.* 2016;263(5):1002–1009. doi:10.1097/SLA.0000000000001447
5. Tan MC, Brennan MF, Kuk D, et al. Histology-based classification predicts pattern of recurrence and improves risk stratification in primary retroperitoneal sarcoma. *Ann Surg.* 2016;263(3):593–600. doi:10.1097/SLA.0000000000001149
6. Rosenberg SA, Tepper J, Glatstein E, et al. The treatment of soft-tissue sarcomas of the extremities: prospective randomized evaluations of (1) limb-sparing surgery plus radiation therapy compared with amputation and (2) the role of adjuvant chemotherapy. *Ann Surg.* 1982;196(3):305–315. doi:10.1097/00000658-198209000-00009
7. Gronchi A, Lo Vullo S, Colombo C, et al. Extremity soft tissue sarcoma in a series of patients treated at a single institution: local control directly impacts survival. *Ann Surg.* 2010;251(3):506–511. doi:10.1097/SLA.0b013e3181cf87fa
8. Gronchi A, Casali PG, Mariani L, et al. Status of surgical margins and prognosis in adult soft tissue sarcomas of the extremities: a series of patients treated at a single institution. *J Clin Oncol.* 2005;23(1):96–104. doi:10.1200/JCO.2005.04.160
9. Pisters PW, Leung DH, Woodruff J, et al. Analysis of prognostic factors in 1,041 patients with localized soft tissue sarcomas of the extremities. *J Clin Oncol.* 1996;14(5):1679–1689. doi:10.1200/JCO.1996.14.5.1679
10. Zagars GK, Ballo MT, Pisters PW, et al. Prognostic factors for patients with localized soft-tissue sarcoma treated with conservation surgery and radiation therapy: an analysis of 1225 patients. *Cancer.* 2003;97(10):2530–2543. doi:10.1002/cncr.11365
11. Gundle KR, Kafchinski L, Gupta S, et al. Analysis of margin classification systems for assessing the risk of local recurrence after soft tissue sarcoma resection. *J Clin Oncol.* 2018;36(7):704–709. doi:10.1200/JCO.2017.74.6941
12. O'Donnell PW, Griffin AM, Eward WC, et al. The effect of the setting of a positive surgical margin in soft tissue sarcoma. *Cancer.* 2014;120(18):2866–2875. doi:10.1002/cncr.28793
13. Gortzak Y, Lockwood GA, Mahendra A, et al. Prediction of pathologic fracture risk of the femur after combined modality treatment of soft tissue sarcoma of the thigh. *Cancer.* 2010;116(6):1553–1559. doi:10.1002/cncr.24949
14. Bishop AJ, Zagars GK, Allen PK, et al. Treatment-related fractures after combined modality therapy for soft tissue sarcomas of the proximal lower extremity: can the risk be mitigated? *Pract Radiat Oncol.* 2016;6(3):194–200. doi:10.1016/j.prro.2015.09.004

15. Dickie CI, Parent AL, Griffin AM, et al. Bone fractures following external beam radiotherapy and limb-preservation surgery for lower extremity soft tissue sarcoma: relationship to irradiated bone length, volume, tumor location and dose. *Int J Radiat Oncol Biol Phys.* 2009;75(4):1119–1124. doi:10.1016/j.ijrobp.2008.12.006
16. Haglund KE, Raut CP, Nascimento AF, et al. Recurrence patterns and survival for patients with intermediate- and high-grade myxofibrosarcoma. *Int J Radiat Oncol Biol Phys.* 2012;82(1):361–367. doi:10.1016/j.ijrobp.2010.08.042
17. Sanfilippo R, Miceli R, Grosso F, et al. Myxofibrosarcoma: prognostic factors and survival in a series of patients treated at a single institution. *Ann Surg Oncol.* 2011;18(3):720–725. doi:10.1245/s10434-010-1341-4
18. Willems SM, Debiec-Rychter M, Szuhai K, et al. Local recurrence of myxofibrosarcoma is associated with increase in tumour grade and cytogenetic aberrations, suggesting a multistep tumour progression model. *Mod Pathol.* 2006;19(3):407–416. doi:10.1038/modpathol.3800550
19. Pearlstone DB, Pisters PW, Bold RJ, et al. Patterns of recurrence in extremity liposarcoma: implications for staging and follow-up. *Cancer.* 1999;85(1):85–92. doi:10.1002/(SICI)1097-0142(19990101)85:1<85::AID-CNCR12>3.0.CO;2-A
20. Schwab JH, Boland P, Guo T, et al. Skeletal metastases in myxoid liposarcoma: an unusual pattern of distant spread. *Ann Surg Oncol.* 2007;14(4):1507–1514. doi:10.1245/s10434-006-9306-3
21. Chung PW, Deheshi BM, Ferguson PC, et al. Radiosensitivity translates into excellent local control in extremity myxoid liposarcoma: a comparison with other soft tissue sarcomas. *Cancer.* 2009; 115(14):3254–3261. doi:10.1002/cncr.24375
22. Evans HL. Low-grade fibromyxoid sarcoma: a clinicopathologic study of 33 cases with long-term follow-up. *Am J Surg Pathol.* 2011;35(10):1450–1462. doi:10.1097/PAS.0b013e31822b3687
23. Smith HG, Memos N, Thomas JM, et al. Patterns of disease relapse in primary extremity soft-tissue sarcoma. *Br J Surg.* 2016;103(11):1487–1496. doi:10.1002/bjs.10227
24. Brennan MF, Antonescu CR, Moraco N, et al. Lessons learned from the study of 10,000 patients with soft tissue sarcoma. *Ann Surg.* 2014;260(3):416–421; discussion 421–422. doi:10.1097/SLA.0000000000000869
25. Berger-Richardson D, Swallow CJ. Needle tract seeding after percutaneous biopsy of sarcoma: risk/benefit considerations. *Cancer.* 2017;123(4):560–567. doi:10.1002/cncr.30370
26. Gronchi A, Lo Vullo S, Fiore M, et al. Aggressive surgical policies in a retrospectively reviewed single-institution case series of retroperitoneal soft tissue sarcoma patients. *J Clin Oncol.* 2009;27(1):24–30. doi:10.1200/JCO.2008.17.8871
27. Bonvalot S, Miceli R, Berselli M, et al. Aggressive surgery in retroperitoneal soft tissue sarcoma carried out at high-volume centers is safe and is associated with improved local control. *Ann Surg Oncol.* 2010;17(6):1507–1514. doi:10.1245/s10434-010-1057-5
28. Bonvalot S, Rivoire M, Castaing M, et al. Primary retroperitoneal sarcomas: a multivariate analysis of surgical factors associated with local control. *J Clin Oncol.* 2009;27(1):31–37. doi:10.1200/JCO.2008.18.0802
29. Trans-Atlantic RPS Working Group. Management of primary retroperitoneal sarcoma (RPS) in the adult: a consensus approach from the Trans-Atlantic RPS Working Group. *Ann Surg Oncol.* 2015;22(1):256–263. doi:10.1245/s10434-014-3965-2
30. Bonvalot S, Raut CP, Pollock RE, et al. Technical considerations in surgery for retroperitoneal sarcomas: position paper from E-Surge, a master class in sarcoma surgery, and EORTC-STBSG. *Ann Surg Oncol.* 2012;19(9):2981–2991. doi:10.1245/s10434-012-2342-2
31. ESMO/European Sarcoma Network Working Group. Soft tissue and visceral sarcomas: ESMO Clinical Practice Guidelines for diagnosis, treatment and follow-up. *Ann Oncol.* 2014;25(suppl 3):iii102–iii112. doi:10.1093/annonc/mdu254
32. Fairweather M, Wang J, Jo VY, et al. Incidence and adverse prognostic implications of histopathologic organ invasion in primary retroperitoneal sarcoma. *J Am Coll Surg.* 2017;224(5):876–883. doi:10.1016/j.jamcollsurg.2017.01.044
33. Fairweather M, Wang J, Jo VY, et al. Surgical management of primary retroperitoneal sarcomas: rationale for selective organ resection. *Ann Surg Oncol.* 2018;25(1):98–106. doi:10.1245/s10434-017-6136-4
34. Bonvalot S, Gronchi A, Le Pechoux C, et al. STRASS (EORTC 62092): *A phase III randomized study of preoperative radiotherapy plus surgery versus surgery alone for patients with retroperitoneal sarcoma. J Clin Oncol.* 2019;37(15):11001. doi:10.1200/JCO.2019.37.15_suppl.11001
35. van Houdt WJ, Westerveld CM, Vrijenhoek JE, et al. Prognosis of solitary fibrous tumors: a multicenter study. *Ann Surg Oncol.* 2013;20(13):4090–4095. doi:10.1245/s10434-013-3242-9
36. Gold JS, Antonescu CR, Hajdu C, et al. Clinicopathologic correlates of solitary fibrous tumors. *Cancer.* 2002;94(4):1057–1068. doi:10.1002/cncr.10328
37. Hirota S, Isozaki K, Moriyama Y, et al. Gain-of-function mutations of c-kit in human gastrointestinal stromal tumors. *Science.* 1998;279(5350):577–580. doi:10.1126/science.279.5350.577
38. Gold JS, Dematteo RP. Combined surgical and molecular therapy: the gastrointestinal stromal tumor model. *Ann Surg.* 2006;244(2):176–184. doi:10.1097/01.sla.0000218080.94145.cf
39. Novelli M, Rossi S, Rodriguez-Justo M, et al. DOG1 and CD117 are the antibodies of choice in the diagnosis of gastrointestinal stromal tumours. *Histopathology.* 2010;57(2):259–270. doi:10.1111/j.1365-2559.2010.03624.x
40. Dematteo RP, Ballman KV, Antonescu CR, et al. Adjuvant imatinib mesylate after resection of localised, primary gastrointestinal stromal tumour: a randomised, double-blind, placebo-controlled trial. *Lancet.* 2009; 373(9669):1097–1104. doi:10.1016/S0140-6736(09)60500-6

41. Joensuu H, Eriksson M, Sundby Hall K, et al. One vs three years of adjuvant imatinib for operable gastrointestinal stromal tumor: a randomized trial. *JAMA*. 2012;307(12):1265–1272. doi:10.1001/jama.2012.347
42. Casali PG, Le Cesne A, Poveda Velasco A, et al. Time to definitive failure to the first tyrosine kinase inhibitor in localized GI stromal tumors treated with imatinib as an adjuvant: a European Organisation for Research and Treatment of Cancer Soft Tissue and Bone Sarcoma Group intergroup randomized trial in collaboration with the Australasian Gastro-Intestinal Trials Group, UNICANCER, French Sarcoma Group, Italian Sarcoma Group, and Spanish Group for Research on Sarcomas. *J Clin Oncol*. 2015;33(36):4276–4283. doi:10.1200/JCO.2015.62.4304
43. Gastrointestinal Stromal Tumor Meta-Analysis Group. Comparison of two doses of imatinib for the treatment of unresectable or metastatic gastrointestinal stromal tumors: a meta-analysis of 1,640 patients. *J Clin Oncol*. 2010;28(7):1247–1253. doi:10.1200/JCO.2009.24.2099
44. Gladdy RA, Qin LX, Moraco N, et al. Predictors of survival and recurrence in primary leiomyosarcoma. *Ann Surg Oncol*. 2013;20(6):1851–1857. doi:10.1245/s10434-013-2876-y
45. Li GZ, Fairweather M, Wang J, et al. Cutaneous radiation-associated breast angiosarcoma: radicality of surgery impacts survival. *Ann Surg*. 2017;265(4):814–820. doi:10.1097/SLA.0000000000001753
46. Barth RJ Jr, Wells WA, Mitchell SE, et al. A prospective, multi-institutional study of adjuvant radiotherapy after resection of malignant phyllodes tumors. *Ann Surg Oncol*. 2009;16(8):2288–2294. doi:10.1245/s10434-009-0489-2
47. Toulmonde M, Bonvalot S, Meeus P, et al. Retroperitoneal sarcomas: patterns of care at diagnosis, prognostic factors and focus on main histological subtypes: a multicenter analysis of the French Sarcoma Group. *Ann Oncol*. 2014;25(3):735–742. doi:10.1093/annonc/mdt577
48. MacNeill AJ, Miceli R, Strauss DC, et al. Post-relapse outcomes after primary extended resection of retroperitoneal sarcoma: a report from the Trans-Atlantic RPS Working Group. *Cancer*. 2017;123(11):1971–1978. doi:10.1002/cncr.30572
49. Chudgar NP, Brennan MF, Munhoz RR, et al. Pulmonary metastasectomy with therapeutic intent for soft-tissue sarcoma. *J Thorac Cardiovasc Surg*. 2017;154(1):319e1–330e1. doi:10.1016/j.jtcvs.2017.02.061
50. Billingsley KG, Burt ME, Jara E, et al. Pulmonary metastases from soft tissue sarcoma: analysis of patterns of diseases and postmetastasis survival. *Ann Surg*. 1999;229(5):602–610; discussion 610–612. doi:10.1097/00000658-199905000-00002
51. Jablons D, Steinberg SM, Roth J, et al. Metastasectomy for soft tissue sarcoma. Further evidence for efficacy and prognostic indicators. *J Thorac Cardiovasc Surg*. 1989;97(5):695–705. doi:10.1016/S0022-5223(19)34514-3
52. Blanke CD, Demetri GD, von Mehren M, et al. Long-term results from a randomized phase II trial of standard- versus higher-dose imatinib mesylate for patients with unresectable or metastatic gastrointestinal stromal tumors expressing KIT. *J Clin Oncol*. 2008;26(4):620–625. doi:10.1200/JCO.2007.13.4403
53. Demetri GD, van Oosterom AT, Garrett CR, et al. Efficacy and safety of sunitinib in patients with advanced gastrointestinal stromal tumour after failure of imatinib: a randomised controlled trial. *Lancet*. 2006;368(9544):1329–1338. doi:10.1016/S0140-6736(06)69446-4
54. Demetri GD, Reichardt P, Kang YK, et al. Efficacy and safety of regorafenib for advanced gastrointestinal stromal tumours after failure of imatinib and sunitinib (GRID): an international, multicentre, randomised, placebo-controlled, phase 3 trial. *Lancet*. 2013;381(9863):295–302. doi:10.1016/S0140-6736(12)61857-1
55. Fairweather M, Balachandran VP, Li GZ, et al. Cytoreductive surgery for metastatic gastrointestinal stromal tumors treated with tyrosine kinase inhibitors: a 2-institutional analysis. *Ann Surg*. 2018;268(2):296–302. doi:10.1097/SLA.0000000000002281
56. Bauer S, Rutkowski P, Hohenberger P, et al. Long-term follow-up of patients with GIST undergoing metastasectomy in the era of imatinib—analysis of prognostic factors (EORTC-STBSG collaborative study). *Eur J Surg Oncol*. 2014;40(4):412–419. doi:10.1016/j.ejso.2013.12.020
57. Bonvalot S, Eldweny H, Pechoux CL, et al. Impact of surgery on advanced gastrointestinal stromal tumors (GIST) in the imatinib era. *Ann Surg Oncol*. 2006;13(12):1596–1603. doi:10.1245/s10434-006-9047-3
58. DeMatteo RP, Maki RG, Singer S, et al. Results of tyrosine kinase inhibitor therapy followed by surgical resection for metastatic gastrointestinal stromal tumor. *Ann Surg*. 2007;245(3):347–352. doi:10.1097/01.sla.0000236630.93587.59
59. Gronchi A, Fiore M, Miselli F, et al. Surgery of residual disease following molecular-targeted therapy with imatinib mesylate in advanced/metastatic GIST. *Ann Surg*. 2007;245(3):341–346. doi:10.1097/01.sla.0000242710.36384.1b
60. Fairweather M, Cavnar MJ, Li GZ, et al. Prediction of morbidity following cytoreductive surgery for metastatic gastrointestinal stromal tumour in patients on tyrosine kinase inhibitor therapy. *Br J Surg*. 2018;105(6):743–750. doi:10.1002/bjs.10774

3

Pathology of Sarcoma

Julio A. Diaz-Perez and Andrew E. Rosenberg

INTRODUCTION

The word *sarcoma* is derived from the Greek term "sarkoun," which means "fleshy substance or excrescence."[1] Sarcoma is defined as a malignant neoplasm whose phenotype recapitulates cells of mesodermal derivatives including the connective tissue, muscle, and peripheral nerve sheath. Sarcoma arises in any portion of the body; however, most originate in the soft tissues and skeleton.[2] Biologically, sarcomas have the potential to progressively enlarge, grow with an infiltrative pattern, and metastasize.[3] Most sarcomas disseminate via the vascular system, with the lungs being the most common site for metastatic disease.[4] Lymph node metastases from sarcomas are uncommon and occur in approximately 3.5% of cases.[5] Tumors associated with the greatest risk of spread to lymph nodes include epithelioid sarcoma and clear cell sarcoma followed by angiosarcoma and synovial sarcoma.[6] The defining biologic behavior of sarcoma dictates treatment, which includes surgery, radiation, and systemic therapy.

CLASSIFICATION

The current 2013 World Health Organization (WHO) classification recognizes more than 100 soft tissue and bone tumor entities, and more than 70 are sarcomas.[7] The features used to classify sarcomas are their normal tissue counterpart, and this group accounts for the vast majority (Table 3.1). A comparatively smaller number of sarcomas have consistent and distinctive clinicopathologic features, but lack an identified normal tissue counterpart, and their classification is based on their morphologic features (spindle cell sarcoma, small round cell sarcoma)[7,8] and their molecular aberrations (*EWSR1/FUS–NFATc2*-rearranged round cell sarcoma).[9]

EPIDEMIOLOGY

Sarcomas are relatively infrequent compared to carcinomas.[10] In 2018, sarcomas represented approximately 1% of all cancers in the United States, with approximately 13,000 to 16,000 new cases and an overall incidence of 7.1 cases per 100,000 people. They are among the top five causes of cancer deaths for those under 20 years of age, and approximately 5,000 to 6,000 patients die of their sarcomas annually in the United States.[11] Most cases are high grade (33.6%) and >5 cm (51.3%), and the 5-year survival rate is estimated to be 71.4%.[11,12]

CLINICAL MANIFESTATIONS

Clinical features associated with sarcoma depend on their location, size, and rate of growth. Common findings are a progressively growing, deep-seated, firm, and fixed mass that is often associated with pain of varying degrees of severity (Figures 3.1 and 3.2). Some tumors may be superficial, mobile, and asymptomatic. Sarcomas arising in the retroperitoneum, abdomen, or pelvis may achieve enormous size before they produce symptoms (Figure 3.3). Tumors developing in bone may present with a devastating pathologic fracture.[13] Occasionally, sarcomas are associated with symptoms secondary to the effects of their metabolic products that cause fever, anemia, lethargy, weight loss, and histamine-like reactions.[14]

TABLE 3.1 Major Groups of Sarcoma

Phenotype	Type
Adipocytic	Atypical lipomatous tumor/well-differentiated liposarcoma Dedifferentiated liposarcoma Myxoid liposarcoma Pleomorphic liposarcomas
Fibroblastic/myofibroblastic	Low-grade myofibroblastic sarcoma Myxoinflammatory fibroblastic sarcoma Infantile fibrosarcoma Adult fibrosarcoma Infantile fibrosarcoma Myxofibrosarcoma Low-grade fibromyxoid sarcoma Sclerosing epithelioid fibrosarcoma
So-called fibrohistiocytic tumors	Malignant giant cell tumor of soft tissue
Smooth muscle/pericytic	Leiomyosarcoma Malignant PEComa
Skeletal muscle	Embryonal rhabdomyosarcoma Alveolar rhabdomyosarcoma Pleomorphic rhabdomyosarcoma Spindle cell/sclerosing rhabdomyosarcoma
Vascular	Retiform hemangioendothelioma Papillary intralymphatic angioendothelioma Composite hemangioendothelioma Kaposi sarcoma Pseudomyogenic hemangioendothelioma Epithelioid hemangioendothelioma Angiosarcoma
Bone forming	Conventional osteosarcoma Well-differentiated intramedullary osteosarcoma Parosteal osteosarcoma Periosteal osteosarcoma High-grade surface osteosarcoma Secondary osteosarcoma Extraskeletal osteosarcoma
Cartilage forming	Conventional chondrosarcoma Dedifferentiated chondrosarcoma Clear cell chondrosarcoma Mesenchymal chondrosarcoma
Gastrointestinal stromal tumor	Malignant gastrointestinal stromal tumor
Nerve sheath	Malignant peripheral nerve sheath tumor Malignant granular cell tumor Ectomesenchymoma
Small round cell sarcoma	Ewing sarcoma and related tumors Melanotic neuroectodermal tumor
Notochordal tumors	Chordoma
Undifferentiated sarcoma	Round cell sarcoma Pleomorphic spindle cell sarcoma Epithelioid cell sarcoma

PEComa, perivascular epithelioid cell tumor.

DIAGNOSIS

Preoperative Biopsy

Primary diagnosis usually requires tissue biopsy to obtain samples of the tumor for histologic, immunohistochemical, and molecular analysis.[15,16] The biopsy site should be selected such that subsequent management of the tumor is not affected. A minimally invasive technique to obtain diagnostic tissue is needle biopsy and this procedure may need to be performed under radiologic guidance—areas of suspected tumor necrosis should be avoided. A minimum of three tumor-bearing cores of tissue is usually

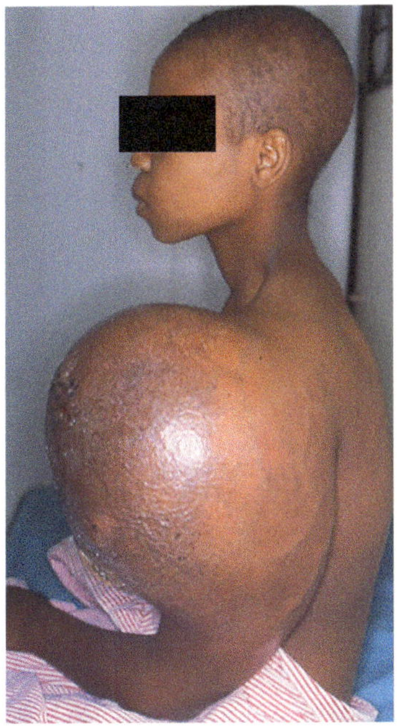

FIGURE 3.1 Large osteosarcoma of proximal humerus presenting as painful mass.

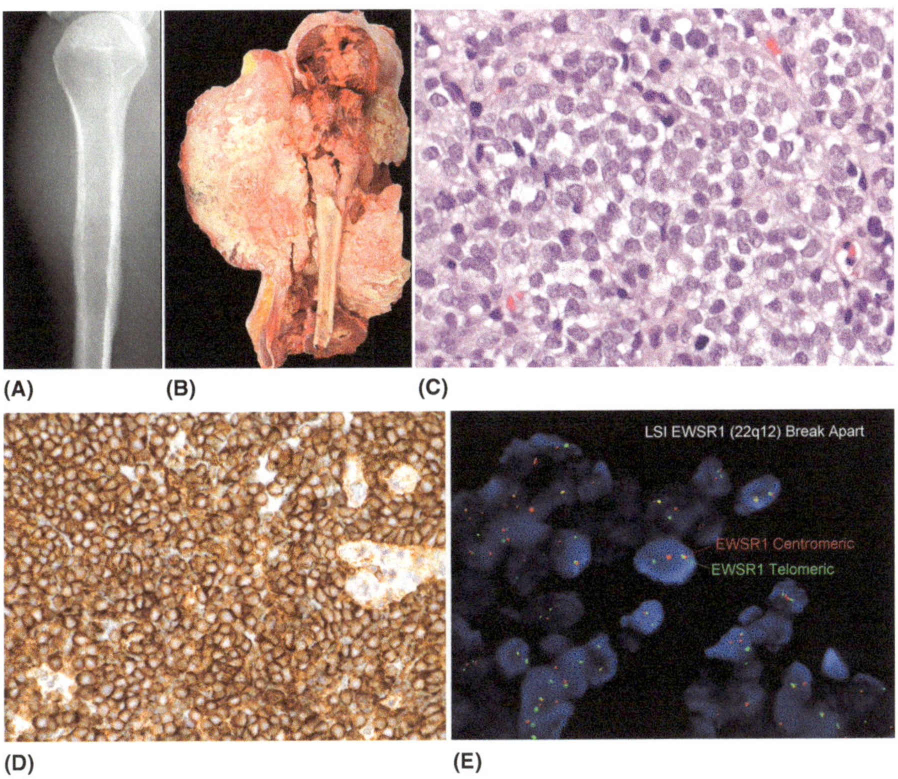

FIGURE 3.2 (A) Radiograph of Ewing sarcoma showing poorly defined mass in proximal diaphysis of humerus. (B) Resected tumor is pink, tan, and fleshy, and destroys the bone and extends into the soft tissues. (C) Tumor is composed of sheets of small round cells with little cytoplasm. (D) Immunohistochemical stain for CD99 shows that tumor cells exhibit strong membranous staining. (E) FISH using EWSR1 break-apart probe shows separation of signals indicative of rearrangement.

FISH, fluorescence in situ hybridization.

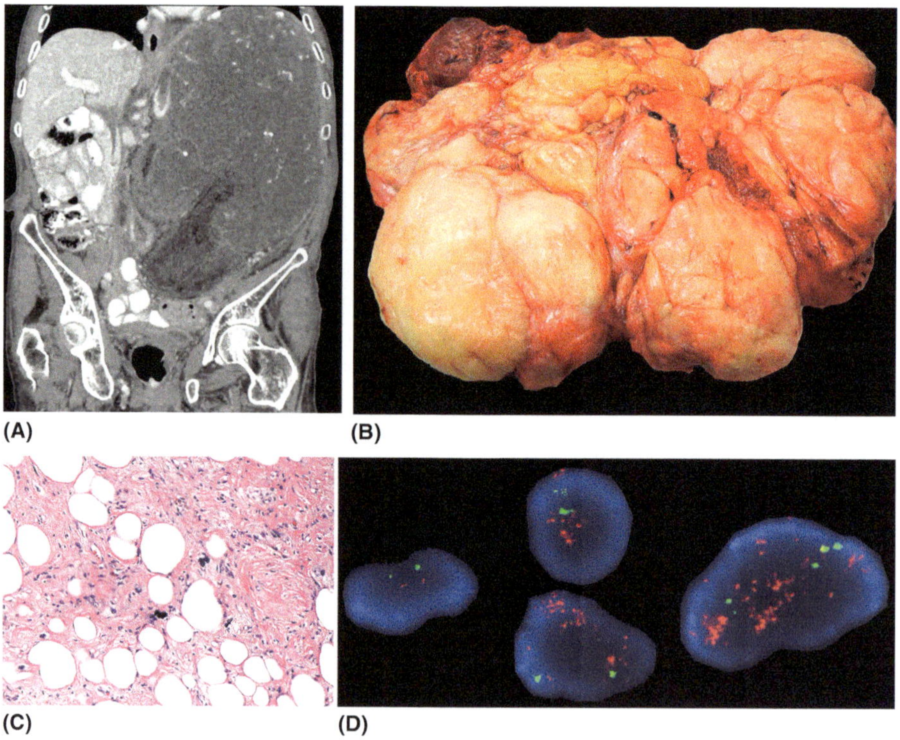

FIGURE 3.3 (A) Reformatted coronal CT image of large well-differentiated liposarcoma filling the left side of retroperitoneum and pelvis. (B) Resected tumor composed of lobule of soft yellow fat. (C) Neoplastic cells are adipocytes with enlarged hyperchromatic nuclei. (D) FISH for amplification of *MDM2* shows numerous copies of the gene.

FISH, fluorescence in situ hybridization.

sufficient, and there should be consideration for performing frozen section analysis on a portion of one core while the patient is still available to confirm that the diagnostic tissue is retrieved; this can also expedite tissue testing (touch preps for fluorescent in situ hybridization [FISH]) and patient triage.[16,17] Fine-needle aspiration cytologic biopsy is usually reserved for documenting recurrence or metastasis. It should be kept in mind that sarcomas are notoriously heterogeneous, and there is a significant potential for sampling error. A minority of tumors may require open biopsy because of failed attempts at needle biopsy, and small superficial tumors may be adequately removed with excisional biopsy by an experienced sarcoma surgeon.[17,18]

Resection Specimens

Surgically excised specimens should be sent to the pathology laboratory in a fresh state directly after removal from the patient. Ideally, the surgeon and pathologist review the specimen together to clarify orientation and proximity of tumor to important anatomic structure, and to identify and assess surgical margins. This can be performed in real time, so that preliminary margin status can be determined and the surgical team can decide whether or not additional tissue removal is necessary to achieve a negative margin. The resected tumor should be cut along its longest axis (Figure 3.4), photographed, and the margins serially sectioned in a perpendicular plane. A small sample of tumor and normal tissue can be collected for biobanking.[19] The specimen should then be thinly bread-loafed at 0.5 to 1 cm intervals; described, indicating color, consistency, presence of cysts, hemorrhage, and necrosis; and placed in formalin in an adequately sized container and allowed to fix for at least 12 hours. The guideline for tumor sampling is one block of tissue per centimeter of greatest tumor dimension.[20] Bone tumors should be decalcified after fixation, and a portion of viable tumor should be decalcified in an agent that does not damage RNA or DNA, such as EDTA.[21]

Resected tumors that have been treated with preoperative chemotherapy (osteosarcoma, Ewing sarcoma, dedifferentiated chondrosarcoma, mesenchymal chondrosarcoma, high-grade fibrosarcoma, and high-grade soft tissue sarcomas) require determination of percent tumor necrosis. To accomplish

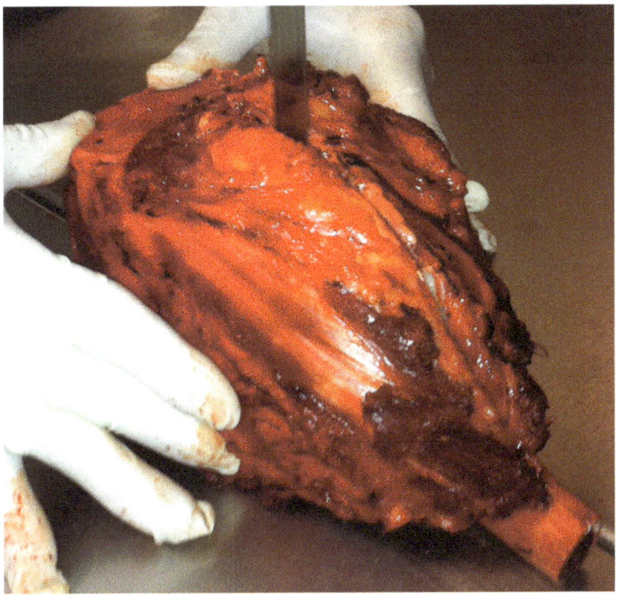

FIGURE 3.4 Osteosarcoma being cut through its long axis parallel to the underlying bone.

this, the central slab of tumor can be mapped and blocked out in its entirety (Figure 3.5). A section of tumor per centimeter (as determined by its greatest dimension) should be processed from each of the remaining two hemispheres of the specimen. During histologic review, the amount of tumor necrosis on each slide can be estimated and these scores can then be averaged to calculate the overall percentage of tumor necrosis (Figure 3.6). The areas of viable and necrotic tumor can then be located on the map of the slab section, if necessary.

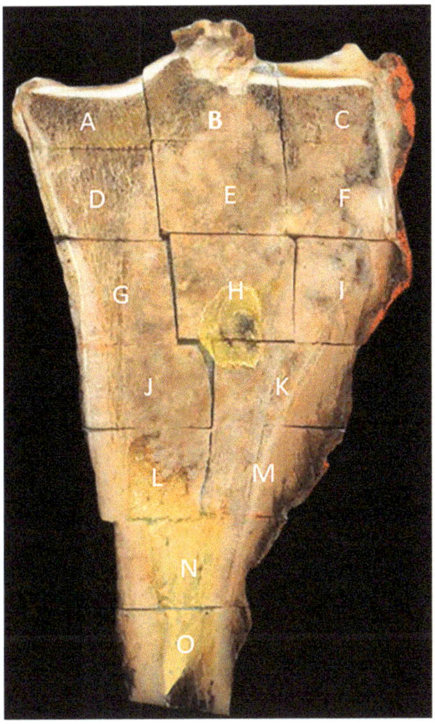

FIGURE 3.5 Central slab of resected osteosarcoma mapped prior to processing.

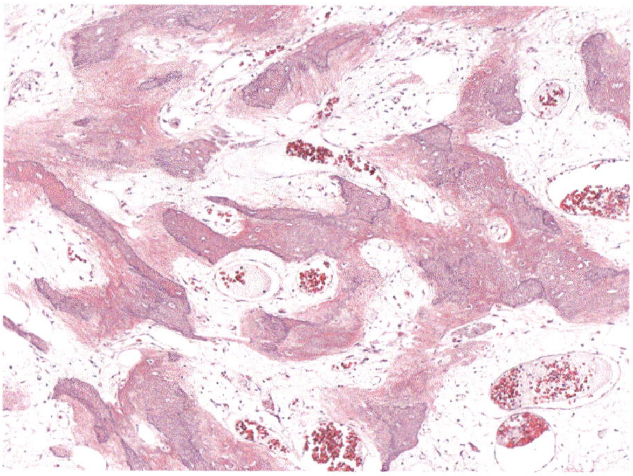

FIGURE 3.6 Osteosarcoma treated with neoadjuvant therapy producing 100% necrosis. The residual trabeculae of neoplastic bone are devoid of tumor cells.

Microscopic Examination

Accurate diagnosis depends on having an adequate quantity of viable tumor to assess architecture, relationship to nonneoplastic tissue, cytologic features, and mitotic activity including atypical forms and necrosis.[22] Criteria of malignancy commonly include hypercellularity, nuclear pleomorphism and hyperchromasia, abundant mitotic activity with structurally atypical forms, necrosis, vascular invasion, and the presence of metastasis.[22,23] An additional feature of bone tumors is the presence of an infiltrative growth pattern within the medullary cavity with encasement of preexisting bone trabeculae (Figure 3.7). An experienced pathologist can differentiate benign from malignant tumors with a sensitivity of 99.4% and a specificity of 98.7%.[24] Once a differential diagnosis is made, immunohistochemistry, cytogenetics, and molecular studies can be performed to establish a precise diagnosis.[14,23,25]

Grading of Bone and Soft Tissue Sarcomas

The pathologist's attempt to predict the biologic behavior of sarcoma is reflected in the histologic grade and this is translated into the biologic grades of low and high.[15] In other words, grading assesses the aggressiveness of the sarcoma and its risk of metastasis. Histologic grading is the single most significant prognostic factor of sarcoma and, as such, is a major independent predictor of metastasis[26] (Table 3.2). Histologic typing alone provides sufficient information for predicting the clinical course in

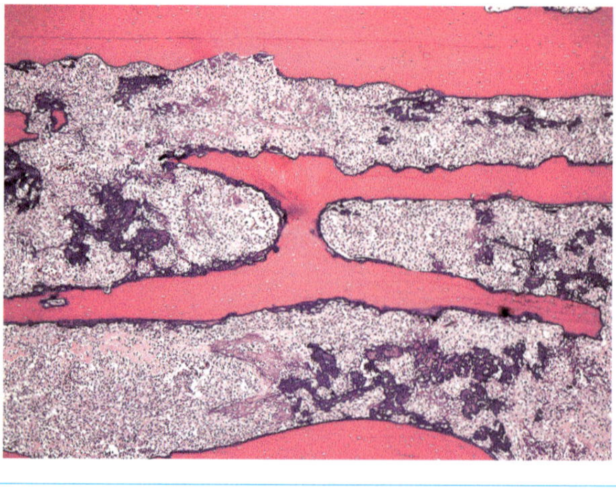

FIGURE 3.7 Osteosarcoma infiltrating the marrow cavity and surrounding individual bony trabeculae.

TABLE 3.2 **Grading of Bone and Soft Tissue Sarcoma**

Score	Tumor Differentiation	Mitotic Count	Tumor Necrosis
1	Sarcomas closely resembling normal adult mesenchymal tissue (e.g., low-grade leiomyosarcoma)	0–9 mitoses per 10 HPF	No necrosis
2	Sarcomas for which histologic typing is certain (e.g., myxoid/round cell liposarcoma)	10–19 mitoses per 10 HPF	<50% tumor necrosis
3	Embryonal and undifferentiated sarcomas, sarcomas of doubtful type, synovial sarcomas, soft tissue osteosarcoma, Ewing sarcoma/PNET of soft tissue	≥20 mitoses per 10 HPF	≥50% tumor necrosis

HPF, high-power field; PNET, primitive neuroectodermal tumor.

select sarcomas such as synovial sarcoma, Ewing sarcoma, mesenchymal chondrosarcoma, low-grade fibromyxoid sarcoma, well-differentiated liposarcoma, and so on; however, many require formal histologic grading.

The most widely used and clinically validated grading system for soft tissue sarcomas is the French Federation of Comprehensive Cancer Centers (*Fédération Nationale des Centres de Lutte Contre le Cancer*; FNCLCC) system. It is three tiered (grade 1—low grade, grade 2—intermediate grade, and grade 3—high grade). The FNCLCC grade is based on the parameters of differentiation, mitotic activity, and necrosis. Each of these parameters receives a score: differentiation (1–3), mitotic activity (1–3), and necrosis (0–2). The scores are summed to produce a grade: grade 1, score of 2 or 3; grade 2, score of 4 or 5; and grade 3, score of 6 to 8.[27] Sarcomas that are grade 2 or 3 are considered to be biologically high grade.

There is no standardized grading scheme for bone sarcoma; however, there are systems that some investigators have proposed for specific types of sarcomas, especially chondrosarcoma.[28] The histologic grading scheme currently recommended for bone sarcoma is that espoused by WHO and is a three-tiered system based on the assessment of standard morphologic criteria, including the degree of differentiation, cellularity, cytologic atypia, mitotic activity, and necrosis.

Another means of integrating clinical and pathologic data in a manner that accounts for sarcoma subtypes is the use of nomograms.[29] This method collates multiple clinical and histologic parameters in a given patient and compares the data against a large population of patients with similar parameters whose outcome is known.

Immunohistochemistry

Immunohistochemistry is now an essential adjunct in the evaluation of sarcomas[16,30] (Table 3.3). The use of immunohistochemistry should be performed in conjunction with and is guided by morphology and clinical and radiologic information. Familiarity with the pattern of reactivity for each antibody is needed to avoid diagnostic pitfalls. A growing number of antibodies are available that help determine the cell phenotype and proliferative activity. Some antibodies are molecular surrogates and others assess the immune environment.

Genetics and Genomics

From a molecular genetics perspective, sarcomas have traditionally been classified into two broad categories, each of which includes clinically diverse neoplasms. The first category comprises sarcomas with near-diploid karyotypes and simple genetic alterations, including translocations or specific activating mutations. The second category includes tumors with complex and unbalanced karyotypes. More recently, epigenetic deregulation is emerging as a highly prevalent oncogenic mechanism in a wide variety of tumors. Mutations causing epigenetic deregulation seem to occur as early events, in a background of low mutational rate, and may serve as primary drivers of tumorigenesis.[31] Examples include histone homozygous deletions and mutations in *SMARCB1*, and *SMARCA4* inactivation in *SMARCA4*-deficient thoracic sarcomas and in select succinate dehydrogenase (SDH)-deficient gastrointestinal stromal tumor.[32]

Molecular analysis can be used to identify specific chromosomal abnormalities. Most sarcomas with simple genetic alterations are translocation-associated sarcomas (which account for approximately one-third of all sarcomas).[8,33] An expanding list of mesenchymal tumors contains recurrent balanced chromosomal rearrangements, most often translocations, and most fusion genes produced by these rearrangements encode chimeric transcription factors that cause transcriptional deregulation that can be susceptible to targeted therapy (Table 3.4; Figure 3.8). The best cytogenetic technique to evaluate

TABLE 3.3 Immunohistochemistry: Antibodies Commonly Used in Sarcoma Diagnosis

Category	Use	Antibody
Lineage markers	Epithelial differentiation	Epithelial membrane antigen Keratins
	Smooth muscle differentiation	Desmin Smooth muscle actin Smooth muscle myosin Caldesmon Calponin
	Skeletal muscle differentiation	Desmin Myoglobin MYOD1 Myogenin
	Nerve sheath differentiation	S-100 protein SOX10 CD56 CD57 Claudin-1
	Endothelial differentiation	Factor VIII-related antigen CD34 CD31 FLI1 ERG GLUT-1 PROX1 Claudin-5 Thrombomodulin Podoplanin/D2-40 Wilms tumor 1 Vascular endothelial growth factor receptor 3
	Histiocytic markers	CD68 CD163 Lysozyme Factor XIIIa NKI/C3
	Melanocytic differentiation	HMB-45 Melan A MITF Tyrosinase
	Osteoblastic differentiation	Osteocalcin Osteonectin SATB2 FOS/FOSB
	Round cell tumors	CD99 WT1 TLE1 BCOR ETV4 NKX2-2 PAX-7
Therapy markers	Immunotherapy (pembrolizumab)	PD-L1
	ALK inhibitors (crizotinib)	ALK
	Tyrosine kinase inhibitors (imatinib)	C-kit DOG1
	Trk inhibitors (larotrectinib)	Pan-TRK
Other useful markers		Beta-catenin Brachyury NB84 TFE3

(continued)

TABLE 3.3 Immunohistochemistry: Antibodies Commonly Used in Sarcoma Diagnosis (*continued*)

Category	Use	Antibody
		MDM2 CDK4 Retinoblastoma SMARCB1 STAT6 BCL2 MUC4 CAMTA1 H3K27me3 Olig-2 Ki67 (MIB1)

ALK, anaplastic lymphoma kinase.

TABLE 3.4 Sarcomas With Simple Genetic Alterations

Sarcoma	Genetic Alteration	Detection Method	Targeted Therapy
Ewing sarcoma	*EWSR1–FLI1* *EWSR1–ERG* *EWSR1–ETV1* *EWSR1–ETV4* *EWSR1–FEV* *EWSR–ZSG* *EWSR1–PATZ1* *FUS–ERG* *FUS–FEV*	IHC (FLI1) Karyotype FISH RT-PCR NGS	
Ewing-like sarcoma	*EWSR1–NFATc2* *CIC–DUX4* *CIC–DUX4L* *CIC–FOX04* *BCOR–CCNB3* *BCOR–MAML3* *ZC3H7B–BCOR*	FISH RT-PCR NGS	
Desmoplastic small round cell tumor	*EWSR1–WT1* *EWSR1–ERG*	IHC (c-WT1) Karyotype FISH PCR NGS	Olaratumab
Clear cell sarcoma	*EWSR1–ATF1* *EWSR1–CREB1* *IRX2–TERT*	FISH PCR NGS	Vemurafenib
Extraskeletal myxoid chondrosarcoma	*EWSR1–NR4A3* *TAF2N–NR4A3* *TCF12–NR4A3* *TFG–NR4A3* *HSPA8–NR4A3*	FISH PCR NGS	
Myxoid/round cell liposarcoma	*FUS–DDIT3* *EWSR1–DDIT3*	FISH NGS	Trabectedin
Dermatofibrosarcoma protuberans	*COL1A1–PDGFB*	FISH PCR NGS	Imatinib mesylate
Gastrointestinal stromal tumor	*KIT* *PDGFRA*	IHC FISH NGS	Imatinib mesylate
Solitary fibrous tumor	*NAB2–STAT6*	IHC FISH NGS	Sunitinib
Low-grade fibromyxoid sarcoma	*FUS–CREB3L2* *FUS–CREB3L1*	FISH PCR NGS	

(*continued*)

TABLE 3.4 **Sarcomas With Simple Genetic Alterations (*continued*)**

Sarcoma	Genetic Alteration	Detection Method	Targeted Therapy
Sclerosing epithelioid fibrosarcoma	*FUS–CREB3L2* *FUS–CREB3L1* *EWSR1–CREBL1* *YAP1–KMT2A*	FISH PCR NGS	
Congenital fibrosarcoma	*ETV6–NTRK3*	FISH PCR NGS	Larotrectinib Entrectinib
Myxoinflammatory fibroblastic sarcoma/hemosiderotic fibrolipomatous tumor	*MGEA5–TGFBR3*	PCR NGS	
Pleomorphic hyalinizing angiectatic tumor	*FBXW4–TGFBR3*	PCR NGS	
Inflammatory myofibroblastic tumor	*TPM3–ALK* *TPM4–ALK* *CLTC–ALK* *RANBP2–ALK* *CLTC–ALK* *CARS–ALK* *SEC31A–ALK* *ATIC–ALK*	FISH PCR NGS	Crizotinib Alectinib Ceritinib
Synovial sarcoma	*SS18–SSX1* *SS18–SSX2* *SS18–SSX4* *SS18L1–SSX1* *SS18–NEDD4*	IHC FISH PCR NGS	CMB305 Adaptimmune
Myxofibrosarcoma	*KIAA2026–NUDT11* *CCBL1–ARL1* *AFF3–PHF1*	PCR NGS	
Tenosynovial giant cell tumor	*COL6A3–CSF1*	PCR NGS	Pexidartinib
Alveolar rhabdomyosarcoma	*PAX3–FOXO1* *PAX7–FOXO1* *PAX3–FOXO4* *PAX3–NCOA1* *PAX3–NCOA2* *FOXO1–FGFR1*	IHC FISH PCR NGS	
Biphenotypic sinonasal sarcoma	*PAX3–MAML3* *PAX3–NCOA1* *PAX3–FOXO1*	PCR NGS	
Alveolar soft part sarcoma	*ASPCR1–TFE3*	IHC FISH PCR NGS	Cediranib
Spindle cell rhabdomyosarcoma	*SRF–NCOA2* *TEAD1–NCOA2*	FISH PCR NGS	
Ossifying fibromyxoid tumor	*EP400–PHF1* *MEAF6–PHF1* *ZC3H3–BCOR*	IHC FISH PCR NGS	
Mesenchymal chondrosarcoma	*HEY1–NCOA2*	FISH PCR	
Epithelioid hemangioendothelioma	*WWTR1–CAMTA1* *YAP1–TFE3*	IHC FISH PCR NGS	
Pseudomyogenic hemangioendothelioma	*SERPINE1–FOSB* *ACTB–FOSB*	IHC FISH PCR	

FISH, fluorescence in situ hybridization; IHC, immunohistochemistry; NGS, next-generation sequencing; PCR, polymerase chain reaction; RT-PCR, reverse transcription polymerase chain reaction.

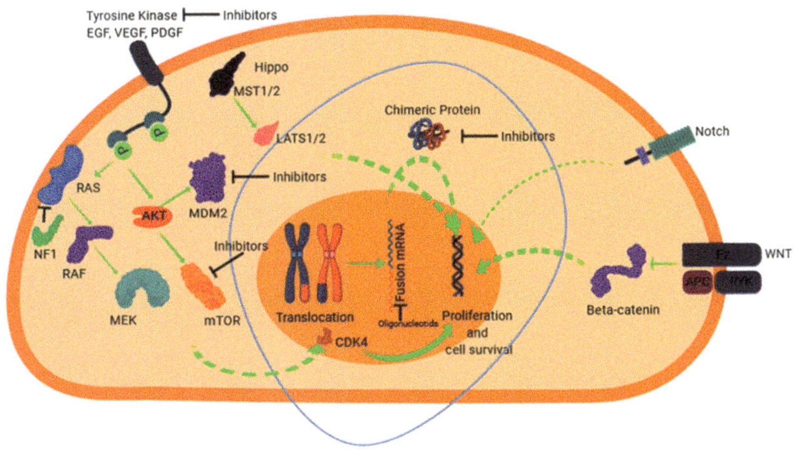

FIGURE 3.8 Graphic of tumor cell with gene fusion.

translocation-associated sarcomas is FISH using specific probes. The chimeric gene fusions can also be identified using molecular genetic techniques, including polymerase chain reaction (PCR) and sequence analysis. It should be noted that there is promiscuity among translocations, in that the same genetic rearrangement can be found in different tumors. Therefore, genetic information must always be integrated with clinical, radiologic, morphologic, and immunohistochemical data. Translocation-associated sarcomas tend to arise de novo and, in some cases, harbor only a single defining cytogenetic abnormality that is present at initiation and retained throughout their clonal evolution. Amplifications of specific genes are also of diagnostic and therapeutic importance. As an example, *MDM2* and *CDK4* amplification provides a useful diagnostic marker for well-differentiated/dedifferentiated liposarcoma and osteosarcoma.

Most high-grade, karyotypically complex sarcomas present de novo; a small minority arise in association with an antecedent lower-grade lesion (dedifferentiated liposarcoma, chondrosarcoma, and osteosarcoma)[8,34] (Table 3.5). They differ from translocation-associated sarcomas by their wide range of genetic complexity, DNA copy number alterations, deletions, insertions, and mutations. These

TABLE 3.5 Sarcomas With Complex Genetic Alterations

Sarcoma	Genetic Alteration	Detection Method	Targeted Therapy
Well-differentiated/ dedifferentiated liposarcoma	12q13–15 rings *MDM2* amplification *CDK4* amplification *FRS2* amplification *HMGA2*	IHC, FISH, NGS	Palbociclib
Pleomorphic liposarcoma	*RB1*	RB1 IHC, NGS	
Leiomyosarcoma	*TP53*, *ATRX*, and *MED12*	NGS	
Malignant peripheral nerve sheath tumor	*NF1*, *SMARCB1*	NF1, SMARCB1 IHC	
Fibrosarcoma	*NTRK* rearrangements	Pan-TRK IHC, NGS	Larotrectinib, entrectinib
Dedifferentiated osteosarcoma	*MDM2* and *CDK4* amplification	IHC, FISH, NGS	
Chondrosarcoma	*IDH1/2*	IHC, FISH, NGS	Ivosidenib
Angiosarcoma	*PTPRB* and *KDR* *ROS1* rearrangements	NGS	
Epithelioid sarcoma	*SMARCB1*	IHC, NGS	Tazemetostat
Undifferentiated sarcoma	*NOTCH1/2* *FAT1* *PRDM10* fusions	NGS	

FISH, fluorescence in situ hybridization; IHC, immunohistochemistry; NGS, next-generation sequencing.

sarcomas are usually high grade and aggressive. Examples include high-grade leiomyosarcoma, osteosarcoma, fibrosarcoma, myxofibrosarcoma, angiosarcoma, pleomorphic and dedifferentiated liposarcoma, and undifferentiated pleomorphic sarcoma. The high mutational load in these tumors potentially makes them good candidates for immunotherapy, with drugs such as immune checkpoint inhibitors.[3,34,35]

Targeted Therapy Assessment

Cytotoxic chemotherapy remains the standard of care for most locally advanced and metastatic sarcomas. However, the treatment of patients with sarcoma has entered a period of rapid evolution, and numerous targeted drugs are being approved for use (see Table 3.4). A careful evaluation should be done to assess if a particular tumor is a candidate for precision targeted therapy. Immunohistochemical markers have been developed as surrogates of genomic alterations and activated cell pathways, and the results can be helpful in therapy selection.

PROGNOSIS

The prognosis of sarcoma depends on a variety of aspects including tumor type, grade, size, location, stage, and patient age and medical condition. Sarcomas can be described as being localized (tumor is limited to the site of origin), locally advanced (tumor involves adjacent structures or organs), and metastatic (the sarcoma has spread to a separate part [local or distant] at the time of diagnosis). The overall 5-year survival rate for sarcoma is approximately 71.4%. Most sarcomas (58%) are localized at diagnosis and the 5-year survival rate is 81%. Approximately 18% of sarcomas are locally advanced at diagnosis and have a 5-year survival rate of 58%. Lastly, 14% of sarcomas are metastatic at diagnosis and have a 5-year survival rate of only 16%.[11,12,36]

STAGING SYSTEMS

In the United States, the American Joint Committee on Cancer (AJCC) Eighth Edition is the major staging system for bone and soft tissue sarcoma.[27,28,36] The pathologic staging system is based on the location, size, and extent of the tumor (Table 3.6). Pathologic staging (pTNM) includes data obtained from examination of the resected tumor, such as the size, location, histopathologic type, regional lymph node status, multicentricity, and the presence of distant metastasis.

REPORTING

Several guidelines for reporting sarcomas have been published.[35,36] The information generally included in the final report includes the tumor type, grade, immunohistochemical profile, genetic profile, percent necrosis, margin status, presence of lymphovascular invasion, and presence of metastasis to lymph nodes or other sites as appropriate (Table 3.7).

SUMMARY

The clinical and morphologic diversity observed in sarcoma is challenging. The diagnosis, classification, prognostication, identification of important biomarkers, and staging of these neoplasms require the integration of radiologic, morphologic, immunohistochemical, and molecular analyses. The identification of genetic abnormalities, biomarkers, susceptibility to immune therapy, and assessment of treatment effect are becoming increasingly important in the management of these neoplasms. The experience and skills required to optimally manage patients with sarcoma reside in the dedicated sarcoma multidisciplinary team.

TABLE 3.6 Pathologic Staging System

Bone primary tumor (T) staging system							
Body site	**Appendicular skeleton, trunk, skull, facial bones**	**Spine**			**Pelvis**		
T category	*T criteria*	*T criteria*			*T criteria*		
TX	Primary tumor cannot be assessed	Primary tumor cannot be assessed			Primary tumor cannot be assessed		
T0	No evidence of primary tumor	No evidence of primary tumor			No evidence of primary tumor		
T1	Tumor ≤8 cm in greatest dimension	Tumor confined to one vertebral segment or two adjacent vertebral segments			Tumor confined to one pelvic segment with no extraosseous extension	T1a	Tumor ≤8 cm in greatest dimension
						T1b	Tumor >8 cm in greatest dimension
T2	Tumor >8 cm in greatest dimension	Tumor confined to three adjacent vertebral segments			Tumor confined to one pelvic segment with extraosseous extension or two segments without extraosseous extension	T2a	Tumor ≤8 cm in greatest dimension
						T2b	Tumor >8 cm in greatest dimension
T3	Discontinuous tumors in the primary bone site	Tumor confined to four or more adjacent vertebral segments, or any nonadjacent vertebral segments			Tumor spanning two pelvic segments with extraosseous extension	T3a	Tumor ≤8 cm in greatest dimension
						T3b	
T4		Extension into the spinal canal or great vessels	T4a	Extension into the spinal canal	Tumor spanning three pelvic segments or crossing the sacroiliac joint	T4a	Tumor involves sacroiliac joint and extends medial to the sacral neuroforamen
			T4b	Evidence of gross vascular invasion or tumor thrombus in the great vessels		T4b	Tumor encasement of external iliac vessels or presence of gross tumor thrombus in major pelvic vessels

(continued)

TABLE 3.6 Pathologic Staging System (*continued*)

Soft tissue primary tumor (T) staging system					
Body site	**Head and neck**	**Trunk and extremities**	**Abdomen and thoracic visceral organs**		
T category	*T criteria*	*T criteria*	*T criteria*		
TX	Primary tumor cannot be assessed	Primary tumor cannot be assessed	Primary tumor cannot be assessed		
T0		No evidence of primary tumor			
T1	Tumor ≤2 cm	Tumor 5 cm or less in greatest dimension	Organ confined		
T2	Tumor >2 to ≤4 cm	Tumor >5 cm and ≤10 cm in greatest dimension	Tumor extension into tissue beyond organ	T2a	Invades serosa or visceral peritoneum
				T2b	Extension beyond serosa (mesentery)
T3	Tumor >4 cm	Tumor >10 cm and ≤15 cm in greatest dimension	Invades another organ		
T4	Tumor with invasion of adjoining structures	Tumor >15 cm in greatest dimension	Multifocal involvement	T4a	Multifocal (two sites)
				T4b	Multifocal (three to five sites)
				T4c	Multifocal (more than five sites)

Regional lymph node (N) staging system		
Body site	**Bone**	**Soft tissue**
N category	*N criteria*	*N criteria*
NX	Regional lymph nodes cannot be assessed	Primary tumor cannot be assessed
N0	No regional lymph node metastasis	No regional lymph node metastases or unknown lymph node status
N1	Regional lymph node metastasis	Regional lymph node metastasis

Distant metastasis (M) staging system				
Body site	**Bone**			**Soft tissue**
M category	*M criteria*			*M criteria*
M0	No distant metastasis			No distant metastasis
M1	Distant metastasis	M1a	Lung	Distant metastasis
		M1b	Bone or other distant sites	

TABLE 3.7 Reporting System

Procedure	Core-needle biopsy
	Curettage
	Excisional biopsy
	Marginal resection
	Wide resection
	Radical resection
Tumor site	
Tumor location and extent	
Tumor size	
Histologic type	
Mitotic rate	
Necrosis	
Histologic grade	
Lymphovascular invasion	
Margins	
Lymph node examination	
Ancillary studies	Immunohistochemistry
	Cytogenetics
	Molecular pathology
Radiographic findings	
Pathologic stage classification	
Previous treatment	
Treatment effect	
Comments	

REFERENCES

1. Helman LJ, Meltzer P. Mechanisms of sarcoma development. *Nat Rev Cancer*. 2003;3(9):685–694. doi:10.1038/nrc1168
2. Antonescu CR. The role of genetic testing in soft tissue sarcoma. *Histopathology*. 2006;48(1):13–21. doi:10.1111/j.1365-2559.2005.02285.x
3. Tang YJ, Huang J, Tsushima H, et al. Tracing tumor evolution in sarcoma reveals clonal origin of advanced metastasis. *Cell Rep*. 2019;28(11):2837.e5–2850.e5. doi:10.1016/j.celrep.2019.08.029
4. Digesu CS, Wiesel O, Vaporciyan AA, Colson YL. Management of sarcoma metastases to the lung. *Surg Oncol Clin North Am*. 2016;25(4):721–733. doi:10.1016/j.soc.2016.05.005
5. Keung EZ, Chiang YJ, Voss RK, et al. Defining the incidence and clinical significance of lymph node metastasis in soft tissue sarcoma. *Eur J Surg Oncol*. 2018;44(1):170–177. doi:10.1016/j.ejso.2017.11.014
6. Sherman KL, Kinnier CV, Farina DA, et al. Examination of national lymph node evaluation practices for adult extremity soft tissue sarcoma. *J Surg Oncol*. 2014;110(6):682–688. doi:10.1002/jso.23687
7. Fletcher CD. The evolving classification of soft tissue tumours—an update based on the new 2013 WHO classification. *Histopathology*. 2014;64(1):2–11. doi:10.1111/his.12267
8. Mariño-Enríquez A, Bovée JV. Molecular pathogenesis and diagnostic, prognostic and predictive molecular markers in sarcoma. *Surg Pathol Clin*. 2016;9(3):457–473. doi:10.1016/j.path.2016.04.009
9. Diaz-Perez JA, Nielsen GP, Antonescu C, et al. EWSR1/FUS-NFATc2 rearranged round cell sarcoma: clinicopathological series of 4 cases and literature review. *Hum Pathol*. 2019;90:45–53. doi:10.1016/j.humpath.2019.05.001
10. Feng L, Wang M, Yibulayin F, et al. Spindle cell sarcoma: a SEER population-based analysis. *Sci Rep*. 2018;8(1):5024. doi:10.1038/s41598-018-23145-4
11. Gage MM, Nagarajan N, Ruck JM, et al. Sarcomas in the United States: recent trends and a call for improved staging. *Oncotarget*. 2019;10(25):2462–2474. doi:10.18632/oncotarget.26809
12. Jacobs AJ, Michels R, Stein J, Levin AS. Improvement in overall survival from extremity soft tissue sarcoma over twenty years. *Sarcoma*. 2015;2015:279601. doi:10.1155/2015/279601
13. Salunke AA, Chen Y, Tan JH, et al. Does a pathological fracture affect the prognosis in patients with osteosarcoma of the extremities? A systematic review and meta-analysis. *Bone Joint J*. 2014;96-B(10):1396–1403. doi:10.1302/0301-620X.96B10.34370

14. Dancsok AR, Asleh-Aburaya K, Nielsen TO. Advances in sarcoma diagnostics and treatment. *Oncotarget*. 2017;8(4):7068–7093. doi:10.18632/oncotarget.12548
15. Siegel GW, Biermann JS, Chugh R, et al. The multidisciplinary management of bone and soft tissue sarcoma: an essential organizational framework. *J Multidiscip Healthc*. 2015;8:109–115. doi:10.2147/JMDH.S49805
16. Rosenberg AE. Bone sarcoma pathology: diagnostic approach for optimal therapy. *Am Soc Clin Oncol Educ Book*. 2017;37:794–798. doi:10.14694/EDBK_174697
17. Ayala AG, Ro JY, Fanning CV, et al. Core needle biopsy and fine-needle aspiration in the diagnosis of bone and soft-tissue lesions. *Hematol Oncol Clin North Am*. 1995;9(3):633–651. doi:10.1016/S0889-8588(18)30088-1
18. Papke DJ Jr, Jo VY. Practical application of cytology and core biopsy in the diagnosis of mesenchymal tumors. *Surg Pathol Clin*. 2019;12(1):227–248. doi:10.1016/j.path.2018.11.002
19. Zhou JH, Sahin AA, Myers JN. Biobanking in genomic medicine. *Arch Pathol Lab Med*. 2015;139(6):812–818. doi:10.5858/arpa.2014-0261-RA
20. Shah C, Wang J, Mubako T, et al. Gross examination and reporting of soft tissue tumours: evaluation of compliance with the UK Royal College of Pathologists soft tissue sarcoma dataset. *J Clin Pathol*. 2016;69(9):761–766. doi:10.1136/jclinpath-2015-203495
21. Singh VM, Salunga RC, Huang VJ, et al. Analysis of the effect of various decalcification agents on the quantity and quality of nucleic acid (DNA and RNA) recovered from bone biopsies. *Ann Diagn Pathol*. 2013;17(4):322–326. doi:10.1016/j.anndiagpath.2013.02.001
22. Rubin BP, Fletcher CD, Inwards C, et al. Protocol for the examination of specimens from patients with soft tissue tumors of intermediate malignant potential, malignant soft tissue tumors, and benign/locally aggressive and malignant bone tumors. *Arch Pathol Lab Med*. 2006;130(11):1616–1629. doi:10.1043/1543-2165(2006)130[1616:PFTEOS]2.0.CO;2
23. Rubin BP, Cooper K, Fletcher CD, et al. Protocol for the examination of specimens from patients with tumors of soft tissue. *Arch Pathol Lab Med*. 2010;134(4):e31–e39. doi:10.1043/1543-2165-134.4.e31
24. Hoeber I, Spillane AJ, Fisher C, Thomas JM. Accuracy of biopsy techniques for limb and limb girdle soft tissue tumors. *Ann Surg Oncol*. 2001;8(1):80–87. doi:10.1007/s10434-001-0080-y
25. Dantey K, Schoedel K, Yergiyev O, et al. Correlation of histological grade of dedifferentiation with clinical outcome in 55 patients with dedifferentiated liposarcomas. *Hum Pathol*. 2017;66:86–92. doi:10.1016/j.humpath.2017.02.015
26. Coindre JM. Grading of soft tissue sarcomas: review and update. *Arch Pathol Lab Med*. 2006;130(10):1448–1453. doi:10.1043/1543-2165(2006)130[1448:GOSTSR]2.0.CO;2
27. Coindre JM. Recommendations for anatamo-pathologic management of soft tissue sarcomas in the adult. Pathologists of the FNCLCC Sarcoma Group (Fédération Nationale des Centres de Lutte Contre le Cancer). *Ann Pathol*. 1998;18(6):505–511. PMID:10349487
28. Inwards CY, Unni KK. Classification and grading of bone sarcomas. *Hematol Oncol Clin North Am*. 1995;9(3):545–569. doi:10.1016/S0889-8588(18)30084-4
29. Callegaro D, Miceli R, Mariani L, et al. Soft tissue sarcoma nomograms and their incorporation into practice. *Cancer*. 2017;123(15):2802–2820. doi:10.1002/cncr.30721
30. Schaefer IM, Hornick JL. Diagnostic immunohistochemistry for soft tissue and bone tumors: an update. *Adv Anat Pathol*. 2018;25(6):400–412. doi:10.1097/PAP.0000000000000204
31. Soini Y. Epigenetic and genetic changes in soft tissue sarcomas: a review. *APMIS*. 2016;124(11):925–934. doi:10.1111/apm.12600
32. Pawel BR. SMARCB1-deficient tumors of childhood: a practical guide. *Pediatr Dev Pathol*. 2018;21(1):6–28. doi:10.1177/1093526617749671
33. Suurmeijer AJH, Kao YC, Antonescu CR. New advances in the molecular classification of pediatric mesenchymal tumors. *Genes Chromosomes Cancer*. 2019;58(2):100–110. doi:10.1002/gcc.22681
34. Lam SW, van IJzendoorn DGP, Cleton-Jansen AM, et al. Molecular pathology of bone tumors. *J Mol Diagn*. 2019;21(2):171–182. doi:10.1016/j.jmoldx.2018.11.002
35. Fisher SB, Chiang YJ, Feig BW, et al. Comparative performance of the 7th and 8th editions of the American Joint Committee on cancer staging systems for soft tissue sarcoma of the trunk and extremities. *Ann Surg Oncol*. 2018;25(5):1126–1132. doi:10.1245/s10434-018-6378-9
36. Cates JM. Reporting surgical resection margin status for osteosarcoma: comparison of the AJCC, MSTS, and Margin Distance Methods. *Am J Surg Pathol*. 2017;41(5):633–642. doi:10.1097/PAS.0000000000000815

4

Radiation Oncology

Jessica W. Lee and David G. Kirsch

INTRODUCTION

In 1921, James Ewing described his eponymous tumor as a *diffuse endothelioma of bone*. In contrast to osteosarcoma, he reported that Ewing sarcoma appeared in adolescents, favored long and flat bones, involved most of the bone shaft while sparing the ends, showed no bone production, and responded exquisitely to radiation.[1] The following year, in his 1922 presentation of the Mütter lecture, *An Analysis of Radiation Therapy in Cancer*, he noted that "basal cell carcinomas," "endothelioma of lymph nodes, endothelioma of bone and myeloma," and other rapidly growing tumors were all "peculiarly susceptible to radiation."[2] Under the microscope, he observed that irradiated tumor cells developed "swelling, hyperchromatism, vacuolar degeneration, and solution of fragmentation of nuclei."

A century later, Ewing's remarks on the relationship between radiation and cancer cells remain relevant. Radiation therapy (RT) uses ionizing radiation (IR), which damages DNA to exert the end effect of cell death that Ewing described. IR is a type of radiation that contains enough energy to ionize or eject orbital electrons from an atom and may take the form of particles or electromagnetic waves. Ionizing electromagnetic waves include x-rays, which are produced when high-energy electrons hit a target atom such as tungsten or gold, and gamma rays, which are produced by nuclear decay of radioactive isotopes such as iodine-125, iodine-131, and iridium-192. Ionizing particles include electrons, protons, and alpha particles. The susceptibility of cancer cells to IR relies mainly on DNA damage, which results from direct action on DNA or occurs through indirect effects. In direct action, IR directly ionizes the DNA molecule, causing structural damage to DNA bases or the sugar–phosphate backbone that causes single-stranded DNA breaks or double-stranded DNA breaks, which are especially lethal to cells. In indirect action, radiation interacts with water or other organic molecules, which results in free radicals such as hydroxyl and alkoxy molecules, which then subsequently react with and ionize DNA. In most normal cells, DNA damage activates the DNA damage response that can lead to repair of DNA damage and survival after exposure to IR. However, in cancer cells, mutations in genes that regulate the DNA damage response or that drive DNA synthesis and mitosis even in the presence of unrepaired DNA double-strand breaks result in cell death. Broadly speaking, IR can selectively kill cancer cells over normal tissue, though the therapeutic ratio varies for different cancer cells and normal tissues.

In addition to the biologic basis (i.e., cancer-specific mutations) for a therapeutic ratio for IR, RT also achieves a therapeutic ratio from physically delivering more radiation to the tumor than to normal tissue. RT can be delivered either from a radiation source outside the patient, referred to as external beam RT, or from a source adjacent to or inside the patient, in the form of brachytherapy or radionuclide therapy. External beam RT is commonly delivered with a medical linear accelerator (LINAC), which produces a beam of x-ray photons or electrons directed at the tumor within the patient. The x-ray photons are deeply penetrating and are used most frequently to treat sarcomas. The x-rays enter the patient and deposit their maximum energy at a specific depth, which depends on the energy of the x-rays, before exiting out of the patient. Electrons are superficially penetrating, with the depth of penetration proportional to their energy, and may be delivered en face to the patient to treat cancers up to approximately 4 cm in depth. External beam RT can also be delivered using a beam of protons, which like x-rays can deeply penetrate tissue to a specific depth based on energy, but then rapidly deposit all of the remaining energy without exiting out of the patient. Protons may be particularly useful when a sarcoma is adjacent to a critical normal tissue, such as a chondrosarcoma in the skull base.

Since the inception of LINAC-based external beam RT in the 1950s, refinements in treatment planning have improved coverage, conformity, and homogeneity of radiation dose to the tumor.

Three-dimensional conformal RT (3D-CRT), first used in the 1980s, starts with creating a 3D model of the patient via CT or MRI. Tumor target volumes and normal tissues are then delineated slice by slice, and radiation beams are manually optimized to achieve the prescribed tumor dose to the tumor target volumes while minimizing dose to normal tissues. In the 1990s, treatment planning advanced with intensity-modulated RT (IMRT), in which computerized optimization of multiple radiation beams as well as nonuniform intensity within each beam provide even more conformal and homogeneous coverage, especially for tumors with complex shapes. Modern 3D-CRT or IMRT is often image guided with x-ray or low-dose CT imaging in the treatment room prior to each fraction, to optimize patient position before treatment and thereby improve accuracy. Improved accuracy of radiation delivery also results from advances in patient immobilization, so that the patient is in the same treatment position each day and in approaches to minimize tumor motion, such as respiratory gating strategies.

Another important consideration of RT is fractionation and total dose. Radiation dose is prescribed in gray (Gy) and the unit of absorbed IR in joules per kilogram. Conventional fractionation is typically 1.8 to 2 Gy/day to a total dose of about 50 to 70 Gy in the curative setting. Stereotactic radiosurgery (SRS), which was developed in the 1950s, is used for brain tumors, and it describes a single highly conformal fraction of approximately 18 to 24 Gy. Over the past two decades, this technology has been applied to other sites and termed stereotactic body RT (SBRT) or stereotactic ablative RT (SABR), in which one to five large fractions are delivered with highly accurate stereotactic guidance to target extracranial tumors, such as pulmonary or spine metastases from sarcomas.

In contrast to external beam RT, brachytherapy places a sealed radioactive isotope such as iridium-192 directly within or adjacent to the tumor for a specified period of time. In this setting, the radiation acts over a short distance because the dose falls off with the square of the distance from the radiation source(s). Brachytherapy is typically used following surgery for soft tissue sarcomas (STSs) when catheters can be placed in the tumor bed to facilitate delivery of the radioactive isotope.

In radionuclide therapy, an unsealed radioactive isotope is ingested by or injected into the patient. Examples include iodine-131, which accumulates in thyroid cells and is used to treat hyperthyroidism and thyroid cancer; yttrium-90–labeled rituximab in non-Hodgkin lymphoma; and transarterial radioembolization with yttrium-90 in liver metastases.

Intraoperative RT (IORT), which is a single fraction delivered at the time of surgery, can use either external beam RT with electrons or brachytherapy with radioactive isotopes. IORT has been used to treat extremity and retroperitoneal sarcomas. An advantage of IORT is direct target visualization and physical manipulation of normal tissues, such as the intestine, away from the target.

SOFT TISSUE SARCOMA

The cornerstone of curative treatment for localized STS is surgery with negative margins. Historically, local control rates following local excision alone were 10% to 50%. Thus, radical resection or amputation was often favored over local excision, which could improve local control rates to >80% at the cost of limb function. Adjuvant RT enhances local control after limb-sparing surgery and is typically employed for large (>5 cm), intermediate, or high-grade sarcomas located deep to the fascia. RT may be delivered preoperatively, intraoperatively, or postoperatively, and the timing of RT with respect to surgery can be tailored to individual patients. Preoperative RT generally allows for smaller radiation field size, lower total radiation dose, and improved functional outcomes, however, with higher rates of acute wound complications. Thus, preoperative RT may be favored for young patients, who would likely recover well from an acute wound complication and who, if cured of their tumor, would be expected to live for many years and would benefit from the anticipated reduction in late radiation toxicity with preoperative RT. In contrast, postoperative RT may be preferable for elderly patients with multiple comorbid conditions, who may be at higher risk for significant morbidity from a wound complication and for whom late radiation effects may be a lesser concern. Current guidelines from the National Comprehensive Cancer Network recommend 50 Gy in the preoperative setting, with postoperative boost reserved for positive margins only.[3] Fifty gray is also utilized in the postoperative setting; however, a tumor bed boost of at least 10 Gy is given for negative margins, 16 to 18 Gy for microscopically positive margins, and 20 to 26 Gy for gross residual disease. Ultimately, the decision of preoperative versus postoperative RT should be made with the patient in a multidisciplinary evaluation involving the surgeon and radiation oncologist, taking into account clinical features such as size and grade of the sarcoma, type and extent of surgery required, patient comorbid conditions, and the potential consequences of a wound complication and late effects of radiation.

Postoperative RT

In the 1970s, external beam RT was advocated as a means to improve local control following local excision of STSs. In 1982, the National Cancer Institute (NCI) published a prospective randomized trial of 43 patients with high-grade STS, comparing amputation to wide local excision with adjuvant RT.[4] Both groups received adjuvant chemotherapy with doxorubicin, cyclophosphamide, and methotrexate. RT dose was 50 Gy to the area at risk for microscopic spread and an additional 10 to 20 Gy tumor bed boost. On multivariate analysis, positive margins were associated with increased local recurrence. Local recurrence was observed in 4/27 patients who underwent limb-sparing surgery and in 0/16 patients who underwent amputation. No difference in 5-year disease-free survival (71% vs. 78%) or overall survival (83% vs. 88%) was seen between the limb-sparing versus amputation groups. This study concluded that the local excision with postoperative RT was an acceptable alternative to amputation.

Following the 1982 NCI study, the benefit of postoperative RT after limb-sparing surgery was directly tested in another NCI study published in 1998.[5] This trial randomized 141 patients, 50 patients with low-grade STS and 91 patients with high-grade STS, to receive postoperative RT of 45 Gy to a wide field and an additional 18 Gy tumor bed boost. Patients with high-grade STS also received postoperative chemotherapy with doxorubicin and cyclophosphamide, either alone or concurrently with radiation. At a median 9.6 years of follow-up, in the high-grade STS group, local recurrence was observed in 9/47 patients who received postoperative chemotherapy alone and 0/44 patients who received postoperative chemotherapy and RT ($p = .003$). In the low-grade STS group, local recurrence was observed in 8/24 patients who received no adjuvant therapy and 1/26 patients who received postoperative RT ($p = .016$). No difference in distant metastases or overall survival was seen with the addition of RT. A concurrent quality-of-life study demonstrated that patients who received RT had transient worsening of muscle strength and edema in the first year after surgery as well as decreased joint motion up to 3 years after surgery, though no significant differences in global quality of life or performance of activities of daily living were seen. Long-term outcomes from this randomized trial were assessed after a median follow-up of 17.9 years.[6] Twenty-year overall survival rate was similar for both groups: 64% for the limb-sparing surgery group and 71% for the limb-sparing surgery plus RT group. Although there was a trend to more edema and functional limb deficits in patients treated with RT, this study established that the addition of postoperative RT to limb-sparing surgery improves local control with acceptable treatment-related morbidity.

Retrospective studies have attempted to define a subgroup of surgical patients in which RT improves survival. A 1998 to 2005 Surveillance, Epidemiology, and End Results (SEER) database analysis suggested benefit was confined to high-grade tumors.[7] This analysis included 6,960 patients with extremity STS who underwent limb-sparing surgery; 47% of patients received RT, of whom 13.5% received preoperative RT. In low-grade tumors, no difference was seen in overall survival at 3 years. In high-grade tumors, patients who received radiation had improved 3-year overall survival versus patients who did not receive radiation (73% vs. 63%, $p < .001$). A retrospective matched-pair analysis from the National Cancer Database (NCDB) of patients with high-grade extremity sarcoma treated from 2004 to 2013 also concluded that patients treated with limb-sparing surgery and postoperative or preoperative RT had improved overall survival (hazard ratio [HR]: approximately 0.7) compared to patients treated with limb-sparing surgery alone.[8]

Preoperative RT

A comparison of preoperative versus postoperative RT was addressed in the SR2 trial by the NCI of Canada Clinical Trials Group.[9] This trial randomized 190 patients with extremity STS to 50 Gy of preoperative RT or postoperative RT. Patients in the preoperative group with tumor cells at the resection margin also received a 16 to 20 Gy boost. All patients in the postoperative group received a 16 to 20 Gy boost. The primary endpoint was wound complications. Major wound complications included secondary operation or invasive procedure for wound repair, deep wound packing, and readmission for wound care. The rate of major wound complications was higher in the preoperative group compared to the postoperative group (35% vs. 17%, $p = .01$), which suggests that preoperative RT does not cause wound complications, but instead exacerbates the underlying risk by approximately twofold. The most common site of wound complications was the upper leg followed by the lower leg. Interestingly, wound complications in the upper extremity were rare: 0/11 patients in the postoperative group and 1/10 patients in the preoperative group. In addition to preoperative RT and anatomic site, maximum tumor size >10 cm was also associated with wound complications on logistic regression. No difference in local control (approximately 90%) or overall survival was observed between the groups. An analysis of late effects found that a greater proportion of patients who received postoperative RT had grade 2 or greater fibrosis compared to the preoperative arm (48% vs. 32%, $p = .07$), which was likely due to larger radiation field size and larger radiation dose.[10] Joint stiffness and edema were also more frequent in the postoperative arm, though the difference was not statistically significant.

RTOG 0630 was a multi-institutional Phase 2 clinical trial of reduced target volume preoperative image-guided RT for extremity STS.[11] Local control for the 79 eligible patients was 93%, and all five local treatment failures were in the radiation field. Of the 57 patients assessed for late toxicities at 2 years, 10.5% experienced at least one grade ≥2 toxicity, as compared with 37% of patients from the preoperative arm of the SR2 trial by the NCI of Canada.

A meta-analysis of 1,098 patients also addressed the question of preoperative versus postoperative RT.[12] This analysis found that a higher proportion of patients who underwent preoperative RT had an initial tumor size >10 cm. The risk of local recurrence was lower in patients who had received preoperative radiation (odds ratio: approximately 0.66). The average survival rate was 76% for patients who received preoperative RT and 67% in patients who received postoperative RT. This meta-analysis concluded that the delay in surgery inherent in preoperative radiation did not appear to adversely affect survival and may even be associated with decreased local recurrence.

The feasibility of preoperative RT with chemotherapy was evaluated in a single-arm, multi-institutional Phase 2 study in RTOG 9514.[13] In this study, 66 patients with high-grade STS ≥8 cm received neoadjuvant chemotherapy (three cycles of modified mesna, doxorubicin, ifosfamide, and dacarbazine), split course 44 Gy RT interdigitated between chemotherapy cycles 1 and 2 and between cycles 2 and 3, as well as three cycles of postoperative chemotherapy. Also, 61/66 patients underwent surgery and 58 had R0 resections including five amputations, while three had R1 resections. The 3-year local–regional failure rate was 17.6% (including amputation as failure), disease-free survival rate was 57%, and overall survival rate was 75%.

Intraoperative RT

IORT may also be used as a boost in addition to preoperative or postoperative RT. IORT is typically delivered using an electron beam from a LINAC or with high dose rate (HDR) brachytherapy. Current National Comprehensive Cancer Network (NCCN) guidelines recommend 10 to 12.5 Gy for microscopic disease and 15 Gy for gross residual disease following preoperative RT, and 10 to 16 Gy boost prior to postoperative RT. The decision to administer IORT is made following multidisciplinary evaluation by the surgeon and radiation oncologist, and may be considered when surgery is likely to leave microscopic residual or gross disease that cannot be adequately treated with conventional external beam RT owing to nearby dose-limiting normal tissue. IORT may be especially useful for certain anatomic sites such as the retroperitoneum, where the radiation dose tolerance of adjacent bowel may limit the amount of radiation that can be delivered safely to a large field. In IORT, bowel or other dose-limiting normal tissues may be manually displaced or shielded during radiation delivery.

Data on IORT with external beam RT are mostly limited to small series. A tumor bed boost with IORT appears to provide similar local control as boosting with external beam RT, with 5-year local control rates of 82% to 97% in IORT series and 93% to 93% in non-IORT series.[14] One prospective randomized trial has examined the use of IORT. In this trial, 35 patients with resected retroperitoneal sarcomas were randomized to 20 Gy IORT with 35 to 40 Gy postoperative radiation or to 50 to 55 Gy postoperative radiation. Six of 15 patients who received IORT developed locoregional recurrences, while 16 of 20 patients who received external beam RT alone developed locoregional recurrences. The IORT group also had lower rates of radiation-related enteritis but, however, had higher rates of peripheral neuropathy. Median overall survival was similar between the two groups.[15]

Brachytherapy

Brachytherapy can be used as a boost in conjunction with preoperative RT. In this case, brachytherapy can be given during or after surgery. However, brachytherapy alone can also be used as adjuvant therapy after surgery (i.e., no external beam RT). A single-institution randomized trial of 164 patients with completely resected sarcomas compared limb-sparing surgery alone to surgery plus adjuvant brachytherapy.[16] Brachytherapy technique consisted of percutaneous catheters placed intraoperatively in the tumor bed in a single plane. Catheters were loaded with low dose rate (LDR) iridium-192, which was designed to deliver 42 to 45 Gy over the course of 4 to 6 days. Five-year local control was 82% in the patients who received brachytherapy and 69% in the patients who received no further therapy ($p = .04$). This benefit was limited to patients with high-grade sarcomas. This local control rate is lower than that reported in studies with external beam RT, which may reflect the challenge in using a single plane of brachytherapy catheters to cover the volume at risk for large sarcomas.[9] No difference was observed in distant metastases or disease-specific survival. Initially, patients who received brachytherapy had a significantly higher risk of wound complications. As an interim analysis demonstrated a relationship between early catheter loading and wound complications, the trial was amended such that catheters were loaded at least 6 days after surgery. After this adjustment, no significant difference in wound complications was observed between the patients who received brachytherapy and those who received no further treatment.

In LDR brachytherapy, the patient is hospitalized while an implanted radioactive source delivers radiation at a rate of 0.4 to 2.0 Gy/hour over several days. Healthcare staff may be at risk of radiation exposure during this period. In contrast, HDR brachytherapy delivers radiation at a rate of >12 Gy/hour, which allows for treatment delivery in minutes, reducing the need for hospitalization and virtually eliminating radiation exposure to healthcare personnel. A comparison of LDR versus HDR brachytherapy in 37 patients with STS showed no significant difference in 2-year local control rates or wound complications.[17]

Definitive RT

Surgery is generally the backbone of definitive treatment of sarcoma. However, in patients with unacceptable medical comorbid conditions or unresectable tumors, definitive RT alone may be considered. Massachusetts General Hospital has published a series of 112 patients with STS who received a median dose of 64 Gy for gross disease, either following biopsy or attempted radical surgery.[18] Twenty-one percent of patients received chemotherapy. Overall, 5-year local control rate and overall survival rate were 45% and 35%, respectively. On multivariate analysis, local control was related to the tumor size, total dose, and stage, but not chemotherapy, grade, age, or location. Tumor sizes of <5, 5 to 10, and >10 cm had 5-year local control rates of 51%, 45%, and 9%, respectively, while radiation doses of <63 and ≥63 Gy had 5-year local control rates of 22% and 60%, respectively. Major complications, the most common of which was wound healing disease requiring major surgery, were seen in 14% of patients and were positively correlated with increased radiation dose. The addition of concurrent chemotherapy to definitive RT as a radiosensitizer has also been examined in a series from Germany.[19] In this retrospective analysis, 11 patients with macroscopic sarcoma received a median of 60 Gy RT, mostly conventionally fractionated, with a single agent ifosfamide at 1.0 or 1.5 g/m^2 during the first and fifth weeks of radiation. Overall, the 2- and 5-year local control rate was 70%; both the patients with local failures had tumors >10 cm. The results from this small series appear to compare favorably to the larger series from Massachusetts General Hospital, where patients were mostly treated with RT alone.

Omitting RT

In addition to the trials of limb- or function-sparing surgery with adjuvant RT described in the preoperative and postoperative RT sections, several series have also sought to characterize the risk of local recurrence following function-sparing surgery alone, in order to define a cohort of favorable-risk patients who may not need adjuvant RT. To that end, a retrospective series published in 1999 reported outcomes of 74 patients who received function-sparing surgery alone for trunk or extremity sarcomas.[20] The median tumor size was 4 cm and the majority were low grade. Ninety-two percent of patients had negative margins, 7% had microscopically positive margins, and one patient had grossly positive margins. Seven patients received adjuvant doxorubicin-based chemotherapy, and none received adjuvant radiation. The 10-year actuarial local control rate and survival rate were 93% and 73%, respectively. Margin status was the most significant predictor of local control, with a local control rate of 100% when the margins were at least 1 cm wide. However, in this patient cohort, tumor size, grade, site, and depth were not significantly associated with local control. This study demonstrated that function-sparing surgery alone with wide negative margins can achieve local control in highly selected patients with STSs.

A recently published nomogram estimating risk of 3- and 5-year local recurrence after function-sparing surgery may also help inform patient and provider decisions on adjuvant RT.[21] The authors analyzed 684 patients who underwent limb-sparing surgery alone without adjuvant chemotherapy or RT from 1982 to 2006 at Memorial Sloan Kettering Cancer Center. The 3- and 5-year actuarial risks of local recurrence were 11% and 13%, respectively. On multivariate analysis, age ≥50, size >5 cm, close or positive margins, high grade, and histologic types other than well-differentiated liposarcoma and atypical lipomatous tumor were all associated with increased risk of local recurrence; patient sex and depth were not significant.

The decision of whether to treat a patient with STS with surgery alone or with surgery and RT should be made after the patient is evaluated by a surgeon and a radiation oncologist with expertise in the care of STSs and after discussion at a multidisciplinary tumor board.[22] Remarkably, the French Sarcoma Group has found that referral to a multidisciplinary tumor board with expertise in sarcomas prior to initial treatment increased the rate of local relapse-free survival and distant relapse-free survival on multivariate analysis.[23] At our multidisciplinary tumor board, we consider treatment of STSs with surgery alone for small (<5 cm), low-grade, superficial tumors, particularly in an anatomic location where salvage surgery and RT for a future local recurrence would not lead to unacceptable morbidity.

Special Considerations

Myxoid Liposarcoma

While most STSs do not shrink during a course of RT, myxoid liposarcomas, which frequently harbor a *FUS–DDIT3* translocation t(12;16)(q13;p11), are exquisitely radiosensitive. In a retrospective analysis of 691 patients with extremity STS who received surgery and RT, patients with myxoid liposarcoma compared to other subtypes had improved local recurrence-free survival, improved metastasis-free survival, and improved overall survival.[24] The radiosensitivity of myxoid liposarcomas has been documented by quantifying the tumor size before and after RT. A study of 16 patients with myxoid liposarcomas who underwent preoperative radiation found mean pre- and postradiation tumor volumes of 415 and 199 cm^3, respectively, for a proportional reduction of 59% following radiation.[25] In contrast, a control group of patients with malignant fibrous histiocytoma (now referred to as undifferentiated pleomorphic sarcoma or pleomorphic fibrosarcoma) had mean pre- and postradiation volumes of 264 and 273 cm^3, respectively, for a proportional increase in 7%.

Lymph Node Metastases

Most STS histologic types rarely metastasize to lymph nodes (<1% risk), and elective radiation of lymph nodes is not recommended. However, synovial sarcoma, clear cell sarcoma, angiosarcoma, rhabdomyosarcoma, and epithelioid sarcoma histologic types are associated with 10% to 20% rates of lymph node metastases.[26] Clinically suspicious lymph nodes may be included in the preoperative radiation volume. Clinically or pathologically involved lymph node stations may also be included in the postoperative radiation volume, especially in the setting of limited lymph node dissection or extracapsular extension. However, the potential benefit of extending the radiation field to cover draining lymph nodes must be considered within the context of potential increased toxicity. While PET/CT[27] and sentinel node biopsies[28] have been assessed for their utility in staging sarcoma patients, their role for determining lymph node metastases remains uncertain.

Angiosarcoma of the Scalp

Surgery can be utilized for angiosarcoma of the scalp. However, local failure rates after surgery alone are high. In retrospective series, use of RT and multimodality therapy has been associated with improved local control.[29] The optimal radiation dose and field size are not well established. Our practice is to manage most patients with scalp angiosarcoma without surgery. We administer total scalp irradiation with bilateral neck lymph node irradiation using a shrinking field technique with concurrent paclitaxel chemotherapy. Total dose to the primary angiosarcoma is typically 70 to 74 Gy.

BONE SARCOMA

Ewing Sarcoma

Following standard induction chemotherapy for Ewing sarcoma, localized disease is treated with surgery and/or RT. As in STSs, RT may be preoperative, postoperative, or definitive. Preoperative RT may be considered when close or positive margins are expected. Postoperative RT is indicated for close margins, poor histologic response, or tumor spill. Definitive RT may be offered when function-preserving surgery is not an option, such as tumors of the acetabulum or pelvis. Chemotherapy is routinely administered during RT. Surgery and radiation have not been compared head-to-head in prospective, randomized studies. A retrospective analysis of local control in pelvic Ewing sarcoma from INT-0091 found no significant differences in local control between surgery and RT.[30] Another retrospective analysis of patients treated on CESS 81, CESS 86, and EICESS 92 trials suggested that postoperative RT improved local control compared to surgery alone for intralesional resections and poor histologic response. In this analysis, definitive RT had higher local failure rates than surgery, though the authors note that these RT-only patients represented a negatively selected subgroup, with comparatively more paraspinal and pelvic tumors and fewer limb tumors than the surgical patients.[31]

For metastatic Ewing sarcoma, RT may have a role along with surgery for local control of primary tumor and for patients with limited pulmonary, soft tissue, or bone metastases. For pulmonary metastases, whole lung irradiation may be considered even after patients have had resection of limited pulmonary metastases or have shown an excellent response to chemotherapy. Retrospective analysis of cooperative group trials have found improved event-free survival in patients who received low-dose whole lung irradiation.[32]

Use of RT in pediatric patients with Ewing sarcoma is balanced against the risk of second malignancy from irradiation of normal tissue. The most common second malignancy is osteosarcoma. Use of IMRT can reduce the amount of normal tissue exposed to high-dose radiation (45–54 Gy), and proton therapy can also reduce the amount of normal tissue exposed to low-dose radiation (<20 Gy).

Osteosarcoma

Osteosarcoma is routinely treated with induction chemotherapy, surgical resection, and adjuvant chemotherapy. However, RT can be utilized to treat osteosarcoma, but high radiation doses are needed to impact local control. Adjuvant RT can be utilized for close or positive surgical margins and inoperable tumors. A retrospective study of 41 patients who received RT for osteosarcoma suggested that local control was improved for doses ≥55 Gy.[33]

Chordoma and Chondrosarcoma

Chordoma, a malignant bone neoplasm arising from notochord remnants, and chondrosarcoma, a malignant bone neoplasm with production of chondroid matrix, both tend to recur locally, particularly when arising in the mobile spine, sacrum, skull base, or pelvis. En bloc resection is recommended, and a systematic review has found decreased local recurrence and mortality following wide or marginal margins en bloc.[34] However, resection may be limited by patient comorbid conditions, surgical access, and proximity to critical structures. Definitive or adjuvant radiation may, therefore, be considered in the setting of absent or incomplete resection. Historically, conventional radiation doses (<60 Gy) of adjuvant RT resulted in poor local control. The same systematic review suggested that radiation doses of >60 to 65 Gy may improve local control. However, as with surgery, proximity and radiation dose constraints of critical structures, especially the brainstem and spinal cord, may limit the radiation plan. Particle RT with protons or carbon ions has been utilized in this setting, especially for the base of skull chordomas and chondrosarcomas, to achieve favorable dosimetry to spare critical structures.

RE-IRRADIATION

Radiation-associated sarcomas arise within a previously irradiated field. Undifferentiated sarcoma, angiosarcoma, or osteosarcoma, or less commonly, other sarcoma subtypes are also seen in patients who have received radiation, particularly among survivors of childhood cancers. Radiation-associated angiosarcomas are recognized as a complication following breast or chest wall radiation for breast cancer.

The mainstay of treatment for sarcomas arising within a previously irradiated field, either for locally recurrent or radiation-associated sarcomas, is wide local excision with or without systemic therapy. When wide margins cannot be achieved, adjuvant or definitive re-irradiation may be considered. The potential benefit of re-irradiation must be balanced by the potential toxicity because of dose tolerance of adjacent normal tissues such as brainstem, spinal cord, brachial plexus, and other major nerves, blood vessels, and bowel. Potential complications of re-irradiation are similar to those of upfront radiation, but the risk and severity increase; of utmost concern are impaired wound healing or nonhealing wounds, tissue necrosis, fistulas, bowel perforation, vascular blowout, and neuropathy.

Retrospective series and single-arm prospective trials have examined re-irradiation with either external beam RT or brachytherapy. A retrospective analysis of 10 patients with locally recurrent limb sarcoma who received electron or photon external beam re-irradiation reported adequate local control, with a median survival of 14 months after re-irradiation. Radionecrosis was seen in a single patient who had received a total dose of 145 Gy.[35] Another retrospective analysis of patients with locally recurrent sarcoma who received re-irradiation with perioperative brachytherapy reported adequate local control with a 5-year local recurrence-free rate of 52% and an overall survival rate of 33%. Complication rates were deemed acceptable, with wound breakdown or osteonecrosis or neuropathy occurring in 5/26 patients.[36] Re-irradiation with proton therapy has also been utilized and may provide favorable dosimetry in respecting adjacent normal tissue constraints.

Hyperfractionated, accelerated RT with smaller fraction sizes delivered two to three times per day rather than once daily can also be used for re-irradiation. A retrospective series of 14 patients who developed angiosarcoma following whole breast radiation for breast cancer used photon and/or electron external beam re-irradiation with adequate local control and limited toxicity.[37] The re-irradiation regimen used was 1 Gy three times per day to total doses of 45, 60, or 75 Gy for low-risk subclinical, high-risk subclinical, and gross disease. All patients received mastectomy for angiosarcoma either before or after RT. The 5- and 10-year overall survival rates were 79% and 63%, respectively, and overall toxicity appeared to be acceptable, with three patients developing lymphedema, one patient developing recurrent benign pleural effusion, and four patients developing self-limited rib fractures.

SBRT FOR METASTASES FROM SARCOMAS

For several decades, surgical metastasectomy has been used for palliative and local control of sarcoma metastases. Some retrospective studies have suggested a longer disease-free interval or even survival benefit in carefully selected patients, typically with a limited number of metastatic sites and/or indolent disease, where resection of all metastatic sites is feasible.[38] In patients unfit for surgery, SBRT has also been used for the local control of metastatic disease to the lungs and spine. Several institutions have published experiences with pulmonary and spine SBRT for sarcoma, with a local control rate >85% and minimal toxicity.

A retrospective series from the University of Rochester examined 52 patients with pulmonary metastases from STS (median four lesions; range 1–16 lesions); 31% had surgical metastasectomy, while 29% received SBRT.[39] No grade ≥3 toxicities were observed with SBRT. Also, 7/74 pulmonary metastases treated with SBRT progressed, with a 3-year local lesion control rate of 82% with SBRT. The median and mean survival for patients who received SBRT was 2.1 years. Another prospective observational study from Milan of 28 patients who received SBRT for pulmonary metastases reported a 5-year local control rate of 96%, also without grade ≥3 toxicity.[40] Five-year overall survival for this cohort was 60.5%. A retrospective analysis from Memorial Sloan Kettering Cancer Center of 88 patients who received SBRT for spinal metastases from STS reported a 12-month local failure-free survival rate of 85.9%.[41,42] Also, 83.3% of local failures failed distantly. The 12-month overall survival rate was 62.1%, and the median overall survival was 18.9 months. No grade >3 toxicities were observed; 1% had acute grade 3 toxicity and 4.5% had chronic grade 3 toxicity.

SUMMARY

RT uses IR to kill sarcoma cells, primarily through DNA damage. RT is typically delivered via external beam RT or brachytherapy. Advances including image-guided RT, IMRT, and particle therapy with protons or carbon ions can improve the therapeutic ratio by maximizing the tumor dose while minimizing the dose to adjacent normal tissues. In localized STS, the backbone of curative treatment is surgery with wide negative margins. Preoperative, intraoperative, or postoperative RT can maximize local control, though omission of radiation may be considered in select cases, particularly for small (<5 cm), low-grade, superficial tumors. Compared to postoperative RT, preoperative RT typically uses a lower total radiation dose and a smaller radiation field size, which causes less late effects. However, the rates of wound complications increase approximately twofold. IORT may also be utilized as a tumor bed boost when normal tissue is displaced out of the radiation field. Brachytherapy is typically used in the setting of an intraoperative or postoperative boost to the tumor bed or as adjuvant postoperative RT. Myxoid liposarcoma is especially radiosensitive, and a significant reduction in tumor volume can occur following RT. Scalp angiosarcoma has a propensity for local, cervical nodal, and distant recurrence. RT to the total scalp with bilateral neck node irradiation has been advocated to decrease the risk of recurrence.

In Ewing sarcoma, RT may be used to treat localized disease when wide margins cannot be achieved with surgery or if surgery would impair function, though the risk of radiation-associated malignancy, especially in pediatric patients, must be considered. In Ewing sarcoma for limited pulmonary metastases, whole lung irradiation can also be considered. In chordoma and chondrosarcoma, RT may also have a role when wide local resection cannot be achieved. Particle therapy with protons has also been utilized, especially at the skull base, to adequately cover the tumor while minimizing the dose to critical structures such as brainstem and spinal cord. Re-irradiation for radiation-associated sarcomas or locally recurrent sarcomas provides local control; however, feasibility depends on dose tolerance of adjacent normal tissues. Complications of re-irradiation include impaired wound healing, soft tissue necrosis or osteonecrosis, fistulas, and neuropathy. Hyperfractionated RT and/or particle therapy with protons have been used to limit normal tissue toxicity for re-irradiation. SBRT may be used for local control of metastatic sites in appropriately selected patients with few metastases and/or indolent disease. Local control rates are typically >85% with minimal grade >3 toxicity.

REFERENCES

1. Ewing J. Diffuse endothelioma of bone. *Proc NY Pathol Soc.* 1921;21:17–24.
2. Ewing J. An analysis of radiation therapy in cancer: the Mütter Lecture. *Trans Coll Phys Phila.* 1922;44:190–235.
3. National Comprehensive Cancer Network. *Soft Tissue Sarcoma.* https://www.nccn.org/professionals/physician_gls/
4. Rosenberg SA, Tepper J, Glatstein E, et al. The treatment of soft-tissue sarcomas of the extremities: prospective randomized evaluations of (1) limb-sparing surgery plus radiation therapy compared with amputation and (2) the role of adjuvant chemotherapy. *Ann Surg.* 1982;196(3):305–315. doi:10.1097/00000658-198209000-00009
5. Yang JC, Chang AE, Baker AR, et al. Randomized prospective study of the benefit of adjuvant radiation therapy in the treatment of soft tissue sarcomas of the extremity. *J Clin Oncol.* 1998;16(1):197–203. doi:10.1200/JCO.1998.16.1.197
6. Beane JD, Yang JC, White D, et al. Efficacy of adjuvant radiation therapy in the treatment of soft tissue sarcoma of the extremity: 20-year follow-up of a randomized prospective trial. *Ann Surg Oncol.* 2014;21(8):2484–2489. doi:10.1245/s10434-014-3732-4
7. Koshy M, Rich SE, Mohiuddin MM. Improved survival with radiation therapy in high-grade soft tissue sarcomas of the extremities: a SEER analysis. *Int J Radiat Oncol Biol Phys.* 2010;77(1):203–209. doi:10.1016/j.ijrobp.2009.04.051
8. Ramey SJ, Yechieli R, Zhao W, et al. Limb-sparing surgery plus radiotherapy results in superior survival: an analysis of patients with high-grade, extremity soft-tissue sarcoma from the NCDB and SEER. *Cancer Med.* 2018;7(9):4228–4239. doi:10.1002/cam4.1625
9. O'Sullivan B, Davis AM, Turcotte R, et al. Preoperative versus postoperative radiotherapy in soft-tissue sarcoma of the limbs: a randomised trial. *Lancet.* 2002;359(9325):2235–2241. doi:10.1016/S0140-6736(02)09292-9
10. Davis A, O'Sullivan B, Turcotte R, et al. Late radiation morbidity following randomization to preoperative versus postoperative radiotherapy in extremity soft tissue sarcoma. *Radiother Oncol.* 2005;75(1):48–53. doi:10.1016/j.radonc.2004.12.020
11. Wang D, Zhang Q, Eisenberg BL, et al. Significant reduction of late toxicities in patients with extremity sarcoma treated with image-guided radiation therapy to a reduced target volume: results of Radiation Therapy Oncology Group RTOG-0630 Trial. *J Clin Oncol.* 2015; 33(20):2231–2238. doi:10.1200/JCO.2014.58.5828
12. Al-Absi E, Farrokhyar F, Sharma R, et al. A systematic review and meta-analysis of oncologic outcomes of preversus postoperative radiation in localized resectable soft-tissue sarcoma. *Ann Surg Oncol.* 2010;17(5):1367–1374. doi:10.1245/s10434-009-0885-7
13. Kraybill WG, Harris J, Spiro IJ, et al. Phase II study of neoadjuvant chemotherapy and radiation therapy in the management of high-risk, high-grade, soft tissue sarcomas of the extremities and body wall: Radiation Therapy Oncology Group Trial 9514. *J Clin Oncol.* 2006;24(4):619–625. doi:10.1200/JCO.2005.02.5577
14. Roeder F, Timke C, Oertel S, et al. Intraoperative electron radiotherapy for the management of aggressive fibromatosis. *Int J Radiat Oncol Biol Phys.* 2010;76(4):1154–1160. doi:10.1016/j.ijrobp.2009.03.067
15. Sindelar WF, Kinsella TJ, Chen PW, et al. Intraoperative radiotherapy in retroperitoneal sarcomas. Final results of a prospective, randomized, clinical trial. *Arch Surg.* 1993;128(4):402–410. doi:10.1001/archsurg.1993.01420160040005
16. Pisters PW, Harrison LB, Leung DH, et al. Long-term results of a prospective randomized trial of adjuvant brachytherapy in soft tissue sarcoma. *J Clin Oncol.* 1996;14(3):859–868. doi:10.1200/JCO.1996.14.3.859
17. Pohar S, Haq R, Liu L, et al. Adjuvant high-dose-rate and low-dose-rate brachytherapy with external beam radiation in soft tissue sarcoma: a comparison of outcomes. *Brachytherapy.* 2007;6(1):53–57. doi:10.1016/j.brachy.2006.11.004
18. Kepka L, DeLaney TF, Suit HD, Goldberg SI. Results of radiation therapy for unresected soft-tissue sarcomas. *Int J Radiat Oncol Biol Phys.* 2005;63(3):852–859. doi:10.1016/j.ijrobp.2005.03.004
19. Eckert F, Matuschek C, Mueller AC, et al. Definitive radiotherapy and single-agent radiosensitizing ifosfamide in patients with localized, irresectable soft tissue sarcoma: a retrospective analysis. *Radiat Oncol.* 2010;5:55. doi:10.1186/1748-717X-5-55
20. Baldini EH, Goldberg J, Jenner C, et al. Long-term outcomes after function-sparing surgery without radiotherapy for soft tissue sarcoma of the extremities and trunk. *J Clin Oncol.* 1999;17(10):3252–3259. doi:10.1200/JCO.1999.17.10.3252
21. Cahlon O, Brennan MF, Jia X, et al. A postoperative nomogram for local recurrence risk in extremity soft tissue sarcomas after limb-sparing surgery without adjuvant radiation. *Ann Surg.* 2012;255(2):343–347. doi:10.1097/SLA.0b013e3182367aa7

22. Derbel O, Heudel PE, Cropet C, et al. Survival impact of centralization and clinical guidelines for soft tissue sarcoma (a prospective and exhaustive population-based cohort). *PLoS One*. 2017;12(2):e0158406. doi:10.1371/journal.pone.0158406
23. Blay JY, Soibinet P, Penel N, et al. Improved survival using specialized multidisciplinary board in sarcoma patients. *Ann Oncol*. 2017;28(11):2852–2859. doi:10.1093/annonc/mdx484
24. Chung PW, Deheshi BM, Ferguson PC, et al. Radiosensitivity translates into excellent local control in extremity myxoid liposarcoma: a comparison with other soft tissue sarcomas. *Cancer*. 2009;115(14):3254–3261. doi:10.1002/cncr.24375
25. Pitson G, Robinson P, Wilke D, et al. Radiation response: an additional unique signature of myxoid liposarcoma. *Int J Radiat Oncol Biol Phys*. 2004;60(2):522–526. doi:10.1016/j.ijrobp.2004.03.009
26. Fong Y, Coit DG, Woodruff JM, Brennan MF. Lymph node metastasis from soft tissue sarcoma in adults. Analysis of data from a prospective database of 1772 sarcoma patients. *Ann Surg*. 1993;217(1):72–77. doi:10.1097/00000658-199301000-00012
27. Volker T, Denecke T, Steffen I, et al. Positron emission tomography for staging of pediatric sarcoma patients: results of a prospective multicenter trial. *J Clin Oncol*. 2007;25:5435–5441. doi:10.1200/JCO.2007.12.2473
28. Maduekwe UN, Hornicek FJ, Springfield DS, et al. Role of sentinel lymph node biopsy in the staging of synovial, epithelioid, and clear cell sarcomas. *Ann Surg Oncol*. 2009;16(5):1356–1363. doi:10.1245/s10434-009-0393-9
29. Patel SH, Hayden RE, Hinni ML, et al. Angiosarcoma of the scalp and face: the Mayo Clinic experience. *JAMA Otolaryngol Head Neck Surg*. 2015;141(4):335–340. doi:10.1001/jamaoto.2014.3584
30. Yock TI, Krailo M, Fryer CJ, et al. Local control in pelvic Ewing sarcoma: analysis from INT-0091—a report from the Children's Oncology Group. *J Clin Oncol*. 2006;24(24):3838–3843. doi:10.1200/JCO.2006.05.9188
31. Schuck A, Ahrens S, Paulussen M, et al. Local therapy in localized Ewing tumors: results of 1058 patients treated in the CESS 81, CESS 86, and EICESS 92 trials. *Int J Radiat Oncol Biol Phys*. 2003;55(1):168–177. doi:10.1016/S0360-3016(02)03797-5
32. Paulussen M, Ahrens S, Burdach S, et al. Primary metastatic (stage IV) Ewing tumor: survival analysis of 171 patients from the EICESS studies. European Intergroup Cooperative Ewing Sarcoma Studies. *Ann Oncol*. 1998;9(3):275–281. doi:10.1023/A:1008208511815
33. DeLaney TF, Park L, Goldberg SI, et al. Radiotherapy for local control of osteosarcoma. *Int J Radiat Oncol Biol Phys*. 2005;61(2):492–498. doi:10.1016/j.ijrobp.2004.05.051
34. Boriani S, Saravanja D, Yamada Y, et al. Challenges of local recurrence and cure in low grade malignant tumors of the spine. *Spine*. 2009;34(22 suppl):S48–S57. doi:10.1097/BRS.0b013e3181b969ac
35. Graham JD, Robinson MH, Harmer CL. Re-irradiation of soft-tissue sarcoma. *Br J Radiol*. 1992;65(770):157–161. doi:10.1259/0007-1285-65-770-157
36. Pearlstone DB, Janjan NA, Feig BW, et al. Re-resection with brachytherapy for locally recurrent soft tissue sarcoma arising in a previously radiated field. *Cancer J Sci Am*. 1999;5(1):26–33.
37. Smith TL, Morris CG, Mendenhall NP. Angiosarcoma after breast-conserving therapy: long-term disease control and late effects with hyperfractionated accelerated re-irradiation (HART). *Acta Oncol*. 2014;53(2):235–241. doi:10.3109/0284186X.2013.819117
38. Blackmon SH, Shah N, Roth JA, et al. Resection of pulmonary and extrapulmonary sarcomatous metastases is associated with long-term survival. *Ann Thorac Surg*. 2009;88(3):877–884; discussion 84–85. doi:10.1016/j.athoracsur.2009.04.144
39. Dhakal S, Corbin KS, Milano MT, et al. Stereotactic body radiotherapy for pulmonary metastases from soft-tissue sarcomas: excellent local lesion control and improved patient survival. *Int J Radiat Oncol Biol Phys*. 2012;82(2):940–945. doi:10.1016/j.ijrobp.2010.11.052
40. Navarria P, Ascolese AM, Cozzi L, et al. Stereotactic body radiation therapy for lung metastases from soft tissue sarcoma. *Eur J Cancer*. 2015;51(5):668–674. doi:10.1016/j.ejca.2015.01.061
41. Leeman JE, Bilsky M, Laufer I, et al. Stereotactic body radiotherapy for metastatic spinal sarcoma: a detailed patterns-of-failure study. *J Neurosurg Spine*. 2016;25(1):52–58. doi:10.3171/2015.11.SPINE151059
42. Folkert MR, Bilsky MH, Tom AK, et al. Outcomes and toxicity for hypofractionated and single-fraction image-guided stereotactic radiosurgery for sarcomas metastasizing to the spine. *Int J Radiat Oncol Biol Phys*. 2014;88(5):1085–1091. doi:10.1016/j.ijrobp.2013.12.042

5

Surgical Approach and Surgical Reconstruction Options in Treatment of Bone Sarcomas

Erika L. Garbrecht, Motasem Al Maaieh, Sheila Ann Conway, and Juan A. Pretell

INTRODUCTION

Patients with sarcoma of the musculoskeletal system require complex care through an extensive multidisciplinary team. One critical component of this care team is an orthopedic surgeon with specialization in musculoskeletal oncology. Orthopedic oncologists provide surgical oncologic expertise and have proficiency in the various limb reconstruction techniques utilized to optimize patient outcome and function. Whether the surgical approach is limb salvage or amputation, sarcoma patients have unique lifelong musculoskeletal needs. These patients often require extensive physical therapy, prosthetics, orthotics, and possibly revision surgery. Therefore, a basic familiarity with these complex surgical procedures and their potential complications will assist all practitioners in optimizing patient care in sarcoma treatment.

The primary goal of this chapter is to familiarize healthcare providers with the critical components of the initial evaluation, biopsy, and surgical treatment options used to treat patients with bone sarcomas. We also review some of the critical tumor characteristics, patient-specific factors, and the procedure-specific rehabilitative requirements that can impact these complex surgical decisions.

INITIAL EVALUATION

The initial evaluation of a patient with a suspected bone sarcoma begins with a relevant history and physical exam. Though simple and easily performed, the importance of this step can often be overlooked. Imaging assessment of a bone sarcoma typically begins with a radiograph followed by a variety of advanced imaging modalities. Each imaging modality can provide different information regarding the tumor. Following adequate imaging, a well-planned and executed biopsy is the next step in the diagnosis. The goal of this biopsy is establishing a definitive diagnosis, subtype, and grade, while providing adequate specimen for any additional pathologic testing. While the staging process begins with the physical exam, this should be completed with appropriate body imaging when a diagnosis of sarcoma is confirmed.

History

The history of present illness and past medical history of the patient is critical in the initial evaluation. This begins with patient-derived history regarding duration of symptoms, intensity and characteristics of pain, growth rate, and functional limitations. A history of any local trauma or injury should be elicited, as well as associated systemic symptoms, such as fevers and weight loss. The history should also include all comorbid conditions, relevant previous procedures (including biopsy), and medications. A personal and/or familial history of cancer may be contributive and should be noted.

A thorough understanding of the patient's baseline functional status is critical and should include any preexisting limitations or perceived dysfunction. At this first encounter, the surgeon should inquire about the patient's current activity level and occupation. As musculoskeletal sarcoma frequently occurs in adolescents and young adults, it is also critical to explore their physical and occupational goals, as this may be impacted by the planned surgery and/or reconstructive option.

Physical Examination

While the focus of physical examination will be the mass or painful extremity, some general exam findings are critical. Body habitus, gait patterns, need for assistive device, and patient affect are immediately apparent examination findings and can impact surgical decision-making. Pathologic fractures can occur in association with bone sarcomas. Pathologic fractures at diagnosis or during neoadjuvant treatment have a prevalence of 5% to 10% in relation to osteosarcoma.[1] Therefore, any deformity and/or significant change in pain symptoms should be evaluated with radiographs both on initial evaluation and throughout neoadjuvant treatments. If present, palpable masses should be well characterized with regard to firmness, mobility, compressibility, and temperature. Previous scars and biopsy sites should be carefully examined, with the orientation, length, and location well documented. Any skin changes (erythema, fungation, telangiectasias, seromas, or hematomas) associated with the tumor or biopsy site should be noted. A comprehensive vascular, lymphatic, and neurologic examination of the affected extremity may reveal edema, lymphadenopathy, vascular findings, or neurologic findings associated with tumor involvement or mass effect.

Imaging

Comprehensive imaging of the involved extremity plus appropriate staging studies should be performed during initial evaluation of all bone sarcomas. As imaging is covered in detail in Chapter 7, Radiologic Evaluation of Bone and Soft Tissue Sarcoma at Diagnosis and Follow-Up, the role of imaging is addressed subsequently as it relates to surgical planning.

Imaging begins with orthogonal radiographs of the entire bone involved with the joint above and below. Orthogonal radiographs that are well taken can allow localization of bone tumors, while also providing information on aggressiveness and matrix formation. Aggressive bone lesions are characterized by a wide zone of transition with possible cortical destruction and intense periosteal reaction.[2] This contrasts with less aggressive lesions, which have narrow zone of transition with little to no effect on the cortex and nonaggressive or absent periosteal reaction.[2] Complete radiographic imaging of the bone allows for evaluation of preexisting deformity of the bone, osteoarthritis, osteopenia, or other musculoskeletal pathologic changes that may affect surgical planning.

Although one can gain significant information from radiographs, additional cross-sectional imaging is still needed. MRI with and without contrast is used for further detailed localization of the tumor, evaluation of any possible soft tissue components, tumor heterogeneity, and relative location to vital structures including neurovascular structures.[3] It is felt that unenhanced T1-weighted sequences are most suitable for evaluation of the tumor margins within the bone without clinically significant under- or overestimation.[4] Obtaining an MRI scan of the entire bone involved is also important for evaluation of skip lesions or a discontinuous lesion within the same bone.[3] MRI allows for detailed evaluation of any vessel encasement or infiltration that may preclude limb-salvage surgery. CT scan is an additional cross-sectional imaging technique that can aid the surgeon in preoperative evaluation, with additional bone detail needed for surgical planning.

BIOPSY

After all initial local imaging studies have been completed, a biopsy is performed for tissue diagnosis. A biopsy is viewed as the final diagnostic procedure, not a shortcut to a diagnosis.[5] In this section are discussed specific principles that should be followed when performing a biopsy for musculoskeletal sarcoma. When a biopsy is improperly performed, it can have significant negative effects to the patient and can alter his or her surgical options.[6–8] Biopsy-related errors are minimized through discussion of a multidisciplinary team, especially involving the orthopedic oncologist.[6,9,10] Various effective biopsy techniques for the management of sarcoma have been described, including office-based biopsy, image-guided biopsy, and open biopsy in the surgical suite. Image-guided biopsy is typically performed by musculoskeletal radiologists, and prior to this biopsy, there should be discussion between the radiologist and the orthopedic oncologist regarding the location of biopsy. Communication with the pathology department is also important, as the pathologist has critical insight regarding the biopsy technique, tumor volume, and special tissue processing needs. As more targeted medical strategies are employed, the role of the treating medical oncologist in biopsy planning becomes more apparent. Nonroutine tumor testing, additional tumor volume, or specific tissue processing may be requested by the medical oncologist, particularly for resistant tumors or patients eligible for novel therapies or clinical trials.

Biopsy Principles

Biopsy should be performed after all imaging studies have been completed, so two important questions can be addressed prior to biopsy: (a) What portion of the sarcoma should be biopsied? and (b) What is the safest anatomic route to the location?[11]

The biology of sarcomas, which are mesenchymal based, is much different from that of carcinomas. Sarcomas usually possess regional morphologic variations.[12–14] Sarcomas grow in a centripetal fashion, with the most immature portion in the peripheral portion and often a central necrotic portion. This immature portion is also surrounded by a reactive zone of tissue.[11] After meticulous imaging review by a radiologist and an orthopedic oncologist, who are familiar with the characteristics of sarcoma, usually viable and diagnostic portion of the tumor can be identified for biopsy. Given the heterogeneous nature of sarcoma, multiple biopsy samples are taken to help reduce the chances of "sampling error." The extraosseous portion of the bony sarcoma is representative of the primary pathology and should be biopsied, if it exists.[8] If no extraosseous portion exists, a cortical window can be created to obtain adequate tissue; if this is done poorly, it can place the patient at increased risk for pathologic fracture due to weakening of the structural integrity of the bone.[15]

After a specific portion of the tumor has been identified for biopsy, the approach to that portion must be identified. Traditional teaching has stressed the following two main principles: (a) The biopsy tract should be in line with the planned incision of definitive surgery. This allows for excision of the biopsy tract during definitive surgery. The thought is that the biopsy tract is seeded with tumor and should be excised to decrease the risk of local recurrence.[8] (b) The biopsy tract should be the shortest route to the tumor, violate only one compartment, and be as distant as possible from vital neurovascular structures.[16]

Evidence has proposed that biopsy of musculoskeletal sarcoma should be performed at the institution of planned definitive treatment. This can decrease morbidity to the patient, can avoid treatment interruption, and can limit delays in diagnosis.[6,17] Mankin et al. reviewed the complications with biopsies for sarcoma performed at referring centers as compared to treating centers.[6] Biopsies for sarcoma performed at referral centers led to 27.4% errors in diagnosis, 13.9% were nonrepresentative, 36.3% led to change in treatment plan, and 17.4% changed the course or outcome of treatment. This is in stark contrast to biopsies performed at the treatment center, where 12.3% led to an error in diagnosis, 3.5% were nonrepresentative, 4.1% led to a change in treatment plan, and 3.5% changed the course or outcome of treatment.

Biopsy Technique

After anatomic location of the biopsy is determined, quality tissue must be obtained to allow for tissue diagnosis. There are various ways to obtain tissue with differences in accuracy. The diagnostic accuracy of fine-needle aspiration (FNA), core-needle biopsy, and open biopsy has been investigated. After review of the literature, Traina et al. found that core-needle biopsy was more accurate than FNA, and open or incisional biopsy showed the highest accuracy of all.[8] Core-needle biopsies allow for better preservation of tumor architecture, leading to increased information from the biopsy tissue, as compared to FNA.[11] Percutaneous core-needle biopsies have the advantage of decreased cost and lower risk of contamination, while providing diagnostic accuracy between 74% and 100%.[8,18] Percutaneous core-needle biopsies appear to be most suitable for diagnosis of bone tumors. The use of image-guided biopsy can also increase diagnostic accuracy in deep musculoskeletal tumors.[19] In the setting of a palpable sarcomatous mass, office-based core-needle biopsies have shown an accuracy of 91% and were found to be safe and well tolerated.[20] If diagnosis cannot be obtained from percutaneous biopsy, an open incisional biopsy is indicated.[21] Recent literature has also questioned the traditional teaching that the biopsy track must be excised and must not cross multiple compartments when performing coaxial core needle biopsies.[22] Binitie et al. reviewed 59 soft tissue sarcoma patients who had undergone core-needle biopsies without excision of biopsy track at definitive treatment and saw no increase in local recurrence or rates of metastasis.[23] As compared to percutaneous biopsy tracks, open incisional biopsy track scars are more clear and usually excised on definitive surgical treatment.[22]

SURGICAL TREATMENT

The primary goal of surgical treatment is complete sarcoma resection with negative margins. The risk of local recurrence in osteosarcoma is significantly increased in patients who undergo resection with inadequate margins.[24–26] While negative margin status is the primary surgical oncologic goal, there remains debate on the optimal size of this margin. In the current literature, this margin can vary between specific bone sarcomas, tumor grade, and tumor location.[27,28] The secondary goal of surgery is to preserve and/or restore optimal function for the patient. The surgeons should be mindful to ensure it is the patients' definition of optimal function that guides this critical discussion. During surgical planning, the patient and his or her support system should be educated about the realistic expectations of the postoperative course and resulting function of the limb. Furthermore, the patient's ability or willingness to comply with postoperative precautions or rehabilitative requirements may influence the planned surgery or the favored reconstructive option.

Complete resection with negative margins can be achieved through amputation or tumor resection followed by reconstruction (limb-salvage surgery). Prior to the 1970s, most primary bone sarcomas were treated with amputation.[29,30] With the limited availability of adjuvant treatments and modern surgical techniques, this provided the patient with the best functional and clinical outcome. The 5-year survival rates were approximately 10% to 20%,[30,31] with a vast majority of these patients succumbing to metastatic disease.[29] With advancements in adjuvant treatment, there has been significant improvement in survival rates and a paradigm shift to limb-salvage surgery (LSS), with approximately 90% of primary bone sarcoma patients undergoing LSS.[32] The following sections discuss the surgical approach to bone sarcomas, followed by a brief synopsis of the most common surgical procedures utilized in bone sarcoma limb-salvage reconstruction and their associated complications.

Preoperative Considerations

A multitude of factors help determine the optimal surgical procedure for the individual patient. Many of these are patient-specific factors discovered during the focused history and physical examinations. Various preexisting medical conditions (diabetes, autoimmune diseases, degenerative joint disease, vasculopathies, coagulopathies) may impact a patient's ability to tolerate a major oncologic procedure or his or her ability to heal and rehabilitate. Behavioral (smoking) and/or psychological factors can also impact the patient's ability to heal or comply with specific postoperative precautions or anticipated deficiencies. Many oncologic surgeries are extensive, and any bleeding or coagulopathy disorders should be elicited preoperatively and could require special treatment during invasive procedures and/or surgical treatment. All modifiable risk factors should be addressed prior to surgical intervention and medical conditions optimized in a timely fashion, so as to not delay treatment. Select patients with significant medical comorbid conditions and poor overall health may be better treated nonsurgically, particularly if they are at an unacceptable risk of mortality or morbidity with an extensive oncologic surgery. In certain instances, limb or osseous reconstruction may be associated with an unacceptable risk, and amputation or sarcoma excision without complex reconstruction is offered.

Tumor-specific factors are also considered in developing a surgical plan for the sarcoma patient. Many pathologic factors impact the patient's overall oncologic care, including the surgical plan. Specific tumor diagnoses and higher-grade tumors may necessitate a larger tumor margin or introduce alternative local control options. For example, extended intralesional curettage has become an acceptable treatment approach for low-grade chondrosarcomas, while high-grade tumors require wide resection.[27] In unresectable Ewing sarcoma, radiation therapy is often implemented for local control owing to this tumor's radiosensitivity.[27] Many of the most critical factors that guide the planned surgery are interpreted from the preoperative imaging and biopsy results, making the quality and interpretation of these studies paramount. In many sarcoma centers, this is completed in a multidisciplinary sarcoma board to optimize the information gathered and to apply this information appropriately to treatment decisions.[33] Critical tumor characteristics gleamed from radiographs include the location and size of the tumor, the mineralization pattern, and the osseous reaction to the tumor. MRI provides detailed information on the marrow extent of the tumor, including identification of skip metastasis, soft tissue extension, and the tumor relationship to (or involvement of) neurovascular structures. Interval MRIs often allow for estimation of neoadjuvant treatment response and can alter planned surgical resections.[34] CT scan may be used an alternative when MRI is contraindicated or as an adjunct to radiographs in tumors involving complex bones (pelvis).

En Bloc Resection

The goal of sarcoma resection traditionally involves resection with a wide margin or en bloc resection.[27] This is defined as a resection with a cuff of normal tissue. Ultraradical resections, which involve sacrificing vital structures to extend the margin, show no significant benefits from wide resection.[27] The exact size of this wide margin has not been fully elicited from literature. In regard to high-grade, nonmetastatic osteosarcoma, Bertrand et al. found that the presence of a positive margin, compared to a negative margin >1 mm, was the only independent predictor of local recurrence after controlling for relevant confounding variables.[35] Li et al. and Bispo et al. also investigated close margins, a margin 5 mm or less compared to >5 mm and margins <2 mm and >2 mm, respectively, and found no difference in likelihood of local recurrence in osteosarcoma patients.[36,37] At this time point, no specific measurement could be borne out from the literature regarding margins, but local recurrence has been shown to be increased in osteosarcoma patients with positive margins.[24] It appears that having a negative margin is an important factor in reducing local recurrence and increasing survival.[27]

When considering the goals of en bloc resection, it is important to consider that the majority of bone sarcomas present with soft tissue extension, requiring resection of associated muscle and soft tissues to achieve negative margins. Once the extent of resection is planned, the function of the residual limb can be estimated based on the residual functional tissue. If adequate margins require resection of critical structures, the anticipated function of the residual extremity will be impacted. While some critical structures are routinely reconstructed in an effort for limb salvage, the loss of multiple critical neurovascular structures often results in impaired neurologic or vascular function of the residual limb. Furthermore, large soft tissue defects may require secondary procedures, such as skin grafts and muscle flaps, to ensure a functional soft tissue envelope. The following sections provide overviews of the major surgical procedures employed in the treatment of bone sarcomas, commonly associated complications, and specific rehabilitation implications.

Endoprosthetic Reconstruction

Endoprosthetic reconstruction involves restoration of structural stability after skeletal resection through the use of a metal alloy implant and polyethylene at gliding surfaces. These are commonly used around periarticular or metaphyseal resections. Various endoprostheses are available for reconstruction throughout both upper and lower extremities. Most contemporary endoprostheses are modular and available in a range of sizes to restore a wide array of osseous defects. A distal femoral endoprosthetic reconstruction is seen in Figure 5.1. Depending on the surgical technique, many endoprosthetic reconstructions can allow for immediate weight bearing and mobilization. This is an advantage, as a subset of patients will be unable to ambulate in a non–weight-bearing fashion owing to comorbid conditions. For example, a patient with severe contralateral arthritis or poor overall condition may become bedridden in the absence of a construct that allows immediate weight bearing.

Although it is a readily available method of reconstruction in limb-salvage surgery, endoprosthetic reconstruction is not without complications. Failures can occur from various methods, including soft tissue failures, aseptic loosening, structural failure, infection, and tumor progression. Henderson et al. performed a retrospective review of the modes of failure of large endoprosthetic reconstructions done after tumor resections.[38] The authors identified a total of 6,533 patients who underwent large endoprosthetic reconstructions done after tumor resections; 2,174 reconstructions came from review of operative databases from five institutions and 4,359 reconstructions from review of the literature. Failure occurred in 27.6% of the reconstructions, with the most common mode of failure being aseptic loosening at 8.2%, followed by infection at 8.0%. Large endoprosthetic reconstructions are exposed

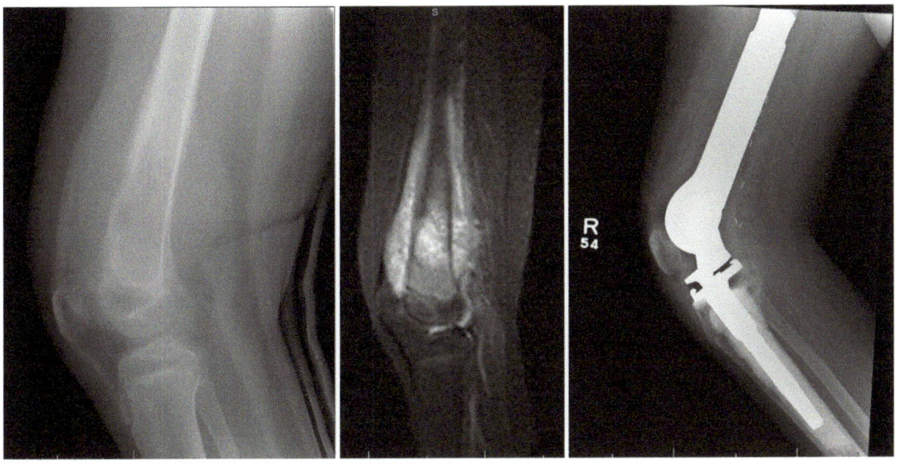

(A) (B) (C)

FIGURE 5.1 Endoprosthetic reconstruction of distal femur. Pre- and postoperative images of a 14-year-old male with right distal femur osteosarcoma. (A) Preoperative radiograph showing a large distal femoral lesion with laminated periosteal reaction and anterior and cortical breakthrough. (B) Also evident is a large soft tissue mass, better seen on the sagittal T2-weighted MRI. (C) Postoperative radiograph after endoprosthetic reconstruction.

to high stress at the bone–implant interface, given long lever arms and concentration of stress at the areas,[39] which could contribute to this relatively high rate of failure. Also, patients undergoing orthopedic oncologic surgeries with reconstruction can be at higher risk for surgical site infection owing to extensive surgical dissection with longer operative times, adjuvant chemotherapy, and adjuvant radiation.[40–42] Infection rate (8%) of large endoprosthetic reconstruction following tumor resection is notably higher than that for a primary total knee or total hip replacement for osteoarthritis, which have infection rates of 1.52% and 0.83%, respectively.[43] Tumor progression was a mode of failure in only 4.9% of patients. Other modes of failure evaluated were soft tissue failure and structural failure, with failure rates of 1.5% and 4.9%, respectively. Henderson et al. also subdivided modes of failure by anatomic location. Proximal tibia endoprosthetic reconstructions had a failure rate of 39%, with infection being the most common mode of failure. Distal femur reconstructions had a failure rate of 26.8%, as compared to proximal femur reconstructions with a failure rate of 18.1%. Continued review of outcomes shows the trend that as the extent of resection and size of endoprosthesis increase, so does the rate of complications.[44]

Endoprosthetic reconstruction options continue to progress. Given the significant heterogeneity of the defect left after tumor resection, some defects may not be easily reconstructable with common modular endoprostheses. With technological advancements in computer-aided design and computer-aided manufacturing, custom-made implants to fill specific resection defects have become possible.[45] The custom implant can also be coupled with custom cutting guides to aid match between bony resection and custom prosthesis. Custom cutting guides have allowed for decreased operative time, decreased intraoperative blood loss, and more accurate margin resection in pelvis surgeries, as compared to surgeries without the use of custom cutting guides.[46] The optimal indications for this technology are not clear, and current investigations have focused on short-term complications after complex reconstructions of the pelvis following resection. Early and small sample size studies have shown acceptable complications rates similar to other methods of reconstruction.[47,48] Further investigation on these implants is necessary to determine if these techniques improve oncologic and/or functional outcomes.

Skeletally immature patients undergoing bone resection near or involving the physeal growth plate add a unique challenge to surgical planning and reconstruction. One solution to this difficult situation is an expandable endoprosthesis. These endoprostheses can be lengthened incrementally over time, in an attempt to maintain length equality to the contralateral limb. Noninvasive expandable prosthesis can be lengthened through a mechanism that is activated by an external electromagnetic coil,[49] eliminating the need to return to the operating room for frequent expansions. Although expandable endoprosthesis is one method that helps resolve the issue of physeal growth plate resection, it is not without complications. These complications are similar to those seen in the adult endoprosthetic reconstruction (soft tissue failures, aseptic loosening, structural failure, infection, and tumor progression), but occur at a much higher rate.[44,49–51] Expandable prosthesis reconstruction can also be complicated by failure of the noninvasive expansion mechanism, which was seen in approximately 10% in one study.[52] At this time, the literature does not support this technique over other reconstructions in the pediatric population.

Although advancements in endoprosthetic design and surgical technique continue, the patient needs to be made aware of the failure and complications rates. Although dependent on the operating surgeon, patients with endoprosthetic reconstruction are given restrictions on activity, including running and other impact activities. Patients with endoprosthetic reconstructions require routine long-term prosthetic surveillance for structural integrity, even well after cancer remission. Survivors of bone sarcoma with limb-salvage reconstruction often require revision surgery for late complications, including mechanical failures such as aseptic loosening and delayed infections.

Optimal functional recovery requires extensive physical and/or occupational therapy, as these patients have often lost significant muscle mass from the required tumor resection. As with all surgical reconstructions, deep infection is a dreaded complication often requiring complex surgical revisions. In some cases, these acute complications can delay adjuvant chemotherapy and/or radiotherapy.

Bulk Allograft Reconstruction

Tissue obtained from another individual is termed an allograft. In the orthopedic oncologic case, this is usually in the form of bulk allograft, which includes a significant portion of segmental bone that allows for restoration of structure.[53,54] Soft tissue components can also be included in the bulk allograft, which can assist in soft tissue reconstruction.[53,54] A variety of allograft types are available for both bony and soft tissue defects after resection. Figure 5.2 shows a bulk allograft reconstruction of the elbow. These allografts are usually in the form of fresh frozen cadaver from tissue bank services. Bulk allograft does

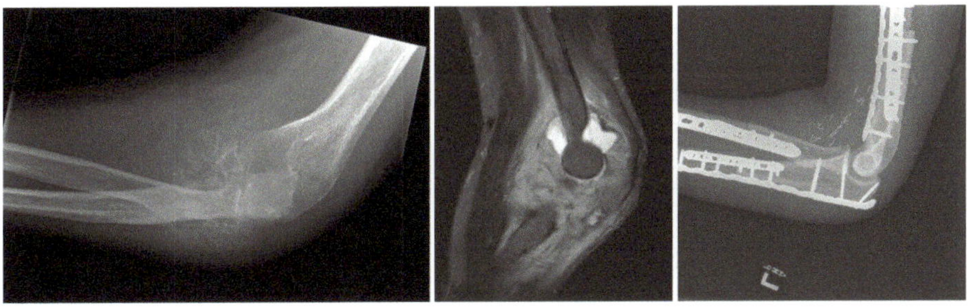

(A) (B) (C)

FIGURE 5.2 Bulk allograft reconstruction of elbow. Pre- and postoperative images of a 22-year-old male with a locally aggressive proximal left ulna cellular osteoblastoma. (A) Preoperative radiograph showing a mass in the anterolateral elbow, originating from the proximal ulna with cortical irregularities and cloud-like periosteal reaction. (B) A T2-weighted sagittal MRI in which the hyperintense mass is more clearly seen with large elbow effusion. (C) A postoperative radiograph after resection and bulk allograft reconstruction.

allow for incorporation into host tissue, such as healing of host bone to allograft, although it does take time. Some common cases of failure are nonunion at graft–host interface, graft fracture, resorption, subchondral fragmentation, and cartilage degeneration.[53]

Bulk allograft reconstruction is often associated with prolonged periods on limited weight bearing, given the time it takes for allograft incorporation. Secondary procedures for nonunions, delayed unions, and infection can also complicate the rehabilitative course. Delayed fractures through nonvascularized allograft bone and late mechanical failures may require delayed revisions. Therefore, long-term clinical and radiologic surveillance of the allograft reconstruction is essential.

Allograft Prosthetic Composite Reconstruction

Allograft prosthetic composite (APC) is a combination of endoprosthetic with bulk allograft. This combination of reconstruction techniques has been shown in some instances to have better function than allograft reconstruction alone.[53,55] APCs are commonly used around joints where along with bone resection, there is soft tissue resection involving important stabilizers of the joint. Examples are the extensor mechanism in proximal tibia resection, rotator cuff in proximal humerus resection, and abductors in proximal femur resection. An example of an APC used in reconstruction after proximal tibia resection is seen in Figure 5.3. These reconstructions are also not without potential complications, including periprosthetic bone resorption, infection, and nonunion of the host–graft bone junction.[56,57]

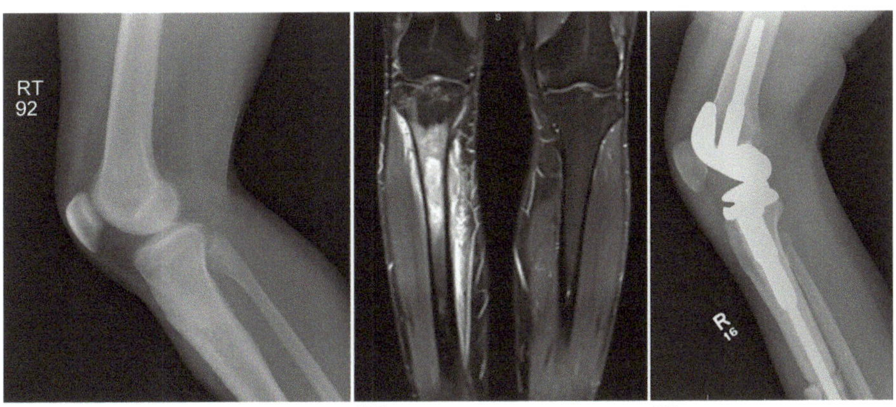

(A) (B) (C)

FIGURE 5.3 APC reconstruction of proximal tibia. Pre- and postoperative images of a 23-year-old male with right proximal tibia Ewing sarcoma. (A) Radiograph showing an ill-defined blastic-type lesion of the proximal tibia. (B) A T2-weighted MRI of the same patient where the lesion is better seen along with the soft tissue component. (C) A postoperative radiograph after APC reconstruction using a proximal tibia allograft with extensor mechanism.

APC, allograft prosthetic composite.

APCs share some of the advantages and the disadvantages of endoprosthetic and graft reconstruction. These constructs attempt to optimize the immediate structural integrity of the endoprosthesis with the biologic advantages of the allograft. Weight-bearing status will vary with the specific construct, and specific restrictions may be placed to protect soft tissue reconstructions. For example, patients undergoing a proximal tibia APC reconstruction require immobilization in extension to allow for healing of the extensor mechanism. Such immobilization may cause arthrofibrosis and/or muscle atrophy, which will ultimately prolong the rehabilitative course.

Autograft Reconstruction

Autograft is tissue removed from one area of the body and grafted into an area of previous resection in the same individual. Autografts can be obtained from iliac crest, tibia, rib, or fibula. These grafts can add structural support, while also bringing the potential for biologic healing. Autograft reconstructions can be used in isolation or in combination with structural allografts to improve immediate structural integrity. Fixation can be accomplished through a variety of techniques with variable degrees of immediate stability. Figure 5.4 shows the use of a vascularized fibula autograft to reconstruct a humeral diaphyseal defect after sarcoma resection. This graft has the ability to bring blood supply to the resection area and osteogenic cells, which allows for bone remodeling and healing, while offering structural support.[58] Autograft reconstruction can have additional complications regarding donor site morbidity, which is not seen in the other reconstruction techniques.

Time to complete healing of autograft reconstructions is variable, resulting in variable restrictions and lengths of rehabilitation. Furthermore, donor site morbidity may alter patient's postoperative course, with fibula being the frequent donor site choice.

Bone Transport

Primary bone sarcomas can involve any portion of the bone, but sarcomas involving the metaphysis and/or diaphysis may be amenable to bone transport to fill the defect after resection.[59] Bone transport, also termed distraction osteogenesis, involves guiding the growth of a desired bone through gradual distraction of osteotomy site. Over time, this allows new bone to fill the defect with living bone with sufficient strength.[60–62] Figure 5.5 shows bone transport after resection of a tibial adamantinoma. Distraction is performed at a rate of 1 mm/day[63] and can fill defects as large as 15 cm.[59] By transporting bone to fill the intercalary defect created by resection, the native joints can be preserved. After successful completion of bone transport, the reconstruction has biologic activity and can be expected to be permanent.[60–62] This can prevent some of the complications seen in endoprosthetic reconstruction, such as aseptic loosening and structural failure. No negative effects on distraction osteogenesis are seen with common chemotherapeutic regimens including methotrexate, doxorubicin, combination of bleomycin, cyclophosphamide, and dactinomycin, and caffeine-potentiated chemotherapy.[60,61,64–66] Bone transport can be performed using special intramedullary nails or external fixators.[59] Bone remodeling after

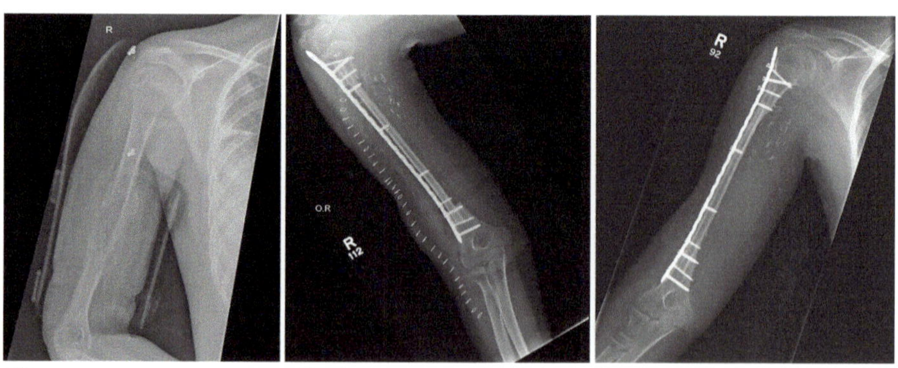

(A) (B) (C)

FIGURE 5.4 **Autograft reconstruction using vascularized fibular autograft of humeral shaft.** Preoperative, postoperative, and maturation images of a 14-year-old male with osteosarcoma of the right humerus. (A) A preoperative radiograph showing pathologic fracture of the midshaft humerus through an aggressive permeative and destructive lytic lesion. (B) Immediate postoperative radiograph after resection with reconstruction using vascularized free fibula autograph with plate fixation. (C) Radiograph taken 2 years postoperatively with complete healing of the graft at both the proximal and distal ends.

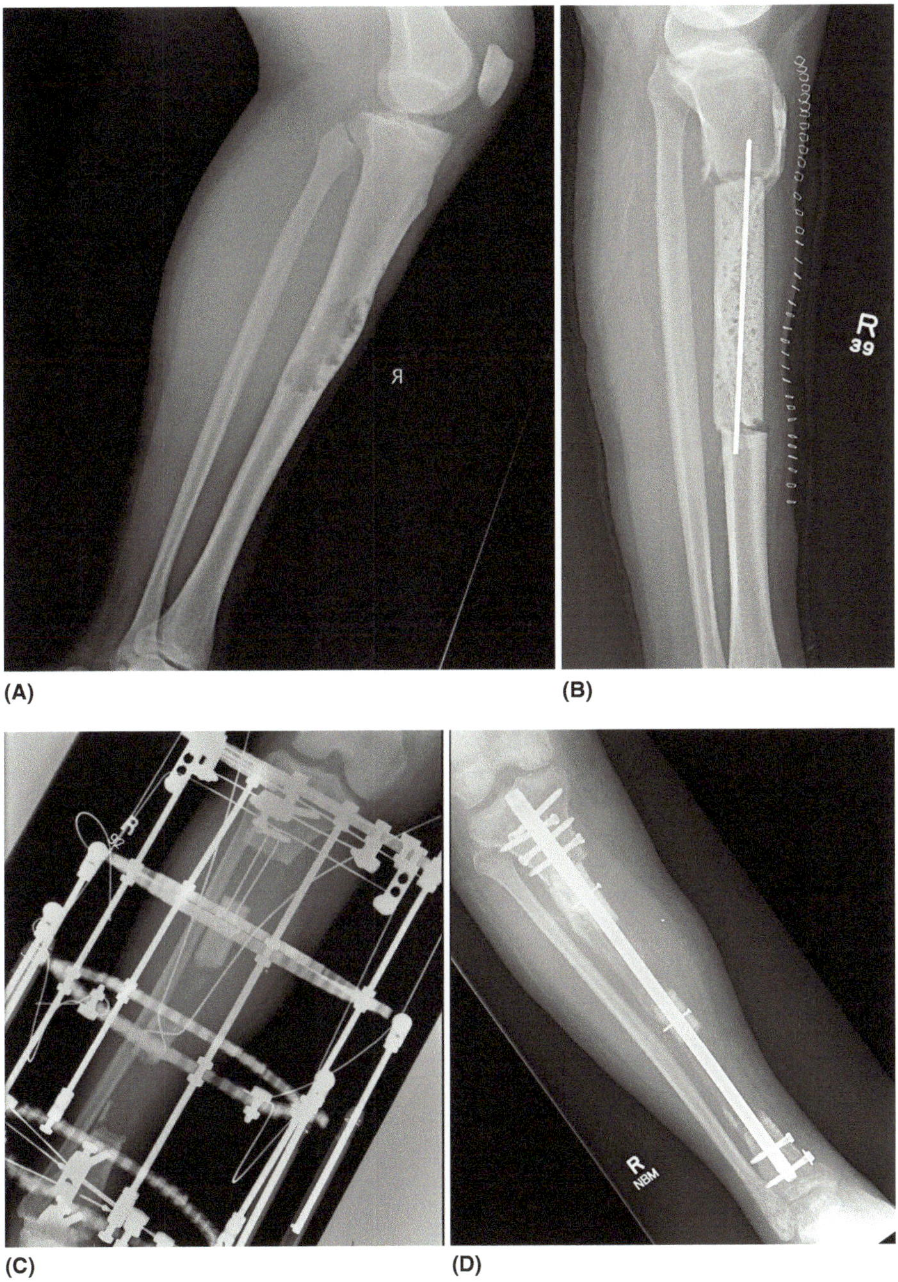

FIGURE 5.5 Bone transport after resection of tibial adamantinoma. Preoperative and postoperative images of a 27-year-old male undergoing bone transport after right tibia adamantinoma resection. (A) Radiograph of the right tibia with a mid-diaphyseal lytic lesion with endosteal scalloping. (B) Postoperative radiograph after intercalary resection of the adamantinoma of the right tibia with placement of temporary antibiotic cement spacer. (C) Radiograph taken during the transport phase. Bone transport is being performed with a ringed external fixator using cables. (D) Radiograph taken after completion of bone transport with removal of ringed external fixator and placement of intramedullary nail. The patient is currently in the consolidation phase as seen by the early mineralization of the new bone formation.

Source: Reproduced with permission from Stephen Quinnan, MD.

completion of bone transport is expected to be structurally sound at a mean of 14.4 months.[60,61] Like many other reconstruction techniques, complications have a high rate and include delayed ossification and maturation, nonunion at the docking site, deformity, and infections.[60,61,67,68]

The process of bone transport is labor-intensive in the postoperative period as the technique and rate of expansion are critical and require patient engagement and participation. Bone transport is more of a process than a single surgical intervention and requires a level of commitment from the patient and physician. Some of these devices are external and require specific care instructions. Weight bearing may be delayed until the desired reconstruction is achieved and will impact the therapy needs and duration.

Amputation

Although approximately 90% of patients undergo LSS, amputation remains a viable option. Amputation may be the only recommended oncologic surgery if limb salvage is not an option secondary to vital structure involvement, pathologic fracture, contamination from unplanned excision, or if significant limb function is threatened or lost.[69–73] Patients may also consider amputation if they wish to participate in specific athletic endeavors, which would be prohibited by concerns of structural integrity in many limb-salvage reconstruction surgeries. With appropriate prosthetic restoration, amputees can participate in physically intense activities including sports and running. Amputation is typically a definitive procedure and avoids some of the complications and revision surgeries needed in complex reconstructions.[74] Amputation can also be a palliative surgery in instances of tumor-related intractable pain, wound complications, and failure of limb-salvage procedure.[75] Multidisciplinary rehabilitation, both physical and emotional, can improve function in patients who have undergone amputation for sarcoma.[76,77] In the modern era of limb-salvage surgery, patients who had undergone primary amputation have been found to have worse survival rates.[72,78] It has been established in the literature that it is likely based on the biology of the tumor requiring amputation, as the local recurrence rates remain lower.[79]

New surgical techniques have been developed for improving the function of prosthetic wear and fit. Specialized centers are investigating the osseointegrated prosthesis in which an intraosseous stem exits transcutaneously, allowing for mechanical connection of the prosthesis to the residual limb.[80,81] Although the intraosseous metallic prosthesis exits the skin, one center has found the risk of osteitis and osteomylelitis is low in patients with amputations secondary to trauma or tumor.[82] Problematic complications in amputees, such as phantom limb pain, painful neuromas, pressure sores, and inability to tolerate a prosthesis, can complicate rehabilitation and function. Prosthesis modifications are frequently required, and revision amputation may be recommended for highly symptomatic patients.

Rotationplasty

Rotationplasty is a reconstructive, limb-sparing technique that is used as an alternative to above-knee amputation. Rotationplasty involves an intercalary resection, traditionally of the knee joint, while preserving the neurovascular bundle. This is followed by 180-degree rotation of the distal limb, allowing the ankle to function as the knee joint. This does require a modified below-knee prosthesis.[72] The preservation of the ankle joint, functioning as the new knee joint, decreases the amount of energy expenditure with ambulation as compared to traditional above-knee amputation.[83] Functional outcome scores of rotationplasty, as measured by the Musculoskeletal Tumor Society Score (MSTS Score) and the functional Motor Assessment Scale, are superior as compared to above-knee amputation.[84] Two authors have found superior MSTS scores with rotationplasty as compared to amputations or endoprosthesis reconstruction in a total of 27 patients.[85,86] Advantages of rotationplasty, as compared to endoprosthetics, include decreased need for revision surgery due to loosening or failure of the endoprosthesis reconstruction.[58] The primary drawback of rotationplasty is appearance of the limb and patient acceptance. Forni et al. did show that patients had relational and emotional difficulties in adolescence, but that these were overcome in adulthood. They also stressed the importance of a cosmetic and functional prosthesis with family support.[87]

Patient adaptation to this unusual surgical procedure requires extensive rehabilitation in addition to psychological and emotional adaptations. Many individuals find the physical appearance after rotationplasty unacceptable, and it may be considered an unacceptable surgical option for this reason alone. These concerns need to be balanced with the potential functional benefits of this surgery for each patient.

SUMMARY

Orthopedic oncologic surgical procedures in the treatment of bone sarcoma are variable and include amputations and limb-salvage surgery with complex reconstructive needs. Optimizing oncologic resection and limb reconstruction requires complex surgical planning and is impacted by a multitude of patient- and tumor-related factors. One such critical factor is the execution of a well-performed biopsy, as a poorly executed biopsy can impact surgical and oncologic outcomes. The goals of surgery are straightforward—prioritizing complete tumor excision and optimizing patient function. However, application of these surgical principles is complex and optimized by a highly specialized orthopedic surgeon and a comprehensive multidisciplinary sarcoma team. The essential information required to make a surgical recommendation comes from a variety of sources, but begins with the initial patient encounter. Patient involvement in this decision should begin early and should guide the establishment of oncologic and functional goals. An understanding of the advantages and drawbacks of the reconstructive options will facilitate the healthcare providers' ability to counsel patients effectively and establish realistic lifetime expectations. Furthermore, anticipating postoperative rehabilitative needs, physical limitations, and potential complications will enhance the provider's ability to provide comprehensive patient-centric care.

REFERENCES

1. Scully SP, Ghert MA, Zurakowski D, et al. Pathologic fracture in osteosarcoma: prognostic importance and treatment implications. *J Bone Joint Surg Am.* 2002;84(1):49–57. doi:10.2106/00004623-200201000-00008
2. Stacy GS, Mahal RS, Peabody TD. Staging of bone tumors: a review with illustrative examples. *AJR Am J Roentgenol.* 2006;186(4):967–976. doi:10.2214/AJR.05.0654
3. Gemescu IN, Thierfelder KM, Rehnitz C, Weber MA. Imaging features of bone tumors: conventional radiographs and MR imaging correlation. *Magn Reson Imaging Clin North Am.* 2019;27(4):753–767. doi:10.1016/j.mric.2019.07.008
4. Putta T, Gibikote S, Madhuri V, Walter N. Accuracy of various MRI sequences in determining the tumour margin in musculoskeletal tumours. *Pol J Radiol.* 2016;81:540–548. doi:10.12659/PJR.898108
5. Jaffe HL. Problems of classification and diagnosis. In: Jaffe HL, ed. *Tumors and Tumorous Conditions of Bone and Joints.* Philadelphia, PA: Lea & Febiger; 1958:9–17.
6. Mankin HJ, Mankin CJ, Simon MA. The hazards of the biopsy, revisited. Members of the Musculoskeletal Tumor Society. *J Bone Joint Surg Am.* 1996;78(5):656–663. doi:10.2106/00004623-199605000-00004
7. Mesko NW, Wilson RJ, Lawrenz JM, et al. Pre-operative evaluation prior to soft tissue sarcoma excision—why can't we get it right? *Eur J Surg Oncol.* 2018;44(2):243–250. doi:10.1016/j.ejso.2017.11.001
8. Traina F, Errani C, Toscano A, et al. Current concepts in the biopsy of musculoskeletal tumors. *J Bone Joint Surg Am.* 2015;97(1):e7. doi:10.2106/JBJS.N.00661
9. Mulder AH, Wardeh G, Hogenboom F, Frankhuyzen AL. Selectivity of various opioid peptides towards delta-, kappa; and mu-opioid receptors mediating presynaptic inhibition of neurotransmitter release in the brain. *Neuropeptides.* 1989;14(2):99–104. doi:10.1016/0143-4179(89)90065-6
10. Pretell-Mazzini J, Barton MD Jr, Conway SA, Temple HT. Unplanned excision of soft-tissue sarcomas: current concepts for management and prognosis. *J Bone Joint Surg Am.* 2015;97(7):597–603. doi:10.2106/JBJS.N.00649
11. Bickels J, Jelinek JS, Shmookler BM, Malawer MM. Biopsy of musculoskeletal tumors. In: Malawer MM, Sugarbaker PH, eds. *Musculoskeletal Cancer Surgery: Treatment of Sarcomas and Allied Diseases.* Dordrecht, The Netherlands: Springer; 2001:37–45.
12. Chang AE, Sondak VK. Clinical evaluation and treatment of soft tissue tumors. In: Enzinger FM, Weiss SW, eds. *Soft Tissue Tumors.* St Louis, MO: Mosby; 1995:17–38.
13. Enneking WF. General principles of musculoskeletal tumor surgery. In: Enneking WF, ed. *Musculoskeletal Tumor Surgery.* New York, NY: Churchill-Livingstone; 1983:3–27.
14. Dorfman HD, Czerniak B. General considerations. In: Dorfman HD, Czerniak B, eds. *Bone Tumors.* St. Louis, MO: Mosby; 1988:1–33.
15. Clark CR, Morgan C, Sonstegard DA, Matthews LS. The effect of biopsy-hole shape and size on bone strength. *J Bone Joint Surg Am.* 1977;59(2):213–217. doi:10.2106/00004623-197759020-00014
16. Bickels J, Jelinek JS, Shmookler BM, et al. Biopsy of musculoskeletal tumors. Current concepts. *Clin Orthop Relat Res.* 1999(368):212–219. doi:10.1097/00003086-199911000-00026
17. Mankin HJ, Lange TA, Spanier SS. The hazards of biopsy in patients with malignant primary bone and soft-tissue tumors. *J Bone Joint Surg Am.* 1982;64(8):1121–1127. doi:10.2106/00004623-198264080-00002
18. Liu PT, Valadez SD, Chivers FS, et al. Anatomically based guidelines for core needle biopsy of bone tumors: implications for limb-sparing surgery. *Radiographics.* 2007;27(1):189–205; discussion 206. doi:10.1148/rg.271065092
19. Issakov J, Flusser G, Kollender Y, et al. Computed tomography-guided core needle biopsy for bone and soft tissue tumors. *Isr Med Assoc J.* 2003;5(1):28–30.
20. Adams SC, Potter BK, Pitcher DJ, Temple HT. Office-based core needle biopsy of bone and soft tissue malignancies: an accurate alternative to open biopsy with infrequent complications. *Clin Orthop Relat Res.* 2010;468(10):2774–2780. doi:10.1007/s11999-010-1422-5
21. Gilbert NF, Cannon CP, Lin PP, Lewis VO. Soft-tissue sarcoma. *J Am Acad Orthop Surg.* 2009;17(1):40–47. doi:10.5435/00124635-200901000-00006
22. Seeger LL. Revisiting tract seeding and compartmental anatomy for percutaneous image-guided musculoskeletal biopsies. *Skeletal Radiol.* 2019;48(4):499–501. doi:10.1007/s00256-018-3127-x
23. Binitie O, Tejiram S, Conway S, et al. Adult soft tissue sarcoma local recurrence after adjuvant treatment without resection of core needle biopsy tract. *Clin Orthop Relat Res.* 2013;471(3):891–898. doi:10.1007/s11999-012-2569-z

24. He F, Zhang W, Shen Y, et al. Effects of resection margins on local recurrence of osteosarcoma in extremity and pelvis: systematic review and meta-analysis. *Int J Surg*. 2016;36(Pt A):283–292. doi:10.1016/j.ijsu.2016.11.016
25. Bacci G, Ferrari S, Mercuri M, et al. Predictive factors for local recurrence in osteosarcoma: 540 patients with extremity tumors followed for minimum 2.5 years after neoadjuvant chemotherapy. *Acta Orthop Scand*. 1998;69(3):230–236. doi:10.3109/17453679809000921
26. Picci P, Sangiorgi L, Rougraff BT, et al. Relationship of chemotherapy-induced necrosis and surgical margins to local recurrence in osteosarcoma. *J Clin Oncol*. 1994;12(12):2699–2705. doi:10.1200/JCO.1994.12.12.2699
27. Durr HR, Bakhshai Y, Rechl H, Tunn PU. Resection margins in bone tumors: what is adequate? *Unfallchirurg*. 2014;117(7):593–599. doi:10.1007/s00113-013-2475-1
28. Tsuda Y, Evans S, Stevenson JD, et al. Is the width of a surgical margin associated with the outcome of disease in patients with peripheral chondrosarcoma of the pelvis? A multicenter study. *Clin Orthop Relat Res*. 2019;477(11):2432–2440. doi:10.1097/CORR.0000000000000926
29. Dhammi IK, Kumar S. Osteosarcoma: a journey from amputation to limb salvage. *Indian J Orthop*. 2014;48(3): 233–234. doi:10.4103/0019-5413.132486
30. DiCaprio MR, Friedlaender GE. Malignant bone tumors: limb sparing versus amputation. *J Am Acad Orthop Surg*. 2003;11(1):25–37. doi:10.5435/00124635-200301000-00005
31. Yang Y, Han L, He Z, et al. Advances in limb salvage treatment of osteosarcoma. *J Bone Oncol*. 2018;10:36–40. doi:10.1016/j.jbo.2017.11.005
32. Chauhan A, Joshi GR, Chopra BK, et al. Limb salvage surgery in bone tumors: a retrospective study of 50 cases in a single center. *Indian J Surg Oncol*. 2013;4(3):248–254. doi:10.1007/s13193-013-0229-8
33. Biermann JS, Adkins DR, Agulnik M, et al. Bone cancer. *J Natl Compr Cancer Netw*. 2013;11(6):688–723. doi:10.6004/jnccn.2013.0088
34. Caracciolo JT, Letson GD. Radiologic approach to bone and soft tissue sarcomas. *Surg Clin North Am*. 2016;96(5):963–976. doi:10.1016/j.suc.2016.05.007
35. Bertrand TE, Cruz A, Binitie O, et al. Do surgical margins affect local recurrence and survival in extremity, nonmetastatic, high-grade osteosarcoma? *Clin Orthop Relat Res*. 2016;474(3):677–683. doi:10.1007/s11999-015-4359-x
36. Li X, Moretti VM, Ashana AO, Lackman RD. Impact of close surgical margin on local recurrence and survival in osteosarcoma. *Int Orthop*. 2012;36(1):131–137. doi:10.1007/s00264-011-1230-x
37. Bispo Junior RZ, Camargo OP. Prognostic factors in the survival of patients diagnosed with primary non-metastatic osteosarcoma with a poor response to neoadjuvant chemotherapy. *Clinics (Sao Paulo)*. 2009;64(12):1177–1186. doi:10.1590/S1807-59322009001200007
38. Henderson ER, Groundland JS, Pala E, et al. Failure mode classification for tumor endoprostheses: retrospective review of five institutions and a literature review. *J Bone Joint Surg Am*. 2011;93(5):418–429. doi:10.2106/JBJS.J.00834
39. Taylor SJ, Walker PS, Perry JS, et al. The forces in the distal femur and the knee during walking and other activities measured by telemetry. *J Arthroplasty*. 1998;13(4):428–437. doi:10.1016/S0883-5403(98)90009-2
40. Berbari EF, Hanssen AD, Duffy MC, et al. Risk factors for prosthetic joint infection: case-control study. *Clin Infect Dis*. 1998;27(5):1247–1254. doi:10.1086/514991
41. Hanssen AD, Rand JA. Evaluation and treatment of infection at the site of a total hip or knee arthroplasty. *Instr Course Lect*. 1999;48:111–122. PMID:10098033.
42. McDonald DJ, Capanna R, Gherlinzoni F, et al. Influence of chemotherapy on perioperative complications in limb salvage surgery for bone tumors. *Cancer*. 1990;65(7):1509–1516. doi:10.1002/1097-0142(19900401)65:7<1509::AID-CNCR2820650710>3.0.CO;2-I
43. Maradit Kremers H, Larson DR, Crowson CS, et al. Prevalence of total hip and knee replacement in the United States. *J Bone Joint Surg Am*. 2015;97(17):1386–1397. doi:10.2106/JBJS.N.01141
44. Smolle MA, Andreou D, Tunn PU, Leithner A. Advances in tumour endoprostheses: a systematic review. *EFORT Open Rev*. 2019;4(7):445–459. doi:10.1302/2058-5241.4.180081
45. Angelini A, Trovarelli G, Berizzi A, et al. Three-dimension-printed custom-made prosthetic reconstructions: from revision surgery to oncologic reconstructions. *Int Orthop*. 2019;43(1):123–132. doi:10.1007/s00264-018-4232-0
46. Liu X, Liu Y, Lu W, et al. Combined application of modified three-dimensional printed anatomic templates and customized cutting blocks in pelvic reconstruction after pelvic tumor resection. *J Arthroplasty*. 2019;34(2):338–345.e331. doi:10.1016/j.arth.2018.10.001
47. Liang H, Ji T, Zhang Y, et al. Reconstruction with 3D-printed pelvic endoprostheses after resection of a pelvic tumour. *Bone Joint J*. 2017;99-B(2):267–275. doi:10.1302/0301-620X.99B2.BJJ-2016-0654.R1
48. Wang B, Hao Y, Pu F, et al. Computer-aided designed, three dimensional-printed hemipelvic prosthesis for peri-acetabular malignant bone tumour. *Int Orthop*. 2018;42(3):687–694. doi:10.1007/s00264-017-3645-5
49. Henderson ER, Pepper AM, Marulanda G, et al. Outcome of lower-limb preservation with an expandable endoprosthesis after bone tumor resection in children. *J Bone Joint Surg Am*. 2012;94(6):537–547. doi:10.2106/JBJS.I.01575
50. Neel MD, Wilkins RM, Rao BN, Kelly CM. Early multicenter experience with a noninvasive expandable prosthesis. *Clin Orthop Relat Res*. 2003;415:72–81. doi:10.1097/01.blo.0000093899.12372.25
51. Kenan S, Bloom N, Lewis MM. Limb-sparing surgery in skeletally immature patients with osteosarcoma. The use of an expandable prosthesis. *Clin Orthop Relat Res*. 1991;270:223–230. doi:10.1097/00003086-199109000-00029

52. Gilg MM, Gaston CL, Parry MC, et al. What is the morbidity of a non-invasive growing prosthesis? *Bone Joint J*. 2016;98-B(12):1697–1703. doi:10.1302/0301-620X.98B12.BJJ-2016-0467
53. Fritz J, Fishman EK, Corl F, et al. Imaging of limb salvage surgery. *AJR Am J Roentgenol*. 2012;198(3):647–660. doi:10.2214/AJR.11.7286
54. Ayerza MA, Piuzzi NS, Aponte-Tinao LA, et al. Structural allograft reconstruction of the foot and ankle after tumor resections. *Musculoskelet Surg*. 2016;100(2):149–156. doi:10.1007/s12306-016-0413-4
55. Gilbert NF, Yasko AW, Oates SD, et al. Allograft-prosthetic composite reconstruction of the proximal part of the tibia. An analysis of the early results. *J Bone Joint Surg Am*. 2009;91(7):1646–1656. doi:10.2106/JBJS.G.01542
56. Gautam D, Malhotra R. Megaprosthesis versus allograft prosthesis composite for massive skeletal defects. *J Clin Orthop Trauma*. 2018;9(1):63–80. doi:10.1016/j.jcot.2017.09.010
57. Unwin PS, Cannon SR, Grimer RJ, et al. Aseptic loosening in cemented custom-made prosthetic replacements for bone tumours of the lower limb. *J Bone Joint Surg Br*. 1996;78(1):5–13. doi:10.1302/0301-620X.78B1.0780005
58. Levin AS, Arkader A, Morris CD. Reconstruction following tumor resections in skeletally immature patients. *J Am Acad Orthop Surg*. 2017;25(3):204–213. doi:10.5435/JAAOS-D-15-00619
59. Panagopoulos GN, Mavrogenis AF, Mauffrey C, et al. Intercalary reconstructions after bone tumor resections: a review of treatments. *Eur J Orthop Surg Traumatol*. 2017;27(6):737–746. doi:10.1007/s00590-017-1985-x
60. Tsuchiya H, Tomita K, Minematsu K, et al. Limb salvage using distraction osteogenesis. A classification of the technique. *J Bone Joint Surg Br*. 1997;79(3):403–411. doi:10.1302/0301-620X.79B3.0790403
61. Tsuchiya H, Abdel-Wanis ME, Sakurakichi K, et al. Osteosarcoma around the knee. Intraepiphyseal excision and biological reconstruction with distraction osteogenesis. *J Bone Joint Surg Br*. 2002;84(8):1162–1166. doi:10.1302/0301-620X.84B8.0841162
62. Tsuchiya H, Tomita K, Shinokawa Y, et al. The Ilizarov method in the management of giant-cell tumours of the proximal tibia. *J Bone Joint Surg Br*. 1996;78(2):264–269. doi:10.1302/0301-620X.78B2.0780264
63. Ilizarov GA. Clinical application of the tension-stress effect for limb lengthening. *Clin Orthop Relat Res*. 1990;250:8–26. doi:10.1097/00003086-199001000-00003
64. Jarka DE, Nicholas RW, Aronson J. Effect of methotrexate on distraction osteogenesis. *Clin Orthop Relat Res*. 1998;354:209–215. doi:10.1097/00003086-199809000-00025
65. Subasi M, Kapukaya A, Kesemenli C, et al. Effect of chemotherapeutic agents on distraction osteogenesis. An experimental investigation in rabbits. *Arch Orthop Trauma Surg*. 2001;121(7):417–421. doi:10.1007/s004020000241
66. Minematsu K, Tsuchiya H, Taki J, Tomita K. Blood flow measurement during distraction osteogenesis. *Clin Orthop Relat Res*. 1998;347:229–235. doi:10.1097/00003086-199802000-00028
67. Ozaki T, Nakatsuka Y, Kunisada T, et al. High complication rate of reconstruction using Ilizarov bone transport method in patients with bone sarcomas. *Arch Orthop Trauma Surg*. 1998;118(3):136–139. doi:10.1007/s004020050333
68. Kapukaya A, Subasi M, Kandiya E, et al. Limb reconstruction with the callus distraction method after bone tumor resection. *Arch Orthop Trauma Surg*. 2000;120(3–4):215–218. doi:10.1007/s004020050048
69. Clark MA, Thomas JM. Amputation for soft-tissue sarcoma. *Lancet Oncol*. 2003;4(6):335–342. doi:10.1016/S1470-2045(03)01113-6
70. Ferrone ML, Raut CP. Modern surgical therapy: limb salvage and the role of amputation for extremity soft-tissue sarcomas. *Surg Oncol Clin North Am*. 2012;21(2):201–213. doi:10.1016/j.soc.2011.11.001
71. Puhaindran ME, Chou J, Forsberg JA, Athanasian EA. Major upper-limb amputations for malignant tumors. *J Hand Surg Am*. 2012;37(6):1235–1241. doi:10.1016/j.jhsa.2012.02.004
72. Ghert MA, Abudu A, Driver N, et al. The indications for and the prognostic significance of amputation as the primary surgical procedure for localized soft tissue sarcoma of the extremity. *Ann Surg Oncol*. 2005;12(1):10–17. doi:10.1007/s10434-004-1171-3
73. Ferguson PC. Surgical considerations for management of distal extremity soft tissue sarcomas. *Curr Opin Oncol*. 2005;17(4):366–369. doi:10.1097/01.cco.0000166651.38417.c8
74. Smith SR. Rehabilitation strategies and outcomes of the sarcoma patient. *Phys Med Rehabil Clin North Am*. 2017;28(1):171–180. doi:10.1016/j.pmr.2016.08.008
75. Parsons CM, Pimiento JM, Cheong D, et al. The role of radical amputations for extremity tumors: a single institution experience and review of the literature. *J Surg Oncol*. 2012;105(2):149–155. doi:10.1002/jso.22067
76. Kauzlaric N, Kauzlaric KS, Kolundzic R. Prosthetic rehabilitation of persons with lower limb amputations due to tumour. *Eur J Cancer Care (Engl)*. 2007;16(3):238–243. doi:10.1111/j.1365-2354.2006.00727.x
77. Punzalan M, Hyden G. The role of physical therapy and occupational therapy in the rehabilitation of pediatric and adolescent patients with osteosarcoma. *Cancer Treat Res*. 2009;152:367–384. doi:10.1007/978-1-4419-0284-9_20
78. Williard WC, Hajdu SI, Casper ES, Brennan MF. Comparison of amputation with limb-sparing operations for adult soft tissue sarcoma of the extremity. *Ann Surg*. 1992;215(3):269–275. doi:10.1097/00000658-199203000-00012
79. Erstad DJ, Ready J, Abraham J, et al. Amputation for extremity sarcoma: contemporary indications and outcomes. *Ann Surg Oncol*. 2018;25(2):394–403. doi:10.1245/s10434-017-6240-5
80. Aschoff HH. Transcutaneous osseointegration after limb amputation: a review over 27 years. *Unfallchirurg*. 2017;120(4):278–284. doi:10.1007/s00113-017-0329-y
81. Thomson S, Lu W, Zreiqat H, et al. Proximal bone remodeling in lower limb amputees reconstructed with an osseointegrated prosthesis. *J Orthop Res*. 2019;37(12):2524–2530. doi:10.1002/jor.24445

82. Frolke JP, Leijendekkers RA, van de Meent H. Osseointegrated prosthesis for patients with an amputation: multidisciplinary team approach in the Netherlands. *Unfallchirurg*. 2017;120(4):293–299. doi:10.1007/s00113-016-0302-1
83. van der Windt DA, Pieterson I, van der Eijken JW, et al. Energy expenditure during walking in subjects with tibial rotationplasty, above-knee amputation, or hip disarticulation. *Arch Phys Med Rehabil*. 1992;73(12):1174–1180.
84. Ginsberg JP, Rai SN, Carlson CA, et al. A comparative analysis of functional outcomes in adolescents and young adults with lower-extremity bone sarcoma. *Pediatr Blood Cancer*. 2007;49(7):964–969. doi:10.1002/pbc.21018
85. Akahane T, Shimizu T, Isobe K, et al. Evaluation of postoperative general quality of life for patients with osteosarcoma around the knee joint. *J Pediatr Orthop B*. 2007;16(4):269–272. doi:10.1097/BPB.0b013e3280925670
86. Lindner NJ, Ramm O, Hillmann A, et al. Limb salvage and outcome of osteosarcoma. The University of Muenster experience. *Clin Orthop Relat Res*. 1999(358):83–89. doi:10.1097/00003086-199901000-00011
87. Forni C, Gaudenzi N, Zoli M, et al. Living with rotationplasty—quality of life in rotationplasty patients from childhood to adulthood. *J Surg Oncol*. 2012;105(4):331–336. doi:10.1002/jso.22088

6

Pediatric Oncology

Sara E. Helmig and Alberto Pappo

INTRODUCTION

Pediatric sarcomas are a heterogeneous group of diseases that can arise in bone or soft tissue and account for approximately 12% of all cancers in patients younger than 20 years of age (see Figure 6.1).[1] New insight into the biology of these tumors has led to the development of more precise risk-based classifications that directly impact treatment. The two most common pediatric bone sarcomas are osteosarcoma (OS) and Ewing sarcoma (EWS). OS accounts for about 3% of all childhood cancers, whereas EWS accounts for only about 2% of all cases. Clinical outcomes for these two sarcomas have dramatically improved over time, with the survival rates exceeding 70% for those with localized disease. Pediatric soft tissue sarcomas include two main types: rhabdomyosarcoma (RMS), which accounts for about 40% of all cases of soft tissue sarcomas in children, and the so-called non-rhabdomyosarcomatous soft tissue sarcomas (NRSTSs), which encompass many different histologic types including synovial sarcoma, malignant peripheral nerve sheath tumor, and fibrosarcoma. This chapter describes the salient clinical and biologic features of these tumors and summarizes the current diagnostic and treatment strategies for these pediatric sarcomas.

EWING SARCOMA

This tumor can arise in the bone and soft tissue and was previously called peripheral primitive neuroectodermal tumor, Askin's tumor (EWS of the chest wall), and extraosseous EWS. However, all of these terms reflect the same tumor entity, which is characterized by recurrent translocations that most commonly involve the *ERWSR1* gene (Table 6.1).[2] Current 5-year overall survival rate for patients with localized disease at diagnosis ranges from 65% to 75%, whereas patients with metastatic disease at diagnosis have survival rates of <30%.[3]

Epidemiology

EWS is the second most common tumor in children and adolescents with approximately 200 cases diagnosed annually in the United States and an annual incidence of approximately one case per million each year.[4,5] This tumor more commonly affects male Caucasian adolescents and young adults with a median age at presentation of 15 years and shows male predominance compared to females, with a ratio of 1.5:1.[6] Caucasians have a ninefold increased incidence of disease compared to Africans.[5] The differences in racial distribution among those with African heritage have been attributed in part to the presence of fewer Alu elements in intron 6 near the *EWSR1* breakpoint, theoretically decreasing the sites for gene recombination.[7] Another group of investigators found two small-nucleotide polymorphisms (SNPs) associated with EWS on chromosomes 1 and 10 (*TARDBP* and *EGR2*, respectively), which are less prevalent in Africans, suggesting that they may contribute to the differences in incidence in the latter population.[8] A third observation that may account for differences in the incidence if EWS in Caucasian and African populations involves greater diversity in GGAA motifs at certain microsatellite loci in African populations, which may negatively impact the expression of *EWS–FLI*.[9]

Molecular Pathology

EWS is characterized by a *EWS–ETS* fusion (Table 6.1), which in part functions as a rogue transcription factor that drives oncogenesis through deregulation of gene expression.[10] *EWS* can bind multiple

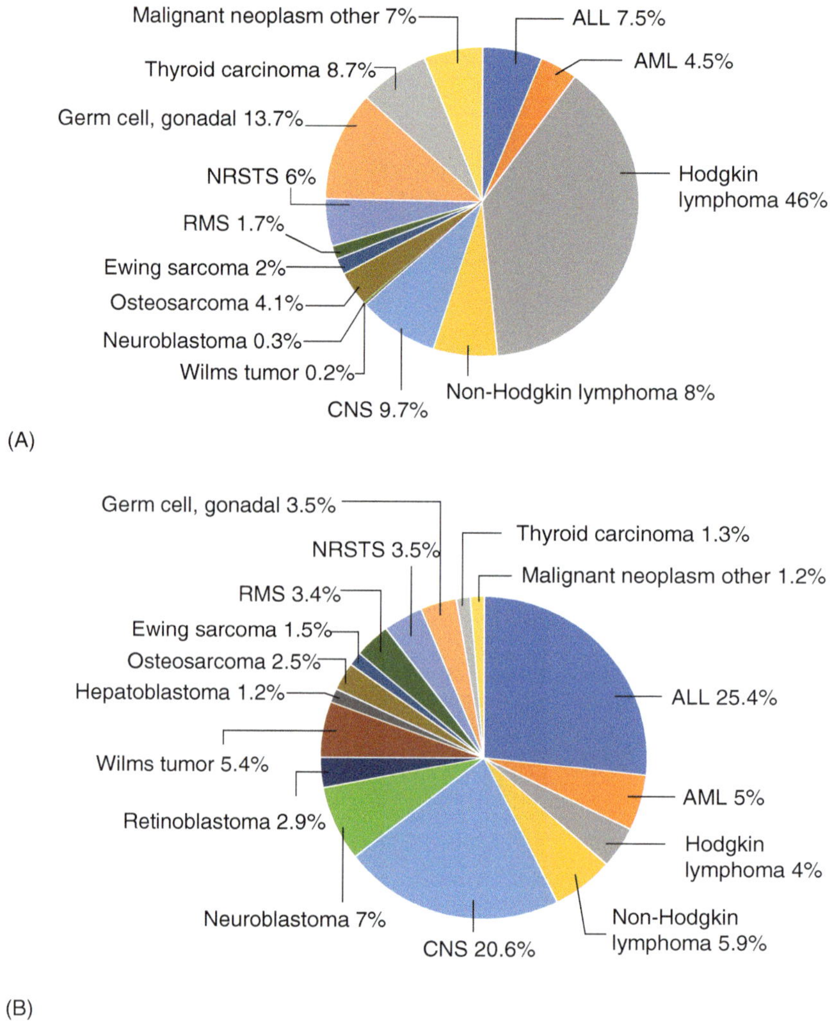

FIGURE 6.1 Percent incidence by age and type of pediatric cancer. (A) Cancer by type for patients 15–19 years of age. (B) Cancer by type for patients <15 years of age.

ALL, acute lymphocytic leukemia; AML, acute myeloid leukemia; CNS, central nervous system; NRSTS, non-rhabdomyosarcomatous soft tissue sarcomas; RMS, rhabdomyosarcoma.

Source: Adapted from Howlader N, Noone AM, Krapcho M, et al, eds. *SEER Cancer Statistics Review, 1975-2010.* Bethesda, MD: National Cancer Institute. https://seer.cancer.gov/archive/csr/1975_2010.

TABLE 6.1 Translocations in ESFT Across All Age Groups

Translocation	Fusion Gene	Percent Positive
t(11;22)(q24;q12)	*EWS–FLI1*	>85
t(21;22)(q22;q12)	*EWS–ERG*	5–10
t(19;der)inv(21;22)	*EWS–ERG*	<1
t(7;22)(p22;q12)	*EWS–ETV1*	<1
t(17;22)(q12;q12)	*EWS–ETV4*	<1
t(2;22)(q33;q12)	*EWS–FEV*	<1
t(16;21)(p11;q22)	*FUS–ERG*	<1
t(2;16)(q35;p11)	*FUS–FEV*	<1

ESFT, Ewing sarcoma family of tumors.
Source: Adapted from Pinto A, Dickman P, Parham D. Pathobiologic markers of the Ewing sarcoma family of tumors: state of the art and prediction of behaviour. *Sarcoma*. 2011;2011:856190. doi:10.1155/2011/856190.

members of the ETS family of transcription factors listed in Table 6.1, all of which are associated with EWS.[2] Sequencing studies have demonstrated that EWS has a low mutational burden. The most commonly mutated gene seen in about 17% of cases is *STAG2;* other less frequently mutated genes include *TP53, EZH2, BCOR,* and *ZMYM*.[11] Homozygous *CDKN2A* deletions are seen in about 13% of the cases,[12] and the presence of *STAG2* and *TP53* mutations has been associated with poor clinical outcomes.[11] Similarly, another group of investigators have found that *TP53* and *16/p14ARF* mutations are associated with poor response to therapy.[13] While EWS is not one of the more common pediatric cancers historically seen in familial cancer syndromes, it has recently been reported that about 10% of patients with EWS have germline mutations in a cancer predisposition gene such as *TP53, RET,* and *PMS2*.[14]

Clinical Presentation

Patients usually present with a palpable mass and pain that can be of several months' duration. In one study, the median time to diagnosis was 70 days, and longer time to diagnosis was more commonly seen in older patients with tumors in the pelvis and extremities; however, the interval to diagnosis did not influence survival.[15] Systemic symptoms, such as fever, were more commonly seen in EWS, when compared to the most common bone tumor in this age group, OS. A German retrospective study found that patients younger than 9 years of age usually presented with less metastatic disease (23.8% compared to 32.3%, $p = .009$) and sites of the primary tumor differed with a decreased incidence of pelvic primary tumors in this younger cohort.[16] Overall, in this German cohort across ages, lungs were the most common site of metastatic disease (ranging from 56.4% to 74.6%) and extrapulmonary metastases increased with age for both bony and soft tissue metastases. Older patients have an increased incidence of extraskeletal EWS, with the average age at presentation being 19.5 years. The extraskeletal location most commonly occurs in females (63.3% of extraskeletal EWS patients and 53.4% of skeletal EWS patients are females) and non-whites.[17]

Diagnosis and Imaging

Initial evaluation should include a complete history with physical exam and laboratory evaluation including a complete blood count (CBC) with differential, blood chemistry tests, and lactate dehydrogenase (LDH). On plain film, EWS of the bone may have a permeative appearance and laminated periosteal reaction of the bone that is commonly referred to as onion skin appearance. The tumor may cause the periosteum to separate from the bone (Codman triangle[18]; see Figure 6.2). EWS and OS may have similar appearances on plain films, and many times, location is the hint to the diagnosis, with EWS primary tumors more commonly found in the diaphysis of long bones compared to the metaphysis in OS. Additional imaging should include an MRI of the primary site including the whole extremity when indicated. The biopsy should involve the surgeon who will be performing surgery when definitive local control is needed. For patients having closed biopsies, several core biopsies may be required for obtaining adequate tissue for pathologic diagnosis.[19]

Following confirmation of diagnosis, a thorough staging assessment is required prior to starting therapy. Traditionally, this involves evaluation of common metastatic sites for EWS, including the chest, bone marrow, and other bony sites. A chest CT is required to assess pulmonary disease and bone scintigraphy to detect bony metastases; however, some centers have opted to use fluorodeoxyglucose (FDG)-PET scan to evaluate bony and soft tissue metastases. The latter modality is preferred at many centers because it may offer improved specificity for identifying bony metastases in EWS when compared to bone scintigraphy.[20] Finally, bilateral bone marrow aspirates and biopsies should always be performed to exclude disease in the bone marrow. It is expected that these additional diagnostic procedures will identify patients with metastases in about 20% to 25% of the cases.[19]

TREATMENT

EWS is treated with a multimodal approach that uses chemotherapy and local control with surgery, radiation therapy (RT), or both. Prior to the introduction of chemotherapy, only 10% of patients with EWS survived. In fact, in the first Intergroup Ewing Sarcoma Study (IESS-I), one of the randomized arms included chemotherapy versus observation following surgery, but this randomization was quickly discontinued when two of three patients who were randomized to no chemotherapy relapsed.[21] With the use of combined modality therapy, over 75% of patients with localized disease are expected to survive; however, patients who present with metastatic disease continue to have poor

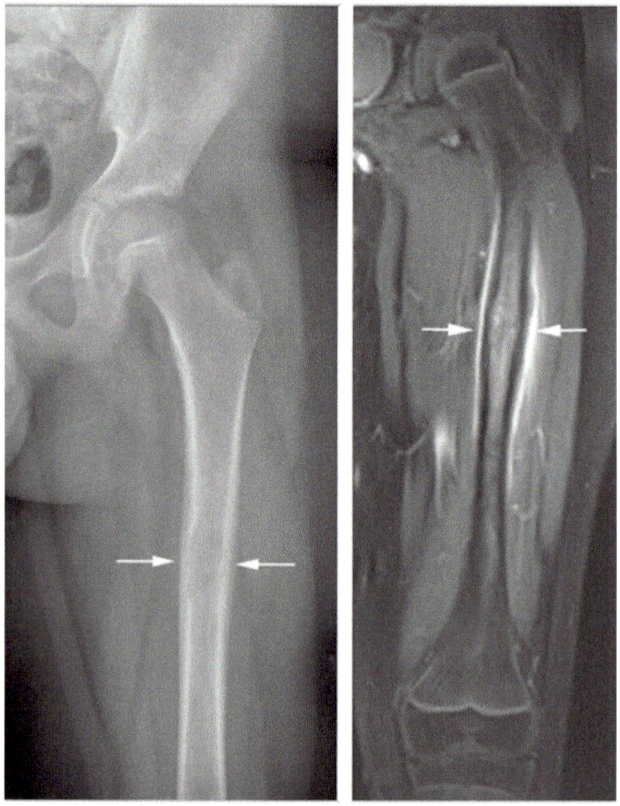

(A) (B)

FIGURE 6.2 An 11-year-old boy with Ewing sarcoma. (A) Anterior–posterior x-ray study showing smooth periosteal reaction and subtle permeative lucency in the femoral diaphysis (arrows). (B) Post-contrast T1-weighted coronal MRI showing permeative lesion in the diaphysis with smooth surrounding periosteal reaction (arrows).

outcomes with <30% expected to survive long term.[19,22,23] The Intergroup trials for localized disease conducted in the United States over the past several decades are summarized in Table 6.2. The first two studies demonstrated the importance of adding doxorubicin to a standard vincristine, actinomycin D, and cyclophosphamide (VAC) backbone and the advantage of giving more intense high-dose intermittent therapy.[21,24] The third Intergroup trial randomized patients to a standard VAC doxorubicin backbone with or without the drug pair ifosfamide and etoposide (IE). The 5-year event-free survival (EFS) rate for those receiving IE was 69% compared to 54% in the standard arm, and median overall survival was also significantly better among patients who received IE (72% vs. 61%).[25] This trial established the five-drug combination as the standard of care for patients with EWS in the United States. A subsequent trial failed to demonstrate any benefit of intensifying the total dose of cyclophosphamide.[26] More recently, the Children's Oncology Group (COG) conducted a randomized trial in which dose intensification was achieved through interval compression by decreasing the period between cycles from 21 to 14 days. This regimen proved to be feasible and the 5-year EFS rates were significantly better for the patients who were randomized to an interval-compressed schedule (73% vs. 65%).[22] This regimen has now become the standard of care for EWS in the United States. The most recent COG study investigated the value of adding another drug pair, cyclophosphamide and topotecan, to this backbone, but the results of this trial are not currently available. The outcomes for patients with metastatic disease remain poor, and several studies have failed to impact the outcomes of these patients.[23] Based on some preliminary evidence of the modest activity of insulin-like growth factor-1 receptor (IGF1R) inhibitors in EWS,[27,28] the COG is evaluating the addition of IGF1R monoclonal antibody, ganitumab, to chemotherapy in patients with disseminated disease. The Euro-Ewing 99 trial attempted to further optimize therapy by randomizing patients with metastatic disease and high-risk localized disease to either standard chemotherapy (with pulmonary radiation therapy [RT] for metastatic patients) or high-dose chemotherapy with stem cell rescue. The results of this study were

TABLE 6.2 Historical Trials and Outcomes in Ewing Sarcoma

Study	Observed Results	
Local disease		
IESS-I (*n* = 342)	VAC versus VACD versus VAC + lung RT	*5-y RFS* 24% 60% 44%
IESS-II (*n* = 214)	VACD q3 weeks versus moderate-dose chemo weekly	*5-y RFS* 73% 56% *p* = .04
INT-0091 (*n* = 518)	VDC versus VDC + IE	*5-y EFS* 54% 69% *p* = .005
INT0154/POG9354 (*n* = 518)	VDC + IE (standard) versus VDC + IE (high dose)	*5-y EFS* 72.1% 70.1% *p* = .005
COG AEWS0031 (*n* = 568)	VDC + IE (3 weeks) versus VDC + IE (2 weeks)	*5-y EFS* 65% 73% *p* = .05
Metastatic disease		
INT-0091	VDC versus VDC + IE	*5-y EFS* 22% 22% (NS)
EE99	VIDE + VAC then HD Bu-Mel w/rescue versus VIDE + VAI then VAI + lung RT	*8-y EFS* 60.7% 46.3% *p* = .032

A, actinomycin D; C, cyclophosphamide; D, doxorubicin; E, etoposide; EFS, event-free survival; HD Bu-Mel, high-dose busulfan-melphalan; I, ifosfamide; RFS, relapse-free survival; RT, radiation therapy; V, vincristine.

Sources: Data from Burgert EO Jr, Nesbit ME, Garnsey LA, et al. Multimodal therapy for the management of nonpelvic, localized Ewing's sarcoma of bone: intergroup study IESS-II. *J Clin Oncol*. 1990;8(9):1514–1524. doi:10.1200/JCO.1990.8.9.1514; Grier HE, Krailo MD, Tarbell NJ, et al. Addition of ifosfamide and etoposide to standard chemotherapy for Ewing's sarcoma and primitive neuroectodermal tumor of bone. *N Engl J Med*. 2003;348(8):694–701. doi:10.1056/NEJMoa020890; Juergens C, Weston C, Lewis I, et al. Safety assessment of intensive induction with vincristine, ifosfamide, doxorubicin, and etoposide (VIDE) in the treatment of Ewing tumors in the EURO-E.W.I.N.G. 99 clinical trial. *Pediatr Blood Cancer*. 2006;47(1):22–29. doi:10.1002/pbc.20820; Nesbit ME Jr, Perez CA, Tefft M, et al. Multimodal therapy for the management of primary, nonmetastatic Ewing's sarcoma of bone: an intergroup Study. *Natl Cancer Inst Monogr*. 1981(56):255–262. PMID:7029293; Womer RB, West DC, Krailo MD, et al. Randomized controlled trial of interval-compressed chemotherapy for the treatment of localized Ewing sarcoma: a report from the Children's Oncology Group. *J Clin Oncol*. 2012;30(33):4148–4154. doi:10.1200/JCO.2011.41.5703.

recently published, with the high-dose chemotherapy with stem cell rescue improving EFS compared to the standard chemotherapy with pulmonary RT at 8 years from randomization (see Table 6.2).[29,30]

Radiation is universally recommended in the case of a positive margin and for patients in whom surgery is not advised; however, in Europe, patients who have a poor histologic response and a negative margin also receive RT.[31] Local control is usually performed at week 12 and is achieved with the use of surgery, RT, or both. A recent review of 1,031 patients treated for EWS demonstrated that patients who received RT alone had decreased overall survival rates at 5 years when compared to those who were treated with surgery alone or surgery plus RT (52.5% vs. 77.2% vs. 64.7%, $p < .001$), although the underlying prognostic factors related to the choice of treatment modality likely contribute to these differences.[32] Radiation to metastatic sites is recommended after completion of chemotherapy; stereotactic body radiation therapy (SBRT) and whole lung irradiation (15 Gy) are used for patients who present with pulmonary metastases.

Sequelae of Therapy

Improved outcomes have resulted in higher numbers of EWS survivors and, therefore, a higher population at risk for developing long-term sequelae after therapy. In one study from the Childhood Cancer Survivor Study (CCSS), the cumulative mortality rate at 25 years following entry into the study was 25%.[33] The most common cause of death was disease recurrence, followed by subsequent malignant neoplasms, cardiac disease, other medical causes, and pulmonary disease. It is recommended that patients be followed with routine imaging scans and laboratory work (CBC with differential and blood chemistry tests) every 3 to 4 months typically in the first year from completion of treatment, followed thereafter by increasing intervals of every 4 to 6 months for 2 to 4 years after finishing therapy and annually thereafter.

Treatment of Recurrence

Patients who experience a recurrence have poor long-term survival rates of about 20%.[34] The most commonly used regimens for relapse include cyclophosphamide with topotecan and temozolomide with irinotecan, with or without vincristine. These regimens have response rates in the range of 32% to 68%.[35,36] High-dose chemotherapy with stem cell rescue has also been used in the setting of recurrent disease to consolidate patients who experience a response to therapy, but its role in this setting remains controversial.[3,37]

EWS has elevated levels of expression of *SLFN11*, a direct transcriptional target of *EWS–FLI* and a determinant of response to several drugs such as camptothecins and poly ADP ribose polymerase (PARP) inhibitors.[38] Several ongoing trials are currently using PARP inhibitors in combination with irinotecan and temozolomide. EWS also has high expression of *LSD1*, and preclinical studies show that *LSD1* inhibition blocks the function of EWS–ETS proteins, therefore making this enzyme an attractive target for treating EWS.[39] Another group is investigating a small-molecule inhibitor called YK-4-279, which is involved in blocking RNA helicase A that partners with *EWS–FLI1*.[10,40] Finally, several trials using drugs targeting IGF1R have demonstrated modest activity with single agents and how these drugs are being used in combination with chemotherapy in frontline COG trials for patients with metastatic disease.[3,27,28]

OSTEOSARCOMA

Epidemiology

OS is the most common bone tumor in children and adolescents, with an age-adjusted incidence rate of 5.4 per million in patients younger than 20 years of age and a slight male predominance compared to females in this age group (1.34:1).[4,41] OS has a bimodal age distribution, peaking in adolescence and after the age of 60 years.[41,42] Although mostly sporadic, OS can be associated with various genetic predisposition syndromes (Table 6.3).[43,44] For example, survivors of retinoblastoma are at the highest risk for developing OS with a standardized incidence ratio of 41.[45] In one study, nearly 10% of younger patients with OS had a Li–Fraumeni-associated *TP53* mutation or a rare exonic *TP53* variant.[46]

TABLE 6.3 Genetic Predisposition Syndromes Associated With Osteosarcoma

Syndrome	Location in Genome	Gene	Function
Bloom syndrome	15q26.1	*BLM (RecQL3)*	DNA helicase
Diamond–Blackfan anemia		Ribosomal proteins	Ribosome production
Li–Fraumeni syndrome	17p13.1	*P53*	DNA damage response
Paget disease	18q21–qa22/5q31/5q35-qter	*LOH18CR1*	IL-1 TNF signaling; RANKL pathway
Hereditary retinoblastoma	13q14.2	*RB1*	Cell cycle checkpoint
Rothmund–Thomson syndrome	8q24.3	*RTS (RecQL4)*	DNA helicase
Werner syndrome	8p12–p11.2	*WRN (RecQL2)*	DNA helicase, exonuclease activity

IL-1, interleukin 1; RANKL, receptor activator of nuclear factor-κB ligand; TNF, tumor necrosis factor.
Sources: Data from Kansara M, Thomas DM. Molecular pathogenesis of osteosarcoma. *DNA Cell Biol*. 2007;26(1):1–18. doi:10.1089/dna.2006.0505

Biology

OS is characterized by multiple chromosomal aberrations including copy number variations and structural variations. Molecular profiling of this tumor has revealed *TP53* pathway aberrations in virtually all of the tumors, either as a result of sequence mutations or structural variations that more commonly involve translocations within the first intron of the gene.[47] In addition, a distinct phenomenon of hypermutation known as kataegis has been reported in up to 50% of the samples analyzed. Other recurrently mutated genes include *RB1*, *ATRX*, and *DLG2*. Pathway analysis has identified the phosphoinositide 3-kinase (PI3K)/mechanistic target of rapamycin (mTOR) pathway as a potential therapeutic vulnerability.[48]

Clinical Presentation

OS usually presents with pain and swelling of the affected area. It most commonly arises in long bones and about 50% of the cases originate around the knee. The next most common site is the proximal humerus, which is involved in about 10% of the cases.[49] In North America, the median duration of symptoms prior to establishing a diagnosis is 2 to 4 months.[50] Most patients present with localized disease, but about 20% have metastases most commonly confined to the lungs.[49]

Diagnosis and Imaging

For all pediatric sarcomas, the initial evaluation is similar, involving imaging of the primary tumor and evaluation for the presence of metastatic disease. After physical exam and history, laboratory studies should be obtained, which include a CBC with differential and blood chemistry tests including LDH and alkaline phosphatase (the latter might be increased in patients with primary bone tumors or metastases). The primary tumor is best imaged with an MRI and plain films. Primary anatomic imaging should include the whole limb to look for skip metastases (Figure 6.3). Chest CT should be obtained as the lungs are the most common site of metastases in 85% of the cases of metastatic disease, and a bone scan or PET should be performed to evaluate for the presence of distant bone

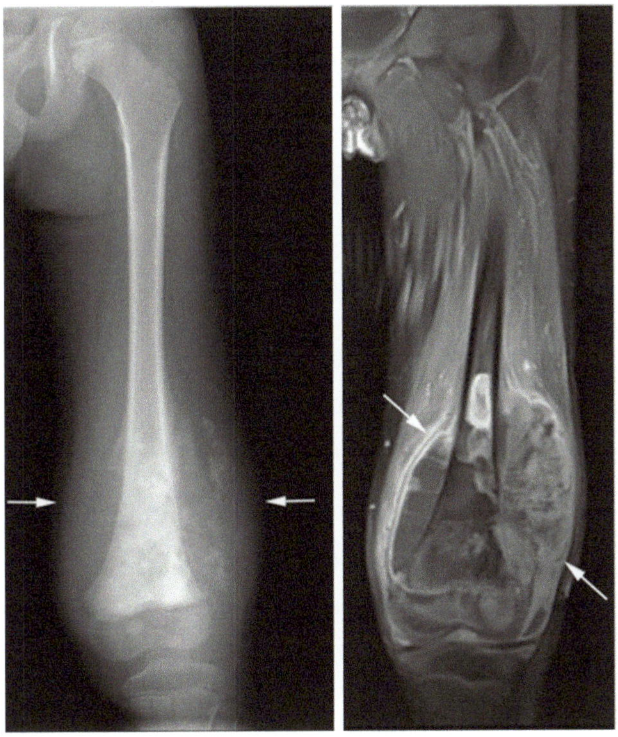

(A) (B)

FIGURE 6.3 A 6-year-old boy with osteosarcoma. (A) Anterior–posterior x-ray study shows typical aggressive bone-forming tumor (arrows) with sunburst periosteal reaction, calcified soft tissue mass, and Codman triangle. (B) Post-contrast T1-weighted coronal MRI shows a large soft tissue mass (arrows) surrounding the tumor involving the marrow of the distal femur.

metastases.[49,51] Biopsy should be carefully planned by the primary surgical treatment team, because the biopsy tract in an extremity primary site can affect local control approaches. Some institutions may conduct a biopsy or remove suspicious lung nodules to confirm the diagnosis.

Treatment

Prior to the use of combined modality therapy, which includes chemotherapy and surgery, the relapse-free survival rates for patients with OS were <20%.[52] The landmark study of Link (see Table 6.4) in which patients with localized OS were randomized to receive surgery alone or adjuvant chemotherapy with methotrexate, cisplatin, doxorubicin (MAP), bleomycin, and actinomycin D demonstrated that the 2-year relapse-free survival rates were significantly improved for those patients who were randomized to adjuvant chemotherapy when compared to those who were treated with surgery alone (66% vs. 17%).[52] This study established the definitive role of chemotherapy in this disease. Other studies during the same time period demonstrated that the timing of chemotherapy either prior to or after resection of the primary tumor did not appear to affect survival, although the use of preoperative chemotherapy could potentially allow for a less morbid surgical procedure with limb preservation and good function.[53–55] To confirm this, the Pediatric Oncology Group (POG) conducted a randomized trial to evaluate the outcomes for patients receiving adjuvant versus neoadjuvant chemotherapy. Another landmark study conducted between 1986 and 1993 established the effectiveness of presurgical chemotherapy followed by limb-sparing surgery (LSS) in patients with localized OS.[56] In this trial, 100 patients were randomized to immediate chemotherapy or immediate surgery. At 5 years, the EFS was 65% for immediate surgery patients and 61% for those assigned to presurgical chemotherapy. Thus, these two studies provided the basis for the current standard of treatment for OS in the United States, which includes preoperative chemotherapy with MAP followed by local control with LSS at around week 10 and additional postoperative chemotherapy for a total of 32 weeks of therapy. Other studies have evaluated the addition of other agents to the MAP backbone in an effort to improve outcomes for patients with the highest risk, such as those with a poor histologic response (as defined as <90% tumor

TABLE 6.4 Historical Osteosarcoma Chemotherapy Regimens

Investigator, Year	Protocol/Therapy	RR or EFS (Duration)
Cortes, 1972, 1974 (*n* = 13 and *n* = 21)	Doxorubicin	45% (1–32 mo)
Jaffe, 1974 (*n* = 20)	Methotrexate with vincristine	80% (2–23 mo)
Ochs, 1978 (*n* = 8)	Cisplatin	63% RR
Marti, 1985 (*n* = 18)	Ifosfamide (9 g/m^2 over 5 days)	33% RR
Link, 1986 (*n* = 36 randomized, 77 declined) — MIOS trial	Observation versus bleomycin, cyclophosphamide, actino-mycin D, methotrexate, doxorubicin, cisplatin	17% (2 y)[a] 66% (2 y)[a]
Goorin, 2003	MIOS chemotherapy-neoadjuvant versus MIOS chemotherapy-adjuvant	61% (2 y) 69% (2 y)
Meyers, 2005	MAP versus MAP + I	65% (4 y) 66% (4 y)

[a]For randomized patients.

EFS, event-free survival; I, ifosfamide; MAP, methotrexate, cisplatin, doxorubicin; MIOS, Multi-Institutional Osteosarcoma Study; RR, relapse rate.

Sources: Data from Goorin AM, Schwartzentruber DJ, Devidas M, et al. Presurgical chemotherapy compared with immediate surgery and adjuvant chemotherapy for nonmetastatic osteosarcoma: Pediatric Oncology Group Study POG-8651. *J Clin Oncol.* 2003;21(8):1574–1580. doi:10.1200/JCO.2003.08.165; Meyers PA, Schwartz CL, Krailo M, et al. Osteosarcoma: a randomized, prospective trial of the addition of ifosfamide and/or muramyl tripeptide to cisplatin, doxorubicin, and high-dose methotrexate. *J Clin Oncol.* 2005;23(9):2004–2011. doi:10.1200/JCO.2005.06.031; Cortes EP, Holland JF, Wang JJ, et al. Doxorubicin in disseminated. *JAMA.* 1972;221(10):1132–1138. doi:10.1001/jama.1972.03200230020005; Cortes EP, Holland JF, Wang JJ, et al. Amputation and adriamycin in primary osteosarcoma. *N Engl J Med.* 1974;291(19):998–1000. doi:10.1056/NEJM197411072911903; Jaffe N, Frei E 3rd, Traggis D, Bishop Y. Adjuvant methotrexate and citrovorum-factor treatment of osteogenic sarcoma. *N Engl J Med.* 1974;291(19):994–997. doi:10.1056/NEJM197411072911902; Marti C, Kroner T, Remagen W, et al. High-dose ifosfamide in advanced osteosarcoma. *Cancer Treat Rep.* 1985;69(1):115–117. PMID:3855382; Link MP, Goorin AM, Miser AW, et al. The effect of adjuvant chemotherapy on relapse-free survival in patients with osteosarcoma of the extremity. *N Engl J Med.* 1986;314(25):1600–1606. doi:10.1056/NEJM198606193142502; Ochs JJ, Freeman AI, Douglass HO Jr, et al. Cis-Dichlorodiammineplatinum (II) in advanced osteogenic sarcoma. *Cancer Treat Rep.* 1978;62(2):239–245.

necrosis) after preoperative chemotherapy.[57] A randomized trial conducted by Meyers et al. assigned patients to receive MAP chemotherapy with or without ifosfamide and with or without muramyl tripeptide.[57] This trial achieved a 3-year EFS of 68%. The addition of ifosfamide to cisplatin, doxorubicin, and methotrexate did not improve EFS or overall survival, but the addition of muramyl tripeptide significantly improved survival.[58] Despite the results of this trial, this agent is currently not available in the United States.[59] The most recent randomized trial, EUROAMOS, attempted to answer several questions in patients with localized disease by modifying therapy based on histologic response. Patients who had >90% tumor necrosis (defined as a "good" response) were randomized to receive either standard MAP chemotherapy or MAP with pegylated interferon alfa-2b.[60] No advantage was seen with the addition of interferon, with the 3-year EFS rates being 77% for the MAP arm and 80% for the MAP plus interferon arm. In addition, 23% of patients randomized to the interferon arm never received it and 39% of those who received interferon stopped it early.[60] In this trial, the remaining 618 patients who had a poor histologic response to preoperative chemotherapy defined as ≥10% viable tumor were randomized to receive MAP chemotherapy alone or MAP with three postoperative cycles of IE and two additional cycles of ifosfamide (MAP/IE). The 3-year EFS was 55% for MAP and 53% for MAP/IE. In addition, MAP/IE was associated with more grade 4 nonhematologic toxicity.[61–67]

Local control measures should be determined by an experienced orthopedic oncologist for most cases of OS involving extremity tumors. Currently, about 80% of patients with extremity OS can be treated with LSS for local control.[68] The role of radiation is limited in this disease to axial lesions that are not resectable or that locally recur (in conjunction with surgery when possible); high radiation doses delivered with specialized techniques such as protons are necessary.[69] The importance of complete surgical resection of all sites of resectable OS is key to long-term control and cure.[70] Historically amputation was the only option for many patients, and this was the preferred method to ensure complete resection of the tumor, with local sites being the most common location for relapse. With the use of preoperative chemotherapy, many resections were made easier for surgeons to allow for limb-sparing procedures that historically would have resulted in an amputation.

Patients who present with pulmonary metastatic disease should have their lesions resected in order to potentially achieve cure.[71] Typically, this procedure is performed in a staged fashion with local control of the primary site occurring first. Prognostic factors associated with inferior clinical outcomes in the presence of pulmonary metastatic disease include the number of metastases at diagnosis and macroscopically incomplete resection of all sites of disease.[71]

Sequelae of Therapy

Survivors of OS are at increased risk of developing therapy-related complications. In a study by the CCSS, patients who survived 5 years from their diagnosis had an 88.6% probability of being alive for 20 years from their original diagnosis.[72] However, 87% of survivors experienced at least one chronic medical issue and over half experienced two or more chronic health conditions. The most common cause of death was attributed to tumor recurrence, followed by subsequent malignant neoplasms, cardiac complications, and pulmonary complications. Tinnitus/vertigo and hearing loss requiring a hearing aid were reported in 14% and 7% of survivors, respectively. About 10% of survivors reported adverse general health and 29% reported a physical limitation. Finally, survivors of OS were less likely to be married or to graduate from high school.

Based on these findings, survivors of OS require lifetime follow-up after completion of treatment. Patients should be followed with routine scans and lab work (CBC with differential and blood chemistry tests) every 3 to 4 months during the first year from completion of therapy with routine subspecialty care that may involve specialists from cardiology, nephrology, fertility, and rehabilitation, depending on the needs of the individual. The patient will also require cardiac evaluations with echocardiograms to assess the heart function, depending on the total dose of doxorubicin. Interval assessments after therapy completion can be spread out to every 4 to 6 months for 2 to 4 years from therapy and annually after 5 years, depending on the institutional standards.

Treatment of Recurrence

Clinical outcome following relapse of OS is poor. In one study by the Cooperative Osteosarcoma Study Group, the overall survival rate at 5 years was 23%.[73] Patients with early relapses and a higher disease burden fared worse, as well as those who did not achieve a surgical complete remission. Administration of chemotherapy appeared to correlate with better survival in those who did not achieve a second complete remission.[73] Similarly, the COG found that survival after recurrence was poor, with 17% of patients being alive at 5 years. Outcome was better for those who were <10 years of age at the time of initial treatment and presented with localized disease, had a longer interval to time of first relapse (>2 years), and had isolated lung or bone relapse.[74] About 50% of all relapses occur within 18 months from the end of initial treatment and another 5% of patients will have a relapse after 5 years of therapy. As previously mentioned, patients who relapse early (<2 years from the initial diagnosis) have worse outcomes than those who recur later.[75] Regardless of the site of recurrence, surgical resection is key to disease control, with 5-year survival rates being 20% to 45% after resection of lung recurrences and 20% at other sites.[76,77]

Patients who experience isolated lung recurrences should undergo complete resection of recurrent disease. Complete resection can be successful for patients with isolated lung disease without requiring chemotherapy or further treatment.[76–79] A retrospective review of patients treated at major centers showed that chemotherapy following metastasectomy did not improve the long-term survival compared to surgery alone.[80]

For patients who require chemotherapy, multiple regimens have been used, including ifosfamide with etoposide, gemcitabine with docetaxel, and sorafenib with everolimus. A recent randomized, placebo-controlled, Phase 2 trial demonstrated that regorafenib increased the median progression-free survival and overall survival of patients with recurrent OS.[81] Because responses to chemotherapy using the Response Evaluation Criteria in Solid Tumors (RECIST) are infrequent and do not appear to accurately predict survival,[82] the COG embarked on a retrospective analysis assessing the outcome of recurrent OS in patients who were treated in seven Phase 2 trials. They observed a 4-month progression-free survival rate of 12%, which is now used as a benchmark for EFS outcomes that can be used to assess the efficacy of novel agents.[83] Using this model to assess the efficacy of new agents, the COG has evaluated several new agents in the Phase 2 setting, such as eribulin, without evidence of clinical activity.[84] For patients with multiple painful bony metastatic sites at the time of recurrence, samarium-153-ethylene-tetramethylene-phosphonate (^{153}Sm-EDTMP; with or without stem cell support) may help with pain symptoms.[85]

NON-RHABDOMYOSARCOMA SOFT TISSUE SARCOMAS

Epidemiology

NRSTSs encompass a large group of tumor types that have a presumed mesenchymal origin and account for about 4% of all childhood malignancies.[86] There is a slight male predominance in childhood, and the histology distribution of these tumors is dramatically different from the histology seen in adults. In the pediatric population, synovial sarcoma, malignant peripheral nerve sheath tumors, and fibroblastic tumors predominate, while most of these malignancies are seen during the second decade of life. Some genetic predisposition syndromes have been associated with an increased risk for developing particular NRSTS (see Table 6.5)[87–98] and these children should be followed closely for their lifetime risk of developing these cancers.

Biology

The majority of pediatric NRSTSs have unique chromosomal translocations (Table 6.6), and some of them, such as tumors characterized by *NTRK* fusions, are amenable to targeted therapy.[99] Owing to the rarity of these individual tumors, they have been grouped together for treatment purposes, though as seen in Table 6.6, the identified pathways involved are often completely unrelated, which has made studying many of these tumors difficult.[100–102]

Clinical Presentation, Diagnosis, and Imaging

Children usually present with an enlarging soft tissue mass, which is usually painless. Systemic symptoms are uncommon and other symptoms are related to the anatomic location of the tumor. Diagnosis is made in most cases by excisional biopsy, core-needle biopsy, and rarely by complete surgical resection of the mass at the time of presentation. Laboratory studies should include a CBC with differential and a chemistry panel including LDH and urinalysis. An MRI of the primary tumor should be obtained, as well as a CT of the chest with FDG-PET to search for distant metastases.

Treatment

Treatment for this broad group of tumors involves surgery, with or without chemotherapy and with or without radiation. This group of tumors was poorly studied in multi-institutional National Cancer Institute (NCI)-sponsored trials until the most recent trial named ARST0332. ARST0332 was the first trial to use a risk-based approach to assign therapy (see Figure 6.4). In addition, this study incorporated

TABLE 6.5 Genetic Predispositions in NRSTS

Genetic Predisposition to NRSTS	Common Sarcomas
Li–Fraumeni syndrome	NRSTS, osteosarcoma
Familial adenomatous polyposis	Desmoid fibromatosis
RB1 gene	Leiomyosarcoma, osteosarcoma
SMARCB1 gene	Extrarenal rhabdoid tumors, epithelioid sarcoma
Neurofibromatosis type 1	Malignant peripheral nerve sheath tumors, RMS
Werner syndrome	NRSTS, osteosarcoma
Tuberous sclerosis complex	Tumors with perivascular epithelioid cell differentiation (PEComas)
Adenosine deaminase-deficient SCID	Multicentric dermatofibrosarcoma protuberans

NRSTS, non-rhabdomyosarcomatous soft tissue sarcoma; PEComa, perivascular epithelioid cell tumor; RMS, rhabdomyosarcoma; SCID, severe combined immunodeficiency.

Sources: Data from Chang F, Syrjanen S, Syrjanen K. Implications of the *p53* tumor-suppressor gene in clinical oncology. *J Clin Oncol*. 1995;13(4):1009–1022. doi:10.1200/JCO.1995.13.4.1009; Groen EJ, Roos A, Muntinghe FL, et al. Extra-intestinal manifestations of familial adenomatous polyposis. *Ann Surg Oncol*. 2008;15(9):2439–2450. doi:10.1245/s10434-008-9981-3; Wong JR, Morton LM, Tucker MA, et al. Risk of subsequent malignant neoplasms in long-term hereditary retinoblastoma survivors after chemotherapy and radiotherapy. *J Clin Oncol*. 2014;32(29):3284–3290. doi:10.1200/JCO.2013.54.7844; Eaton KW, Tooke LS, Wainwright LM, et al. Spectrum of *SMARCB1/INI1* mutations in familial and sporadic rhabdoid tumors. *Pediatr Blood Cancer*. 2011;56(1):7–15. doi:10.1002/pbc.22831; Rubin BP, Fletcher CDM, Inwards C, et al. Protocol for the examination of specimens from patients with soft tissue tumors of intermediate malignant potential, malignant soft tissue tumors, and benign/locally aggressive and malignant bone tumors. *Arch Pathol Lab Med*. 2006;130(11):1616–1629. doi:10.1043/1543-2165(2006)130[1616:PFTEOS]2.0.CO;2; deCou JM, Rao BN, Parham DM, et al. Malignant peripheral nerve sheath tumors: the St. Jude Children's Research Hospital experience. *Ann Surg Oncol*. 1995;2(6):524–529. doi:10.1007/bf02307086; Stark AM, Buhl R, Hugo HH, Mehdorn HM. Malignant peripheral nerve sheath tumours—report of 8 cases and review of the literature. *Acta Neurochir (Wien)*. 2001;143(4):357–363; discussion 363–364. doi:10.1007/s007010170090; Goto M, Miller RW, Ishikawa Y, Sugano H. Excess of rare cancers in Werner syndrome (adult progeria). *Cancer Epidemiol Biomarkers Prev*. 1996;5(4):239–246. https://www.ncbi.nlm.nih.gov/pubmed/8722214; Fricke BL, Donnelly LF, Casper KA, Bissler JJ. Frequency and imaging appearance of hepatic angiomyolipomas in pediatric and adult patients with tuberous sclerosis. *AJR Am J Roentgenol*. 2004;182(4):1027–1030. doi:10.2214/ajr.182.4.1821027; Hornick JL, Fletcher CDM. PEComa: what do we know so far? *Histopathology*. 2006;48(1):75–82. doi:10.1111/j.1365-2559.2005.02316.x; Kesserwan C, Sokolic R, Cowen EW, et al. Multicentric dermatofibrosarcoma protuberans in patients with adenosine deaminase-deficient severe combined immune deficiency. *J Allergy Clin Immunol*. 2012;129(3):762–769.e1. doi:10.1016/j.jaci.2011.10.028; PDQ® Pediatric Treatment Editorial Board. *PDQ childhood soft tissue sarcoma treatment*. Bethesda, MD: National Cancer Institute. https://www.cancer.gov/types/soft-tissue-sarcoma/hp/child-soft-tissue-treatment-pdq.

for the first time the French Federation of Comprehensive Cancer Centers (*Fédération Nationale des Centres de Lutte Contre le Cancer*; FNCLCC) grading system in addition to the POG system to assign histologic grade.[103] Spunt and colleagues compared these two systems in a cohort of 130 patients from three POG historical trials (8653, 8654, and 9553) and showed they had a correlative value.[104] More importantly, their data showed that mitotic index may have the highest correlative value for pediatric NRSTS. They found 44 patients had discrepant grades between the two systems; but when they further looked at mitotic index using 10 mitotic figures per high-power field (HPF) as a cutoff, these patients' outcomes followed the trend with patients who had <10 mitotic figures per HPF having an EFS close to 70% compared to those with >10 figures per HPF having an EFS of around 15%. These outcomes matched up with those patients who had correlative grades as had been previously said by the two systems. The recently completed ARST0332 study analyzes data using the two systems to determine which one better applies to the pediatric population prospectively.

Spunt et al. reported the preliminary results of the ARST0332 trial. This trial demonstrated that some patients can be treated with surgery alone, while the RT can be spared. In fact, children with synovial sarcoma who have tumors <5 cm can be treated with resection alone without chemotherapy or RT regardless of the grade, with a 3-year EFS rate of 90%.[141] In patients with metastatic disease or large tumors that cannot be resected, the outcomes remain poor.

The currently recommended chemotherapy regimen from ARST0332 for those patients who need chemotherapy is the two-drug combination of ifosfamide and doxorubicin. The most recently completed trial ARST1321 added pazopanib to the ifosfamide/doxorubicin backbone to evaluate the response as defined by the percent necrosis at the time of local control, but results of this trial are currently pending.

Some NRSTS are responsive to specific therapies. For example, alveolar soft part sarcoma (ASPS) is a notoriously chemotherapy-resistant tumor. Surgery is the standard of care for this tumor, but targeted therapies such as pazopanib and sunitinib, both being receptor tyrosine kinase inhibitors that target multiple pathways, have been able to achieve stable disease and partial responses (in the

TABLE 6.6 Selected Chromosomal Aberrations in Non-Rhabdomyosarcomatous Soft Tissue Sarcomas in Pediatric Patients

Histology	Chromosomal Aberrations	Genes Involved
Alveolar soft part sarcoma	t(x;17)(p11.2;q25)	*ASPL/TFE3*
Angiomatoid fibrous histiocytoma	t(12;16)(q13;p11), t(2;22)(q33;q12), t(12;22)(q13;q12)	*FUS/ATF1, EWSR1/CREB1, EWS/ATF1*
BCOR-rearranged sarcomas	Inv(X)(p11.4;p11.2)	*BCOR/CCN83*
CIC-rearranged sarcomas	t(4;19)(q35;q13), t(10;19)(q26;q13)	*CIC–DUX4*
Clear cell sarcoma	t(12;22)(q13;q12), t(2;22)(q33;q12)	*ATF1/EWSR1, EWSR1/CREB1*
Congenital/infantile fibrosarcoma/ mesoblastic nephroma	t(12;15)(p13;q25)	*ETV6–NTRK3*
Desmoid fibromatosis	Trisomy 8 or 20, loss of 5q21	*CTNNB1* or *APC* mutations
Desmoplastic small round cell tumors	t(11;22)(p13;q12)	*EWS/WT1*
Epithelioid hemangioendothelioma	t(1;3)(p36;q25)	*WWTR1/CAMTA1*
Epithelioid sarcoma/rhabdoid tumor	Inactivation of *SMARC81*	*SMARC81*
Extraskeletal myxoid chondrosarcoma	t(9;22)(q22;q12), t(9;17)(q22;q11), t(9;15)(q22;q21), t(3;9)(q11;q22)	*EWSR1/NR4A3, TAF2N/NR4A3, TCF12/NR4A3, TGF/NR4A3*
Inflammatory myofibroblastic tumor	t(1;2)(q23;q23), t(2;19)(q23;q13) t(2;17)(q23;q23), t(2;2)(p23;q13) t(2;11)(p23;p15)	*TPM3/ALK, TPM4/ALK, CLTC/ALK, RANBP2/ALK, CARS/ALK, RAS*
Infantile myofibromatosis		*PDGFRB*
Malignant peripheral nerve sheath tumor	17q11.2, loss or rearrangement of 10p, 11q, 17q, 22q	*NF1*
Myoepithelioma		*EWSR1/ZNF44, EWSR1/PBX1, EWSR1/POU5F1*
Synovial sarcoma	t(x;18)(p11.2;q11.2)	*SYT/SSX*
Giant cell tumor	t(1;2)(p13;q35)	*COL6A3/CSF1*

Sources: Data from Laetsch TW, DuBois SG, Mascarenhas L, et al. Larotrectinib for paediatric solid tumours harbouring *NTRK* gene fusions: phase 1 results from a multicentre, open-label, phase 1/2 study. *Lancet Oncol*. 2018;19(5):705–714. doi:10.1016/S1470-2045(18)30119-0; Slater O, Shipley J. Clinical relevance of molecular genetics to paediatric sarcomas. *J Clin Pathol*. 2007;60(11):1187–1194. doi:10.1136/jcp.2006.040113; Sandberg AA. Translocations in malignant tumors. *Am J Pathol*. 2001;159(6):1979–1980. doi:10.1016/S0002-9440(10)63047-7; Mertens F, Antonescu CR, Hohenberger P, et al. Translocation-related sarcomas. *Semin Oncol*. 2009;36(4):312–323. doi:10.1053/j.seminoncol.2009.06.004.

case of sunitinib) for some patients in several series of patients who had unresectable disease.[105,106] In the adult literature, there is Phase 2 data for cediranib, a small-molecule inhibitor of all three vascular endothelial growth factor receptors, and currently, there is a Phase 2 trial ongoing that compares cediranib with sunitinib for ASPS.[107]

Targeted therapy with anaplastic lymphoma kinase (ALK) inhibitors is extremely effective in inflammatory myofibroblastic tumor.[108,109] Infantile fibrosarcoma is one of the most common tumors in younger children and about 70% carry *ETV6–NTRK3* fusion. The *NTRK* inhibitor larotrectinib was found to be highly effective across tropomyosin receptor kinase (TRK) fusion-positive tumors in both adult and pediatric cancers that harbor the fusion.[99] Desmoid tumors are typically difficult to resect and treat. A 2018 adult trial found that patients, many of whom had been previously treated, had durable responses to sorafenib, with 89% of patients showing stable disease after 12 months of therapy.[110]

Enhancer of zeste homolog 2 (EZH2) inhibitors such as tazemetostat have produced objective responses in about 5% of patients with solid tumors and clinical benefit such as stable disease in about one-third of patients with *INI1*- or *SMARCA4*-negative tumors.[111]

Sequelae of Therapy

Patients who are long-term survivors of NRSTS have many similar issues to the conditions that have been discussed in the previous Sequelae of Therapy sections in this chapter. In 2018, a comparison of survivors who received therapy in different eras of pediatric cancer treatment showed that patients who received NRSTS treatment in 1990 to 1999 compared to 1970 to 1979 had fewer grade 3–5 chronic conditions (28.3% vs. 36.5%, p = .021).[112] In general, this means that, while the outcomes for children

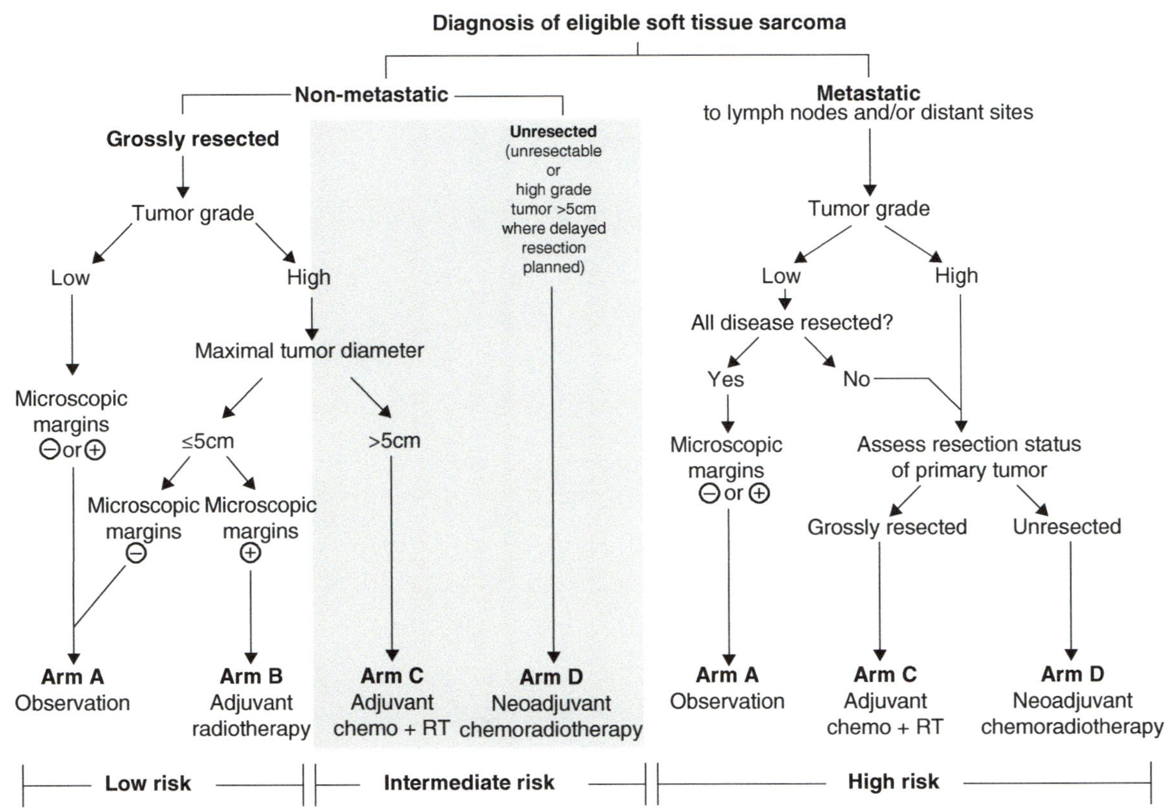

FIGURE 6.4 **Treatment algorithm ARST0332.**

RT, radiation therapy.

Source: Reproduced with permission from Spunt SL, Million L, Anderson JR, et al. Risk-based treatment for nonrhabdomyosarcoma soft tissue sarcomas (NRSTS) in patients under 30 years of age: Children's Oncology Group study ARST0332. *J Clin Oncol*. 2014;32(15_suppl):10008–10008. doi:10.1200/jco.2014.32.15_suppl.10008 and adolescents with NRSTS have improved, we have also been able to reduce long-term morbidity from the treatment. Issues revolve around activity limitations due to surgery to remove the tumor and sequelae from chemotherapy and RT for those treated with them. Follow-up after completion of chemotherapy usually involves many subspecialists specially trained in the treatment of sequelae of pediatric cancer treatment. Initially, the patient is followed with routine scans and lab work (CBC with differential and blood chemistry tests) every 3 to 4 months with routine subspecialty care that may involve specialists from cardiology, nephrology, fertility, and rehabilitation, depending on the individual needs of the child. The patient will need echocardiograms to follow the heart function, depending on the total dose of doxorubicin and the radiation field. This initial interval during follow-up may be spread out to every 4 to 6 months for 2 to 4 years from therapy and annually after 5 years, depending on the institutional standards. Patients who have been exposed to doxorubicin and ifosfamide will need at least an annual CBC with differential to look for any signs of early bone marrow failure that may indicate chemotherapy-related myeloproliferative disorder or even leukemia.

Treatment of Recurrence

Progressive or recurrent NRSTS is very difficult to treat and the prognosis remains poor. Treatment of recurrence or refractory disease should be tailored to the patient when possible, based on the type of tumor, actionable targets in the tumor, individual patient considerations, and open clinical trials. The pediatric Molecular Analysis for Therapy Choice (MATCH) through the COG is currently enrolling patients who have specific actionable targets, and this may be an option for certain patients with relapsed or refractory disease that cannot be resected. Surgery to prevent recurrence should be performed when possible, including isolated pulmonary occurrences. Patients who were able to have second surgical remission have prolonged survival overall, but still have a dismal overall outcome.[113] If the patient has not previously been radiated to the site of recurrence, then radiation is recommended as well. Chemotherapy options for relapsed disease are limited, but several regimens including gemcitabine with docetaxel have produced limited responses.[114] Pazopanib, which was moved into the Phase 3 setting for the most recent NRSTS COG protocol, can be used as monotherapy in the relapsed setting. One adult study showed significant improvement in progression-free survival compared to placebo, and it has been Food and Drug Administration (FDA) approved subsequently for treatment of adult advanced soft tissue sarcoma.[115] Eribulin and trabectedin are two agents that have been approved for treatment of adult soft tissue sarcoma. Trabectedin plus irinotecan has shown some limited but promising results in translocation-positive sarcomas, though larger patient cohorts are needed to determine which translocation-positive patients may be best served by this combination.[116] Eribulin, an antimitotic agent, was tested in the Phase 1 setting in pediatrics with acceptable toxicity, and in this limited population, one patient with sarcoma had a partial response and three more patients received at least three courses of eribulin.[117]

RHABDOMYOSARCOMA

Epidemiology

RMS is the most common soft tissue sarcoma in children and accounts for about 3% of all childhood cancer cases with an incidence of 4.9 cases per 1 million.[118,119] Males have a higher incidence than females. The embryonal rhabdomyosarcoma (eRMS) histologic subtype is more common in young children, whereas alveolar rhabdomyosarcoma (aRMS) is equally distributed among patients under 20 years of age.[119] Several genetic predisposition syndromes are associated with an increased risk of developing RMS, including Li–Fraumeni syndrome, germline *DICER1* mutations, neurofibromatosis type 1, Costello syndrome, Beckwith–Wiedemann syndrome, and Noonan syndrome (see Table 6.7).[119–121]

Molecular Pathology

Embryonal RMS is characterized by a high mutational burden that increases with age. The most common genes mutated in eRMS belong to the *RAS* family and include *HRAS*, *KRAS*, *NRAS*, and *NF1*. Other genes that are less frequently mutated include *PI3KCA*, *BCOR*, *FBXW7*, *TP53*, *CTNNB1*, and *FGFR4*.[12,122]

Alveolar RMS is characterized by a lower background mutation rate and translocations of the *PAX3* or *PAX7* gene to the *FOXO1* gene. Rarely, aRMS has been reported to harbor *PIK3CA* mutations.[12,122]

A rare variant called sclerosing RMS accounts for 5% to 10% of all cases and is genetically heterogeneous. A subgroup of patients who are generally older (median age 19 years) has tumors with spindle

TABLE 6.7 Genetic Syndromes Associated With Rhabdomyosarcoma

Syndrome	Location in Genome	Gene	Function
Beckwith–Wiedemann syndrome	11p15.5, 11p15.4	*CDKN1C, H19, IGF2, KCNQ10T1*	
Costello syndrome	11p15.5	*HRAS*	Cell growth and division
DICER1 syndrome	14q23.13	*DICER1*	Ribonuclease
Gorlin syndrome	9q22.3	*PTCH1*	Tumor suppressor
Li–Fraumeni syndrome	17p13.1	*P53*	DNA damage response
Noonan syndrome	12q24	*PTPN11*	
Neurofibromatosis type 1	17q11.2	*NF1*	Regulator of the RAS system

Sources: Data from Skapek SX, Ferrari A, Gupta AA, et al. Rhabdomyosarcoma. *Nat Rev Dis Primers*. 2019;5(1):1. doi:10.1038/s41572-018-0051-2; Diller L, Sexsmith E, Gottlieb A, et al. Germline *p53* mutations are frequently detected in young children with rhabdomyosarcoma. *J Clin Invest*. 1995;95(4):1606–1611. doi:10.1172/JCI117834.

cell/sclerosing morphology. These tumors have an *MYOD1* (L122R) gene mutation which can coexist with a *PIK3CA* mutation and are associated with very poor clinical outcome.[123] Another subgroup of patients comprising infants who have a predominantly spindle cell histology is characterized by *VGLL2* and *NCOA2* rearrangements and is associated with a favorable clinical outcome.[124]

Clinical Presentation and Diagnosis

Because RMS can arise almost anywhere in the body, symptoms are usually related to the site of primary tumor. The most common sites of RMS include the head or neck (about one-third of the cases), genitourinary tract (23%), extremities (20%), and other sites.[125] RMS is staged using a surgicopathologic (Tables 6.8 and 6.9) staging system, which assigns clinical group based on the extent of initial surgery (Table 6.9), and a pretreatment staging system, which assigns a stage based on the site of disease, nodal status, and the size of the tumor. As shown in Table 6.8, favorable sites include the orbit, other nonparameningeal head and neck tumors, nonbladder prostate tumors, and the biliary tract. Approximately 50% of children with RMS present with group III (unresected) tumors and 16% present with metastases at diagnosis that most commonly involve the lung (39%), bone marrow (32%), and bone (27%).[126] Nodal metastases are particularly prevalent among patients with extremity primary tumors and in patients older than 10 years of age with paratesticular tumors.[127–129]

Diagnosis is made in most cases by excisional biopsy, core-needle biopsy, and rarely by complete resection of the mass at presentation. At presentation, a CT scan or an MRI of the primary tumor should be obtained depending on the location. Once tissue diagnosis is made, further workup should include a CT scan of the chest to look for metastatic disease, a PET scan to identify bone or soft tissue

TABLE 6.8 TNM Staging for Rhabdomyosarcoma

Stage	Site	T	Size	N	M
I	Orbit Head/neck (non-PM), GU-nonbladder/nonprostate, biliary tract	T1 or T2	a or b	N0 or N1 or N2	M0
II	Bladder/prostate, extremity, cranial, PM, other (trunk, retroperitoneum, excludes biliary tract)	T1 or T2	a	N0 or N1	M0
III	Bladder/prostate extremity, cranial, PM, other (trunk, retroperitoneum, excludes biliary tract)	T1 or T2	a b	N1 N0 or N1 or N2	M0
IV	All	T1 or T2	a or b	N0 or N1	M1

Note: M0, no distant metastasis; M1, metastasis present (includes positive cerebrospinal fluid, pleural or peritoneal cytology); N0, regional nodes not involved; N1, regional nodes involved; Nx, status of regional nodes not known; T1, primary tumor confined to the anatomic site of origin; T2, primary tumor with extension and/or fixation to the surrounding tissue. Size (a) indicates primary tumor <5 cm; size (b) indicates primary tumor >5 cm.
GU, genitourinary; PM, parameningeal; TNM, tumor node metastasis.
Source: Adapted from Malempati S, Hawkins DS. Rhabdomyosarcoma: review of the Children's Oncology Group (COG) Soft-Tissue Sarcoma Committee experience and rationale for current COG studies. *Pediatr Blood Cancer*. 2012;59(1):5–10. doi:10.1002/pbc.24118.

TABLE 6.9 Clinical Group Staging for Rhabdomyosarcoma

Clinical Group	Definition
I	Completely resected localized disease
IIa	Tumor grossly resected with R1 margins
IIb	Regional lymph nodes are involved, though primary is completely resected with R0 margins
IIc	Regional lymph nodes are involved, though primary is completely resected with R1 margins
III	Biopsy only, or partial resection only, debulking
IV	Distant metastatic disease

R0, no residual tumor; R1, microscopic residual tumor.

Source: Adapted from Malempati S, Hawkins DS. Rhabdomyosarcoma: review of the Children's Oncology Group (COG) Soft-Tissue Sarcoma Committee experience and rationale for current COG studies. *Pediatr Blood Cancer*. 2012;59(1):5–10. doi:10.1002/pbc.24118.

metastases, as well as bilateral bone marrow aspirates and biopsies. Patients with extremity tumors should undergo sentinel node biopsy, and patients older than 10 years of age with paratesticular tumors should undergo nerve-sparing ipsilateral retroperitoneal node dissection.

Treatment

Combined modality therapy with chemotherapy and surgery and/or RT is used to treat all patients with RMS. Treatment decisions are based on a risk stratification system that takes into consideration the histology of the tumor, the site of the tumor, and the stage and clinical group of the tumor (Table 6.10). In North America, the backbone that has been used for most cases of RMS has been VAC. Addition of other drugs or intensification of cyclophosphamide has not resulted in improved cure rates for patients with intermediate- or high-risk disease.[130–132] As seen in Table 6.10, there is a group of patients designated as low risk who can be treated with a short course of therapy that includes a lower dose of cyclophosphamide with an expected 5-year EFS rate of 89%.[132] Intermediate-risk patients comprise a heterogeneous group with outcomes that range from 65% to 87% and are usually treated with more intensive cyclophosphamide doses or with VAC alternating with vincristine and irinotecan. A 2018 European study EpSSG 2005 evaluated, in a randomized fashion, the addition of six cycles of maintenance therapy with low-dose cyclophosphamide and vinorelbine. The results of this trial demonstrated improved outcomes for those who received maintenance therapy (3-year EFS rate 78.4% vs. 72.3%, $p = .061$ and overall survival rate 87.3% vs. 77.4%, $p = .011$).[133] Based on these results, most trials in Europe and North America will now incorporate a maintenance phase for

TABLE 6.10 Treatment Stratification Using the COG and Oberlin Risk Prognostic Factors

Risk	COG Risk Assignment	EFS Rate (5 Years)
Low	Low risk subset 1: eRMS (*FOXO1* negative) Stages I and II, groups I and II Stage I, group III orbital only	90%
Intermediate	eRMS Stage I, group II (nonorbit) Stage III, groups I and II Stages II and III, group III Stage IV, group IV (age <10 years old) aRMS: Stages I to III, groups I to III	60% to 75%
High	eRMS: Stage IV, group IV (age >10 years old) aRMS: Stage IV, group IV	10% to 20%

aRMS, alveolar rhabdomyosarcoma; eRMS, embryonal rhabdomyosarcoma; COG, Children's Oncology Group; EFS, event-free survival; RMS, rhabdomyosarcoma.

Sources: Data from Pappo AS, Dirksen U. Rhabdomyosarcoma, Ewing sarcoma, and other round cell sarcomas. *J Clin Oncol*. 2018;36(2):168–179. doi:10.1200/JCO.2017.74.7402; Oberlin O, Rey A, Lyden E, et al. Prognostic factors in metastatic rhabdomyosarcomas: results of a pooled analysis from United States and European cooperative groups. *J Clin Oncol*. 2008;26(14):2384–2389. doi:10.1200/JCO.2007.14.7207.

children with intermediate-risk RMS. As previously mentioned, the outcome for patients with high-risk features (Table 6.10) has not improved over the past 30 years, with the 3-year EFS rates being under 20%. Radiation doses usually range from 36 to 50.4 Gy and it is usually administered at week 12 or 20. Currently, metastatic sites should be radiated as well; these are typically addressed at the end of chemotherapy.[134,135]

Sequelae of Therapy

As survival rates for patients with RMS have increased over the past 30 to 40 years, late consequences of therapy have become more obvious. The main long-term issues seem to be associated with exposure to radiation during therapy, including late visual and endocrine effects. Functional impairments similar to those seen with long-term survivors of other types of pediatric sarcomas are also seen and seem possibly related to aggressive surgical procedures, size of the tumor, and the location of primary disease.[136] Follow-up after completion of therapy should include routine scans and lab work (CBC with differential and blood chemistry) initially every 3 to 4 months with routine subspecialty care that may involve specialists from cardiology, nephrology, fertility, and rehabilitation, depending on the individual needs of the child. The patient will need echocardiograms to follow the heart function, depending on the total dose of doxorubicin and the radiation fields. This initial interval of follow-up may be spread out to every 4 to 6 months for 2 to 4 years from therapy and annually after 5 years, depending on the institutional standards. Patients exposed to doxorubicin, cyclophosphamide, and etoposide will need at least an annual CBC with differential to look for any signs of early bone marrow failure that may indicate chemotherapy-related myeloproliferative disorder or even leukemia.

Treatment of Recurrence

Patients who experience a recurrence of their disease have a poor outcome, with only 17% surviving 5 years following their first recurrence.[137] The COG trial ARST0921 was a trial for relapsed RMS patients with randomization to either vinorelbine and cyclophosphamide with either temsirolimus or bevacizumab. Results showed a superior 6-month EFS with temsirolimus (65%) compared to bevacizumab (50%) and a higher proportion of patients with partial responses on the temsirolimus arm as well (33% vs. 18%).[138] Hence, today many would consider this first-line therapy for patients with relapsed RMS. Other regimens include vincristine, irinotecan, temodar (VIT) and irinotecan, temodar, temsirolimus (ITT). High-dose chemotherapy with autologous bone marrow transplant plays has no role in the treatment of recurrent RMS.[139] Promising data in mouse models show that targeting WEE1 kinase may be effective in patients with high-risk RMS, and the COG is conducting a Phase 1 trial of this agent in combination with irinotecan in patients with recurrent RMS.[140]

SUMMARY

This chapter delves into the wide array of pediatric sarcoma diagnoses, their historical treatments, outcomes, and future directions, as we continue to try to find the best way to treat this heterogeneous group of pediatric cancers. The future of pediatric sarcomas will likely be based on the genomic background of each tumor to allow a more individualized approach to patient care, though currently we rely on combination treatment regimens utilizing chemotherapy, radiation, and surgery for most patients. Great improvements in pediatric cancer treatment have been seen in the past 50 years, though for most sarcomas, this improvement has been modest at best with many children still requiring large operations including amputations, harsh treatments, and for those who survive, long-term side effects from treatment as a child or adolescent.

REFERENCES

1. Howlader N, Noone A, Krapcho M, et al. *SEER Cancer Statistic Review, 1975-2010*. Bethesda, MD: National Cancer Institute. http://seer.cancer.gov/csr/1975_2010
2. Pinto A, Dickman P, Parham D. Pathobiologic markers of the Ewing sarcoma family of tumors: state of the art and prediction of behaviour. *Sarcoma*. 2011;2011:856190. doi:10.1155/2011/856190
3. Gaspar N, Hawkins DS, Dirksen U, et al. Ewing sarcoma: current management and future approaches through collaboration. *J Clin Oncol*. 2015;33(27):3036–3046. doi:10.1200/JCO.2014.59.5256
4. Noone AM, Howlander N, Krapcho M, et al. *SEER Cancer Statistics Review*. Bethesda, MD: National Cancer Institute; 1975. https://seer.cancer.gov/csr/1975_2015

5. Jawad MU, Cheung MC, Min ES, et al. Ewing sarcoma demonstrates racial disparities in incidence-related and sex-related differences in outcome. *Cancer*. 2009;115(15):3526–3536. doi:10.1002/cncr.24388
6. Hense HW, Ahrens S, Paulussen M, et al. Deskriptive Epidemiologie der Ewing-Tumoren–Analysen der deutschen Patienten von (EI) CESS 1980-1997. *Klin Padiatr*. 1999;211(4):271–275. doi:10.1055/s-2008-1043799
7. Zucman-Rossi J, Batzer MA, Stoneking M, et al. Interethnic polymorphism of EWS intron 6: genome plasticity mediated by Alu retroposition and recombination. *Hum Genet*. 1997;99(3):357–363. doi:10.1007/s004390050372
8. Postel-Vinay S, Véron AS, Tirode F, et al. Common variants near TARDBP and EGR2 are associated with susceptibility to Ewing sarcoma. *Nat Genet*. 2012;44:323–327. doi:10.1038/ng.1085
9. Beck R, Monument MJ, Watkins WS, et al. EWS/FLI-responsive GGAA microsatellites exhibit polymorphic differences between European and African populations. *Cancer Genet*. 2012;205(6):304–312. doi:10.1016/j.cancergen.2012.04.004
10. Selvanathan SP, Graham GT, Erkizan HV, et al. Oncogenic fusion protein EWS-FLI1 is a network hub that regulates alternative splicing. *Proc Natl Acad Sci U S A*. 2015;112(11):E1307–E1316. doi:10.1073/pnas.1500536112
11. Tirode F, Surdez D, Ma X, et al. Genomic landscape of Ewing sarcoma defines an aggressive subtype with co-association of STAG2 and TP53 mutations. *Cancer Discov*. 2014;4(11):1342–1353. doi:10.1158/2159-8290.CD-14-0622
12. Shern JF, Chen L, Chmielecki J, et al. Comprehensive genomic analysis of rhabdomyosarcoma reveals a landscape of alterations affecting a common genetic axis in fusion-positive and fusion-negative tumors. *Cancer Discov*. 2014;4(2):216–231. doi:10.1158/2159-8290.CD-13-0639
13. Huang HY, Illei PB, Zhao Z, et al. Ewing sarcomas with p53 mutation or p16/p14ARF homozygous deletion: a highly lethal subset associated with poor chemoresponse. *J Clin Oncol*. 2005;23(3):548–558. doi:10.1200/JCO.2005.02.081
14. Zhang J, Walsh MF, Wu G, et al. Germline mutations in predisposition genes in pediatric cancer. *N Engl J Med*. 2015;373(24):2336–2346. doi:10.1056/NEJMoa1508054
15. Brasme JF, Chalumeau M, Oberlin O, et al. Time to diagnosis of Ewing tumors in children and adolescents is not associated with metastasis or survival: a prospective multicenter study of 436 patients. *J Clin Oncol*. 2014;32(18):1935–1940. doi:10.1200/JCO.2013.53.8058
16. Worch J, Ranft A, DuBois SG, et al. Age dependency of primary tumor sites and metastases in patients with Ewing sarcoma. *Pediatr Blood Cancer*. 2018;65(9):e27251. doi:10.1002/pbc.27251
17. Applebaum MA, Worch J, Matthay KK, et al. Clinical features and outcomes in patients with extraskeletal Ewing sarcoma. *Cancer*. 2011;117(13):3027–3032. doi:10.1002/cncr.25840
18. Bernstein M, Kovar H, Paulussen M, et al. Ewing's sarcoma family of tumors: current management. *Oncologist*. 2006;11(5):503–519. doi:10.1634/theoncologist.11-5-503
19. Balamuth NJ, Womer RB. Ewing's sarcoma. *Lancet Oncol*. 2010;11(2):184–192. doi:10.1016/S1470-2045(09)70286-4
20. Franzius C, Sciuk J, Daldrup-Link HE, et al. FDG-PET for detection of osseous metastases from malignant primary bone tumours: comparison with bone scintigraphy. *Eur J Nucl Med*. 2000;27(9):1305–1311. doi:10.1007/s002590000301
21. Nesbit ME Jr, Perez CA, Tefft M, et al. Multimodal therapy for the management of primary, nonmetastatic Ewing's sarcoma of bone: an intergroup study. *Natl Cancer Inst Monogr*. 1981(56):255–262. PMID:7029293
22. Womer RB, West DC, Krailo MD, et al. Randomized controlled trial of interval-compressed chemotherapy for the treatment of localized Ewing sarcoma: a report from the Children's Oncology Group. *J Clin Oncol*. 2012;30(33):4148–4154. doi:10.1200/JCO.2011.41.5703
23. Miser JS, Goldsby RE, Chen Z, et al. Treatment of metastatic Ewing sarcoma/primitive neuroectodermal tumor of bone: evaluation of increasing the dose intensity of chemotherapy—a report from the Children's Oncology Group. *Pediatr Blood Cancer*. 2007;49(7):894–900. doi:10.1002/pbc.21233
24. Burgert EO Jr, Nesbit ME, Garnsey LA, et al. Multimodal therapy for the management of nonpelvic, localized Ewing's sarcoma of bone: intergroup study IESS-II. *J Clin Oncol*. 1990;8(9):1514–1524. doi:10.1200/JCO.1990.8.9.1514
25. Grier HE, Krailo MD, Tarbell NJ, et al. Addition of ifosfamide and etoposide to standard chemotherapy for Ewing's sarcoma and primitive neuroectodermal tumor of bone. *N Engl J Med*. 2003;348(8):694–701. doi:10.1056/NEJMoa020890
26. Granowetter L, Womer R, Devidas M, et al. Dose-intensified compared with standard chemotherapy for nonmetastatic Ewing sarcoma family of tumors: a Children's Oncology Group Study. *J Clin Oncol*. 2009;27(15):2536–2541. doi:10.1200/JCO.2008.19.1478
27. Pappo AS, Patel SR, Crowley J, et al. R1507, a monoclonal antibody to the insulin-like growth factor 1 receptor, in patients with recurrent or refractory Ewing sarcoma family of tumors: results of a phase II Sarcoma Alliance for Research through Collaboration study. *J Clin Oncol*. 2011;29(34):4541–4547. doi:10.1200/JCO.2010.34.0000
28. Juergens H, Daw NC, Geoerger B, et al. Preliminary efficacy of the anti-insulin-like growth factor type 1 receptor antibody figitumumab in patients with refractory Ewing sarcoma. *J Clin Oncol*. 2011;29(34):4534–4540. doi:10.1200/JCO.2010.33.0670
29. Whelan J, Le Deley MC, Dirksen U, et al. High-dose chemotherapy and blood autologous stem-cell rescue compared with standard chemotherapy in localized high-risk Ewing sarcoma: results of Euro-E.W.I.N.G.99 and Ewing-2008. *J Clin Oncol*. 2018;36(31):3110–3119. doi:10.1200/JCO.2018.78.2516

30. Juergens C, Weston C, Lewis I, et al. Safety assessment of intensive induction with vincristine, ifosfamide, doxorubicin, and etoposide (VIDE) in the treatment of Ewing tumors in the EURO-E.W.I.N.G. 99 clinical trial. *Pediatr Blood Cancer*. 2006;47(1):22–29. doi:10.1002/pbc.20820
31. Schuck A, Ahrens S, Paulussen M, et al. Local therapy in localized Ewing tumors: results of 1058 patients treated in the CESS 81, CESS 86, and EICESS 92 trials. *Int J Radiat Oncol Biol Phys*. 2003;55(1):168–177. doi:10.1016/s0360-3016(02)03797-5
32. Miller BJ, Gao Y, Duchman KR. Does surgery or radiation provide the best overall survival in Ewing's sarcoma? A review of the National Cancer Data Base. *J Surg Oncol*. 2017;116(3):384–390. doi:10.1002/jso.24652
33. Ginsberg JP, Goodman P, Leisenring W, et al. Long-term survivors of childhood Ewing sarcoma: report from the childhood cancer survivor study. *J Natl Cancer Inst*. 2010;102(16):1272–1283. doi:10.1093/jnci/djq278
34. Rodríguez-Galindo C, Navid F, Liu T, et al. Prognostic factors for local and distant control in Ewing sarcoma family of tumors. *Ann Oncol*. 2008;19(4):814–820. doi:10.1093/annonc/mdm521
35. Hunold A, Weddeling N, Paulussen M, et al. Topotecan and cyclophosphamide in patients with refractory or relapsed Ewing tumors. *Pediatr Blood Cancer*. 2006;47(6):795–800. doi:10.1002/pbc.20719
36. Raciborska A, Bilska K, Drabko K, et al. Vincristine, irinotecan, and temozolomide in patients with relapsed and refractory Ewing sarcoma. *Pediatr Blood Cancer*. 2013;60(10):1621–1625. doi:10.1002/pbc.24621
37. Gardner SL, Carreras J, Boudreau C, et al. Myeloablative therapy with autologous stem cell rescue for patients with Ewing sarcoma. *Bone Marrow Transplant*. 2008;41(10):867–872. doi:10.1038/bmt.2008.2
38. Tang S-W, Bilke S, Cao L, et al. SLFN11 is a transcriptional target of EWS-FLI1 and a determinant of drug response in Ewing sarcoma. *Clin Cancer Res*. 2015;21(18):4184–4193. doi:10.1158/1078-0432.CCR-14-2112
39. Theisen ER, Pishas KI, Saund RS, Lessnick SL. Therapeutic opportunities in Ewing sarcoma: EWS-FLI inhibition via LSD1 targeting. *Oncotarget*. 2016;7(14):17616–17630. doi:10.18632/oncotarget.7124
40. Zöllner SK, Selvanathan SP, Graham GT, et al. Inhibition of the oncogenic fusion protein EWS-FLI1 causes G-M cell cycle arrest and enhanced vincristine sensitivity in Ewing's sarcoma. *Sci Signal*. 2017;10(499). doi:10.1126/scisignal.aam8429
41. Mirabello L, Troisi RJ, Savage SA. Osteosarcoma incidence and survival rates from 1973 to 2004: data from the Surveillance, Epidemiology, and End Results Program. *Cancer*. 2009;115(7):1531–1543. doi:10.1002/cncr.24121
42. Isakoff MS, Bielack SS, Meltzer P, Gorlick R. Osteosarcoma: current treatment and a collaborative pathway to success. *J Clin Oncol*. 2015;33(27):3029–3035. doi:10.1200/JCO.2014.59.4895
43. Kansara M, Thomas DM. Molecular pathogenesis of osteosarcoma. *DNA Cell Biol*. 2007;26(1):1–18. doi:10.1089/dna.2006.0505
44. PDQ® Pediatric Treatment Editorial Board. *PDQ osteosarcoma and malignant fibrous histiocytoma of bone treatment*. Bethesda, MD: National Cancer Institute. 2002. https://www.cancer.gov/types/bone/hp/osteosarcoma-treatment-pdq
45. Fidler MM, Reulen RC, Winter DL, et al. Risk of subsequent bone cancers among 69 460 five-year survivors of childhood and adolescent cancer in Europe. *J Natl Cancer Inst*. 2018;110(2):183–194. doi:10.1093/jnci/djx165
46. Mirabello L, Yeager M, Mai PL, et al. Germline TP53 variants and susceptibility to osteosarcoma. *J Natl Cancer Inst*. 2015;107(7). doi:10.1093/jnci/djv101
47. Chen X, Bahrami A, Pappo A, et al. Recurrent somatic structural variations contribute to tumorigenesis in pediatric osteosarcoma. *Cell Rep*. 2014;7(1):104–112. doi:10.1016/j.celrep.2014.03.003
48. Perry JA, Kiezun A, Tonzi P, et al. Complementary genomic approaches highlight the PI3K/mTOR pathway as a common vulnerability in osteosarcoma. *Proc Natl Acad Sci U S A*. 2014;111(51):E5564–E5573. doi:10.1073/pnas.1419260111
49. Bielack SS, Kempf-Bielack B, Delling G, et al. Prognostic factors in high-grade osteosarcoma of the extremities or trunk: an analysis of 1,702 patients treated on Neoadjuvant Cooperative Osteosarcoma Study Group Protocols. *J Clin Oncol*. 2002;20(3):776–790. doi:10.1200/JCO.2002.20.3.776
50. Goyal S, Roscoe J, Ryder WD, et al. Symptom interval in young people with bone cancer. *Eur J Cancer*. 2004;40(15):2280–2286. doi:10.1016/j.ejca.2004.05.017
51. Whelan JS, Davis LE. Osteosarcoma, chondrosarcoma, and chordoma. *J Clin Oncol*. 2018;36(2):188–193. doi:10.1200/JCO.2017.75.1743
52. Link MP, Goorin AM, Horowitz M, et al. Adjuvant chemotherapy of high-grade osteosarcoma of the extremity. Updated results of the Multi-Institutional Osteosarcoma Study. *Clin Orthop Relat Res*. 1991;(270):8–14. doi:10.1097/00003086-199109000-00003
53. Rosen G, Carparros B, Huvos AG, et al. Preoperative chemotherapy for osteogenic sarcoma: selection of postoperative adjuvant chemotherapy based on the response of the primary tumor to preoperative chemotherapy. *Cancer*. 1982;49(6):1221–1230. doi:10.1002/1097-0142(19820315)49:6<1221::AID-CNCR2820490625>3.0..CO;2-E
54. Rosen G, Marcove RC, Caparros B, et al. Primary osteogenic sarcoma: the rationale for preoperative chemotherapy and delayed surgery. *Cancer*. 1979;43(6):2163–2177. doi:10.1002/1097-0142(197906)43:6<2163::AID-CNCR2820430602>3.0.CO;2-S
55. Bacci G, Avella M, Capanna R, et al. Neoadjuvant chemotherapy in the treatment of osteosarcoma of the extremities: preliminary results in 131 cases treated preoperatively with methotrexate and cisdiamminoplatinum. *Ital J Orthop Traumatol*. 1988;14(1):23–39.

56. Goorin AM, Schwartzentruber DJ, Devidas M, et al. Presurgical chemotherapy compared with immediate surgery and adjuvant chemotherapy for nonmetastatic osteosarcoma: Pediatric Oncology Group Study POG-8651. *J Clin Oncol*. 2003;21(8):1574–1580. doi:10.1200/JCO.2003.08.165
57. Meyers PA, Schwartz CL, Krailo M, et al. Osteosarcoma: a randomized, prospective trial of the addition of ifosfamide and/or muramyl tripeptide to cisplatin, doxorubicin, and high-dose methotrexate. *J Clin Oncol*. 2005;23(9):2004–2011. doi:10.1200/JCO.2005.06.031
58. Meyers PA, Schwartz CL, Krailo M, et al. Osteosarcoma: the addition of muramyl tripeptide to chemotherapy improves overall survival—a report from the Children's Oncology Group. *J Clin Oncol*. 2008;26(4):633–638. doi:10.1200/JCO.2008.14.0095
59. Lewis IJ, Nooji MA, Whelan J, et al. Improvement in histologic response but not survival in osteosarcoma patients treated with intensified chemotherapy: a randomized phase III trial of the European Osteosarcoma Intergroup. *J Natl Cancer Inst*. 2007;99(2):112–128. doi:10.1093/jnci/djk015
60. Bielack SS, Smeland S, Whelan JS, et al. Methotrexate, doxorubicin, and cisplatin (MAP) plus maintenance pegylated interferon alfa-2b versus MAP alone in patients with resectable high-grade osteosarcoma and good histologic response to preoperative MAP: first results of the EURAMOS-1 Good Response randomized controlled trial. *J Clin Oncol*. 2015;33(20):2279–2287. doi:10.1200/JCO.2014.60.0734
61. Marina NM, Smelan S, Bielack SS, et al. Comparison of MAPIE versus MAP in patients with a poor response to preoperative chemotherapy for newly diagnosed high-grade osteosarcoma (EURAMOS-1): an open-label, international, randomised controlled trial. *Lancet Oncol*. 2016;17(10):1396–1408. doi:10.1016/S1470-2045(16)30214-5
62. Gill J, Ahluwalia MK, Geller D, Gorlick R. New targets and approaches in osteosarcoma. *Pharmacol Ther*. 2013;137(1):89–99. doi:10.1016/j.pharmthera.2012.09.003
63. Cortes EP, Holland JF, Wang JJ, et al. Doxorubicin in disseminated. *JAMA*. 1972;221(10):1132–1138. doi:10.1001/jama.1972.03200230020005
64. Cortes EP, Holland JF, Wang JJ, et al. Amputation and adriamycin in primary osteosarcoma. *N Engl J Med*. 1974;291(19):998–1000. doi:10.1056/NEJM197411072911903
65. Jaffe N, Frei E 3rd, Traggis D, Bishop Y. Adjuvant methotrexate and citrovorum-factor treatment of osteogenic sarcoma. *N Engl J Med*. 1974;291(19):994–997. doi:10.1056/NEJM197411072911902
66. Marti C, Kroner T, Remagen W, et al. High-dose ifosfamide in advanced osteosarcoma. *Cancer Treat Rep*. 1985;69(1):115–117. PMID:3855382.
67. Link MP, Goorin AM, Horowitz M, et al. Adjuvant chemotherapy of high-grade osteosarcoma of the extremity. Updated results of the Multi-Institutional Osteosarcoma Study. *Clin Orthop Relat Res*. 1991;(270):8–14. doi:10.1097/00003086-199109000-00003
68. Bacci G, Ferrari S, Bertoni F, et al. Long-term outcome for patients with nonmetastatic osteosarcoma of the extremity treated at the Istituto Ortopedico Rizzoli according to the Istituto Ortopedico Rizzoli/Osteosarcoma-2 Protocol: an updated report. *J Clin Oncol*. 2000;18(24):4016–4027. doi:10.1200/JCO.2000.18.24.4016
69. Ciernik IF, Niemierko A, Harmon DC, et al. Proton-based radiotherapy for unresectable or incompletely resected osteosarcoma. *Cancer*. 2011;117(19):4522–4530. doi:10.1002/cncr.26037
70. Andreou D, Bielack SS, Carrle D, et al. The influence of tumor- and treatment-related factors on the development of local recurrence in osteosarcoma after adequate surgery. An analysis of 1355 patients treated on neoadjuvant Cooperative Osteosarcoma Study Group protocols. *Ann Oncol*. 2011;22(5):1228–1235. doi:10.1093/annonc/mdq589
71. Kager L, Zoubek A, Pötschger U, et al. Primary metastatic osteosarcoma: presentation and outcome of patients treated on Neoadjuvant Cooperative Osteosarcoma Study Group protocols. *J Clin Oncol*. 2003;21(10):2011–2018. doi:10.1200/JCO.2003.08.132
72. Nagarajan R, Kamruzzaman A, Ness KK, et al. Twenty years of follow-up of survivors of childhood osteosarcoma: a report from the Childhood Cancer Survivor Study. *Cancer*. 2011;117(3):625–634. doi:10.1002/cncr.25446
73. Kempf-Bielack B, Bielack SS, Jürgens H, et al. Osteosarcoma relapse after combined modality therapy: an analysis of unselected patients in the Cooperative Osteosarcoma Study Group (COSS). *J Clin Oncol*. 2005;23(3):559–568. doi:10.1200/JCO.2005.04.063
74. Spraker-Perlman HL, Barkauskas DA, Krailo MD, et al. Factors influencing survival after recurrence in osteosarcoma: A report from the Children's Oncology Group. *Pediatr Blood Cancer*. 2019;66(1):e27444. doi:10.1002/pbc.27444
75. Gelderblom H, Jinks RC, Sydes M, et al. Survival after recurrent osteosarcoma: data from 3 European Osteosarcoma Intergroup (EOI) randomized controlled trials. *Eur J Cancer*. 2011;47(6):895–902. doi:10.1016/j.ejca.2010.11.036
76. Harting MT, Blakely ML, Jaffe N, et al. Long-term survival after aggressive resection of pulmonary metastases among children and adolescents with osteosarcoma. *J Pediatr Surg*. 2006;41(1):194–199. doi:10.1016/j.jpedsurg.2005.10.089
77. Rodriguez-Galindo C, Shah N, McCarville MB, et al. Outcome after local recurrence of osteosarcoma: the St. Jude Children's Research Hospital experience (1970-2000). *Cancer*. 2004;100(9):1928–1935. doi:10.1002/cncr.20214
78. Bacci G, Briccoli A, Longhi A, et al. Treatment and outcome of recurrent osteosarcoma: experience at Rizzoli in 235 patients initially treated with neoadjuvant chemotherapy. *Acta Oncol*. 2005;44(7):748–755. doi:10.1080/02841860500327503

79. Chou AJ, Merola PR, Wexler LH, et al. Treatment of osteosarcoma at first recurrence after contemporary therapy: the Memorial Sloan-Kettering Cancer Center experience. *Cancer*. 2005;104(10):2214–2221. doi:10.1002/cncr.21417
80. Daw NC, Chou AJ, Jaffe N, et al. Recurrent osteosarcoma with a single pulmonary metastasis: a multi-institutional review. *Br J Cancer*. 2015;112(2):278–282. doi:10.1038/bjc.2014.585
81. Duffaud F, Blay J-Y, Mir O, et al. Results of randomized, placebo (PL)-controlled phase II study evaluating efficacy and safety of regorafenib (REG) in patients (pts) with metastatic osteosarcoma (metOS), on behalf of the French Sarcoma Group (FSG) and Unicancer. *J Clin Oncol*. 2018;36(15_suppl):11504–11504.
82. Guenther LM, Rowe RG, Acharya PT, et al. Response Evaluation Criteria in Solid Tumors (RECIST) following neoadjuvant chemotherapy in osteosarcoma. *Pediatr Blood Cancer*. 2018;65(4). doi:10.1002/pbc.26896
83. Lagmay JP, Krailo MD, Dang H, et al. Outcome of patients with recurrent osteosarcoma enrolled in seven Phase II trials through Children's Cancer Group, Pediatric Oncology Group, and Children's Oncology Group: learning from the past to move forward. *J Clin Oncol*. 2016;34(25):3031–3038. doi:10.1200/JCO.2015.65.5381
84. Isakoff MS, Goldsby R, Villauna D, et al. A phase II study of eribulin in recurrent or refractory osteosarcoma: a report from the Children's Oncology Group. *Pediatr Blood Cancer*. 2019;66(2):e27524. doi:10.1002/pbc.27524
85. Anderson PM, Wiseman GA, Dispenzieri A, et al. High-dose samarium-153 ethylene diamine tetramethylene phosphonate: low toxicity of skeletal irradiation in patients with osteosarcoma and bone metastases. *J Clin Oncol*. 2002;20(1):189–196. doi:10.1200/JCO.2002.20.1.189
86. Ries LG, Smith M, Gurney JG, et al, eds. *Cancer Incidence and Survival Among Children and Adolescents: United States SEER Program 1975-1995, National Cancer Institute, SEER Program*. NIH Pub. No. 99-4649. Bethesda, MD: National Cancer Institute; 1999.
87. Chang F, Syrjanen S, Syrjanen K. Implications of the p53 tumor-suppressor gene in clinical oncology. *J Clin Oncol*. 1995;13(4):1009–1022. doi:10.1200/JCO.1995.13.4.1009
88. Groen EJ, Roos A, Muntinghe FL, et al. Extra-intestinal manifestations of familial adenomatous polyposis. *Ann Surg Oncol*. 2008;15(9):2439–2450. doi:10.1245/s10434-008-9981-3
89. Wong JR, Morton LM, Tucker MA, et al. Risk of subsequent malignant neoplasms in long-term hereditary retinoblastoma survivors after chemotherapy and radiotherapy. *J Clin Oncol*. 2014;32(29):3284–3290. doi:10.1200/JCO.2013.54.7844
90. Eaton KW, Tooke LS, Wainwright LM, et al. Spectrum of SMARCB1/INI1 mutations in familial and sporadic rhabdoid tumors. *Pediatr Blood Cancer*. 2011;56(1):7–15. doi:10.1002/pbc.22831
91. Rubin BP, Fletcher CDM, Inwards C, et al. Protocol for the examination of specimens from patients with soft tissue tumors of intermediate malignant potential, malignant soft tissue tumors, and benign/locally aggressive and malignant bone tumors. *Arch Pathol Lab Med*. 2006;130(11):1616–1629. doi:10.1043/1543-2165(2006)130[1616:PFTEOS]2.0.CO;2
92. deCou JM, Rao BN, Parham DM, et al. Malignant peripheral nerve sheath tumors: the St. Jude Children's Research Hospital experience. *Ann Surg Oncol*. 1995;2(6):524–529. doi:10.1007/bf02307086
93. Stark AM, Buhl R, Hugo HH, Mehdorn HM. Malignant peripheral nerve sheath tumours—report of 8 cases and review of the literature. *Acta Neurochir (Wien)*. 2001;143(4):357–363; discussion 363–364. doi:10.1007/s007010170090
94. Goto M, Miller RW, Ishikawa Y, Sugano H. Excess of rare cancers in Werner syndrome (adult progeria). *Cancer Epidemiol Biomarkers Prev*. 1996;5(4):239–246. https://www.ncbi.nlm.nih.gov/pubmed/8722214
95. Fricke BL, Donnelly LF, Casper KA, Bissler JJ. Frequency and imaging appearance of hepatic angiomyolipomas in pediatric and adult patients with tuberous sclerosis. *AJR Am J Roentgenol*. 2004;182(4):1027–1030. doi:10.2214/ajr.182.4.1821027
96. Hornick JL, Fletcher CDM. PEComa: what do we know so far? *Histopathology*. 2006;48(1):75–82. doi:10.1111/j.1365-2559.2005.02316.x
97. Kesserwan C, Sokolic R, Cowen EW, et al. Multicentric dermatofibrosarcoma protuberans in patients with adenosine deaminase-deficient severe combined immune deficiency. *J Allergy Clin Immunol*. 2012;129(3):762–769.e1. doi:10.1016/j.jaci.2011.10.028
98. PDQ® Pediatric Treatment Editorial Board. *PDQ childhood soft tissue sarcoma treatment*. Bethesda, MD: National Cancer Institute. 2002. https://www.cancer.gov/types/soft-tissue-sarcoma/hp/child-soft-tissue-treatment-pdq
99. Laetsch TW, DuBois SG, Mascarenhas L, et al. Larotrectinib for paediatric solid tumours harbouring NTRK gene fusions: phase 1 results from a multicentre, open-label, phase 1/2 study. *Lancet Oncol*. 2018;19(5):705–714. doi:10.1016/S1470-2045(18)30119-0
100. Slater O, Shipley J. Clinical relevance of molecular genetics to paediatric sarcomas. *J Clin Pathol*. 2007;60(11):1187–1194. doi:10.1136/jcp.2006.040113
101. Sandberg AA. Translocations in malignant tumors. *Am J Pathol*. 2001;159(6):1979–1980. doi:10.1016/S0002-9440(10)63047-7
102. Mertens F, Antonescu CR, Hohenberger P, et al. Translocation-related sarcomas. *Semin Oncol*. 2009;36(4):312–323. doi:10.1053/j.seminoncol.2009.06.004
103. Khoury JD, Coffin CM, Spunt SL, et al. Grading of nonrhabdomyosarcoma soft tissue sarcoma in children and adolescents: a comparison of parameters used for the Fédération Nationale des Centers de Lutte Contre le Cancer and Pediatric Oncology Group systems. *Cancer*. 2010;116(9):2266–2274. doi:10.1002/cncr.24929

104. Ferrari A, Chi YY, De Salvo GL, et al. Surgery alone is sufficient therapy for children and adolescents with low-risk synovial sarcoma: a joint analysis from the European Paediatric Soft Tissue Sarcoma Study Group and the Children's Oncology Group. *Eur J Cancer*. 2017;78:1–6. doi:10.1016/j.ejca.2017.03.003
105. Stacchiotti S, Negri T, Zaffaroni N, et al. Sunitinib in advanced alveolar soft part sarcoma: evidence of a direct antitumor effect. *Ann Oncol*. 2011;22(7):1682–1690. doi:10.1093/annonc/mdq644
106. Flores RJ, Harrison DJ, Federman NC, et al. Alveolar soft part sarcoma in children and young adults: a report of 69 cases. *Pediatr Blood Cancer*. 2018;65(5):e26953. doi:10.1002/pbc.26953
107. Kummar S, Allen D, Monks A, et al. Cediranib for metastatic alveolar soft part sarcoma. *J Clin Oncol*. 2013;31(18):2296–2302. doi:10.1200/JCO.2012.47.4288
108. Sasaki T, Okuda K, Zheng W, et al. The neuroblastoma-associated F1174L ALK mutation causes resistance to an ALK kinase inhibitor in ALK-translocated cancers. *Cancer Res*. 2010;70(24):10038–10043. doi:10.1158/0008-5472.CAN-10-2956
109. Mossé YP, Voss SD, Lim MS, et al. Targeting ALK with crizotinib in pediatric anaplastic large cell lymphoma and inflammatory myofibroblastic tumor: a Children's Oncology Group study. *J Clin Oncol*. 2017;35(28):3215–3221. doi:10.1200/JCO.2017.73.4830
110. Gounder MM, Mahoney MR, Van Tine BA, et al. Sorafenib for advanced and refractory desmoid tumors. *N Engl J Med*. 2018;379(25):2417–2428. doi:10.1056/NEJMoa1805052
111. Italiano A, Soria J-C, Toulmonde M, et al. Tazemetostat, an EZH2 inhibitor, in relapsed or refractory B-cell non-Hodgkin lymphoma and advanced solid tumours: a first-in-human, open-label, phase 1 study. *Lancet Oncol*. 2018;19(5):649–659. doi:10.1016/S1470-2045(18)30145-1
112. Gibson TM, Mostoufi-Moab S, Stratton KL, et al. Temporal patterns in the risk of chronic health conditions in survivors of childhood cancer diagnosed 1970-99: a report from the Childhood Cancer Survivor Study cohort. *Lancet Oncol*. 2018;19(12):1590–1601. doi:10.1016/S1470-2045(18)30537-0
113. Bergamaschi L, Bisogno G, Manzitti C, et al. Salvage rates and prognostic factors after relapse in children and adolescents with malignant peripheral nerve sheath tumors. *Pediatr Blood Cancer*. 2018;65(2):e26816. doi:10.1002/pbc.26816
114. Seddon B, Strauss SJ, Whelan J, et al. Gemcitabine and docetaxel versus doxorubicin as first-line treatment in previously untreated advanced unresectable or metastatic soft-tissue sarcomas (GeDDiS): a randomised controlled phase 3 trial. *Lancet Oncol*. 2017;18(10):1397–1410. doi:10.1016/S1470-2045(17)30622-8
115. van der Graaf WT, Blay JY, Chawla SP, et al. Pazopanib for metastatic soft-tissue sarcoma (PALETTE): a randomised, double-blind, placebo-controlled phase 3 trial. *Lancet*. 2012;379(9829):1879–1886. doi:10.1016/S0140-6736(12)60651-5
116. Herzog J, von Klot-Heydenfeldt F, Jabar S, et al. Trabectedin followed by irinotecan can stabilize disease in advanced translocation-positive sarcomas with acceptable toxicity. *Sarcoma*. 2016;2016:7461783. doi:10.1155/2016/7461783
117. Schafer ES, Rau RE, Berg S, et al. A phase 1 study of eribulin mesylate (E7389), a novel microtubule-targeting chemotherapeutic agent, in children with refractory or recurrent solid tumors: a Children's Oncology Group Phase 1 consortium study (ADVL1314). *Pediatr Blood Cancer*. 2018;65(8):e27066. doi:10.1002/pbc.27066
118. Casillas J, Ross J, Keohan, ML. Soft tissue sarcomas. In: Bleyer A, Barr R, Ries LAG, eds. *Cancer Epidemiology in Older Adolescents and Young Adults 15 to 29 Years of Age, Including SEER Incidence and Survival: 1975-2000*. Bethesda, MD: National Cancer Institute; 1975:81–96.
119. Ognjanovic S, Linabery AM, Charbonneau B, Ross JA. Trends in childhood rhabdomyosarcoma incidence and survival in the United States, 1975–2005. *Cancer*. 2009;115(18):4218–4226. doi:10.1002/cncr.24465
120. Skapek SX, Ferrari A, Gupta AA, et al. Rhabdomyosarcoma. *Nat Rev Dis Primers*. 2019;5(1):1. doi:10.1038/s41572-018-0051-2
121. Diller L, Sexsmith E, Gottlieb A, et al. Germline p53 mutations are frequently detected in young children with rhabdomyosarcoma. *J Clin Invest*. 1995;95(4):1606–1611. doi:10.1172/JCI117834
122. Chen X, Stewart E, Shelat AA, et al. Targeting oxidative stress in embryonal rhabdomyosarcoma. *Cancer Cell*. 2013;24(6):710–724. doi:10.1016/j.ccr.2013.11.002
123. Agaram NP, LaQuaglia MP, Alaggio R, et al. MYOD1-mutant spindle cell and sclerosing rhabdomyosarcoma: an aggressive subtype irrespective of age. A reappraisal for molecular classification and risk stratification. *Mod Pathol*. 2019;32(1):27–36. doi:10.1038/s41379-018-0120-9
124. Alaggio R, Zhang L, Sung Y-S, et al. A molecular study of pediatric spindle and sclerosing rhabdomyosarcoma: identification of novel and recurrent VGLL2-related fusions in infantile cases. *Am J Surg Pathol*. 2016;40(2):224–235. doi:10.1097/PAS.0000000000000538
125. Crist W, Gehan EA, Ragab AH, et al. The Third Intergroup Rhabdomyosarcoma Study. *J Clin Oncol*. 1995;13(3):610–630. doi:10.1200/JCO.1995.13.3.610
126. Breneman JC, Lyden E, Pappo AS, et al. Prognostic factors and clinical outcomes in children and adolescents with metastatic rhabdomyosarcoma—a report from the Intergroup Rhabdomyosarcoma Study IV. *J Clin Oncol*. 2003;21(1):78–84. doi:10.1200/JCO.2003.06.129
127. Walterhouse DO, Barkauskas DA, Hall D, et al. Demographic and treatment variables influencing outcome for localized paratesticular rhabdomyosarcoma: results from a pooled analysis of North American and European Cooperative Groups. *J Clin Oncol*. 2018;36(35):3466–3476. doi:10.1200/JCO.2018.78.9388

128. La TH, Wolden SL, Rodeberg DA, et al. Regional nodal involvement and patterns of spread along in-transit pathways in children with rhabdomyosarcoma of the extremity: a report from the Children's Oncology Group. *Int J Radiat Oncol Biol Phys*. 2011;80(4):1151–1157. doi:10.1016/j.ijrobp.2010.03.050
129. Malempati S, Hawkins DS. Rhabdomyosarcoma: review of the Children's Oncology Group (COG) Soft-Tissue Sarcoma Committee experience and rationale for current COG studies. *Pediatr Blood Cancer*. 2012;59(1):5–10. doi:10.1002/pbc.24118
130. Malempati S, Weigel BJ, Chi YY, et al. The addition of cixutumumab or temozolomide to intensive multiagent chemotherapy is feasible but does not improve outcome for patients with metastatic rhabdomyosarcoma. *Cancer*. 2019;125(2):290–297. doi:10.1002/cncr.31770
131. Spunt SL, Smith LM, Ruymann FB, et al. Cyclophosphamide dose intensification during induction therapy for intermediate-risk pediatric rhabdomyosarcoma is feasible but does not improve outcome: a report from the Soft Tissue Sarcoma Committee of the Children's Oncology Group. *Clin Cancer Res*. 2004;10(18 Pt 1):6072–6079. doi:10.1158/1078-0432.CCR-04-0654
132. Walterhouse DO, Pappo AS, Meza JL, et al. Shorter-duration therapy using vincristine, dactinomycin, and lower-dose cyclophosphamide with or without radiotherapy for patients with newly diagnosed low-risk rhabdomyosarcoma: a report from the Soft Tissue Sarcoma Committee of the Children's Oncology Group. *J Clin Oncol*. 2014;32(31):3547–3552. doi:10.1200/JCO.2014.55.6787
133. Bisogno G, De Salvo GL, Bergeron C, et al. Maintenance low-dose chemotherapy in patients with high-risk (HR) rhabdomyosarcoma (RMS): a report from the European Paediatric Soft Tissue Sarcoma Study Group (EpSSG). *J Clin Oncol*. 2018;36(18_suppl):LBA2–LBA2. doi:10.1200/JCO.2018.36.18_suppl.LBA2
134. Pappo AS, Dirksen U. Rhabdomyosarcoma, Ewing sarcoma, and other round cell sarcomas. *J Clin Oncol*. 2018;36(2):168–179. doi:10.1200/JCO.2017.74.7402
135. Oberlin O, Rey A, Lyden E, et al. Prognostic factors in metastatic rhabdomyosarcomas: results of a pooled analysis from United States and European cooperative groups. *J Clin Oncol*. 2008;26(14):2384–2389. doi:10.1200/JCO.2007.14.7207
136. Punyko JA, Mertens AC, Gurney JG, et al. Long-term medical effects of childhood and adolescent rhabdomyosarcoma: a report from the childhood cancer survivor study. *Pediatr Blood Cancer*. 2005;44(7):643–653. doi:10.1002/pbc.20310
137. Pappo AS, Anderson JR, Crist WM, et al. Survival after relapse in children and adolescents with rhabdomyosarcoma: a report from the Intergroup Rhabdomyosarcoma Study Group. *J Clin Oncol*. 1999;17(11):3487–3493. doi:10.1200/JCO.1999.17.11.3487
138. Mascarenhas L, Meyer WH, Lyden E, et al. Randomized phase II trial of bevacizumab and temsirolimus in combination with vinorelbine (V) and cyclophosphamide (C) for first relapse/disease progression of rhabdomyosarcoma (RMS): a report from the Children's Oncology Group (COG). *J Clin Oncol*. 2014;32(15_suppl):10003. doi:10.1200/jco.2014.32.15_suppl.10003
139. Mackall CL, Helman LJ. High-dose chemotherapy for rhabdomyosarcoma: where do we go from here. *J Pediatr Hematol Oncol*. 2001;23(5):266–267. doi:10.1097/00043426-200106000-00005
140. Stewart E, McEvoy J, Wang H, et al. Identification of therapeutic targets in rhabdomyosarcoma through integrated genomic, epigenomic, and proteomic analyses. *Cancer Cell*. 2018;34(3):411.e19–426.e19. doi:10.1016/j.ccell.2018.07.012
141. Spunt SL, Million L, Anderson JR, et al. Risk-based treatment for nonrhabdomyosarcoma soft tissue sarcomas (NRSTS) in patients under 30 years of age: Children's Oncology Group study ARST0332. *J Clin Oncol*. 2014;32(15_suppl):10008–10008. doi:10.1200/jco.2014.32.15_suppl.10008

7

Radiologic Evaluation of Bone and Soft Tissue Sarcoma at Diagnosis and Follow-Up

Ty K. Subhawong and Felipe F. de Souza

INTRODUCTION

Radiology encompasses a diverse practice ranging from diagnostic imaging to definitive interventional treatments. While the field has become increasingly subspecialized by imaging modality and anatomic domains, sarcoma cuts across multiple subspecialty fields even within radiology. Because sarcomas arise in bone and soft tissue, musculoskeletal radiologists play a particularly prominent role in the diagnosis and management of sarcoma patients.

This chapter focuses on the radiologic evaluation of both bone and soft tissue sarcomas. The most common imaging modalities are reviewed, with an emphasis on understanding the language radiologists use to describe key features of disease. Characteristic radiographic findings that indicate biologic aggressiveness and matrix composition of bone sarcomas, distinguishing features of soft tissue sarcomas, and issues regarding initial staging are described. The chapter also discusses imaging follow-up pertaining to criteria for assessment of treatment response and guidelines for both local and distant disease surveillance.

IMAGING MODALITIES

A brief review of common radiology imaging modalities highlights a few basic principles that may provide a broader understanding of each modality's advantages and drawbacks, as well as a primer for commonly used terminology.

Radiographs

Radiographs are the diagnostic images resulting from exposure of a film (nowadays, digital imaging panel) to x-rays that have passed through a bone and soft tissue. It is interesting to think that little has changed in the basic physics of this modality since Röntgen first published the phenomenon in 1895 (a discovery for which he earned the first Nobel Prize in Physics in 1901); few other medical technologies from that era have endured essentially unaltered. The terms "plain film," "x-ray," and "radiograph" all refer to these two-dimensional clinical images. Denser material (metal, bone) attenuates the x-ray beam and appears white, whereas less dense tissue (e.g., lung) allows the x-rays to pass through unimpeded to expose the film/plate, appearing black (radiolucent). X-ray exposure results in a small dose of ionizing radiation, but the biologic risk of this exposure varies with the anatomic site being imaged and is generally negligible in the extremities at diagnostic imaging dosage. Radiographs are absolutely essential in the evaluation of any osseous abnormality, be it traumatic, neoplastic, developmental, or infectious. This is because of the wealth of information gleaned from this simple and ubiquitous examination: size and location of the lesion, presence and character of tumor mineralization, and biologic aggressiveness.

Computed Tomography

In the early 1970s, Sir Godfrey Hounsfield developed a method for reconstructing images based on three-dimensional exposure to rotating x-rays, revolutionizing medical imaging and sharing the 1979 Nobel Prize in Medicine with Allan Cormack. Differences in tissue density determine tissue contrast and are measured in Hounsfield units (HU). By convention, the scale is set with water at 0 HU, air at −1,000 HU, and fatty tissue between −40 and −120 HU; normal cortical bone is generally >800 HU and healthy muscle is typically around 30 to 40 HU. Lesions may be described as hyperdense, isodense, or hypodense relative to normal muscle or water. Iodinated contrast material may be injected intravenously to improve lesion conspicuity or delineate vascular anatomy. The degree of tumor enhancement with intravenous (IV) contrast material is often used as a surrogate marker for tumor viability, and nonenhancing regions of tumor are assumed to reflect tumor necrosis. Assessing the proportions of enhancing viable tumor and nonenhancing necrotic tumor, and how these proportions change over time, is as critical as measuring changes in tumor dimension when determining sarcoma treatment efficacy.

Magnetic Resonance Imaging

A discussion of the physics of nuclear magnetic resonance, which forms the basis for MRI, is beyond the scope of this chapter. The basic premise is that hydrogen protons (mainly in water) in the body are aligned by a strong magnetic field (clinical strengths commonly at 1.5 and 3.0 T). The protons are spinning, and precess (much like a spinning top) with a specific Larmor frequency. To get signal, the protons must first be energized or "excited" by a radiofrequency (RF) pulse. The RF pulse also brings the proton into phase coherence. The protons then release that energy, or "relax" also by means of radiation. For their work in developing MRI, Peter Mansfield and Paul Lauterbur were awarded the 2003 Nobel Prize in Medicine.

On T1-weighted images, tissue contrast is generated by exploiting differences in the rate at which the protons in different tissues relax to their ground state; for example, protons in fat relax faster than those in free water. A second type of image (T2-weighted) is dependent upon the rate at which the protons dephase; protons in fat and muscle dephase much faster than those in free water. T1-weighted, fat-suppressed T2 (or sometimes proton density [PD])-weighted, and contrast-enhanced T1-weighted (frequently also fat-suppressed) sequences form the standard sequences around which most orthopedic oncology MRI protocols are built.

In this clinically oriented review, we focus on explaining terminology frequently used in clinical radiology reports. With T1 weighting, fat is hyperintense (white) compared to skeletal muscle, and water is dark. T1-weighted images are helpful in evaluating bone marrow, because most marrow in adults (particularly appendicular) comprises yellow or "fatty" marrow; because cellular tissue contains more water, hematopoietic "red" marrow is variably darker (more hypointense) on T1-weighted images than yellow marrow. In T2-weighted images, both fat and water are hyperintense (relative to skeletal muscle); but in many situations, the signal from fat is suppressed, such that only water or tissues containing high water content are bright. We often refer to these as "fluid-sensitive" sequences, and the term "T2 hyperintensity" invariably refers to water-like signal (see Figure 7.1).

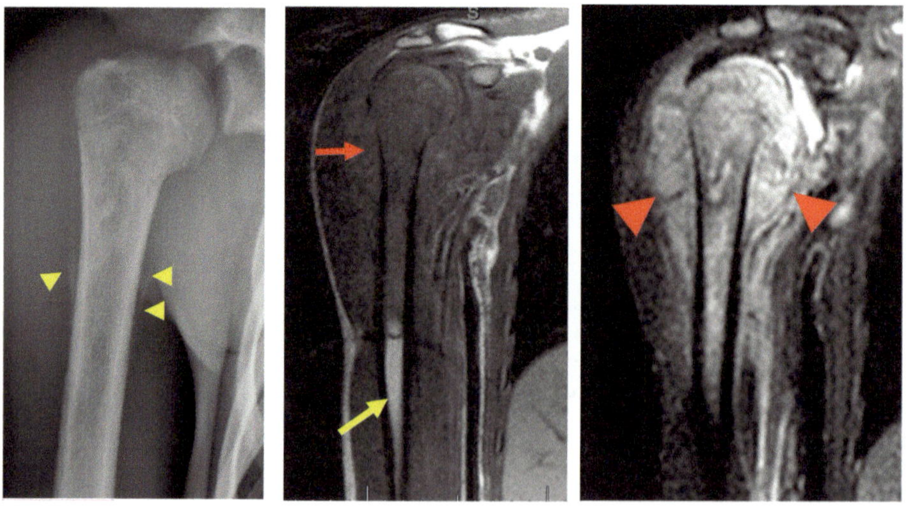

FIGURE 7.1 (A) Frontal radiograph shows a conventional osteosarcoma in the proximal humerus with periosteal reaction (arrowheads) indicative of an aggressive lesion. (B) On the coronal T1-weighted image, note the normal T1-hyperintense signal in the more distal humeral diaphysis (yellow arrow), while the osteosarcoma obliterates the normal proximal humeral marrow (red arrow). (C) The coronal STIR, a fluid-sensitive sequence, depicts the tumor's T2 hyperintensity as well as the extraosseous component both medially and laterally (arrowheads). The glenohumeral joint effusion is suggestive of intra-articular extension.

STIR, short-tau inversion recovery.

Because tumors are hypercellular, and cellular tissue is composed mostly of water, musculoskeletal neoplasms are generally hyperintense on T2-weighted images, though the presence of other components (e.g., evolving blood products) will alter the relaxation parameters. Hemosiderin, as a superparamagnetic material, accumulating at the periphery of a hemorrhagic or necrotic tumor component, will substantially shorten T2 relaxation times and may result in a rim of T2-hypointense signal at the margins. Solid viable tumor components will enhance with gadolinium-based contrast agent; nonenhancing components (e.g., tumor necrosis) will manifest as areas of hypointensity on the post-contrast sequences. Because changes in the amount or proportion of viable tumor may supersede dimensional changes in clinical decision-making, it is sometimes useful to obtain "subtraction" images, where the precontrast images are subtracted from the postcontrast images, which aids in discriminating true tissue enhancement from areas of tumor hemorrhage that are often intrinsically T1 hyperintense.

Like CT, MRI does utilize electromagnetic radiation; however, the radiation employed is "nonionizing" and poses no known carcinogenic threat (although the U.S. Food and Drug Administration [FDA] does place limits on the amount of RF energy to be delivered). Intrinsic tissue contrast, that is, conspicuity of soft tissue planes and the ability to distinguish substances such as blood from fat, muscle, and fibrous tissue, is superior to that of CT and can be improved even further with administration of gadolinium-based contrast agents. MR images are arbitrarily assigned pixel values based on signal strength; thus, unlike HUs in CT, it is impossible to quantify absolute tissue signal in a given region of interest; only relative signal strengths (to muscle by convention) can be evaluated. Whereas a CT scan of the entire body may take only several seconds on modern multirow detector machines, MRI is generally much more time-consuming, in part because standard MRI sequences are acquired separately in a single plane (coronal, axial, and sagittal), although some MRI sequences permit isotropic resolution, so that the acquired data set can be reformatted into any desired image plane. Routine protocols may require anywhere between 30 and 60 minutes, depending on the extent of anatomic coverage. Finally, patients must be screened for MRI because of the possibility of fatal implant migration (e.g., non–MR-compatible brain aneurysm clips, cardiac pacing implants, or other metals that are not MR compatible).

Ultrasound

Ultrasound exploits the piezoelectric effect that allows certain solid crystals to translate mechanical motion into small electrical charges. The ultrasound probe is essentially an array of these crystals that transmits mechanical wave energy (insonation) into tissue and then detects the reflected waves that are converted into electronic signals, eventually formed into a gray scale image. The insonated sound waves are reflected and refracted based on a number of factors including tissue composition, orientation, and tissue boundaries/interfaces. Because water transmits the sound waves efficiently, simple fluid-filled cysts reflect back little acoustic energy, and thus appear "anechoic." Solid soft tissue neoplasms typically appear hypoechoic to adjacent adipose tissue, but may also result in attenuation of sound wave transmission to deeper tissues. Ultrasound also detects blood flow within a lesion using the Doppler effect (see Figure 7.2); echoes reflected from the moving intravascular blood will be phase shifted by the direction of blood flow, either toward the transducer (frequency is compressed) or away from the transducer (frequency is stretched). This allows one to calculate both the velocity and directionality of

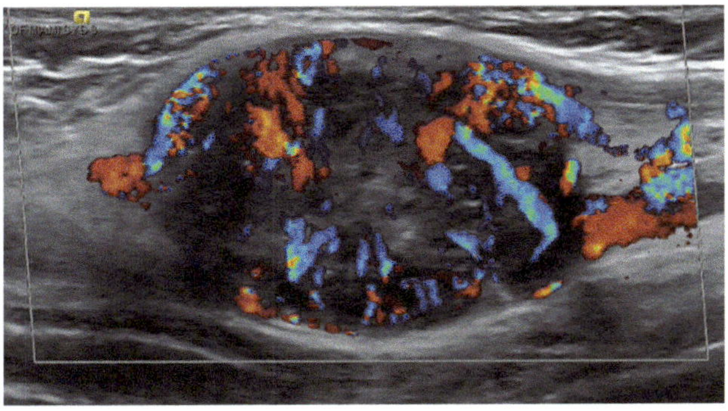

FIGURE 7.2 Ultrasound shows that the lesion is hypervascular, with markedly increased internal blood flow on Doppler interrogation, typical of alveolar soft part sarcoma. The red and blue coloring reflects blood moving away from or toward the probe.

blood flow. Doppler interrogation is particularly useful when seeking to target viable solid tumor components in an otherwise cystic/necrotic mass, assessing tumor relationships to the neurovascular bundle, and in distinguishing high- from low-flow vascular neoplasms and malformations. Ultrasound is generally well suited to localized exams of more superficial soft tissue masses. Lower-frequency sound waves can interrogate deeper soft tissues, but at the cost of decreased spatial resolution.

Positron Emission Tomography

The basis for most PET imaging is use of a radiolabeled glucose analog—fluorodeoxyglucose (^{18}F), often abbreviated FDG—that becomes concentrated in metabolically active tissues. ^{18}F decays by emitting a positron, which self-annihilates with its electron antiparticle, thus releasing two gamma rays that travel in opposite directions. A ring of scintillators and photomultiplier tubes surrounds the patient to detect and spatially localize only photons arriving simultaneously at the detector, that is, coincidence events. CT scanning of the patient is either performed on a dual PET–CT machine or the CT may be acquired on a separate machine with the images anatomically registered to the PET images to create a fused PET–CT series. The CT portion of the exam serves two key roles—one is to create an attenuation map that corrects for undercounting of true coincidence events that arise because of photon absorption in the bones, soft tissues, or metallic implants and the other purpose is to refine anatomic localization of the site of increased tissue metabolism. PET–CT plays important roles in initial staging by identifying distant sites of disease and in characterizing morphologically indeterminate lesions as either metabolically active or relatively quiescent. Generally, lung nodules <1 cm in size are not well characterized by PET–CT and are said to be below the threshold for reliable determination of FDG avidity. It should also be pointed out that some benign tumors may show surprisingly high levels of FDG avidity and may be detected incidentally on staging PET–CT, for example, intra-articular tenosynovial giant cell tumor.[1] On the other hand, some malignant tumors may show little FDG uptake relative to background. While there are a variety of ways FDG uptake may be quantified, most radiologists and nuclear medicine physicians will report a lesion's maximum standardized uptake value in a given region of interest (SUVmax). PET–CT may be an excellent problem-solving tool in circumstances in which identifying viable residual tumor would mandate a change in treatment; but one must be aware of nonspecificity of FDG uptake in any postinfectious/inflammatory setting, which limits PET–CT's role in early postoperative surveillance.

BONE TUMORS

General Considerations

Radiography plays a central role in the initial evaluation of any bone lesion. While the reader is referred to other sources for a full discussion of the radiographic differential for bone tumors,[2] we focus on providing a brief primer for nonradiologists in a basic interpretative approach. During initial evaluation of a bone lesion, one should attempt to answer several key questions in determining its likelihood of being neoplastic, its malignant potential, and any impending fracture risk:

- Where is the lesion: which bone and where in the bone?
- What is the structural effect on the bone?
- How is the bone responding?
- What is in the lesion (any clues to the histology)?

Answers to these questions, coupled with a few demographic and clinical details, can lead to a confident diagnosis in many cases. Even if the likely histology cannot be determined, the radiographs will elucidate a lesion's biologic aggressiveness and whether it should be biopsied.

Where Is the Lesion?

The skeletal location of a tumor is a particularly helpful discriminator of tumor subtypes. While most bone tumors may occur in or near the metaphysis of long bones, particularly around the knees and proximal humerus, other locations favor a few diagnoses, for example, Ewing sarcoma and chondrosarcoma in the flat bones such as the iliacs or ribs, adamantinoma in the tibial shaft and mandible, and chordoma in the skull base or sacrum. The location of the tumor in a long bone—epiphysis, metaphysis, or diaphysis—is helpful in further narrowing the differential considerations. Osteosarcoma usually occurs in the metaphysis, while Ewing sarcoma is known to occur in the diaphysis. A large majority of giant cell tumors of bone are subarticular and generally extend into the metaphysis. Osteolytic tumors that involve only the epiphysis include chondroblastoma and clear cell chondrosarcoma.

What Is the Structural Effect on the Bone?

Some tumors are osteolytic and others are osteoblastic. Some, notably breast carcinoma metastases, can be mixed. Osteolysis caused by tumor is, at a cellular level, performed by osteoclasts and not the tumor cells themselves; while tumor cells cannot resorb bone, they can upregulate the osteoclasts via the RANK (receptor activator of nuclear factor-κB) ligand pathway. Note that for a lytic lesion to be seen on a radiograph, at least 50% of the bone matrix (compared to the surrounding bone) must be resorbed.

As described by Lodwick,[3] there are three classic patterns of bone destruction that give a clue to the aggressive nature of an osteolytic lesion and predict tumor growth rate (see Figure 7.3):

- "Geographic bone destruction" implies a lesion with a sharply defined border. This can also be described as a narrow zone of transition between pathologic and normal bone. A geographic appearance implies a benign or less aggressive tumor, particularly when a thick sclerotic rim is present, as this implies sufficiently slow growth as to allow osteoblasts to deposit bone around the tumor margin.
- "Moth-eaten appearance" refers to areas of bone destruction with ragged edges. This is indicative of a malignant process rapidly expanding in the bone, resulting in mottled appearance. Metastatic disease, myeloma, lymphoma, and Ewing sarcoma commonly have a moth-eaten appearance.
- "Permeative appearance" implies that the tumor is moving through the bone without destroying all the trabeculae, resulting in numerous tiny "holes" in the bone that may become confluent in larger areas of destruction. There is, therefore, an ill-defined wide zone of transition between pathologic and normal bone. This classically is characteristic of round cell tumors such as lymphoma, leukemia, Ewing sarcoma, myeloma, osteomyelitis, and neuroblastoma. From a practical standpoint, moth-eaten and permeative appearances are distinctions without a clinically meaningful difference as they may coexist in a lesion and both mark a biologically aggressive process.

Recognizing such realities, Caracciolo et al. have proposed a modified Lodwick–Madewell grading system that groups geographic lesions with a well-defined margin (sclerotic or not) as grade I; geographic lesion with partial or circumferential ill-defined margins as grade II; and moth-eaten/permeative appearance, lesions exhibiting changes in margin or progressive endosteal scalloping, or radiographically occult lesions (but seen as marrow infiltrative processes on advanced modalities such as PET or MRI) as grade III.[4] Of 183 lytic bone tumors, 76 of 81 (94%) grade I lesions were confirmed histologically as benign and 39 of 48 grade III lesions (81%) were malignant; however, grade II lesions were nearly as likely to be benign as malignant.

How Is the Bone Responding?

This question is closely related to the above issues of what the lesion is doing, but focuses on how the bone and specifically the periosteum are reacting to the lesion. The universal response of periosteum to disease or injury is to make more bone. With slower-growing lesions, the periosteum is raised off the cortex, but has sufficient time to lay down new bone, resulting in solid periosteal mineralization. With

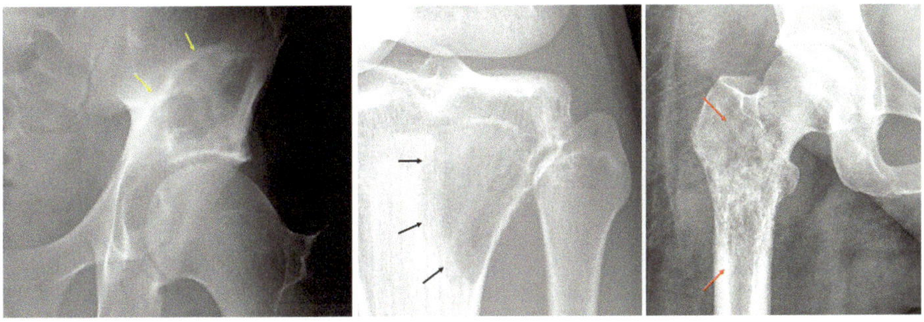

FIGURE 7.3 Geographic lytic lesions depicting a range of biologic aggressiveness that can be inferred from the pattern of osteolysis. (A) Fibrous dysplasia in the left iliac bone shows a grade I pattern with thick sclerotic margins. (B) Giant cell tumor of bone in the proximal tibia shows a grade Ib pattern with narrow zone of transition. (C) Metastatic Ewing sarcoma to the proximal femur shows a grade III pattern with permeative lucency and wide zone of transition.

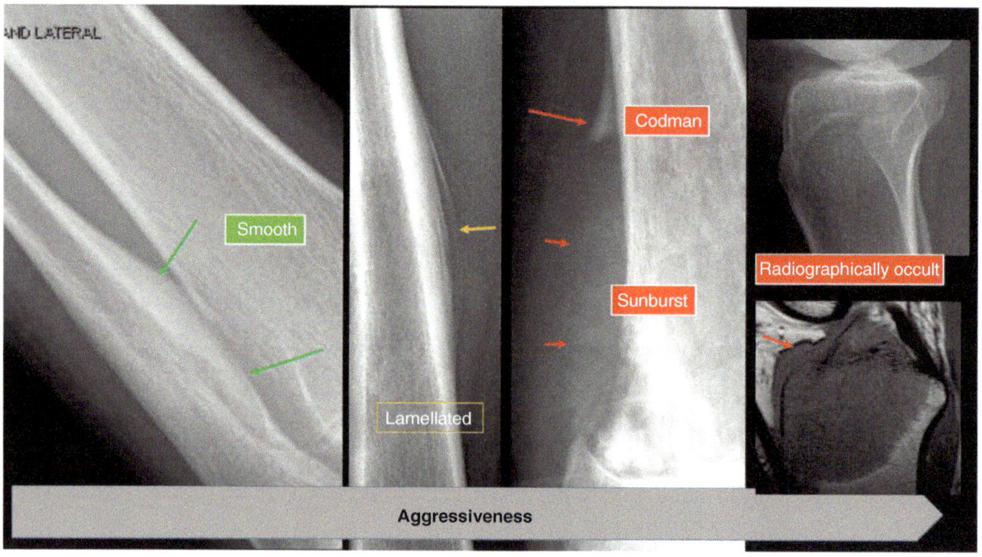

FIGURE 7.4 Patterns of periosteal reaction that correlate with tumor growth rates. Examples in this figure include an osteoid osteoma with smooth dense cortical reaction, periosteal osteosarcoma with lamellated periosteal reaction ("onion skinning"), conventional osteosarcoma with both Codman triangle and a sunburst pattern of mineralization along Sharpey's fibers, and lymphoma with tumor growth outstripping ability of periosteum to lay down layers of surrounding bone.

slightly faster growth, a smooth line of mineralization may form a shell around the lesion. "Onion-skinning" or lamellated periosteal reaction occurs when the periosteum lays down bone between sporadic intervals of more rapid tumor growth. Tumors that are rapidly increasing in size outstrip the periosteum's ability to lay down surrounding bone and stretch the small orthogonally oriented Sharpey's fibers between the periosteum and cortex; ossification along these perpendicular fibers results in a "sunburst" or "hair-on-end" appearance of periosteal reaction (see Figure 7.4). In some highly aggressive lesions, ossification may occur only at the margins of the lesion where the periosteum is lifted off the bone, resulting in the appearance of a Codman triangle when viewed tangentially at radiography. Finally, and perhaps counterintuitively, the most aggressive lesions may perforate the cortex and enlarge so rapidly that the periosteum has no time to lay down new bone; this type of growth is classically seen in primary bone lymphoma or very aggressive osteosarcoma.

What Is in the Lesion?

An assessment of the matrix of a lesion can give a clue to the histologic diagnosis. An osseous matrix appears fluffy and white on a radiograph. Often, radiologists may refer to this as an "osteoid matrix," and it should be pointed out that use of the term "osteoid" in this context is distinct from pathologists' usage, which denotes an absence of mineralization. The term "ground glass" matrix has been used to refer to the smooth increased mineralization pattern observed in fibrous dysplasia, although this can also be seen in low-grade central osteosarcoma. A chondroid matrix has a classical appearance of "rings and arcs" on plain films, reflecting the lobular growth pattern of the underlying cartilage-forming neoplasm. Fat-containing lesions, such as intraosseous lipoma or liposclerosing myxofibrous tumor, will exhibit intralesional fat, although the quantity may vary, depending on the extent of cystic involutional changes.

Osteosarcoma

Osteosarcoma (OS) is the most common primary bone sarcoma, typically occurring during childhood and adolescence. In patients over the age of 40, it is more often associated with a preexistent condition such as Paget's disease or irradiated bone.[5] Between 80% and 90% of the tumors occur in the metaphysis of long bone, with the most common sites being the distal femur, proximal tibia, and proximal humerus. The hallmark radiographic features of conventional osteosarcoma include production of neoplastic bone, which manifests radiologically as dense or calcifications, and aggressive periosteal reaction indicative of rapid tumor growth.[6,7] Cross-sectional imaging studies may reveal centrally necrotic components in particularly aggressive lesions.

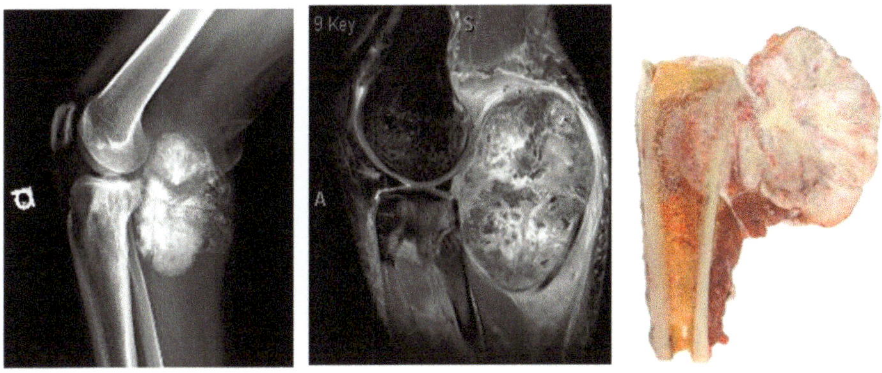

(A) (B) (C)

FIGURE 7.5 (A) Lateral radiograph in a 25-year-old man with a grade 3 dedifferentiated parosteal osteosarcoma shows a large ossifying tumor centered on the posterior cortex of the proximal tibia, with a "stuck-on" type of appearance. (B) Sagittal T2-weighted, fat-suppressed MRI reveals extensive peritumoral edema, suggesting a higher-grade malignancy than typical low-grade parosteal osteosarcoma. (C) Gross resection specimen.

Juxtacortical Osteosarcoma

Juxtacortical osteosarcoma refers to OS originating from the surface of bone. It is primarily associated with the periosteum, with medullary canal involvement observed with higher grades and dedifferentiation. Juxtacortical OS is classified into three main subtypes—parosteal, periosteal, and high-grade surface OS. Parosteal OS is the most common type of juxtacortical OS, and the posterior aspect of the distal femur is the most commonly encountered site of disease.[8] Anatomically, parosteal OS putatively originates from the outer fibrous layer of the periosteum and is usually low grade, appearing as a lobulated and exophytic mass with central dense ossification adjacent to the bone, in what has been described as a "stuck-on" appearance (Figure 7.5). At cross-sectional imaging, invasion into the medullary canal can be seen in both low-grade (41%) and high-grade (50%) lesions, but its prognostic implications are unclear.[8] Dedifferentiation of low-grade parosteal OS to high-grade disease has been reported in approximately 25% of cases.[9]

Periosteal OS is the second most common type of juxtacortical OS, accounting for 1.5% of all OS cases.[10] It typically affects patients in the second or third decade of life, with a characteristic location along the diaphyses of long bones, most commonly the tibia, and a general prognosis intermediate between parosteal and conventional osteosarcoma.[11] Periosteal OS arises from the inner, germinative layer of periosteum, and common radiographic findings include a soft tissue mass with periosteal reaction, cortical erosion, and cortical thickening (Figure 7.6)

Differentiation of high-grade surface OS from periosteal OS may be difficult at imaging, as both can occur in diaphyses and cause periosteal reaction and bone destruction. However, high-grade surface OS often involves the entire circumference of the cortex and is more likely to show medullary invasion.[12] Furthermore, the presence of a high histologic grade, identical to that of conventional OS, throughout the entire tumor is diagnostic of high-grade surface OS.

Telangiectatic Osteosarcoma

Telangiectatic OS accounts for <5% of all OS cases; it most frequently occurs in long bone metaphyses, particularly the femur. Characteristic radiographic appearances of telangiectatic OS include asymmetric aneurysmal bone expansion, geographic osteolysis, and an aggressive growth pattern with cortical destruction and minimal peripheral sclerosis.[7] Common features at CT and MRI include soft tissue mass, osteoid matrix mineralization, fluid levels, and thick peripheral and nodular septal enhancement. Osteoid matrix mineralization is often subtle on radiographs and of limited extent because viable tumor cells make up only a small amount of the lesion compared with the volume of cystic spaces. At MRI, hemorrhage and fluid–fluid levels are frequently identified, although this is a nonspecific finding shared with aneurysmal bone cysts and giant cell tumors of bone. The presence of nodular septal thickening, osteoid matrix mineralization in a soft tissue mass, and an aggressive growth pattern can aid in distinguishing telangiectatic OS from aneurysmal bone cyst (Figure 7.7).

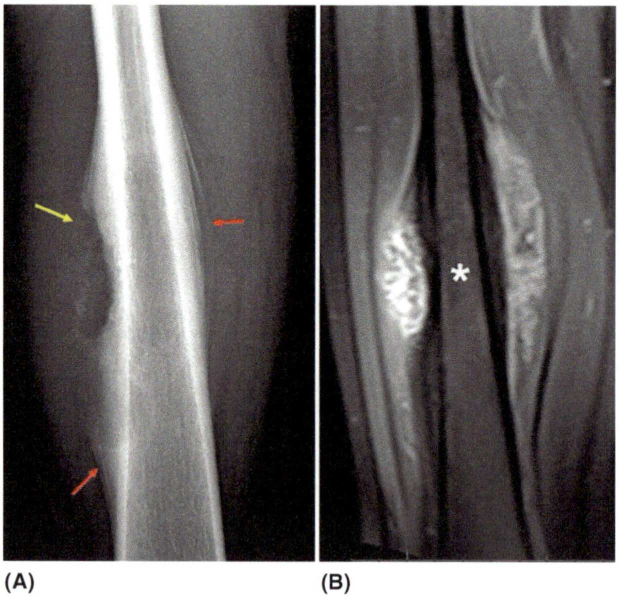

FIGURE 7.6 Periosteal osteosarcoma in the femoral diaphysis of a 17-year-old female. (A) Note the lamellated periosteal reaction (red arrows) and faintly mineralized more superior component that erodes the underlying thickened cortex (yellow arrow). (B) Contrast-enhanced MRI shows the enhancing tumor growing along the surface of the femoral shaft, but sparing the intramedullary canal (asterisk).

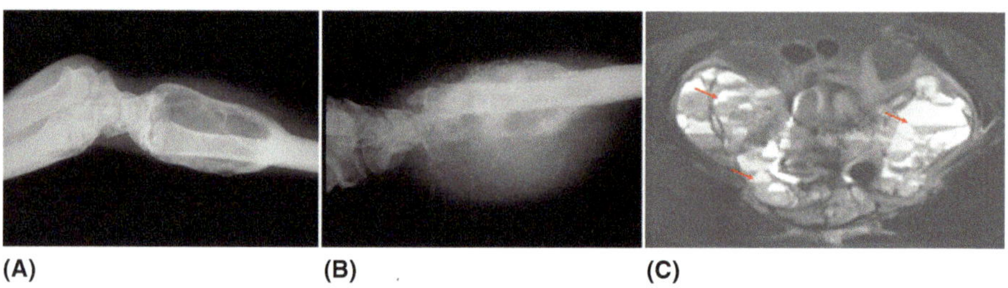

FIGURE 7.7 (A) Initial radiograph shows an expansile osteolytic lesion of the distal radius with internal septations, thought to represent an ABC. (B) Fourteen months after the initial radiograph, there is increased expansion and frank cortical destruction of the distal radius, aggressive periosteal reaction, and increased soft tissue swelling in this telangiectatic OS. (C) Axial fat-suppressed, proton density–weighted MRI through the lower lumbar spine reveals dependent layering of numerous fluid–fluid levels (arrows) in this recurrent vertebral body telangiectatic OS.

ABC, aneurysmal bone cyst; OS, osteosarcoma.

Chondrosarcoma

Chondrosarcoma is a malignant tumor that produces cartilage matrix. Primary chondrosarcoma constitutes 20% to 27% of all primary malignant osseous neoplasms. There are numerous types of primary chondrosarcomas, including conventional intramedullary, clear cell, juxtacortical, myxoid, mesenchymal, extraskeletal, and dedifferentiated. Early diagnosis and treatment of chondrosarcomas are paramount to achieving a better prognosis. Multiple imaging modalities have been used for the purpose of initial detection, characterization, and staging, as well as for the performance of image-guided biopsies.

The difficulties that clinicians, radiologists, and pathologists face in the differentiation of enchondroma from low-grade chondrosarcoma and the difficulty in uniform histologic grading of chondrosarcoma have been emphasized in two studies that evaluated the interobserver variability in the diagnosis and histologic grading of cartilaginous tumors. Both studies demonstrated low reliability in the distinction between enchondroma and low-grade chondrosarcoma and a low reliability in the histologic grading of chondrosarcoma among bone tumor pathologists.[13–15] Furthermore, the Skeletal Lesions Interobserver Correlation among Expert Diagnosticians (SLICED) study group also demonstrated significant variation among radiologists in differentiating enchondroma from low-grade chondrosarcoma

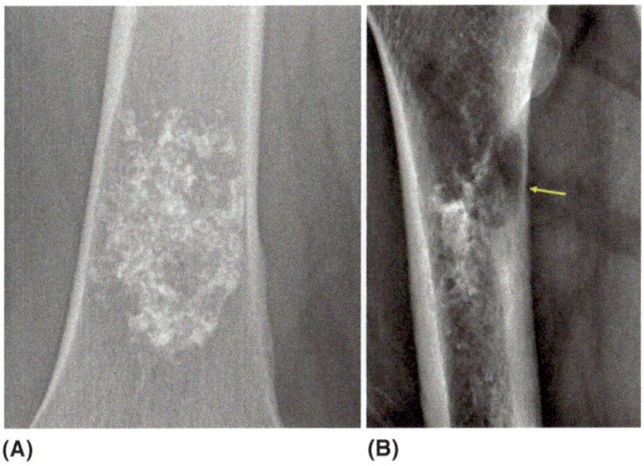

FIGURE 7.8 (A) Enchondroma in the distal femur displaying classic chondroid mineralization pattern of "rings and arcs," recapitulating the lobular growth of this cartilage-forming tumor. (B) Chondrosarcoma in the proximal femur showing high-grade (more than two-thirds of the cortical depth) endosteal scalloping (arrow).

and a low reliability in the grading of chondrosarcoma based on radiography or CT, with slightly improved agreement among radiologists when MRI was used.[14] As Roitman et al. observed, concordance with respect to histologic grade between initial needle biopsy and final resection specimen was only 67% for pelvic chondrosarcomas,[16] further supporting a multidisciplinary team strategy that incorporates clinical, imaging, and histologic findings in the diagnosis and management of patients with these types of lesions.

Imaging features directly reflect this pathologic appearance, and the various subtypes often show distinctive features. Radiographic findings often suggest the diagnosis of chondrosarcoma because of identification of typical "ring-and-arc" chondroid matrix mineralization (representing the enchondral ossification) and aggressive features of deep endosteal scalloping and soft tissue extension (Figure 7.8). These latter features are usually best assessed, as is lesion staging, with CT or MRI. Radiographs of central long bone chondrosarcoma (CS) typically show a region of mixed lysis and sclerosis, with the sclerotic areas representing classical rings and arcs of chondral matrix mineralization, which are seen in 60% to 78% of cases. The degree of calcification is variable, but higher-grade tumors tend to show less mineralization. Low-grade tumors classically demonstrate a geographic, lobular margin, while moth-eaten or permeative bone destruction is indicative of higher-grade lesions or possible dedifferentiation. Deep endosteal scalloping (more than two-thirds of the depth of the cortex) and cortical thickening are the morphologic features of central CS that aid to discriminate it from enchondroma.

PET–CT has been used to improve diagnostic accuracy of chondroid tumors; a recent systematic literature review of 166 total lesions confirmed that SUVmax was lower for benign compared to malignant tumors, with mean values of 1.6 versus 4.4, respectively.[17] Moreover, SUVmax correlated with tumor grade, and SUVmax ≥4.4 was 99% specific for grade 2/3 chondrosarcoma. However, it remains to be established whether metabolic activity, as quantified by F-18 FDG PET, meaningfully correlates with the clinical outcome measures such as disease-free survival or overall survival.

Peripheral Chondrosarcomas

Peripheral chondrosarcomas may arise from the cartilaginous cap of a preexisting osteochondroma. Patients with multiple hereditary exostoses (MHE) are particularly prone to this complication, as already indicated. The risk of malignant transformation in a solitary osteochondroma is very low but has been estimated to be between 1% and 2%. The radiographic signs of malignant progression in an osteochondroma include increased growth after skeletal maturity, or irregularity and thickening of the cartilage cap or destruction of the stalk radiographically (Figure 7.9).

Juxtacortical Chondrosarcoma

Juxtacortical chondrosarcoma, which arises on the surface of bone, has also been referred to as periosteal and parosteal chondrosarcoma. Juxtacortical chondrosarcoma most frequently affects adults in the third to fourth decades of life and has a mild male predilection. Lesions are most frequently seen

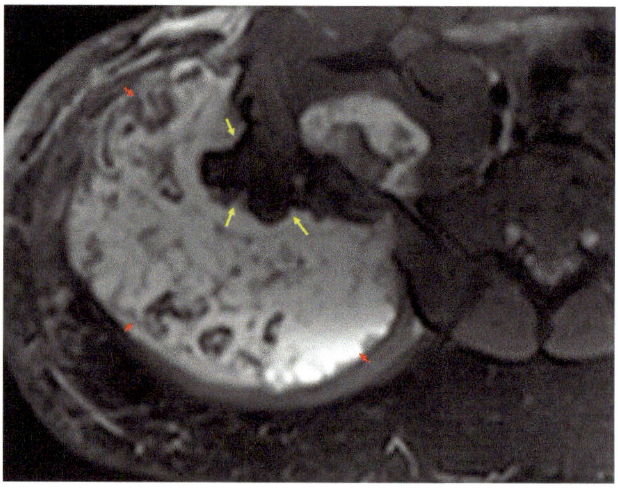

FIGURE 7.9 Axial proton density–weighted, fat-suppressed image shows a large chondrosarcoma arising from a preexisting osteochondroma of the right iliac bone; note the corticomedullary continuity of the underlying osteochondroma (yellow arrows) with the iliac bone. The large tumor demonstrates a hyperintense lobular, cartilaginous matrix (red arrows) on this fluid-sensitive sequence.

on the surface of long bones, particularly the posterior distal femoral metaphysis or diaphysis, but can arise anywhere. Typical chondroid matrix mineralization is usually present. In addition, metaplastic ossification is often apparent to a variable extent.

Chondrosarcoma Variants

Clear Cell Chondrosarcoma

Clear cell chondrosarcoma is a rare variant of chondrosarcoma, which is characterized by tumor cells with an abundant clear or ground glass cytoplasm and sharply defined borders. It has overlapping clinical and radiographic features with chondroblastoma, and some have proposed that it may represent its malignant counterpart. Most patients are older than those affected by chondroblastoma. Radiographically, the lesion is usually entirely radiolucent, often sharply circumscribed, and may be complicated by pathologic fracture. Most cases involve the proximal femoral or humeral epiphysis, and the behavior is generally that of a low-grade malignancy, with some outstanding exceptions.

Dedifferentiated Chondrosarcoma

The term "dedifferentiated chondrosarcoma" refers to the phenomenon of conventional chondrosarcoma undergoing malignant transformation after acquiring additional genetic mutations. The dedifferentiated component may comprise a number of different tissue types, such as fibroblastic, spindle cell, or osteosarcoma lines of heterologous differentiation (Figure 7.10); it most commonly occurs as central chondrosarcoma but features of peripheral dedifferentiated chondrosarcomas have also been described.[18] Usually, a discrete soft tissue mass apart from the underlying chondrosarcoma is radiologically evident, but an admixture of dedifferentiated components interspersed in a mosaic pattern with the preexisting lower-grade lesion has recently been recognized.[19] Dedifferentiation is accompanied by a marked deterioration of the patient's clinical course and a decidedly worse prognosis.

Chordoma

Chordoma is a rare primary bone sarcoma that is thought to arise from transformed residual notochordal cells. Thus, chordomas may occur anywhere in the spine, though there is a propensity for skull base (e.g., clivus) and sacral locations (see Figure 7.11). Their cell of origin also explains why they occur in the midline, in contrast to other primary bone tumors that may occur in these locations, such as giant cell tumor of bone or chondrosarcoma. Chordomas result in osteolysis and commonly have exophytic soft tissue components that show variable degrees of internal punctate calcifications.[20] While biopsy is required for definitive diagnosis, recent attempts to use machine learning algorithms to distinguish chordomas from other diagnostic possibilities have seen early success.[21] Surgery and adjuvant radiation therapy are advocated for achieving optimal survival outcomes.[22]

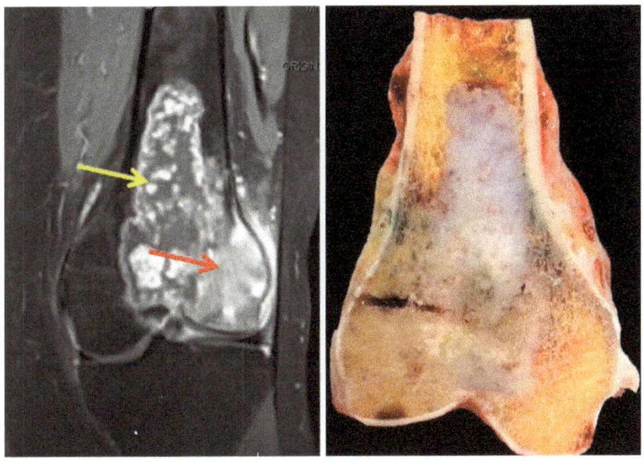

(A) (B)

FIGURE 7.10 (A) Coronal contrast-enhanced MRI highlights the difference between the lower-grade chondroid component (yellow arrow) and the dedifferentiated component (red arrow) that has lost the lobular chondroid architecture. (B) Gross specimen shows the lower-grade component with typical lobular chondroid matrix and higher-grade chondrosarcoma inferolaterally (note prior percutaneous needle biopsy tract).

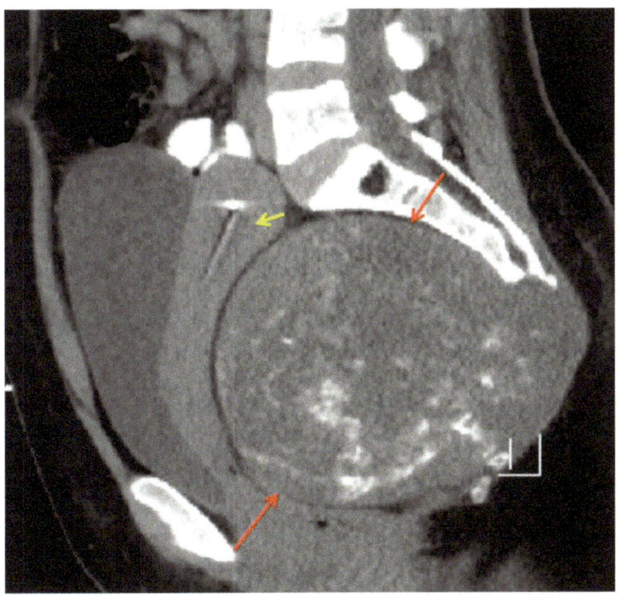

FIGURE 7.11 Sagittal CT shows a large midline eroding posteriorly through the sacrum at S3 to the coccyx, with large anterior exophytic soft tissue component (red arrows), and numerous coarse calcifications. The uterus is displaced anteriorly (yellow arrow) and contains an intrauterine contraceptive implant.

Ewing Sarcoma

Osseous Ewing sarcoma represents the second most common primary malignant tumor of bone in children and adolescents.[10] There is a wide skeletal distribution for Ewing sarcoma, but the most commonly affected sites are the femur (21% of cases), ilium (12%–13%), tibia (8%–11%), humerus (10%), fibula (7%–9%), ribs (8%), and sacrum (6%). At radiography, osseous Ewing sarcoma reveals aggressive features; bone destruction with a moth-eaten to permeative pattern is seen in approximately 80% of lesions and a wide zone of transition (poor margination) is almost uniformly observed.[23,24] Geographic bone destruction with a wide zone of transition may be seen in a minority of cases. Cortical destruction (19%–42%) with an associated soft tissue mass (56%–80%) is also common. Periosteal reaction

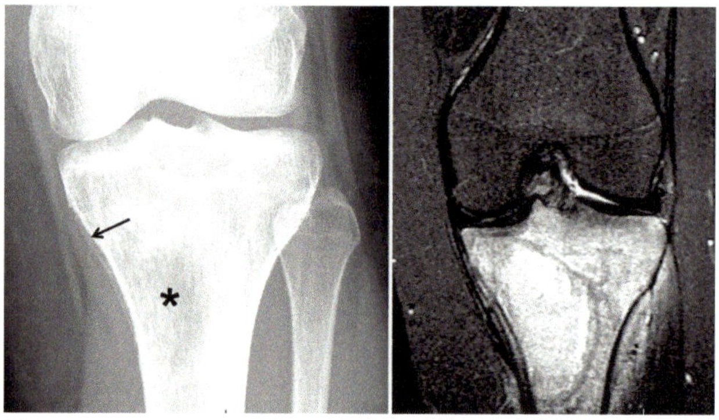

FIGURE 7.12 (A) Ewing sarcoma in a 15-year-old female appears as a permeative lytic lesion (asterisk) in the proximal tibia, with periosteal reaction identified medially (arrow). (B) Coronal STIR MRI shows the extensive and confluent involvement of the proximal tibia, with extraosseous component laterally.

STIR, short-tau inversion recovery.

is frequent (58%–84%) and almost always aggressive (94%), with either lamellated (onionskin) or spiculated ("sunburst" or "hair-on-end") pattern.[23,24] MRI of Ewing sarcoma of bone reveals marrow infiltration and cortical breakthrough, with an associated soft tissue mass in the majority of cases.[25] The soft tissue mass is commonly circumferential, but asymmetric about the osseous involvement (Figure 7.12).

SOFT TISSUE TUMORS

Benign soft tissue masses vastly outnumber malignant soft tissue tumors, but the majority of benign soft tissue masses are probably not referred for imaging evaluation. The American College of Radiology (ACR) has proposed guidelines for appropriate diagnostic imaging tests for various clinical scenarios.[26] Briefly, these guidelines suggest that radiographs should be the initial diagnostic modality for evaluation of soft tissue masses. Radiographs are easily obtained and may be diagnostic, for example, in the case of an osteochondroma presenting as a palpable mass, obviating the need for more advanced imaging. Important information regarding tumor mineralization and relationships to adjacent bones can also be obtained. But while it is a good initial step, radiographs are usually indeterminate, and further cross-sectional imaging is required. Generally, MRI is advocated[26] because it allows excellent assessment of soft tissue composition, often being definitive for simple lipomas or other low-grade lipomatous neoplasms; reveals key anatomic relationships to adjacent tendons, bone, vessels, and nerves; and delivers a relatively operator-independent set of images of the abnormality.

Diagnostic Approach to Soft Tissue Tumors

Many lesions may be referred to an orthopedic oncology clinic, such as juxta-articular ganglia or cysts (e.g., paralabral cysts in the hip or shoulder, parameniscal cysts in the knee), muscle herniations, or even accessory muscles, which might simulate soft tissue neoplasms. Distinguishing benign hematoma from a hemorrhagic soft tissue sarcoma is always problematic, if not impossible, as clinical history is often unreliable in both situations—some patients with benign hematoma report no trauma and some patients with hemorrhagic sarcoma recall direct trauma. Because the imaging features of benign and malignant soft tissue tumors overlap to a great degree, many soft tissue masses have indeterminate imaging findings and require either biopsy or clinical follow-up depending on the clinical context.

Matrix

Lipomatous

Leaving aside the nonneoplastic diagnoses that may enter into clinical differential diagnosis (e.g., abscess, hematoma), we may focus on a few key aspects of indeterminate soft tissue tumors that suggest a tumor subtype or hint at tumor grade. First, one needs to try to determine the tumor matrix. Lipomatous tumors are the most common soft tissue neoplasms to come to radiologic attention and are readily identifiable when containing macroscopic fat (Figure 7.13). While histologically identical,

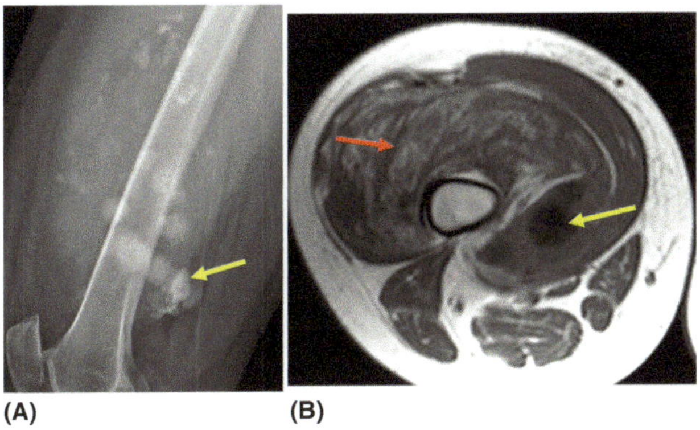

FIGURE 7.13 (A) Lateral radiograph of atypical lipomatous tumor in the thigh, partially encompassing the mid to distal femur, with coarse calcifications (yellow arrows in A and B). (B) Note the intratumoral macroscopic fat content (red arrow) which follows the same signal as subcutaneous fat.

the term "well-differentiated liposarcoma" (WDL) is reserved for those tumors occurring intra-abdominally or intrathoracically, where resection with negative surgical margins is difficult, if not impossible, to achieve and there is substantial risk of subsequent dedifferentiation. "Atypical lipomatous tumor" (ALT) is used for tumors in the extremities, where the term "sarcoma" is avoided, given their excellent prognosis and minimal risk of subsequent dedifferentiation and metastatic spread. The key to identifying low-grade lipomatous tumors from their high-grade counterparts is the amount of nonlipomatous tissue found within them. Simple lipomas manifest as solid tumors of similar signal to normal subcutaneous fat—in fact, these tumors may appear "clean" in that they often lack the thin septa that mark normal subcutaneous fat. The best sequences to evaluate tumor fat content are the non–fat-suppressed, T1-weighted images and the fat-suppressed, T2/PD (fluid-sensitive) sequences, which should confirm homogeneous signal matching that of normal subcutaneous fat across all pulse sequences.

The presence of thick (>2 mm) septations, areas of hyperintensity on the fluid-sensitive sequences, or small nodular areas of nonadipocytic soft tissue signal raises the possibility of WDL/ALT. However, it should be noted that many fatty tumors with these features suspected of being WDL/ALT turn out to be simple lipoma variants, because internal fat necrosis or inflammatory change results in T2 hyperintensity.[27] Other lipoma variants, such as pleomorphic lipoma, may also show ill-defined internal T2 hyperintensity but have a demographic/anatomic propensity for the upper back, neck, and shoulders in older males. Myxoid and pleomorphic liposarcoma may present without identifiable macroscopic fat visible on MRI (Figure 7.14). Dedifferentiated liposarcoma, in contrast, typically arises in a background of WDL, although the well-differentiated component can be difficult to distinguish from nonneoplastic adipose tissue other than its ability to "push" organs such as kidney and intestine away from the normal location, particularly in the peritoneum and retroperitoneum. The dedifferentiated component manifests as a solid, nonlipomatous soft tissue mass distinct from adjacent fat.[28]

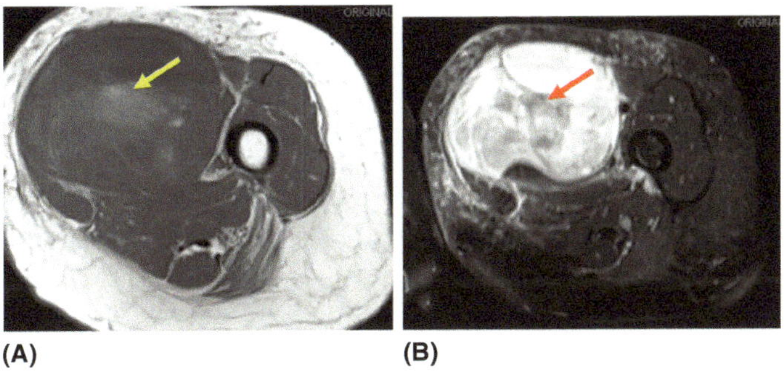

FIGURE 7.14 (A) Axial T1-weighted and (B) proton density fat-suppressed MR images of dedifferentiated liposarcoma in the medial thigh. Note the relatively small amounts of macroscopic fat (yellow arrow in A, red arrow in B).

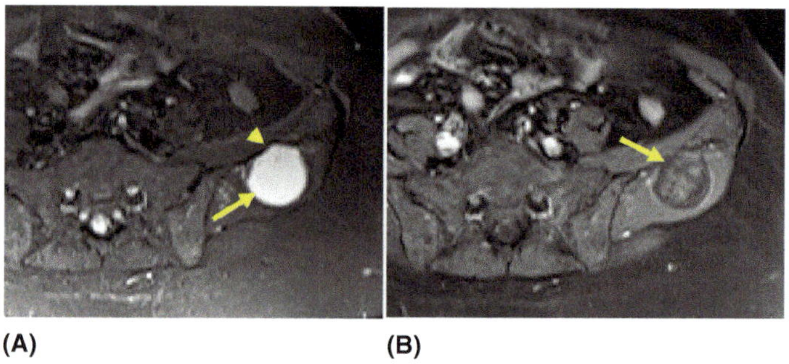

FIGURE 7.15 (A) Axial fat-suppressed, T2-weighted, and (B) contrast-enhanced MR images reveal a homogeneous T2-hyperintense mass with heterogeneous low-level enhancement (arrows) in the left gluteus maximus muscle, subsequently confirmed by percutaneous biopsy to be a myxoma. The high water content in myxoid stroma results in striking T2 hyperintensity on fluid-sensitive sequences and variable enhancement after intravenous contrast agent is used. Note the smooth scalloping of the adjacent iliac cortex (arrowhead in A), a finding that suggests an indolent process, allowing the bone sufficient time to remodel around the tumor.

Myxoid

The high water content of the matrix of myxoid soft tissue tumors results in these tumors appearing T2 hyperintense and T1 hypointense on MRI and hypodense on CT. Contrast-enhanced scans show variable enhancement; hypoenhancing tumors reflect the abundance of myxoid stroma with little vascularity (Figure 7.15). Benign myxomas often occur within the muscle belly and show little peritumoral edema or adjacent soft tissue reactive changes. Because they are usually well marginated and homogeneously T2 hyperintense, they may be mistaken for cysts if no IV contrast agent is given (or no enhancement is seen). Histologic low-grade myxoid tumors, such as low-grade fibromyxoid sarcoma (Evan's tumor; Figure 7.16), also show little central enhancement because of the nonenhancing myxoid stroma. Radiologically, these lesions often appear centrally necrotic, mimicking higher-grade sarcomas that are marked by central necrosis, with thicker enhancing rinds of tissue made up of more cellular tumor elements. Higher-grade myxoid sarcomas, such as myxofibrosarcoma, often grow in an infiltrative fashion, with T2-hyperintense tails radiating from the tumor margins.[29] Radiologically, it is virtually impossible to distinguish whether these T2-hyperintense tails comprise infiltrating tumor or form part of a zone of reactive peritumoral edema,[30] but it is common practice to consider these tails as containing tumor in known or suspected myxofibrosarcoma. Their identification is critical in determining the extent of local surgical resection, radiation therapy, and the corresponding need for soft tissue coverage.

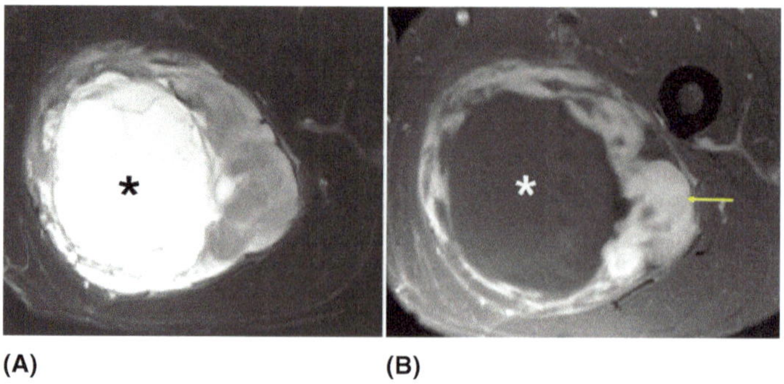

FIGURE 7.16 (A) Axial fat-suppressed, T2-weighted, and (B) contrast-enhanced MR images demonstrate a predominantly T2-hyperintense mass with heterogeneous peripheral enhancement (arrow) in the left posteromedial thigh, subsequently confirmed by percutaneous biopsy to be a low-grade fibromyxoid sarcoma (Evan's tumor). Note the central T2 hyperintensity (asterisk) reflecting the tumor's myxoid stroma.

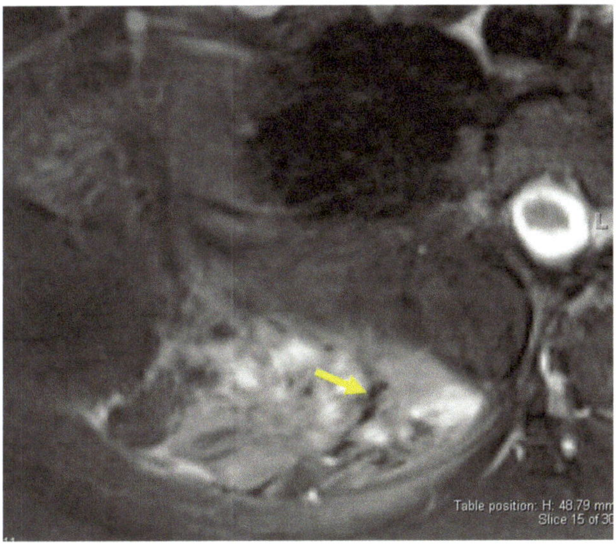

FIGURE 7.17 Axial T2-weighted MRI depicts a heterogeneous hyperintense mass in the right paraspinal muscles, with linear bands of hypointensity coursing through the mass. While not entirely specific, this finding is characteristic of desmoid-type fibromatosis.

Fibrous

Normal fibrous tissue in ligaments and tendons appears hyperdense on CT and uniformly hypointense on all standard MR pulse sequences. Similarly, the fibrous or collagenous hypocellular component of soft tissue tumors appears hypointense on MRI. Generally, the contrast between collagenous components and more cellular fibroblastic tumor components is best appreciated on fluid-sensitive and contrast-enhanced sequences. Desmoid-type fibromatosis exemplifies how imaging characteristics correlate with tumor composition and histology, as infiltrating tendrils of collagen deposited by the tumor extend into the adjacent soft tissues and muscle (Figure 7.17). It has been shown that maturing desmoids exhibit increases in T2 hypointensity,[31,32] reflecting increased collagen deposition.

Necrosis or Hemorrhage

Spontaneous intratumoral coagulative necrosis is a marker of biologic aggressiveness, indicating rapid tumor growth that outstrips tumor blood supply and generally portends poorer clinical outcomes. For this reason, tumor necrosis is an element considered in the French Federation of Comprehensive Cancer Centers (*Fédération Nationale des Centres de Lutte Contre le Cancer*; FNCLCC) grading system and an important feature to evaluate when imaging soft tissue tumors. A fluid–fluid level is nearly pathognomonic for intratumoral hemorrhage and necrosis, the effect due to the gravity-dependent settling of denser blood components, appropriately termed a "hematocrit effect." This phenomenon is modality independent and may be observed on ultrasound, CT, or MRI. The sharp linear interfaces of layering fluid evolve depending on the age of the hemorrhage. Heterogeneity in the T2 signal of a tumor is the basis for the "triple sign," a nonspecific finding related to the presence of mixed T2 signal intensities (hypo-, iso-, and hyperintense components, all within the same tumor) of which hemorrhage is a component and which has been described as occurring with some frequency (though not exclusively) in synovial sarcoma. On contrast-enhanced imaging, differentiation between viable and necrotic tumors is readily accomplished by identifying enhancing tumor components (Figure 7.18). Fat-suppressed, T1-weighted sequences are the best to highlight areas of gadolinium enhancement; enhancement can be made even more conspicuous by postprocessing techniques such as digitally subtracting the precontrast from the postcontrast images. While this technique reduces the overall image signal, it can be particularly helpful when trying to ascertain whether lesions are truly enhancing or simply intrinsically bright on T1, as can happen in the presence of evolving blood products or proteinaceous debris.

Mineralization

The most common causes of soft tissue calcifications have a benign cause and are usually related to old trauma, tissue necrosis, or infection/inflammation. However, some patterns of calcification deserve

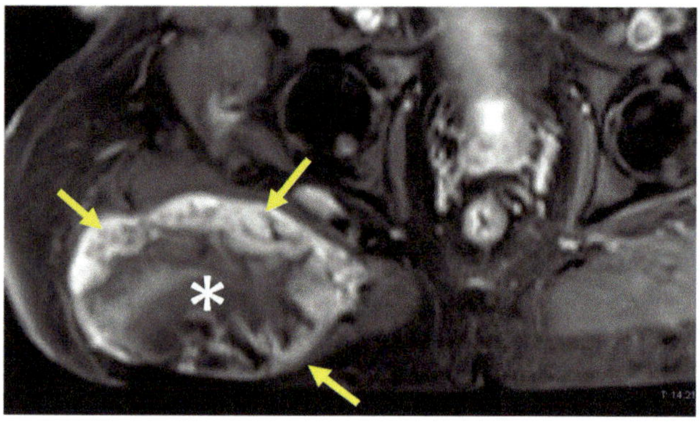

FIGURE 7.18 Contrast-enhanced MRI shows a high-grade pleomorphic fibroblastic tumor with a thick rind of enhancing viable tumor (arrows) surrounding a necrotic tumor center (asterisk). It is important for surgeons and radiologists performing percutaneous needle biopsies to identify and adequately sample the solid, viable tumor components, which are at the tumor periphery rather than the core of necrotic sarcomas. Biopsy deep in the center of such masses would yield nondiagnostic material.

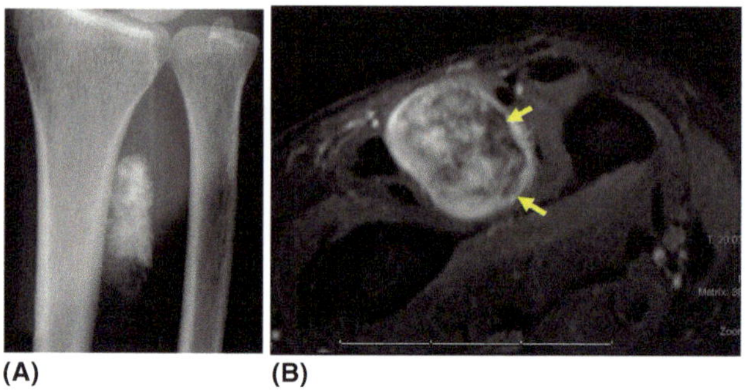

FIGURE 7.19 (A) A calcified soft tissue mass of a 48-year-old woman in the dorsal aspect of the distal forearm. Note the coarse lobular calcifications on radiography, suggestive of an underlying chondroid tumor matrix. (B) The axial fat-suppressed, T2-weighted image shows that the lesion is heterogeneously T2 hyperintense with numerous curvilinear rings and arcs of hypointense signal (arrows) correlating with intratumoral calcification in this extraskeletal mesenchymal chondrosarcoma. Note the adjacent extensor tendons.

special consideration because they are suggestive of, or they mimic, more sinister neoplastic causes. Heterotopic ossification is radiographically marked by the organizational and structural features of trabecular bone and peripheral cortex occurring in the soft tissues, most commonly following trauma. Peripheral mineralization, with an "eggshell"-like appearance, may mark early stages of heterotopic ossification, with denser trabecular bone forming over time. In contradistinction, extraskeletal osteosarcoma and extraskeletal chondrosarcoma may show varying degrees of calcification, but lacking the zonal organization of heterotopic ossification. Extraskeletal osteosarcoma typically shows denser and more mature bone centrally, with the most recent neoplastic bone formation located at the periphery and appearing less heavily mineralized. Extraskeletal chondrosarcoma may show coarse mineralization in rings and arcs, recapitulating the lobular growth pattern of the underlying chondroid matrix (Figure 7.19).

Among other soft tissue sarcoma subtypes, calcifications are most frequently seen in lipomatous neoplasms and synovial sarcoma. It should also be pointed out that, as a general rule, the presence of calcifications is not particularly helpful in determining whether a lipomatous tumor is benign, as simple lipomas and high-grade liposarcomas may both exhibit calcifications.

LOCAL STAGING

Historically, the depth of soft tissue tumor involvement was used in local staging because deeper tumors were associated with more aggressive behavior. However, the American Joint Committee on

Cancer (AJCC) *Cancer Staging Manual*, Eighth Edition has de-emphasized tumor depth, and instead identified tumor maximum diameter as the dominant consideration in local stage: T0, no evidence of primary; T1, ≤5 cm; T2, >5 and ≤10 cm; T3, >10 and <15 cm; and T4 >15 cm.[33] While they are eliminated from the AJCC staging guidelines, tumor depth and compartmental involvement are still critical features to fully characterize because of their surgical implications. A separate staging system for soft tissue sarcomas of the head and neck was also included in the most updated staging guidelines, importantly establishing primary tumor size cut-offs of 2 and 4 cm to better reflect the common tumor size range.[34]

Unlike in bone, the soft tissues surrounding a primary soft tissue mass may offer little insight into the aggressiveness of the neoplasm. High-grade soft tissue sarcomas may exhibit a well-delineated pseudocapsule; benign entities such as nodular fasciitis may be associated with an infiltrative pattern of perifascial soft tissue edema. Despite these exceptions, peritumoral edema and enhancement have been correlated with sarcoma grade.[35]

DISTANT STAGING

When metastatic, most sarcomas spread hematogenously to the lungs. High-resolution chest CT is the most sensitive imaging modality for identification of lung metastases, although PET–CT may be used in some centers because of its ability to detect metabolically active lesions elsewhere in the body. Chest radiographs may be a cost-effective alternative to serial CT chest scans with lower risk sarcomas,[36] with the caveat that the threshold for reliable prospective detection of lung nodules radiographically is approximately 2 to 3 cm. The typical appearance of lung metastases is that of a solid, spherical nodule of soft tissue density. Uniquely, osteosarcoma metastases are frequently calcified; this can pose a diagnostic dilemma in adults who have a history of old granulomatous disease resulting in punctate calcified lung nodules. Given their organ of origin, gastrointestinal stromal tumors (GISTs) metastasize to the liver or implant in the peritoneum. Unlike in carcinomas of the lung and breast, sarcoma brain metastases are rare with the exception of alveolar soft parts sarcoma.

Several sarcoma subtypes have characteristic patterns of spread that deserve mention. A 2018 review of the National Cancer Database by Keung et al. revealed metastatic spread to lymph nodes in only 3.5% of soft tissue sarcoma at presentation; however, certain histologic types showed a higher likelihood of nodal involvement: angiosarcoma (6%), epithelioid (13%), clear cell sarcoma (16%), and small cell sarcoma (19%).[37] Historically, rhabdomyosarcoma has been included in this list[38]; but it should be pointed out that owing to their much higher prevalence, liposarcoma, fibroblastic/myofibroblastic sarcoma, and leiomyosarcoma account for the greatest absolute number of nodal metastases. Nevertheless, when encountering a primary soft tissue sarcoma of a type more likely to spread lymphatically, lymphoscintigraphy, PET–CT imaging, and sentinel node biopsy can be considered in improving staging accuracy.

Metastatic spread to bones is generally rare for most sarcomas, but is a feature of osteosarcoma, Ewing sarcoma, and myxoid liposarcoma. In addition, myxoid liposarcoma frequently metastasizes to the soft tissues, as does alveolar soft part sarcoma. In fact, myxoid liposarcoma metastasizes to bone and soft tissue more frequently than lung.[39] Knowing these metastatic patterns can guide appropriate staging imaging studies, for example, CT of chest, abdomen, and pelvis in patients with myxoid liposarcoma, or even whole spine MRI in myxoid liposarcoma (Figure 7.20).

RESPONSE ASSESSMENT

Radiologic imaging provides an important noninvasive means of assessing treatment efficacy. Objective response rate and progression-free survival derived from imaging studies are frequently employed as primary endpoints in clinical trials because, compared to survival endpoints, imaging endpoints may significantly shorten the necessary trial duration. It has become part of clinical trial design paradigm that imaging response metrics may serve as good surrogates for survival.

Response Evaluation Criteria in Solid Tumors

The most commonly used of the response criteria is Response Evaluation Criteria in Solid Tumors version 1.1 (RECIST 1.1).[40,41] The reader is referred to these sources for more comprehensive discussion of the criteria, but briefly, RECIST 1.1 defines four types of response: complete response (CR) or partial response (PR), stable disease (SD) and progressive disease (PD). Conditions for PD are met if (a) the

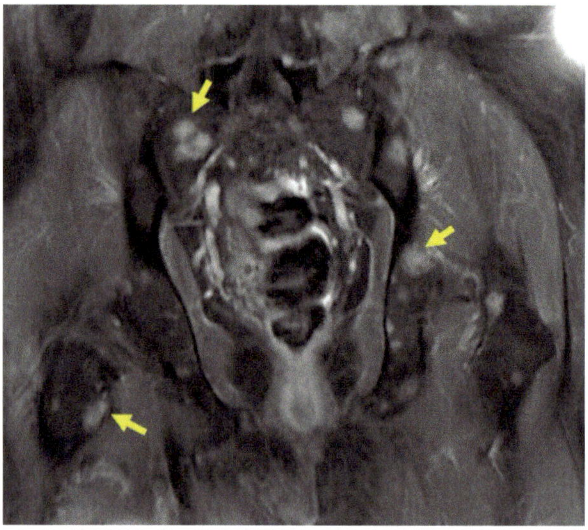

FIGURE 7.20 Myxoid liposarcoma with bone metastases. Coronal fat-suppressed, T2-weighted image of the pelvis shows numerous bone metastases (arrows) in the sacrum, bilateral iliac bones, and proximal femur.

sum of longest diameters of target lesions (up to five) exceeds nadir (not baseline) sum by 20% or (b) unequivocal progression is observed in nontarget lesions or (c) new lesions are present. PR is achieved if the sum of maximum diameters of the target lesion decreases by 30% from baseline. CR describes the disappearance of all target and nontarget lesions; but in our experience, it is rarely seen in sarcoma. SD essentially encompasses all other response scenarios. There are numerous rules and guidelines to adhere to in order to ensure uniform assessments are made between time points and between readers; for example, lymph nodes must be measured in "short axis," must be ≥10 mm to be considered pathologic, and must be ≥15 mm to be a target lesion. Evidence has emerged that PD rendered by appearance of new lesions or unequivocal progression of nontarget lesions may portend worse prognosis than PD marked only by target lesion growth.[42]

RECIST Alternatives

Despite being a powerful instrument to assess radiologic response, RECIST suffers a number of drawbacks that stem from reliance on one-dimensional target lesion assessments. While this approach is straightforward, it fails to account for the imaging manifestations of true biologic activity, which can lead to underestimation of therapeutic efficacy or, worse, mischaracterizing the biologic response as PD. RECIST is particularly ill-suited to assessing bone tumors, and recent evidence has shown that three-dimensional measurements outperform one-dimensional measurements in predicting Ewing sarcoma response.[43] Response of GIST to imatinib serves as the prototypical example of the failure of RECIST to capture treatment response among soft tissue sarcomas, in which biologic response may be manifested radiologically by an increase in tumor size, but a decrease in tumor enhancement (Figure 7.21). Such cases of "pseudoprogression" spurred the development of Choi criteria as a set of alternative response metrics,[44] initially specific to GIST, but later on adopted in several studies for the longitudinal assessment of sarcomas.[45,46] The Choi criteria use lesion density on contrast-enhanced CTs as a biomarker of tumor viability; decreases in tumor density over time are evidence of decreased tumor blood flow and correlate with decreases in FDG activity and increases in histologic necrosis.[47]

When quantifying changes in tumor enhancement by measuring HU, care must be taken to ensure comparisons are being made in similar contrast-enhancement phases (i.e., arterial, portal venous, or late venous). It should be pointed out that a similar phenomenon may be observed when using MRI instead of CT; however, decreased enhancement marking the tumor response is not as easily quantified. Because MRI signal intensity is relative, absolute region of interest (ROI) values cannot be directly compared between scans on conventional sequences. To overcome this limitation, one may use muscle as an internal reference tissue and essentially normalize the intensity of contrast enhancement by obtaining a ratio of tumor:muscle ROIs; this approach has been used to show that therapeutic response in soft tissue sarcomas manifests as decreased tumor enhancement,[45] although clear thresholds have not been established as for GIST (Figure 7.22).

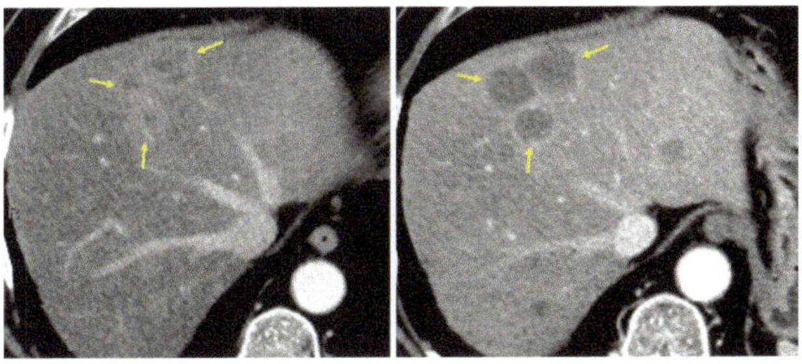

(A) (B)

FIGURE 7.21 (A) Axial contrast-enhanced CT of the abdomen demonstrates a conglomerate of three enhancing liver masses (arrows) in a patient with GIST. (B) After treatment with regorafenib, the masses enlarge, which could be mistaken for disease progression, particularly as smaller lesions become newly conspicuous. However, the masses show considerably less central enhancement than on the pretreatment scan, which is a characteristic of Choi response.

GIST, gastrointestinal stromal tumor.

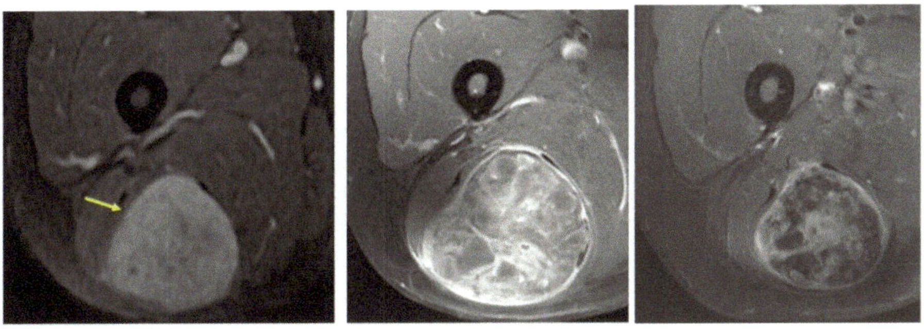

(A) (B) (C)

FIGURE 7.22 (A) Axial contrast-enhanced MRI of high-grade pleomorphic myofibrosarcoma at baseline. (B) After two cycles of neoadjuvant chemotherapy (doxorubicin/ifosfamide), the tumor demonstrated increasing heterogeneity of contrast enhancement and approximately 35% increase in maximum diameter; note that this would constitute RECIST 1.1 progressive disease. (C) After four cycles of neoadjuvant chemotherapy, the tumor regressed in both size and contrast enhancement, indicative of treatment response. The patient subsequently received neoadjuvant radiation therapy; the resected specimen demonstrated 98% histologic necrosis.

RECIST, Response Evaluation Criteria in Solid Tumors.

The advent of immunotherapy has also driven the development of response criteria that modify the basic RECIST framework. Immune-related response criteria (irRC), irRECIST, and iRECIST attempt to better account for the equivocacy of early morphologic changes in target lesions.[48–50] As the antitumor immunogenic response develops, local intratumoral and peritumoral inflammation may cause mass-like areas of consolidation and peritumoral edema that are radiologically indistinguishable from true tumor growth. As a result, additional follow-up scans are required as a confirmatory evidence of PD.

Tumor-Specific Response Patterns

Some tumor types exhibit idiosyncratic response manifestations that reflect underlying changes in tumor biology. For example, giant cell tumor of bone may be treated with denosumab, a RANK-ligand inhibitor that blocks tumoral osteoclastic activity and eliminates ≥90% of tumor giant cells.[51] This permits more net osteoblastic activity and increases bone deposition within the tumor. Treated giant cell tumor of bone may appear radiographically as an increasingly radiodense lesion with a more conspicuous sclerotic margin and slightly thickened bony trabeculae.[52]

In addition to reduction in size, desmoid-type fibromatosis may show increasing collagen deposition as the tumor biologic activity is attenuated. The extent of collagenization correlates with the degree of hypointensity on contrast-enhanced and fluid-sensitive sequences.[31] Moreover, our clinical experience has shown that in some cases, desmoid tumors show size reduction in a minor axis of measurement, rather than the longest tumor diameter, which is used in RECIST. As medical therapy, particularly with targeted agents such as sorafenib,[53] becomes more widely accepted as a first-line therapy for advanced or refractory tumors, these alternative morphologic features may be useful as more sensitive or earlier biomarkers for treatment efficacy.

In many clinical trials, response assessment is carried out locally by the investigator, rather than relying on central radiology review. In these circumstances, close collaboration with radiologists is advised to ensure optimal imaging protocols and consistent target lesion tracking and measurement techniques. The complexity of tracking multiple lesions over time across multiple scans led to the development of dedicated software to help serially track target and nontarget lesions. This greatly facilitates consistent identification of target lesions and conformity in application of response criteria.[54,55] Such software also permits multiple response assessment criteria to be run in parallel, which is particularly important in sarcoma immunotherapy trials where RECIST 1.1, Choi, and irRC/irRECIST/iRECIST criteria all emphasize different relevant features of response.

SURVEILLANCE

The ACR provides recommendations regarding the follow-up of aggressive musculoskeletal tumors after completion of therapy.[26] A few salient points are briefly reviewed here regarding this topic, while acknowledging that surveillance strategies may vary among institutions with sarcoma expertise.[56,57]

For the initial staging of metastatic disease to the lung, the ACR recommends noncontrast chest CT. Lung surveillance is recommended at intervals of every 3 to 4 months after surgery for the first 2 to 3 years after definitive treatment (for high-grade sarcomas), then every 6 months until year 5, and annually thereafter. This mirrors the recommendations made by Cipriano et al. based on recent data for development of lung metastases in bone sarcomas.[58] PET–CT may also be used for this purpose, though it should be pointed out that the imaging resolution of the CT portion of the exam is usually inferior to dedicated chest CT. Staging for osseous metastatic disease from a musculoskeletal primary tumor is optimally carried out with PET–CT, although Tc-99m bone scan or whole body MRI may be used, the latter depending on institutional availability and interpretive expertise.

For local surveillance of treated bone tumors, both radiography and MRI are recommended. When significant metallic hardware has been used in reconstruction, metal artifact reduction techniques are mandatory; specifically requesting these techniques in the order can expedite appropriate protocoling. For soft tissue sarcomas, we advocate contrast-enhanced MRI for local surveillance, in accordance with the ACR guidelines. Because recurrence risk is highest in the first 2 years after definitive STS resection, at our institution, we perform surveillance exams every 3 to 4 months during this early surveillance period, which decreases to every 6 months over the subsequent 3 years and finally to annually in the late 5- to 10-year surveillance period (Figure 7.23). It should be noted that ultrasound may be an appropriate local surveillance modality, particularly if the primary STS was superficial or there is extensive hardware resulting in CT or MRI artifact obscuring the surgical bed. However, these advantages must be considered alongside personnel experience, given the highly operator-dependent nature of ultrasound examinations. The National Comprehensive Cancer Network (NCCN) guidelines for soft tissue sarcomas of the trunk and extremities call for postoperative baseline and periodic imaging of the primary site based on the estimated risk of locoregional recurrence.

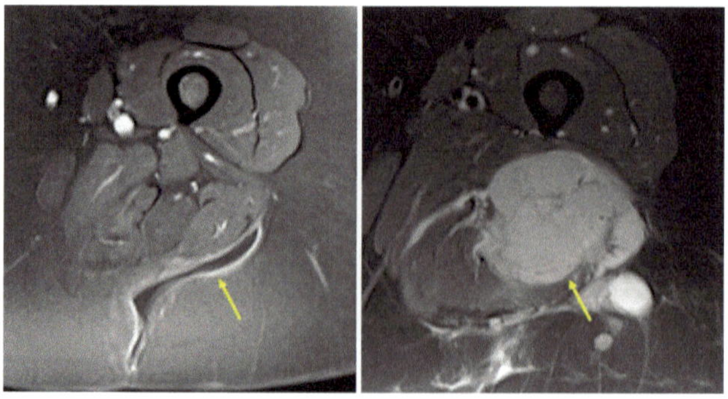

(A) (B)

FIGURE 7.23 (A) Axial contrast-enhanced MRI of the surgical bed in the posterior thigh 9 months after resection of a myxoid liposarcoma shows a postoperative seroma (arrow) that had diminished in size since previous MRI (not shown). (B) Only 3 months later, a large recurrent tumor (arrow) was evident on the surveillance scan.

SAFETY CONCERNS

As the use of CT has increased exponentially in the past two decades, advancements have been made in hardware (e.g., multirow detectors) and the algorithms used to reconstruct images to lower the dose of ionizing radiation without compromising diagnostic accuracy.[59] This is particularly important in pediatric sarcoma patients who may be exposed to serial examinations resulting in substantial cumulative dose; however, when contending with a life-threatening diagnosis, the risk–benefit and cost–benefit analyses of accurate diagnostic imaging must be weighed against other imaging alternatives.

Iodinated contrast agents have, for many years, been withheld because of concerns over nephrotoxicity. However, recent evidence from large retrospective studies well designed to account for potential biases in patient illness severity have shown little impact on renal function[60]; data are also emerging that prophylactic IV hydration confers no benefit in reducing the risk of contrast-induced nephropathy.[61] In a similar vein, gadolinium-based contrast agents have been associated with increased risk of nephrogenic systemic fibrosis in patients with or approaching renal failure. However, this association was strongest with older gadolinium contrast agents, and the number of confirmed cases of nephrogenic systemic fibrosis (NSF) with newer macrocyclic gadolinium-based agents is vanishingly small.[62,63] We emphasize that when treatment decisions stand to be heavily based on accurate imaging, use of IV contrast material should usually be weighed favorably against largely historical or theoretical risks.

ADVANCEMENTS

Radiology is a rapidly advancing discipline, but two of the more interesting developments pertaining to sarcoma imaging concern improvements in MR scanning techniques to reduce metal artifact and in imaging analytics with the increasing prevalence of radiomics.

Metallic implants result in varying degrees of susceptibility artifact based on their size, composition, and orientation in the body. The metal induces heterogeneity in the magnetic field, causing mislocalization of signal and resultant image distortion. In general, techniques used to mitigate the artifact include imaging at lower magnetic field strength (1.5 vs. 3 T), increasing receiver bandwidth, and utilizing spin echo rather than gradient echo pulse sequences. Dedicated pulse sequences designed to minimize metal artifact, such as SEMAC (from Siemens), have further improved image quality when even large metal implants are present.[64] These improvements will undoubtedly enable earlier detection of reconstruction complications such as metal-induced particle disease/osteolysis, infection, and tumor recurrence.

Radiology is currently at the forefront of the sea change in how disease will be diagnosed and monitored in a future increasingly driven by big data and analytics. Radiomics describes an approach to quantifying image texture[65]; these textural parameters can be correlated with outcomes of interest, such as histologic necrosis or survival. Recent data have shown that a radiomics analysis of soft tissue sarcomas can stratify lesions by grade,[66] but more data regarding radiomics' utility in predicting or serving as a biomarker for clinical endpoints in sarcoma are clearly needed.

SUMMARY

For bone tumors, a combination of radiographic and MRI findings often elucidates tumor subtype and biologic aggressiveness. Radiologic findings in soft tissue tumors are generally more indeterminate, though MRI can offer clues to the tumor matrix being lipomatous, myxoid, or collagenous. MRI permits accurate local staging, revealing compartmental and neurovascular involvement critical in operative planning. In the neoadjuvant setting, the degree of tumor enhancement with IV contrast agent is used as a surrogate marker for tumor viability, and changes in the nonenhancing necrotic tumor components are frequently more important than changes in tumor size in assessing therapeutic response. Awareness of particular patterns of metastatic spread (e.g., myxoid liposarcoma → soft tissues and bone) should influence staging and surveillance strategies.

REFERENCES

1. Cohen-Levy WB, Pretell-Mazzini J, Singer AD, et al. Significance of incidental intra-articular and peri-articular FDG avid foci on PET/CT. *Acta Radiol*. 2019;60(1):78–84. doi:10.1177/0284185118770901
2. Miller TT. Bone tumors and tumorlike conditions: analysis with conventional radiography. *Radiology*. 2008;246(3):662–674. doi:10.1148/radiol.2463061038

3. Lodwick GS. Radiographic diagnosis and grading of bone tumors, with comments on computer evaluation. *Proc Natl Cancer Conf*. 1964;5:369–380. PMID:5856167.
4. Caracciolo JT, Temple HT, Letson GD, Kransdorf MJ. A modified Lodwick-Madewell grading system for the evaluation of lytic bone lesions. *AJR Am J Roentgenol*. 2016;207(1):150–156. doi:10.2214/AJR.15.14368
5. Mirabello L, Troisi RJ, Savage SA. Osteosarcoma incidence and survival rates from 1973 to 2004: data from the Surveillance, Epidemiology, and End Results Program. *Cancer*. 2009;115(7):1531–1543. doi:10.1002/cncr.24121
6. Murphey MD, Robbin MR, McRae GA, et al. The many faces of osteosarcoma. *Radiographics*. 1997;17(5):1205–1231. doi:10.1148/radiographics.17.5.9308111
7. Yarmish G, Klein MJ, Landa J, et al. Imaging characteristics of primary osteosarcoma: nonconventional subtypes. *Radiographics*. 2010;30(6):1653–1672. doi:10.1148/rg.306105524
8. Jelinek JS, Murphey MD, Kransdorf MJ, et al. Parosteal osteosarcoma: value of MR imaging and CT in the prediction of histologic grade. *Radiology*. 1996;201(3):837–842. doi:10.1148/radiology.201.3.8939240
9. Bertoni F, Bacchini P, Staals EL, Davidovitz P. Dedifferentiated parosteal osteosarcoma: the experience of the Rizzoli Institute. *Cancer*. 2005;103(11):2373–2382. doi:10.1002/cncr.21039
10. Damron TA, Ward WG, Stewart A. Osteosarcoma, chondrosarcoma, and Ewing's sarcoma: National Cancer Data Base Report. *Clin Orthop*. 2007;459:40–47. doi:10.1097/BLO.0b013e318059b8c9
11. Revell MP, Deshmukh N, Grimer RJ, et al. Periosteal osteosarcoma: a review of 17 cases with mean follow-up of 52 months. *Sarcoma*. 2002;6(4):123–130. doi:10.1080/1357714021000066368
12. Murphey MD, Jelinek JS, Temple HT, et al. Imaging of periosteal osteosarcoma: radiologic-pathologic comparison. *Radiology*. 2004;233(1):129–138. doi:10.1148/radiol.2331030326
13. Eefting D, Schrage YM, Geirnaerdt MJA, et al. Assessment of interobserver variability and histologic parameters to improve reliability in classification and grading of central cartilaginous tumors. *Am J Surg Pathol*. 2009;33(1):50–57. doi:10.1097/PAS.0b013e31817eec2b
14. Skeletal Lesions Interobserver Correlation among Expert Diagnosticians (SLICED) Study Group. Reliability of histopathologic and radiologic grading of cartilaginous neoplasms in long bones. *J Bone Joint Surg Am*. 2007;89(10):2113–2123. doi:10.2106/00004623-200710000-00003
15. Crim J, Schmidt R, Layfield L, et al. Can imaging criteria distinguish enchondroma from grade 1 chondrosarcoma? *Eur J Radiol*. 2015;84(11):2222–2230. doi:10.1016/j.ejrad.2015.06.033
16. Roitman PD, Farfalli GL, Ayerza MA, et al. Is needle biopsy clinically useful in preoperative grading of central chondrosarcoma of the pelvis and long bones? *Clin Orthop*. 2017;475(3):808–814. doi:10.1007/s11999-016-4738-y
17. Subhawong TK, Winn A, Shemesh SS, Pretell-Mazzini J. F-18 FDG PET differentiation of benign from malignant chondroid neoplasms: a systematic review of the literature. *Skeletal Radiol*. 2017;46(9):1233–1239. doi:10.1007/s00256-017-2685-7
18. Henderson ER, Pala E, Angelini A, et al. Dedifferentiated peripheral chondrosarcoma: a review of radiologic characteristics. *Sarcoma*. 2013;2013:505321. doi:10.1155/2013/505321
19. Taylor K, Kransdorf MJ, Schwartz AJ, et al. Mosaic-pattern dedifferentiation in liposarcoma and chondrosarcoma: imaging features of an uncommon form of dedifferentiation. *Skeletal Radiol*. 2018;47(6):877–882. doi:10.1007/s00256-017-2866-4
20. Farsad K, Kattapuram SV, Sacknoff R, et al. Sacral chordoma. *Radiographics*. 2009;29(5):1525–1530. doi:10.1148/rg.295085215
21. Yin P, Mao N, Zhao C, et al. Comparison of radiomics machine-learning classifiers and feature selection for differentiation of sacral chordoma and sacral giant cell tumour based on 3D computed tomography features. *Eur Radiol*. 2019;29(4):1841–1847. doi:10.1007/s00330-018-5730-6
22. van Wulfften Palthe ODR, Tromp I, Ferreira A, et al. Sacral chordoma: a clinical review of 101 cases with 30-year experience in a single institution. *Spine J*. 2018;19(5):869–879. doi:10.1016/j.spinee.2018.11.002
23. Eggli KD, Quiogue T, Moser RP. Ewing's sarcoma. *Radiol Clin North Am*. 1993;31(2):325–337. PMID:8446752.
24. Saifuddin A, Whelan J, Pringle JA, Cannon SR. Malignant round cell tumours of bone: atypical clinical and imaging features. *Skeletal Radiol*. 2000;29(11):646–651. doi:10.1007/s002560000277
25. Murphey MD, Senchak LT, Mambalam PK, et al. From the radiologic pathology archives: Ewing sarcoma family of tumors: radiologic-pathologic correlation. *Radiographics*. 2013;33(3):803–831. doi:10.1148/rg.333135005
26. Roberts CC, Kransdorf MJ, Beaman FD, et al. ACR appropriateness criteria follow-up of malignant or aggressive musculoskeletal tumors. *J Am Coll Radiol*. 2016;13(4):389–400. doi:10.1016/j.jacr.2015.12.019
27. Gaskin CM, Helms CA. Lipomas, lipoma variants, and well-differentiated liposarcomas (atypical lipomas): results of MRI evaluations of 126 consecutive fatty masses. *AJR Am J Roentgenol*. 2004;182(3):733–739. doi:10.2214/ajr.182.3.1820733
28. Rizer M, Singer AD, Edgar M, et al. The histological variants of liposarcoma: predictive MRI findings with prognostic implications, management, follow-up, and differential diagnosis. *Skeletal Radiol*. 2016;45(9):1193–1204. doi:10.1007/s00256-016-2409-4
29. Lefkowitz RA, Landa J, Hwang S, et al. Myxofibrosarcoma: prevalence and diagnostic value of the "tail sign" on magnetic resonance imaging. *Skeletal Radiol*. 2013;42(6):809–818. doi:10.1007/s00256-012-1563-6
30. White LM, Wunder JS, Bell RS, et al. Histologic assessment of peritumoral edema in soft tissue sarcoma. *Int J Radiat Oncol Biol Phys*. 2005;61(5):1439–1445. doi:10.1016/j.ijrobp.2004.08.036
31. Sheth PJ, Del Moral S, Wilky BA, et al. Desmoid fibromatosis: MRI features of response to systemic therapy. *Skeletal Radiol*. 2016;45(10):1365–1373. doi:10.1007/s00256-016-2439-y

32. Gondim Teixeira PA, Chanson A, Verhaeghe J-L, et al. Correlation between tumor growth and hormonal therapy with MR signal characteristics of desmoid-type fibromatosis: a preliminary study. *Diagn Interv Imaging*. 2019;100(1):47–55. doi:10.1016/j.diii.2018.06.007
33. Amin MB, Edge S, Greene F, et al., eds. AJCC Cancer Staging Manual. 8th ed. Berlin, Germany: Springer; 2017.
34. Hahn E, Huang SH, Hosni A, et al. Ending 40 years of silence: rationale for a new staging system for soft tissue sarcoma of the head and neck. *Clin Transl Radiat Oncol*. 2019;15:13–19. doi:10.1016/j.ctro.2018.11.009
35. Zhao F, Ahlawat S, Farahani SJ, et al. Can MR imaging be used to predict tumor grade in soft-tissue sarcoma? *Radiology*. 2014;272(1):192–201. doi:10.1148/radiol.14131871
36. Royce TJ, Punglia RS, Chen AB, et al. Cost-effectiveness of surveillance for distant recurrence in extremity soft tissue sarcoma. *Ann Surg Oncol*. 2017;24(11):3264–3270. doi:10.1245/s10434-017-5996-y
37. Keung EZ, Chiang Y-J, Voss RK, et al. Defining the incidence and clinical significance of lymph node metastasis in soft tissue sarcoma. *Eur J Surg Oncol*. 2018;44(1):170–177. doi:10.1016/j.ejso.2017.11.014
38. Fong Y, Coit DG, Woodruff JM, Brennan MF. Lymph node metastasis from soft tissue sarcoma in adults. Analysis of data from a prospective database of 1772 sarcoma patients. *Ann Surg*. 1993;217(1):72–77. doi:10.1097/00000658-199301000-00012
39. Dürr HR, Rauh J, Baur-Melnyk A, et al. Myxoid liposarcoma: local relapse and metastatic pattern in 43 patients. *BMC Cancer*. 2018;18(1):304. doi:10.1186/s12885-018-4226-8
40. Eisenhauer EA, Therasse P, Bogaerts J, et al. New response evaluation criteria in solid tumours: revised RECIST guideline (version 1.1). *Eur J Cancer*. 2009;45(2):228–247. doi:10.1016/j.ejca.2008.10.026
41. Schwartz LH, Litière S, de Vries E, et al. RECIST 1.1—update and clarification: from the RECIST committee. *Eur J Cancer*. 2016;62:132–137. doi:10.1016/j.ejca.2016.03.081
42. Litière S, de Vries EGE, Seymour L, et al. The components of progression as explanatory variables for overall survival in the Response Evaluation Criteria in Solid Tumours 1.1 database. *Eur J Cancer*. 2014;50(10):1847–1853. doi:10.1016/j.ejca.2014.03.014
43. Aghighi M, Boe J, Rosenberg J, et al. Three-dimensional radiologic assessment of chemotherapy response in Ewing sarcoma can be used to predict clinical outcome. *Radiology*. 2016;280(3):905–915. doi:10.1148/radiol.2016151301
44. Choi H, Charnsangavej C, Faria SC, et al. Correlation of computed tomography and positron emission tomography in patients with metastatic gastrointestinal stromal tumor treated at a single institution with imatinib mesylate: proposal of new computed tomography response criteria. *J Clin Oncol*. 2007;25(13):1753–1759. doi:10.1200/JCO.2006.07.3049
45. Stacchiotti S, Collini P, Messina A, et al. High-grade soft-tissue sarcomas: tumor response assessment—pilot study to assess the correlation between radiologic and pathologic response by using RECIST and Choi criteria. *Radiology*. 2009;251(2):447–456. doi:10.1148/radiol.2512081403
46. Stacchiotti S, Morosi C, Lo Vullo S, et al. Imatinib and everolimus in patients with progressing advanced chordoma: a phase 2 clinical study. *Cancer*. 2018;124(20):4056–4063.doi:10.1002/cncr.31685
47. Choi H, Charnsangavej C, de Castro Faria S, et al. CT evaluation of the response of gastrointestinal stromal tumors after imatinib mesylate treatment: a quantitative analysis correlated with FDG PET findings. *AJR Am J Roentgenol*. 2004;183(6):1619–1628. doi:10.2214/ajr.183.6.01831619
48. Seymour L, Bogaerts J, Perrone A, et al. iRECIST: guidelines for response criteria for use in trials testing immunotherapeutics. *Lancet Oncol*. 2017;18(3):e143–e152. doi:10.1016/S1470-2045(17)30074-8
49. Carter BW, Bhosale PR, Yang WT. Immunotherapy and the role of imaging. *Cancer*. 2018;124(14):2906–2922. doi:10.1002/cncr.31349
50. Wolchok JD, Hoos A, O'Day S, et al. Guidelines for the evaluation of immune therapy activity in solid tumors: immune-related response criteria. *Clin Cancer Res*. 2009;15(23):7412–7420. doi:10.1158/1078-0432.CCR-09-1624
51. Branstetter DG, Nelson SD, Manivel JC, et al. Denosumab induces tumor reduction and bone formation in patients with giant-cell tumor of bone. *Clin Cancer Res*. 2012;18(16):4415–4424. doi:10.1158/1078-0432.CCR-12-0578
52. Engellau J, Seeger L, Grimer R, et al. Assessment of denosumab treatment effects and imaging response in patients with giant cell tumor of bone. *World J Surg Oncol*. 2018;16(1):191. doi:10.1186/s12957-018-1478-3
53. Gounder MM, Mahoney MR, Van Tine BA, et al. Sorafenib for advanced and refractory desmoid tumors. *N Engl J Med*. 2018;379(25):2417–2428. doi:10.1056/NEJMoa1805052
54. Gjolaj L, Dang A, Peck H, et al. System redesign of a radiology research clinic for oncology clinical trial patients. *J Am Coll Radiol*. 2018;15(9):1304–1308. doi:10.1016/j.jacr.2018.04.019
55. Machado LB, Apolo AB, Steinberg SM, Folio LR. Radiology reports with hyperlinks improve target lesion selection and measurement concordance in cancer trials. *AJR Am J Roentgenol*. 2017;208(2):W31–W37. doi:10.2214/AJR.16.16845
56. Patel SA, Royce TJ, Barysauskas CM, et al. Surveillance imaging patterns and outcomes following radiation therapy and radical resection for localized extremity and trunk soft tissue sarcoma. *Ann Surg Oncol*. 2017;24(6):1588–1595. doi:10.1245/s10434-016-5755-5
57. Ezuddin NS, Pretell-Mazzini J, Yechieli RL, et al. Local recurrence of soft-tissue sarcoma: issues in imaging surveillance strategy. *Skeletal Radiol*. 2018;47(12):1595–1606. doi:10.1007/s00256-018-2965-x
58. Cipriano C, Griffin AM, Ferguson PC, Wunder JS. Developing an evidence-based followup schedule for bone sarcomas based on local recurrence and metastatic progression. *Clin Orthop*. 2017;475(3):830–838. doi:10.1007/s11999-016-4941-x

59. Raman SP, Mahesh M, Blasko RV, Fishman EK. CT scan parameters and radiation dose: practical advice for radiologists. *J Am Coll Radiol*. 2013;10(11):840–846. doi:10.1016/j.jacr.2013.05.032
60. Luk L, Steinman J, Newhouse JH. Intravenous contrast-induced nephropathy-the rise and fall of a threatening idea. *Adv Chronic Kidney Dis*. 2017;24(3):169–175. doi:10.1053/j.ackd.2017.03.001
61. Nijssen EC, Rennenberg RJ, Nelemans PJ, et al. Prophylactic hydration to protect renal function from intravascular iodinated contrast material in patients at high risk of contrast-induced nephropathy (AMACING): a prospective, randomised, phase 3, controlled, open-label, non-inferiority trial. *Lancet*. 2017;389(10076):1312–1322. doi:10.1016/S0140-6736(17)30057-0
62. Amet S, Launay-Vacher V, Clément O, et al. Incidence of nephrogenic systemic fibrosis in patients undergoing dialysis after contrast-enhanced magnetic resonance imaging with gadolinium-based contrast agents: the Prospective Fibrose Nephrogénique Systémique study. *Invest Radiol*. 2014;49(2):109–115. doi:10.1097/RLI.0000000000000000
63. Soyer P, Dohan A, Patkar D, Gottschalk A. Observational study on the safety profile of gadoterate meglumine in 35,499 patients: the SECURE study. *J Magn Reson Imaging*. 2017;45(4):988–997. doi:10.1002/jmri.25486
64. Fritz J, Lurie B, Potter HG. MR imaging of knee arthroplasty implants. *Radiographics*. 2015;35(5):1483–1501. doi:10.1148/rg.2015140216
65. Gillies RJ, Kinahan PE, Hricak H. Radiomics: images are more than pictures, they are data. *Radiology*. 2016;278(2):563–577. doi:10.1148/radiol.2015151169
66. Corino VDA, Montin E, Messina A, et al. Radiomic analysis of soft tissues sarcomas can distinguish intermediate from high-grade lesions. *J Magn Reson Imaging*. 2018;47(3):829–840. doi:10.1002/jmri.25791

II

Select Sarcoma Subtypes

8

Leiomyosarcoma

Amanda Parkes and Neeta Somaiah

INTRODUCTION

Leiomyosarcoma (LMS) is a malignant mesenchymal tumor originating from the smooth muscle connective tissue. With a propensity for early hematogenous dissemination, LMS, in general, behaves aggressively, with studies showing higher risk for distant recurrence and poorer disease-specific survival than most other sarcoma subtypes. As in other sarcoma subtypes, histologic grade is a fundamental prognostic indicator, and reports show that up to 90% of LMS are moderate to high grade. This translates into survival differences, with a 5-year survival rate for LMS of 40%, which decreases to 10% to 15% for high-grade LMS. This aggressive behavior is paired with a relatively high frequency of LMS cases relative to other soft tissue sarcoma subtypes, with LMS accounting for approximately 10% of all soft tissue sarcomas. There has been a reported decrease in the overall incidence of LMS since 1970; however, this has been attributed most significantly to the reclassification of some previously classified gastric LMS as gastrointestinal stromal tumors with improved immunohistochemical characterization.

The two broad categories of LMS include uterine leiomyosarcoma (ULMS) and nonuterine leiomyosarcoma (NULMS), with some unique differences that are also incorporated into the current treatment paradigms. ULMS is associated with higher sensitivity to ifosfamide, greater metastatic potential, and lower median survival of approximately 4.2 years, compared with NULMS, which has a median survival of approximately 8 years.[1] Though NULMS can occur in any part of the body with smooth muscle, a common site of origin is the wall of the inferior vena cava in the retroperitoneum. There are also unique molecular aberrations associated with ULMS and NULMS, some of which may influence sensitivity to treatment. Of the three LMS molecular subtypes confirmed by Guo et al. in 2015, types 1 and 2 are linked with extrauterine sites and type 3 is associated with ULMS.[2] In addition to the differing molecular aberrations of ULMS and NULMS that are described in further detail in this chapter, LMS has frequent losses in chromosome 10q, which houses the *PTEN* gene. Loss of *PTEN* expression ultimately leads to constitutive Akt and mTOR (mammalian target of rapamycin) activation, which has been shown to be important in LMS pathology. Given their distinctive behaviors, ULMS and NULMS are described in greater detail under separate sections, and differences are highlighted when applicable all through the chapter.

WORKUP

Presenting symptoms for LMS are often nonspecific, typically caused by the primary tumor displacing normal structures, and hence unique to the location. Alternatively, they may present as a palpable mass, such as with an extremity primary or with subcutaneous metastases. Many times, these tumors are incidental discoveries, either on imaging or as a surprise finding on hysterectomy (ULMS). Certain presenting symptoms are unique to their tumor location, with half of ULMS patients with uterine-confined disease presenting with a solitary, large intramural mass that is often palpable. Other presenting symptoms for ULMS may include uterine bleeding, increased abdominal girth, and pelvic pain or pressure. This is in contrast to the LMS of the inferior vena cava, which is often associated with abdominal or flank pain, with other possible presenting symptoms including abdominal distention, Budd–Chiari syndrome, lower extremity edema, and even deep venous thrombosis.

Initial workup includes imaging approaches to visualize the primary tumor and possible sites of metastatic disease. With regard to primary tumor imaging, typical approaches involve use of MRI with and without contrast for extremity soft tissue tumors and CT with contrast for chest, abdominal, or pelvic masses. Chest and abdominal CT scan is required in the initial workup, given the frequent hematogenous spread seen in LMS, with liver and lung being the common sites of metastatic disease. Other sites of metastatic disease include subcutaneous sites, bone, central nervous system, and rarely, the gastrointestinal system. Morphologic imaging features associated with LMS depend on imaging modality and site of the primary tumor. On CT imaging, LMS is typically heterogeneous with central low attenuation that represents necrosis. Calcification is typically not observed in LMS. MRI shows signal characteristics including T1 isointense to muscle, T2 fat-suppressed predominantly hyperintense, and T2 non–fat-suppressed intermediate to hypointense to surrounding fat. MRI may also show cystic foci within the tumor. As with other soft tissue sarcomas, there are no pathognomonic findings for LMS on imaging, which is why the diagnostic approach for LMS involves pretreatment biopsy with appropriate pathologic review. LMS is typically reactive for smooth muscle actin, h-caldesmon, and desmin on immunohistochemistry; however, none of these markers are specific for smooth muscle differentiation. Pathologic review must also include histologic grading, which, as mentioned above, is an independent indicator of disease-specific survival as well as probability of metastatic disease.

TREATMENT OF LOCALIZED DISEASE

Nuances specific to the treatment of ULMS and NULMS are detailed in their respective sections; however, for both ULMS and NULMS, the cornerstone of treatment is complete surgical excision with wide negative margins, whenever possible. Large NULMS tumors in the retroperitoneum are associated with anatomic constraints that often make complete surgical resection challenging. R0 resection remains the most important prognostic factor associated with survival.

Use of neoadjuvant or adjuvant radiation and chemotherapy should be considered based on unique clinical characteristics similar to other soft tissue sarcomas. Given the high propensity for metastases with high-grade LMS and their relative sensitivity to chemotherapy, it is common clinical practice to consider neoadjuvant or adjuvant chemotherapy in large tumors >5 cm in size, similar to other soft tissue sarcomas.[3] Neoadjuvant/adjuvant chemotherapy use in ULMS is even less standardized, and the approach varies among different centers and whether patients are managed by sarcoma oncologists versus gynecologic oncologists. This is discussed in further detail in the section "Uterine Leiomyosarcoma." Preferred chemotherapy regimens for neoadjuvant or adjuvant treatment differ by LMS subtype with doxorubicin plus dacarbazine used in NULMS and either doxorubicin plus ifosfamide or gemcitabine plus docetaxel used in ULMS.

ULMS has no clear indication for adjuvant radiation, but can be discussed on a case-by-case basis if there is a concern for positive margin surgery or for a localized pelvic recurrence. Neoadjuvant radiation is given as a lower dose than adjuvant radiation, and thus is generally preferred to minimize toxicity to the bowel and other surrounding structures that occupy the resection cavity. For NULMS, radiation has been shown to improve local control with decreased local recurrence rates, but without a proven overall survival benefit. This specifically applies to the extremity and trunk location, where neoadjuvant/adjuvant radiation therapy is standard for intermediate to high-grade, ≥5 cm soft tissue sarcomas.[4] There is a paucity of data regarding its use for primary retroperitoneal soft tissue sarcomas. Ultimately, preoperative or postoperative radiation is the standard of care for LMS patients with intermediate or high-grade, large tumors involving the limbs and trunk, whereas it is not standard for retroperitoneal NULMS or ULMS.

FOLLOW-UP AFTER DEFINITIVE TREATMENT

Following definitive treatment of initial localized disease, surveillance recommendations are similar to other soft tissue sarcomas with history and physical exams taken every 3 to 6 months for 2 to 3 years, which is then lengthened to every 6 months for the next 2 years and then annually. Surveillance imaging is incorporated into these visits to include the primary site and chest imaging. For retroperitoneal or pelvic tumors, imaging should include the entire abdomen and pelvis. The imaging schedule can be altered based on the estimated risk of locoregional recurrence.

TREATMENT OF METASTATIC DISEASE

As previously noted, LMS is a highly aggressive tumor with a propensity for early hematogenous dissemination. Common sites of metastases in both ULMS and NULMS are lung and liver. Liver is a common metastatic site for visceral primaries, whereas lung is the most common site of metastasis in patients with ULMS and NULMS with extremity primary tumors. In addition to this high risk for metastatic disease, LMS is associated with a high risk of relapse. Both relapsed and metastatic disease are associated with a high mortality rate. Treatment intent in metastatic LMS is palliative, with the goals of improving symptoms and quality of life, decreasing the tumor bulk, and improving survival.

Similar to other soft tissue sarcomas, first-line chemotherapy involves anthracycline-based regimens, but the most data are available for doxorubicin-based therapies. Combination chemotherapy with doxorubicin, using either doxorubicin plus ifosfamide or doxorubicin plus dacarbazine, has historically shown improved response rates, but not improved overall survival. Given this, these doxorubicin-based combination therapies are typically utilized when the response is critical, such as in symptomatic disease, potentially resectable disease, or when the tumor threatens the end organ function. The combination of doxorubicin plus olaratumab uniquely did not improve the response rate compared to single-agent doxorubicin, but did improve overall survival in a Phase 2 study. The Phase 3 results of the doxorubicin plus olaratumab combination did not confirm the findings of the Phase 2 study; thus, doxorubicin plus either ifosfamide or dacarbazine remains standard. Uniquely, ULMS has been associated with higher response to ifosfamide, whereas it has limited activity as a single agent in NULMS, suggesting that doxorubicin plus ifosfamide may be a more appropriate frontline regimen for ULMS as compared with NULMS. In NULMS, given the poorer response to ifosfamide, frontline chemotherapy with doxorubicin doublets is now typically doxorubicin plus dacarbazine.

Beyond the first-line treatment with anthracyclines, other active cytotoxic agents for metastatic LMS include gemcitabine with or without docetaxel, pazopanib, and trabectedin. If not given in the first-line setting, dacarbazine (or temozolamide) and ifosfamide (particular to ULMS) also has activity. Gemcitabine plus docetaxel has a higher activity in LMS (50% response rate) compared to most other soft tissue sarcoma subtypes, and hence is often used in the frontline setting for LMS.[5] There has been conflicting evidence regarding the benefit of addition of docetaxel to single-agent gemcitabine, with one trial showing improved efficacy of the combination in the second-line treatment of LMS,[5] but a second randomized trial specific to LMS patients showing no improvement in response rate, progression-free survival, and overall survival in patients treated with gemcitabine plus docetaxel as compared with gemcitabine alone.[6] In healthy patients with a good performance status, the use of gemcitabine plus docetaxel is reasonable; however, gemcitabine single agent is a reasonable treatment strategy, particularly for those patients with poorer performance status or intolerance to the more toxic side effects associated with the gemcitabine plus docetaxel combination.

In further lines of therapy, the multikinase inhibitor pazopanib was approved for treatment of soft tissue sarcomas, including LMS, that have progressed after prior cytotoxic therapy, with improved progression-free survival but not overall survival found in the Phase 3 trial as compared with a control group. The cytotoxic agent trabectedin is also approved for LMS and liposarcomas and should be considered in later lines of therapy. As with other therapies, tumor shrinkage with trabectedin is often preceded by early tissue changes. This can lead to radiographic response in the form of decreasing density, as seen in Figure 8.1, which may not be captured if utilizing only Response Evaluation Criteria in Solid Tumors (RECIST) criteria for response assessments and is an important consideration when assessing individual patients as well as designing clinical trials. Beyond the aforementioned treatments, the Phase 2 REGOSARC trial showed improved progression-free survival with regorafenib in patients with nonadipocytic soft tissue sarcomas including LMS. Additionally, while only approved in liposarcoma, a randomized Phase 3 trial of eribulin versus dacarbazine showed some disease stabilization with eribulin in LMS, but not superior to dacarbazine, suggesting this as a treatment option in later lines of therapy for LMS patients.

Various options are under investigation for LMS, including a multitarget tyrosine kinase inhibitor anlotinib. In the Phase 2 clinical trial of anlotinib in soft tissue sarcoma patients, reported outcomes showed that almost 70% of LMS patients were progression free at 12 weeks with a median progression-free survival of 11.07 months in LMS patients. There is an ongoing randomized study of dacarbazine versus anlotinib in LMS to confirm this activity. Additionally, while not considered the standard of care, mTOR inhibitors can be considered in LMS patients, given the loss of *PTEN* expression in these tumors, leading to Akt and mTOR activation, which is thought to be instrumental in LMS. In a Phase 2 clinical trial in advanced bone and soft tissue sarcomas, ridaforolimus, a second-generation mTOR inhibitor, showed a median progression-free survival of 15.3 weeks and a higher clinical benefit rate in LMS than other cohorts (33.3%).

More recently, immunotherapy combinations have been evaluated, as they were felt to have potential in LMS, given the presence of PD-1 (programmed cell death 1 protein) expression on some tumors, high

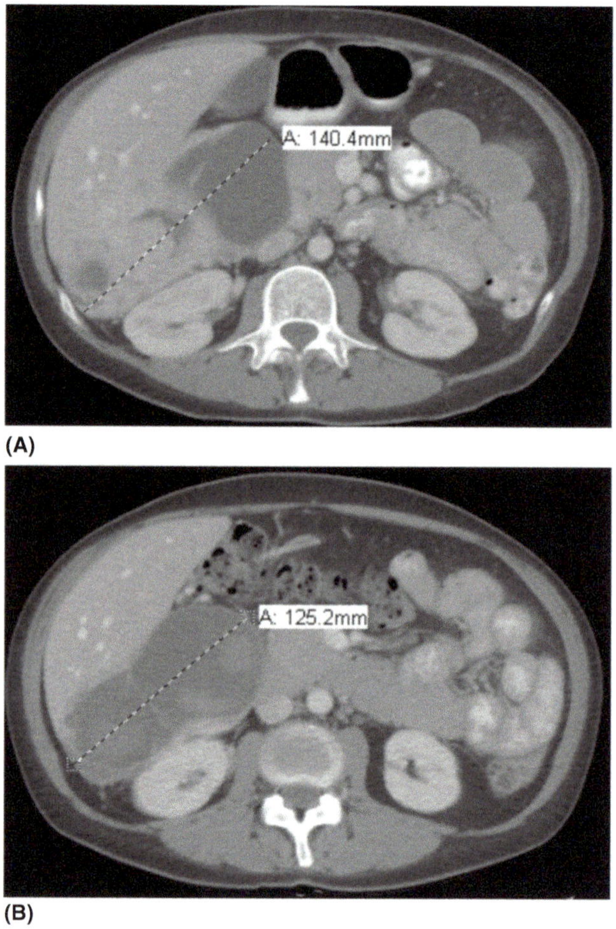

FIGURE 8.1 (A) Pretreatment imaging showing a pathologically confirmed leiomyosarcoma (peritoneal and liver metastases). (B) Imaging following just two cycles of doxorubicin and dacarbazine showed tumor response with increased cystic changes, highlighting that initial radiographic response can be in the form of decreasing density that may not always fulfill the RECIST response criteria.

RECIST, Response Evaluation Criteria in Solid Tumors.

mutation rates, and high levels of T-cell–related gene expression. While these findings would suggest immunogenicity, the SARC028 trial notably showed no objective responses in patients with LMS treated with single-agent pembrolizumab. Additionally, an early Phase 2 trial of nivolimumab in patients with metastatic ULMS also failed to show a response. This suggests that immunotherapy combinations are likely necessary to overcome possible reasons for poor single-agent immunotherapy response, including immunosuppressive tumor-activated macrophages. To this end, Alliance A091401 did show responses in ULMS ($n = 1$) and NULMS ($n = 1$) in the group receiving the nivolumab plus ipilimumab combination. Additionally, molecular analysis has suggested that *PTEN* loss in LMS may lead to resistance to PD1 inhibitors, which may need to be addressed in future immunotherapy treatment paradigms for LMS patients.

Beyond the standard therapies and the clinical trials discussed, patients with reasonable performance status can be evaluated for other available clinical trials. Possible targets include surora kinase A inhibition with or without mTOR inhibition, ROR2, EGFR inhibition, LMP2, HCG/SF, and CD47 inhibition.

For certain patients with advanced disease, surgery, stereotactic radiation, or radiofrequency ablation or cryoablation should be considered in the following circumstances. Patients who develop oligometastatic disease, appearing >6 months after the primary resection, might benefit from surgery alone. In patients with limited lung-only metastases, pulmonary metastatectomy has been associated with improved survival outcomes.[7] In addition, some patients who were initially unresectable, but have a significant response to chemotherapy and can have all visible tumor resected, should also be evaluated in a multidisciplinary setting.

UTERINE LEIOMYOSARCOMA

ULMS is a high-risk malignancy of uterine smooth muscle. While accounting for only 1% of all uterine malignancies, ULMS accounts for approximately 40% of all uterine sarcomas (the remainder is made up of approximately 50% carcinosarcomas followed by 10% of adenosarcomas and endometrial stromal sarcomas). This leads to a quoted incidence of ULMS of 0.36 per 100,000 woman-years. Most commonly, ULMS is seen in women over the age of 40, with the incidence rapidly increasing after age 50. African American females have a twofold higher incidence of ULMS than white females. In addition to race, other risk factors felt possibly associated with increased ULMS risk include obesity, diabetes, and use of tamoxifen for >5 years, which have been reported to increase ULMS risk to 17 per 100,000 woman-years.

Multiple molecular alterations are associated with ULMS. Most ULMS cases show 13q chromosome loss, which contains the tumor suppressor gene *Rb*, while approximately 60% of ULMS cases show loss of 10q, which contains the tumor suppressor gene *PTEN*. Loss of 13q has been shown to be associated with an improved prognosis as compared with 10q loss, which is associated with recurrent and higher-grade tumors. Additionally, almost half of ULMS cases are associated with X-chromosome gains, notably with amplicons located near regions containing the androgen receptor. This has been hypothesized to contribute to ULMS resistance to hormone therapy, which highlights the importance of molecular aberrations that, in the future, might drive treatment decision-making.

ULMS typically occurs de novo; however, there have been reports of transformation from uterine leiomyomas, which are a commonly occurring smooth muscle hyperplasia documented in up to 80% of women. Transformation from uterine leiomyoma to ULMS is very rare (<0.1%).

As noted in the section "Workup," ULMS requires appropriate pathologic diagnosis. This is particularly important as carcinosarcomas, otherwise known as malignant mixed müllerian tumors, are another type of uterine sarcoma that are currently treated according to epithelial uterine cancer paradigms, which are distinctly different from those used for ULMS. Given this, a pathologic review to ensure lack of an epithelial component through proper immunohistochemical analysis is critical. Of note, differentiating between uterine leiomyoma and ULMS is particularly difficult as benign uterine lesions can have high mitotic rate or atypical features. The term "smooth uterine muscle of uncertain malignant potential" (STUMP) is used for uterine smooth muscle tumors that cannot be unequivocally diagnosed as benign or malignant.

Notably, given lack of both clinical and radiologic criteria to differentiate leiomyomas from malignant uterine tumors, procedures such as morcellation that lead to possible tumor spillage are highly discouraged. Instead, standard treatment of uterine fibroids should be en bloc resection of the tumor and, if localized LMS is proved, then a total hysterectomy. The added benefit of bilateral salpingo-oophorectomy is not established, particularly in premenopausal patients, and should be determined on a case-by-case basis. Additionally, lymph node dissection has not demonstrated improved outcomes. Following surgical resection, there is no clear indication for adjuvant radiation, with a prospective randomized trial of adjuvant radiation failing to show improved relapse-free survival or overall survival. Although data are limited, adjuvant chemotherapy is considered at some centers, particularly for high-grade tumors >5 cm. This is, in part, due to the high risk of recurrent disease even in patients with disease limited to the uterus, where there is an estimated 50% to 70% risk for recurrence. A small randomized trial of adjuvant single-agent doxorubicin versus observation did not show a survival benefit to doxorubicin when given without ifosfamide or dacarbazine. This is contrasted by suggestion of improved 2-year progression-free survival with four cycles of adjuvant gemcitabine plus docetaxel or four cycles of adjuvant gemcitabine plus docetaxel followed by four cycles of doxorubicin, compared to historical progression-free survival rates. Notably, these are uncontrolled studies. GOG 277 was a planned randomized trial to answer the question of the role of adjuvant chemotherapy in early-stage ULMS; however, the study was closed owing to accrual futility. The authors did note that the observed survival data did not suggest improved outcomes for patients treated with adjuvant chemotherapy; however, statistical analysis was limited by the small sample size.

In metastatic ULMS, the combination of doxorubicin plus ifosfamide is an appropriate frontline consideration, given the higher response to ifosfamide in ULMS, particularly for patients with good performance status. Doxorubicin plus dacarbazine is also a consideration for first-line treatment. The GeDDiS trial evaluated single-agent doxorubicin versus gemcitabine plus docetaxel as the first-line treatment in metastatic soft tissue sarcomas and found no difference in response rate or progression-free survival in patients, including in subgroup analyses that specifically evaluated ULMS. As noted in the section "Treatment of Metastatic Disease," other therapeutic options include trabectedin and pazopanib.

Uniquely, for ULMS as compared with NULMS, there is activity of endocrine therapy agents in estrogen receptor/progesterone receptor–positive, low–intermediate-grade ULMS. Specifically, aromatase inhibitors have shown low overall response rates in LMS, but are a reasonable consideration in patients with low disease burden with an indolent pace of disease.

NONUTERINE LEIOMYOSARCOMA

As noted in the section "Introduction," LMS accounts for approximately 10% of all soft tissue sarcomas. The most common anatomic location of NULMS is the retroperitoneum, and hence, NULMS constitutes a high percentage of soft tissue sarcomas arising in the retroperitoneum (10%–37%). NULMS is less commonly seen in the extremities and represents only approximately 10% to 15% of sarcomas seen in the extremities. When arising in an extremity, NULMS is most commonly seen in the thigh, often arising from veins. Indeed, LMS is the most common sarcoma arising from large blood vessels; however, LMS of the inferior vena cava is still a rare clinical entity, accounting for only 0.5% of all soft tissue sarcomas in adults. Finally, primary cutaneous and primary bone LMS is a well-documented entity that is, however, fairly infrequent. Uniquely, primary bone LMS, which accounts for <0.7% of all primary bone tumors, is typically treated with bone regimens rather than typical soft tissue sarcoma regimens utilized for other LMS tumors.

As mentioned in the section "Introduction," improved immunohistochemical characterization has led to reclassification of some previously classified gastric LMS as gastrointestinal stromal tumors. True gastrointestinal LMS is rare, but this diagnosis is an important consideration, as gastrointestinal LMS has a less favorable outcome than gastrointestinal stromal tumors. Gastrointestinal LMS is predominantly found in the stomach, while leiomyomas occur most often in the esophagus, colon, and rectum. Location of gastrointestinal LMS correlates with outcomes, with colonic LMS representing aggressive tumors regardless of the tumor size and mitotic activity and rectal LMS typically presenting as smaller tumors with improved prognosis.

Common clinical presentation for retroperitoneal NULMS involves symptoms related to tumor impinging on the surrounding organs and structures. Given this, patients can present with back pain, increased abdominal girth, weight loss, fatigue, and fever or night sweats, which are all nonspecific symptoms that require diligent evaluation in order to lead to an appropriate diagnosis. Notably, given the retroperitoneum is an expansible site, retroperitoneal LMS can be very large at the time of diagnosis with a median size of 15 cm.

In addition to differences in prevalence, tumor location is an independent prognostic factor. LMS arising in the retroperitoneum is associated with poorer outcomes than that arising in the extremity. Cutaneous LMS has decreased risk of metastatic disease compared to other LMS tumors, with 0% to 10% risk of distant metastases and 30% to 50% risk of local recurrence. There are, however, poor prognostic features associated with cutaneous LMS, including tumor size of 5 cm or greater, acral location, high histologic grade, and fascia involvement.

Gender incidence differs based on NULMS tumor location, with most retroperitoneal and inferior vena cava LMS found in females, compared to a mild male predominance in soft tissue and cutaneous LMS. The overall incidence of LMS increases with age, and it is most commonly seen in patients in their 70s.

Unique genetic alterations seen in LMS include genomic imbalances in 88% of LMS patients and aberrant chromosome numbers and structures in 60% of patients, seen particularly in higher-grade tumors. Additionally, *RASSF1A* promoter hypermethylation is seen in 39% of LMS patients and has been associated with poorer prognosis of stage II and III LMS cases.

SUMMARY

LMS is a relatively common type of soft tissue sarcoma, commonly with an aggressive clinical course. Accurate diagnosis and pathologic review are critical, particularly given distinct outcomes based on histology, tumor size, and grade. Multidisciplinary evaluation at a dedicated sarcoma center, involving a team comprising pathologists, radiologists, medical oncologists, radiation oncologists, and surgical oncologists, is paramount for optimal outcomes. This is particularly critical, given the differences in treatment paradigms for ULMS and NULMS, with unique site-specific considerations for NULMS. Pretreatment consideration for possible LMS is critical, particularly in patients with uterine leiomyomas, where morcellation procedures are highly discouraged, given possible tumor spillage. In patients with metastatic LMS, active systemic agents include doxorubicin-based combinations as described in detail in the section "Treatment of Metastatic Disease," gemcitabine ± docetaxel, dacarbazine, ifosfamide (specific to ULMS), trabectedin, and pazopanib.

CASE STUDY

This illustrative case is of a 67-year-old woman who presented in late 2012, approximately 2 months after undergoing resection of a 12.6-cm left retroperitoneal mass along with left nephrectomy and mobilization of splenic flexure. Surgical pathology revealed that the resected left kidney in the adjacent soft tissue was positive for LMS involving perinephric fat, with 10 mitotic figures/10 high-power fields, 20% necrosis, and tumor extending to the resection margins and, as per the French Federation of Comprehensive Cancer Centers (*Fédération Nationale des Centres de Lutte Contre le Cancer*; FNCLCC) guidelines, at least intermediate grade tumor. At the time of initial consultation, her imaging showed indeterminate pulmonary nodules; however, lung biopsy was negative for LMS. After discussion, she opted to receive six cycles of adjuvant doxorubicin (75 mg/m^2) plus dacarbazine (750 mg/m^2) with dexrazoxane. Following completion of adjuvant chemotherapy in early 2013, she was continued on surveillance for approximately 3 years until restaging studies showed an increasing pleural-based nodule in the right upper hemithorax, which was biopsy-proven to be metastatic LMS. While upfront surgical resection was considered, particularly given that she had been without evidence of disease for 3 years, she had a myocardial infarction just prior to this biopsy result. Given this, she went on to receive six cycles of gemcitabine (900 mg/m^2) plus docetaxel (dose reduced to 60 mg/m^2) and had stable disease. She ultimately underwent wedge resection of bilateral pulmonary nodules approximately 1 year after the initial evidence of metastatic disease. Following resection, she has been monitored, and on surveillance, she has been found to be without recurrent disease.

This case reflects several important considerations in the treatment of patients with LMS. Treatment of localized disease involved careful assessment of risk factors including grade, tumor size, location, and margin status, leading to the recommendation for adjuvant chemotherapy. If the patient had presented to the medical oncologist prior to surgery, neoadjuvant chemotherapy could have been considered. Routine surveillance detected pulmonary metastases, which highlights the need for follow-up imaging in order to detect recurrence/metastasis early. Feasibility for oligometastatectomy should be explored upfront, especially if there is a significant interval from initial treatment to the development of lung-only metastases that are slow growing. However, her medical comorbid conditions required delaying surgery. Multidisciplinary care helped achieve the optimal outcome for her recurrence, taking into consideration tumor and patient factors. Other alternatives to consider for oligometastatic disease include stereotactic radiation, radiofrequency ablation or cryoablation, or systemic therapy alone.

REFERENCES

1. Lamm W, Natter C, Schur S, et al. Distinctive outcome in patients with non-uterine and uterine leiomyosarcoma. *BMC Cancer*. 2014;14:981. doi:10.1186/1471-2407-14-981
2. Guo X, Jo VY, Mills AM, et al. Clinically relevant molecular subtypes in leiomyosarcoma. *Clin Cancer Res*. 2015;21(15):3501–3511. doi:10.1158/1078-0432.CCR-14-3141
3. Sarcoma Meta-analysis Collaboration. Adjuvant chemotherapy for localised resectable soft-tissue sarcoma of adults: meta-analysis of individual data. *Lancet*. 1997;350(9092):1647–1654. doi:10.1016/S0140-6736(97)08165-8
4. Yang JC, Chang AE, Baker AR, et al. Randomized prospective study of the benefit of adjuvant radiation therapy in the treatment of soft tissue sarcomas of the extremity. *J Clin Oncol*. 1998;16(1):197–203. doi:10.1200/JCO.1998.16.1.197
5. Maki RG, Wathen JK, Patel SR, et al. Randomized phase II study of gemcitabine and docetaxel compared with gemcitabine alone in patients with metastatic soft tissue sarcomas: results of sarcoma alliance for research through collaboration study 002. *J Clin Oncol*. 2007;25(19):2755–2763. doi:10.1200/JCO.2006.10.4117
6. Pautier P, Floguet A, Penel N, et al. Randomized multicenter and stratified Phase II study of gemcitabine alone versus gemcitabine and docetaxel in patients with metastatic or relapsed leiomyosarcomas: a Fédération Nationale des Centres de Lutte Contre le Cancer (FNCLCC) French Sarcoma Group Study (TAXOGEM study). *Oncologist*. 2012;17(9):1213–1220. doi:10.1634/theoncologist.2011-0467
7. Chudgar NP, Brennan MF, Munhoz RR, et al. Pulmonary metastasectomy with therapeutic intent for soft-tissue sarcoma. *J Thorac Cardiovasc Surg*. 2017;154(1):319-330.e1. doi:10.1016/j.jtcvs.2017.02.061

9

Dedifferentiated Liposarcoma

William W. Tseng, Angelo Paolo Dei Tos, Roberta Giovanna Sanfilippo, Jennifer Wang, and Alessandro Gronchi

INTRODUCTION

Dedifferentiated (DD) liposarcoma is a high-grade, adipocytic malignancy and can be considered a part of a spectrum of diseases that include its low-grade counterpart, well-differentiated (WD) liposarcoma. A patient's tumor can be entirely WD, WD with focal area(s) of DD disease, or rarely, entirely DD without a WD component. The presence of dedifferentiation in a tumor changes the disease biology, making the tumor more aggressive and conferring metastatic potential. WD/DD disease is distinct from other subtypes of liposarcoma, such as myxoid round cell and pleomorphic, which will not be covered in this chapter.

WD/DD liposarcoma is almost exclusively a disease of adults without any gender or race predilection. There are no known risk factors or associated genetic syndromes. For patients with WD/DD liposarcoma, symptoms may vary by body location, but overall, they are frequently vague and nonspecific. Some patients may be completely asymptomatic, their tumors discovered only after imaging is done for another purpose.

On cross-sectional imaging (e.g., MRI or CT), WD/DD liposarcoma appears as a well-defined lipomatous mass with thickened internal fibrous septa. Dedifferentiation is suspected when focal nonlipomatous areas are seen, particularly if these areas have contrast enhancement or necrosis. Ultimately, the gold standard of diagnosis for WD/DD liposarcoma relies on histologic examination of the tissue (e.g., obtained from core-needle biopsy). The diagnosis can be confirmed with fluorescence in situ hybridization (FISH) for chromosomal amplification at 12q13–15, the pathognomonic genetic feature of WD/DD liposarcoma. This amplicon includes several key genes including *MDM2* and *CDK4*. Recently, further genetic differences between WD and DD disease have begun to be elucidated.

WD/DD liposarcoma can occur anywhere in the body, including the extremities, trunk, head/neck, and commonly, the retroperitoneum, where in the latter case, tumors can reach very large size. Tumors with dedifferentiation are far more common in the retroperitoneum, whereas DD liposarcoma is rare elsewhere in the body.

Surgery is the mainstay of treatment for patients with localized disease in WD/DD liposarcoma. Complete resection is the goal but may be challenging, particularly for retroperitoneal tumors, given their large size and potential invasion of major visceral organs and critical structures. The role of radiation therapy to improve local control in WD/DD liposarcoma is controversial. If given, delivery is ideal in the neoadjuvant setting. The role of systemic therapy in localized disease is currently undefined, but may benefit some subsets of patients with high-risk disease. For each patient, the utility and sequence of therapy should be discussed in a multidisciplinary conference at a sarcoma referral center.

Recurrence is a significant risk in patients with WD/DD liposarcoma, especially those with retroperitoneal tumors and DD liposarcoma. Surveillance with serial cross-sectional imaging is important and should be personalized based on each patient's risk and anticipated pattern of recurrence. When recurrence develops, although surgery is an option, the appropriate candidates must be carefully selected. Multimodality therapy is frequently used in these situations.

Overall, DD liposarcoma has an approximately 20% to 30% rate of distant metastasis. For patients with unresectable and distant metastatic disease, systemic therapy options include chemotherapy and targeted therapies. Several newer drugs including immunotherapy are under investigation.

This chapter will focus on DD liposarcoma within the context of WD/DD disease. We highlight the differences that arise with the presence of DD liposarcoma, especially how this may impact decision-making and management. We then conclude with additional pearls and pitfalls, along with a discussion of active issues for further investigation.

ESTIMATED INCIDENCE PER YEAR, GENDER, AND RACE

WD/DD disease represents one subset of liposarcoma, which is itself just one of over 50 to 70 different histologic subtypes of soft tissue sarcoma that together constitute only 1% of all cancers in adults.[1–3] WD/DD liposarcoma is clearly very rare, and to our knowledge, there are no estimates of incidence specific to this disease. WD/DD liposarcoma occurs almost exclusively in middle-aged and elderly adults; in fact, the disease is exceedingly rare in infants, children, and adolescents. There is no gender or race predilection. Furthermore, there are no known risk factors for development of WD/DD liposarcoma, either social or environmental. Although this is a malignancy of fat, there are no clear associations with obesity or high-fat diet. Second primary cancers have been reported in WD/DD liposarcoma[4]; however, there are currently no defined genetic syndromes that predispose to disease development. DD disease tends to occur more frequently at the initial disease presentation (90%), but can also be observed later at recurrence (10%) in previously entirely WD disease.

MOST COMMON PRESENTING SYMPTOMS

WD/DD liposarcoma can occur in any location of the body, and as a result, presenting symptoms may vary. Overall, for most patients, the symptoms are vague and nonspecific. In the retroperitoneum, patients may have abdominal fullness, back pain, early satiety, reflux, or constipation. Unless there is specific nerve impingement (e.g., femoral), pain is otherwise generally mild, chronic, and tolerated. Giant retroperitoneal tumors can impede venous return, causing lower extremity edema in some patients, but this may not occur if collaterals (e.g., in the abdominal wall) have formed. Bowel and biliary obstruction is quite rare for retroperitoneal tumors. In all body locations, a mass lesion may be felt on physical examination. Alternatively, some patients may be completely asymptomatic, with their tumors discovered only after imaging done for another purpose (e.g., kidney stones). Tumors with dedifferentiation can be more locally aggressive compared to entirely WD tumors, but there is no clear association between presence of DD disease and higher frequency of symptoms.

A small proportion of patients affected with WD/DD liposarcoma in the retroperitoneum and pelvis may present with systemic symptoms such as fever, elevated white blood cell count, hypoglycemia, or elevated transaminases. These symptoms may mandate expedited treatment (e.g., surgery), as patients may deteriorate very quickly.

DIAGNOSTIC APPROACH

Accurate diagnosis of WD/DD liposarcoma includes high-quality, contrast-enhanced cross-sectional imaging. In the extremity and trunk, this usually consists of MRI, whereas in the abdomen or retroperitoneum, CT is the most common imaging modality. WD liposarcoma is typically seen as a well-defined lipomatous mass with thickened internal fibrous septa.[5] Presence of DD disease is suspected within a lipomatous tumor when there are focal, nonlipomatous (soft tissue density) areas. Suspicion is higher when these areas are well defined, have vascular contrast enhancement, or have central necrosis.[6,7] Interestingly, DD tumors may also undergo osteogenic differentiation, which can be evident on imaging as focal intratumoral calcification. Overall, with characteristic features, cross-sectional imaging can almost be diagnostic, especially for tumors seen in the retroperitoneum. However, there are pitfalls, and expertise from a radiologist familiar with the disease is critical.

Cross-sectional imaging is also critical for surgical planning purposes. A high-quality imaging study is necessary to adequately plan the surgical approach and anticipate possible complications. Therefore, if the quality of initial studies is poor, repeating the studies for better quality is warranted. Moreover, for patients with suspected or confirmed DD disease, staging should be done with a contrast-enhanced CT of the chest, as the lungs are the most common site of metastatic disease. The role of PET remains to be determined. WD tumors do not have metabolic activity on PET scan. Some, but not all, DD tumors have metabolic activity, but whether this correlates with disease aggressiveness is currently under investigation.

Ultimately, to establish a diagnosis, the gold standard is histologic examination of the tumor tissue. In the preoperative setting, tissue is most commonly obtained through core-needle biopsy. Image (e.g., CT) guidance is recommended and the standard technique is coaxial (one pass of the sheath up to the periphery of the tumor, followed by multiple needle passes through the sheath and sampling of different tumor areas), for which the risk of tumor seeding is minimal.[8,9] With core-needle biopsy, the diagnosis of

WD/DD liposarcoma can typically be made; however, studies have shown relatively low accuracy for the specific diagnosis of DD disease.[10,11] Incisional biopsy is not recommended for WD/DD liposarcoma because it may sample the wrong portion of tumor (without image guidance, e.g., for DD disease) and also disrupt the natural tissue planes, potentially making subsequent surgery more challenging.

Microscopically, WD liposarcoma is characterized by atypical-appearing adipocytes of varying sizes separated by fibrous stroma with the sparse presence of cells with hyperchromatic nuclei. In tumors with DD, an abrupt transition from WD liposarcoma (low grade) to a nonlipogenic (most often, high-grade) sarcoma is seen (Figure 9.1). The morphology of the DD component can frequently overlap with undifferentiated pleomorphic sarcoma or less frequently with high-grade myxofibrosarcoma. Historically, the original definition of dedifferentiation by Evans in 1979 included the abrupt WD transition and within the nonlipogenic component, five or more mitoses per 10 high-power fields (with fewer mitoses being called "cellular" WD disease).[12] To date, Evans' criteria for dedifferentiation are still used, but not universally adopted. It is also now well recognized that the WD to DD transition can actually be more gradual and, in some cases, low-grade and high-grade areas can even appear to be comingled.

"Low-grade dedifferentiation" has been used to describe the presence of fascicles of bland spindle cells with a cellularity somewhat intermediate between sclerosing WD liposarcoma and the typical high-grade areas. This, in part, overlaps with the "cellular" variants of WD liposarcoma described by

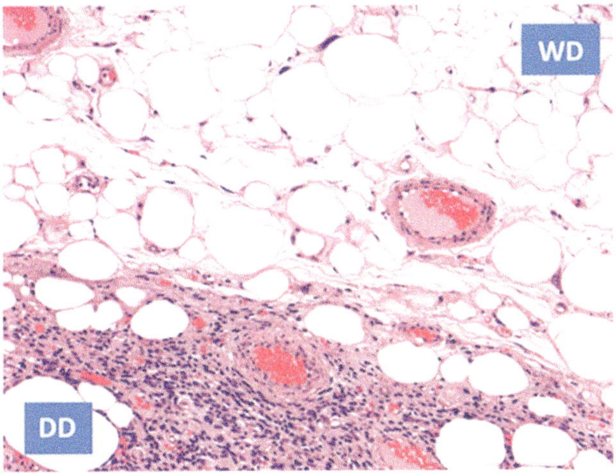

(A)

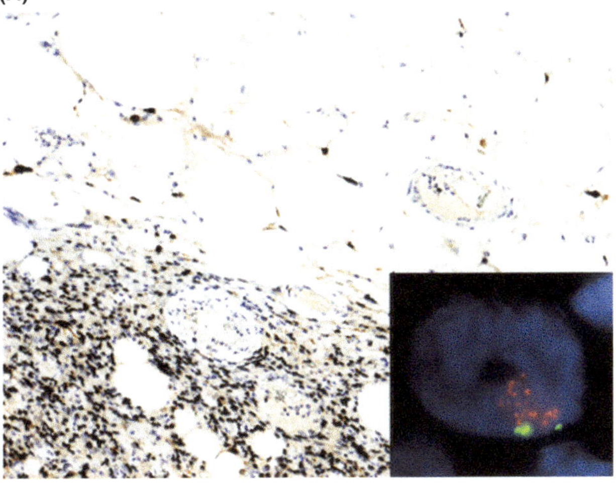

(B)

FIGURE 9.1 Microscopic appearance of liposarcoma with a dedifferentiated component. (A) Hematoxylin and eosin image. The abrupt transition to high-grade disease is clearly shown. (B) Immunohistochemistry demonstrating the expression of *MDM2* (brown). Inset showing fluorescence in situ hybridization, positive for *MDM2* amplification.

DD, dedifferentiated; WD, well differentiated.

Evans.[13–15] Low-grade DD areas can feature variable morphologic features somewhat mimicking desmoid fibromatosis, solitary fibrous tumors, gastrointestinal stromal tumors, and even inflammatory myofibroblastic tumors.

Dedifferentiation can have additional fascinating morphologic features. Heterologous differentiation can be observed in about 5% to 10% of cases, most often myogenic but also osteo- and chondrogenic. This can even be lipogenic in nature (so-called "homologous" dedifferentiation), overlapping morphologically with pleomorphic liposarcoma.[16] Another very peculiar morphologic presentation of DD disease is represented by the presence of whorls of spindle cells mimicking neural or meningothelial structures.[17] Very rarely, an intense inflammatory infiltrate is observed to the extent that it may obscure the lipogenic nature of the neoplasm.

While dedifferentiation in itself is considered high grade, recent work has shown that application of the three-tier French (*Fédération Nationale des Centres de Lutte Contre le Cancer*; FNCLCC) grading system used for soft tissue sarcomas, in general, can be useful to further stratify DD disease in terms of prognosis.[18] Furthermore, data support the association of myogenic differentiation (particularly, rhabdomyoblastic) with remarkably poorer prognosis.[18,19]

The hallmark molecular aberration and pathognomonic genetic feature of WD/DD liposarcoma is chromosomal amplification at 12q13–15. This amplicon includes several key genes including *MDM2* and *CDK4*. In addition to the microscopic appearance on hematoxylin and eosin (H&E) stain, interpreted by an experienced sarcoma pathologist, demonstration of *MDM2* gene amplification by FISH contributes greatly to increased diagnostic accuracy (Figure 9.1). Immunohistochemically, as a result of 12q amplification, DD disease overexpresses both *MDM2* and *CDK4* in both lipogenic and nonlipogenic components.[20,21] The demonstration of *MDM2* nuclear overexpression is of great diagnostic support (Figure 9.1). In our experience, *MDM2* immunohistochemistry exhibits high concordance with FISH analysis of *MDM2* gene status.

Co-amplification of *c-JUN* (mapping at 1p32) and of its activating kinase (mapping at 6q23) is also observed.[22] In fact, it has been suggested that the activation of the c-JUN pathway may be involved in tumor progression from WD to DD liposarcoma; however, this is debated. Recent work has also identified a number of other genetic changes that may support WD to DD progression.[23]

GENERAL THERAPEUTIC APPROACH

WD/DD liposarcoma can occur anywhere in the body, including the extremities, trunk, head and neck, and retroperitoneum. In the latter case, tumors can reach very large sizes (average 20–30 cm), and in fact, retroperitoneal liposarcomas are likely the largest cancers in the human body. Importantly, tumors with presence of dedifferentiation are also more common in the retroperitoneum, whereas dedifferentiation is quite rare elsewhere in the body.

For WD/DD liposarcoma of any location in the body, surgery is the mainstay of treatment in patients with localized disease. Particularly in the retroperitoneum, where the tumors are larger and can abut or invade critical organs and structures (e.g., major vessels), expertise from a surgical oncologist with experience in this disease is critical.[24] For retroperitoneal WD/DD liposarcoma, the goal of surgery is macroscopically complete resection with a single specimen encompassing the tumor and the involved contiguous organs, while attempting to minimize microscopically positive margins.[25] In some cases, resection of adjacent organs or structures even without obvious involvement is necessary.[26,27] Preservation of organs or structures should be made on a case-by-case basis, balancing disease biology and potential for local control versus potential morbidity and dysfunction. In general, tumors with dedifferentiation tend to be locally more invasive, and therefore, multiorgan resection (e.g., kidney, colon) may be anticipated in these cases compared to tumors that are WD only. Except in unique cases of palliative resection,[28] there is no role for piecemeal or grossly incomplete (debulking) resection.

Importantly, resections for retroperitoneal WD/DD liposarcoma can be major operations and patients should be optimized medically (e.g., comorbid conditions) before surgery. Specifically, in many patients, moderate to severe malnutrition may be present. There is some evidence, in fact, that malnutrition is generally underestimated and these patients have more postoperative complications and longer hospitalization.[29]

Surgical expertise and clinical judgment is also important for WD/DD liposarcoma of the extremities, trunk, and head/neck area, where there are arguably less well defined guidelines. If wide margins can be obtained, this is ideal, similar to many other subtypes of soft tissue sarcoma. There is, however, evidence to support that marginal complete resection may be adequate for these tumors in these nonretroperitoneal locations, which are mostly WD.[30–32]

For patients with WD/DD liposarcoma, even after complete resection, there remains the risk for recurrence. This risk varies, but is definitely higher for tumors in the retroperitoneum and those with dedifferentiation.[33] As an example, the 5-year locoregional recurrence rates range from 20% to 30% for extremity and trunk (mostly WD) to up to 50% to 60% for retroperitoneum (WD/DD disease).[30,34–36] Other clinicopathologic factors also impact the risk of locoregional recurrence, including age, tumor size up to a certain extent, and multifocality (more than one tumor), the latter of which can also occur in some patients at the initial disease presentation.[37–39]

In an attempt to optimize local control, radiation therapy may be of benefit; however, this is considered controversial in WD/DD liposarcoma. In the retroperitoneum, if radiation therapy is given, attempts should be made to minimize toxicity to the bowel. Delivery is, therefore, ideal in the neoadjuvant setting with the tumor in place to act as a natural "spacer," displacing the bowel. In the context of the broader group of all retroperitoneal sarcomas, several retrospective studies have shown that, indeed, radiation therapy improves local control compared to surgery alone.[40–43] Recently, a multi-institutional retrospective study specifically focused on retroperitoneal liposarcoma, finding that across all histologic subtypes (WD vs. DD liposarcoma) and grades within DD disease, radiation therapy significantly reduced local recurrence rates on univariate analysis; however, this benefit was lost in all subgroups after multivariate analysis.[44] A recent prospective clinical trial (EORTC 62092-22092 or STRASS)[45] did not seem to support the benefit of radiation therapy for retroperitoneal sarcomas in general; however, further subanalysis by histologic subtype is still pending.

Few data are available to define the benefit of radiation therapy for local control in the extremity and trunk. Without the constraints of adjacent viscera, delivery of radiation therapy may occur in the neoadjuvant or adjuvant setting, similar to other soft tissue sarcomas. One single-institution study showed that in extremity and truncal WD disease, there was significant reduction in 5-year local recurrence-free survival rate with the addition of adjuvant radiation therapy (98% vs. 80%); however, the authors highlighted potential disadvantages, including making subsequent surgery more challenging, and ultimately concluded that the decision should be personalized to each case.[46] Given the rarity of DD disease in non-retroperitoneal sites, there have been no studies exploring the benefit of radiation therapy in this specific situation to date.

The role of systemic therapy (e.g., chemotherapy) in either the adjuvant or neoadjuvant setting for localized WD/DD liposarcoma is currently undefined. There is likely no benefit in patients with WD-only disease; however, there may be benefit of chemotherapy with doxorubicin plus ifosfamide (or dacarbazine if renal dysfunction) for patients with DD disease. Multi-institutional data for retroperitoneal sarcoma suggest that patients with FNCLCC grade 3 DD tumor have a distant metastatic rate of 33% at 5 years after complete resection, which is approximately threefold higher than that seen in patients with grade 2 DD disease.[35] Given the complexity of retroperitoneal surgery and potential for complications, which can delay receipt of systemic therapy in the adjuvant setting, most sarcoma centers prefer to administer drug treatment in the neoadjuvant setting to these patients; however, this remains to be formally studied.

Overall, the utility and sequence of therapy for each patient with WD/DD liposarcoma should be discussed within a multidisciplinary conference at a sarcoma referral center. The vast majority of patients with primary, localized disease will have first-line surgery and this may be the only therapy needed. This is particularly true for patients with nonretroperitoneal (extremity, trunk, head/neck) tumors and those with WD disease only (no evidence of DD disease). Alternatively, in patients with retroperitoneal tumors and those with DD disease, as discussed, some may benefit from multimodality treatment including neoadjuvant radiation therapy and systemic therapy, either before or after surgery. Neoadjuvant therapy (radiation and/or chemotherapy) may facilitate resectability in borderline cases, especially if tumor shrinkage can be achieved; however, to date, no studies have quantitated this potential benefit.

RECOMMENDED FOLLOW-UP

Given the risk of recurrence, close surveillance is important in patients with WD/DD liposarcoma. Although consensus recommendations (National Comprehensive Cancer Network [NCCN], European Society of Medical Oncology [ESMO]) exist for surveillance in soft tissue sarcomas in general, there are no validated guidelines specific for WD/DD liposarcoma. For retroperitoneal tumors, along with history and physical examination, most sarcoma centers recommend initial contrast-enhanced CT of the abdomen and pelvis at 3 to 4 months after surgery to serve as a postoperative baseline. Repeat imaging should then be done every 4 to 6 months for at least 2 to 3 years and up to 5 years.[47] For nonretroperitoneal body locations (extremity, trunk, head/neck), a similar schedule of interval imaging should be followed with contrast-enhanced MRI. For superficial tumors, ultimately, MRI may be replaced with ultrasound scans. In patients with DD disease, chest CT should be added. Surveillance should be modified based on personalized risk and the anticipated pattern of recurrence. Late recurrences can occur, particularly in DD liposarcoma.[30,36] In support of this concept, in the multi-institutional retroperitoneal sarcoma studies, the curves for recurrence do not plateau even up to 8 years after resection.[35]

When recurrence develops (e.g., detected by surveillance imaging), decision-making and overall management can be complex and multimodality therapy is frequently used. Surgery is always an option and is ultimately performed in most patients. In fact, many patients with WD/DD liposarcoma, particularly retroperitoneal, will have multiple resections during their lifetime.[48] An important consideration is that re-resection is often more challenging in comparison to surgery for primary disease owing to scar tissue and distorted tissue planes. Candidates for surgery must, therefore, be carefully selected. One study described a "1 cm per month" rule in which patients with at least this rate of tumor growth on imaging had poor outcomes and would be less likely to benefit from surgery.[49] For patients who are asymptomatic, indeed, a period of observation may be warranted, not only to assess the rate of growth but also to better understand the disease biology, as in some cases, multifocal disease may soon be evident on subsequent imaging.[37,50–52] Interestingly, there may also be a subset of patients (mostly with WD disease) who may remain stable over a prolonged period without any treatment.[53]

Currently, there are no laboratory tests that are useful to detect recurrence in WD/DD liposarcoma, although this is an area under investigation (e.g., serum biomarkers).[54] Patients with retroperitoneal tumors who have had nephrectomy as part of their surgery should have residual kidney function checked and optimized as needed prior to contrast administration done for their imaging.

PROPENSITY TO METASTASIZE

DD liposarcoma has a low/intermediate propensity to metastasize. The overall frequency is approximately 20% to 30%, and the common site of distant metastasis is the lungs. As discussed, however, there are likely subsets within DD liposarcoma (e.g., FNCLCC grade 3 or rhabdomyoblastic differentiation) with a higher metastatic propensity, and in some patients, extrapulmonary sites of distant disease (e.g., liver, bone) may also be seen. In contrast, entirely WD tumors do not metastasize. WD/DD liposarcoma never metastasizes to the locoregional lymph nodes.

THERAPEUTIC APPROACH FOR METASTATIC DISEASE

Treatment options for patients with unresectable and metastatic disease are limited. In soft tissue sarcoma in general, frontline treatment for unresectable/metastatic disease is usually systemic therapy with doxorubicin, alone or in combination with ifosfamide, with a reported objective response rate (ORR) in the range of 20% to 40%.[55] The combination of doxorubicin and ifosfamide is superior to doxorubicin alone in terms of progression-free survival (PFS) and results in a doubling of ORR (26% vs. 14%), but with a trend toward an overall survival (OS) benefit.[56] Therefore, this combination regimen is often used, for example, in symptomatic patients who need tumor shrinkage or in an attempt to facilitate resectability. In contrast, a single-agent regimen can be used in a patient with multiorgan metastasis and poor performance status, with the goal of fewer chemotherapy-related side effects.

In WD/DD liposarcoma specifically, the ORR reported for anthracycline-based chemotherapy is lower, and therefore, traditionally, this is considered to be a poorly chemosensitive subtype of soft tissue sarcoma.[57] As an example, in a retrospective multicenter analysis, the ORR was 12%.[58] More recent single-institution data for WD/DD liposarcoma, however, suggests that the ORR may be higher (up to 21%), especially with combination chemotherapy regimens.[59] It is important to note that treatment is usually given for DD tumors; there are currently no systemic therapies with demonstrated efficacy in WD-only tumors.

At this point, for WD/DD liposarcoma, the first-line treatment remains doxorubicin with or without ifosfamide. In second-line systemic therapy, gemcitabine and docetaxel (Taxotere) are often used.[59] Approved drugs for second, third, and further lines of treatment include trabectedin, high-dose (single agent 14 g/m^2) ifosfamide, and eribulin. After the first-line treatment, the best further line treatment is not established, and of course, performance status and patient preference are included in the decision-making process.

Trabectedin represents a valid second-line treatment for WD/DD liposarcoma, although the ORR of this drug does not exceed 10%.[60] Interestingly, there are reports of greater activity of trabectedin in a subset of "low-grade" DD liposarcoma. One advantage of this drug is that it is well tolerated without cumulative toxicity. In fact, it has been reported that several patients have been treated for >1 year with trabectedin.[60]

Continuous infusion, high-dose ifosfamide (ciHDIFX) is another treatment option. In a retrospective series of advanced WD/DD liposarcoma patients treated with ciHDIFX, the ORR was 26% with an additional 50% of patients achieving disease stabilization.[61] All partial responses in this series occurred in patients with a "high-grade" DD component. Compared with the classic schedule, high-dose (12–14 g/m^2) ifosfamide is given via a portable external device over 14 days with good tolerability. At these dose levels, ifosfamide can be active in patients already exposed to standard dose in combination with doxorubicin.[62–64]

Eribulin was recently approved by the U.S. Food and Drug Administration and the European Medicines Agency as a third-line treatment in liposarcoma. This was based on results from a randomized Phase 3 study comparing eribulin to dacarbazine in advanced liposarcoma and leiomyosarcoma.[65] Although there was no difference in median PFS between the two groups (2.6 vs. 2.6 months, $p = .23$), eribulin demonstrated a statistically significant improvement in OS (13.5 vs. 11.5 months, $p = .0169$). Tumor responses, however, were limited to just two patients. Subgroup analyses suggested that liposarcoma patients benefited the most, with the median OS being 15.6 versus 8.4 months in those who received eribulin versus dacarbazine. Importantly, this benefit was observed irrespective of the liposarcoma subtype (e.g., 18.0 vs. 8.1 months, hazard ratio [HR]: 0.43 in DD liposarcoma).[66]

As discussed in the section "Diagnostic Approach," WD/DD liposarcoma has a distinct genetic signature characterized by amplification of several notable genes including *MDM2* and *CDK4*. Recently, several targeted therapies directed at *MDM2* or *CDK4* have been developed. In the clinical studies conducted so far,[67,68] however, activity has been limited. Disease stabilization is noted in some patients (in some cases, it is prolonged), but tumor response (ORR) is rarely seen.

Among the newer drugs, another targeted therapy under investigation in DD liposarcoma is selinexor, an inhibitor of exportin 1 (XPO1), which is involved in the movement of cargo proteins from the nucleus to the cytoplasm. These proteins include the tumor suppressor proteins, which can be inactivated through nuclear exclusion in the presence of XPO1 overactivity. After promising Phase 1b study results showing improved PFS,[69] a randomized double-blind study versus placebo is now ongoing in the United States and Europe (NCT0260646).

Immune checkpoint inhibitors are not yet the standard treatment in soft tissue sarcoma in general, but several trials are currently ongoing. Specific to DD liposarcoma, the SARC028 trial showed that two of 10 patients treated with pembrolizumab (anti-PD1) showed a partial response (ORR 20%) with a median follow-up period (across all soft tissue sarcoma patients) of 14.5 months.[70] Additional expansion cohort studies for DD and undifferentiated pleomorphic sarcoma (another histologic subtype with tumor response) are ongoing.

SUMMARY

DD liposarcoma can be considered a part of a spectrum of diseases that include WD liposarcoma and, in fact, the two counterparts are often found within the same tumor. Compared to a tumor that is entirely WD, the presence of dedifferentiation changes the disease biology, making it clinically more aggressive and conferring metastatic potential. WD/DD liposarcoma can occur anywhere in the body, but DD disease is more common in the retroperitoneum, where tumors are also larger and surgery is more challenging. As a result, DD disease should be viewed from a different perspective on many levels in comparison to WD-only disease. Several active issues remain.

From a disease biology standpoint, the basis for development of dedifferentiation is currently elusive. Is DD disease truly clonally derived from WD disease and what leads to this transformation? Is this transformation intrinsic to the tumor cell or perhaps related to the microenvironment? For the latter, work has been done describing a unique intratumoral immune response in WD/DD liposarcoma, which has set forth hypotheses to be tested.[71–73] Another unresolved issue is the importance of DD content within a tumor: Are there clinical differences between a microscopic versus macroscopic focus and how do we manage an entirely DD tumor (no evidence of WD disease)? Ultimately, understanding DD development is disease-defining and has significant clinical implications.

Given the importance of recognizing dedifferentiation and the impact on subsequent decision-making and management, the pretreatment diagnosis of DD disease needs to be optimized. As discussed in the section "Diagnostic Approach," the accuracy of core-needle biopsy for diagnosis of DD disease is relatively low, even with standard image guidance.[10] The utility of PET to discern DD disease and specifically identify high-risk disease is being studied. Evaluation of other imaging modalities (e.g., radiomics) is warranted, and in the future, perhaps a serum biomarker will be found that marks the presence of DD disease (vs. WD-only disease).

Greater clarity is also needed with the pathologic diagnosis of DD disease. First, the criteria for diagnosis (FNCLCC vs. Evans) should be unified. This would facilitate research studies and broaden the applicability of study findings to more patients. Second, clearly within DD disease, there is also a spectrum of disease aggressiveness. Although data exist that rhabdomyoblastic differentiation and FNCLCC grade 3 disease are associated with a higher metastatic potential,[19,35] are there other subsets of DD disease with clinical significance that remain to be identified?

With regard to treatment for localized disease, as discussed in the section "General Therapeutic Approach," the true benefit of nonsurgical treatments (radiation and systemic therapy) deserves further study. For radiation therapy, ongoing subgroup analysis of the completed, prospective STRASS trial may hopefully define the subset of patients for whom treatment improves local control. For systemic therapy, the potential for durable locoregional and distant disease remains to be determined. Similar to radiation therapy, the benefit of systemic therapy over surgery alone in patients with localized disease may only be limited to a subset of patients.

For patients with unresectable and metastatic disease, while there are, indeed, several systemic therapy options available, the challenge remains in identifying the appropriate option for the goal of treatment (e.g., rapid tumor shrinkage vs. prolonged disease stabilization), while balancing toxicity. Disease-specific combination therapies with potential synergistic effect in WD/DD liposarcoma should also be explored. After systemic treatment, do select patients benefit from resection, perhaps even metastasectomy, for limited sites of disease?

It is hopeful that all of these active issues with WD/DD liposarcoma—from disease biology to clinical—can be addressed through further investigation, ideally through collaborative research among sarcoma centers.

CASE STUDY

A 42-year-old Hispanic woman presented with a recent history of right-sided abdominal pain and fullness. She also reported decreased appetite and shortness of breath with just walking. On physical examination, an ill-defined palpable mass was detected in the right abdomen. She did not have any lower extremity edema.

Contrast-enhanced CT of the abdomen and pelvis demonstrated a large right retroperitoneal mass extending from under the liver to the pelvic inlet, displacing the right kidney anteriorly and medially and abutting much of the inferior vena cava (Figure 9.2). The mass itself had both lipomatous and nonlipomatous components, and given the body location, it was suspicious for liposarcoma. CT-guided biopsy was performed by interventional radiology using coaxial technique with an 18-gauge core needle. The final pathologic finding was consistent with DD liposarcoma, FNCLCC grade 3. The diagnosis was confirmed with molecular testing that showed amplification of *CDK4* and *MDM2*. Staging was done, including both chest CT and whole-body PET scan, which did not show any gross evidence of distant metastatic disease. The tumor itself had FDG (fluorodeoxyglucose) avidity (Figure 9.2) with a maximum SUV (standardized uptake value) of 11.3.

The patient was discussed at a multidisciplinary sarcoma tumor board. Given the high risk of distant metastatic disease and the potential complexity of resection (including possible caval involvement), the decision was made to give neoadjuvant systemic combination chemotherapy that consisted of doxorubicin plus ifosfamide. After therapy, repeat CT was performed, and there was again no gross evidence to suggest distant metastatic disease. The tumor itself showed slight partial response, but likely not enough to change the proposed extent of resection.

At surgery, tumor resection was performed with en bloc right nephrectomy and colectomy (Figure 9.2). As anticipated based on preoperative imaging, the tumor completely encased the right kidney and the mesocolon was involved. Posteriorly, the tumor was compressing the inferior vena cava and right common iliac vein, but the tissue planes were preserved and vascular resection was not necessary. The patient recovered uneventfully and the overall postoperative

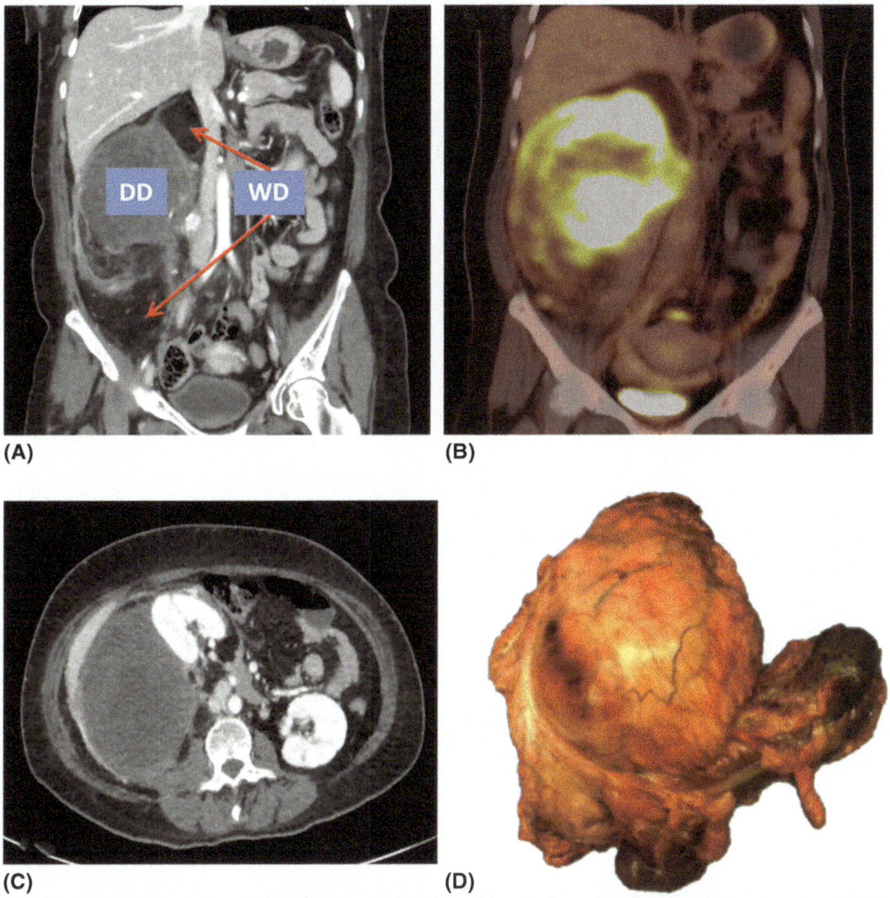

FIGURE 9.2 **Case example of retroperitoneal DD liposarcoma.** (A) Coronal CT image showing large tumor with fatty (well-differentiated, WD) and nonfatty (dedifferentiated, DD) components, abutting the inferior vena cava. (B) PET image demonstrating focal areas of high FDG avidity in this patient's tumor. (C) Axial CT image showing the large tumor displacing the right kidney. (D) Gross appearance of the resected tumor with en bloc colon and right kidney (within tumor).

DD, dedifferentiated; FDG, fluorodeoxyglucose; WD, well differentiated.

course was routine. The final pathologic finding for the resection specimen was consistent with the preoperative biopsy (DD tumor) and had evidence of treatment effect with areas of up to 90% tumor necrosis.

Further adjuvant systemic therapy was given with the same regimen. Baseline postoperative CT showed no evidence to suggest residual disease, and the patient has since been under surveillance with scheduled CT of the chest, abdomen, and pelvis, and clinic visits every 4 to 6 months for 2 to 3 years up to 5 years.

REFERENCES

1. Dei Tos AP. Liposarcomas: diagnostic pitfalls and new insights. *Histopathology*. 2014;64(1):38–52. doi:10.1111/his.12311
2. Thway K, Jones RL, Noujaim J, et al. Dedifferentiated liposarcoma: updates on morphology, genetics, and therapeutic strategies. *Adv Anat Pathol*. 2016;23(1):30–40. doi:10.1097/PAP.0000000000000101
3. Lee ATJ, Thway K, Huang PH, et al. Clinical and molecular spectrum of liposarcoma. *J Clin Oncol*. 2018;36(2):151–159. doi:10.1200/JCO.2017.74.9598
4. Jung E, Fiore M, Gronchi A, et al. Second primary malignancies in patients with well-differentiated/dedifferentiated liposarcoma. *Anticancer Res*. 2018;38(6):3535–3542. doi:10.21873/anticanres.12625

5. Teniola O, Wang KY, Wang WL, et al. Imaging of liposarcomas for clinicians: characteristic features and differential considerations. *J Surg Oncol*. 2018;117(6):1195–1203. doi:10.1002/jso.24949
6. Morosi C, Stacchiotti S, Marchianò A, et al. Correlation between radiological assessment and histopathological diagnosis in retroperitoneal tumors: analysis of 291 consecutive patients at a tertiary reference sarcoma center. *Eur J Surg Oncol*. 2014;40(12):1662–1670. doi:10.1016/j.ejso.2014.10.005
7. Bhosale P, Wang J, Varma D, et al. Can abdominal computed tomography imaging help accurately identify a dedifferentiated component in a well-differentiated liposarcoma? *J Comput Assist Tomogr*. 2016;40(6):872–879. doi:10.1097/RCT.0000000000000462
8. Van Houdt WJ, Schrijver AM, Cohen-Hallaleh RB, et al. Needle tract seeding following core biopsies in retroperitoneal sarcoma. *Eur J Surg Oncol*. 2017;43(9):1740–1745. doi:10.1016/j.ejso.2017.06.009
9. Berger-Richardson D, Swallow CJ. Needle tract seeding after percutaneous biopsy of sarcoma: risk/benefit considerations. *Cancer*. 2017;123(4):560–567. doi:10.1002/cncr.30370
10. Ikoma N, Torres KE, Somaiah N, et al. Accuracy of preoperative percutaneous biopsy for the diagnosis of retroperitoneal liposarcoma subtypes. *Ann Surg Oncol*. 2015;22(4):1068–1072. doi:10.1245/s10434-014-4210-8
11. Almond LM, Tirotta F, Tattersall H, et al. Diagnostic accuracy of percutaneous biopsy in retroperitoneal sarcoma. *Br J Surg*. 2019;106(4):395–403. doi:10.1002/bjs.11064
12. Evans HL. Liposarcoma: a study of 55 cases with a reassessment of its classification. *Am J Surg Pathol*. 1979;3:507–523. doi:10.1097/00000478-197912000-00004
13. Elgar F, Goldblum JR. Well-differentiated liposarcoma of the retroperitoneum: a clinicopathologic analysis of 20 cases, with particular attention to the extent of low-grade dedifferentiation. *Mod Pathol*. 1997;10:113–120. PMID:9127316
14. Henricks WH, Chu YC, Goldblum JR, et al. Dedifferentiated liposarcoma: a clinicopathological analysis of 155 cases with a proposal for an expanded definition of dedifferentiation. *Am J Surg Pathol*. 1997;21:271–281. doi:10.1097/00000478-199703000-00002
15. Evans HL. Atypical lipomatous tumor, its variants, and its combined forms: a study of 61 cases, with a minimum follow-up of 10 years. *Am J Surg Pathol*. 2007;31:1–14. doi:10.1097/01.pas.0000213406.95440.7a
16. Mariño-Enríquez A, Fletcher CD, Dal Cin P, et al. Dedifferentiated liposarcoma with "homologous" lipoblastic (pleomorphic liposarcoma-like) differentiation: clinicopathologic and molecular analysis of a series suggesting revised diagnostic criteria. *Am J Surg Pathol*. 2010;34:1122–1131. doi:10.1097/PAS.0b013e3181e5dc49
17. Nascimento AG, Kurtin PJ, Guillou L, et al. Dedifferentiated liposarcoma. A report of nine cases with a peculiar neural-like whorling pattern associated with metaplastic bone formation. *Am J Surg Pathol*. 1998;22:945–955. doi:10.1097/00000478-199808000-00004
18. Mussi C, Collini P, Miceli R, et al. The prognostic impact of dedifferentiation in retroperitoneal liposarcoma: a series of surgically treated patients at a single institution. *Cancer*. 2008;113(7):1657–1665. doi:10.1002/cncr.23774
19. Gronchi A, Collini P, Miceli R, et al. Myogenic differentiation and histologic grading are major prognostic determinants in retroperitoneal liposarcoma. *Am J Surg Pathol*. 2015;39:383–393. doi:10.1097/PAS.0000000000000366
20. Dei Tos AP, Doglioni C, Piccinin S, et al. Molecular abnormalities of the p53 pathway in dedifferentiated liposarcoma. *J Pathol*. 1997;181:8–13. doi:10.1002/(SICI)1096-9896(199701)181:1<8::AID-PATH700>3.0.CO;2-%23
21. Binh MB, Sastre-Garau X, Guillou L, et al. MDM2 and CDK4 immunostainings are useful adjuncts in diagnosing well-differentiated and dedifferentiated liposarcoma subtypes: a comparative analysis of 559 soft tissue neoplasms with genetic data. *Am J Surg Pathol*. 2005;29:1340–1347. doi:10.1097/01.pas.0000170343.09562.39
22. Snyder EL, Sandstrom DJ, Law K, et al. c-Jun amplification and overexpression are oncogenic in liposarcoma but not always sufficient to inhibit the adipocytic differentiation programme. *J Pathol*. 2009;218:292–300. doi:10.1002/path.2564
23. Beird HC, Wu CC, Ingram DR, et al. Genomic profiling of dedifferentiated liposarcoma compared to matched well-differentiated liposarcoma reveals higher genomic complexity and a common origin. *Cold Spring Harb Mol Case Stud*. 2018;4(2). doi:10.1101/mcs.a002386
24. Tseng WW, Pollock RE, Gronchi A. Retroperitoneal sarcomas: big tumors that involve more than just "getting it out." *J Surg Oncol*. 2018;117(1):5–6. doi:10.1002/jso.24886
25. Trans-Atlantic RPS Working Group. Management of primary retroperitoneal sarcoma (RPS) in the adult: a consensus approach from the Trans-Atlantic RPS Working Group. *Ann Surg Oncol*. 2015;22(1):256–263. doi:10.1245/s10434-014-3965-2
26. Gronchi A, Lo Vullo S, Fiore M, et al. Aggressive surgical policies in a retrospectively reviewed single-institution case series of retroperitoneal soft tissue sarcoma patients. *J Clin Oncol*. 2009;27(1):24–30. doi:10.1200/JCO.2008.17.8871
27. Bonvalot S, Rivoire M, Castaing M, et al. Primary retroperitoneal sarcomas: a multivariate analysis of surgical factors associated with local control. *J Clin Oncol*. 2009;27(1):31–37. doi:10.1200/JCO.2008.18.0802
28. Shibata D, Lewis JJ, Leung DH, et al. Is there a role for incomplete resection in the management of retroperitoneal liposarcomas? *J Am Coll Surg*. 2001;193(4):373–379. doi:10.1016/s1072-7515(01)01024-9
29. Kirov KM, Xu HP, Crenn P, et al. Role of nutritional status in the early postoperative prognosis of patients operated for retroperitoneal liposarcoma (RLS): a single center experience. *Eur J Surg Oncol*. 2019;45(2):261–267. doi:10.1016/j.ejso.2018.07.001
30. Mavrogenis AF, Lesensky J, Romagnoli C, et al. Atypical lipomatous tumors/well-differentiated liposarcomas: clinical outcome of 67 patients. *Orthopedics*. 2011;34(12):e893–e898. doi:10.3928/01477447-20111021-11

31. Arvinius C, Torrecilla E, Beano-Collado J, et al. A clinical review of 11 cases of large-sized well-differentiated liposarcomas. *Eur J Orthop Surg Traumatol*. 2017;27(6):837–841. doi:10.1007/s00590-017-1968-y
32. Kito M, Yoshimura Y, Isobe K, et al. Clinical outcome of dedifferentiated liposarcoma in the extremities: a retrospective case series of 7 patients. *J Orthop Sci*. 2016;21(5):673–677. doi:10.1016/j.jos.2016.05.006
33. Dalal KM, Kattan MW, Antonescu CR, et al. Subtype specific prognostic nomogram for patients with primary liposarcoma of the retroperitoneum, extremity, or trunk. *Ann Surg*. 2006;244(3):381–391. doi:10.1097/01.sla.0000234795.98607.00
34. Vos M, Koseła-Paterczyk H, Rutkowski P, et al. Differences in recurrence and survival of extremity liposarcoma subtypes. *Eur J Surg Oncol*. 2018;44(9):1391–1397. doi:10.1016/j.ejso.2018.03.028
35. Gronchi A, Strauss DC, Miceli R, et al. Variability in patterns of recurrence after resection of primary retroperitoneal sarcoma (RPS): a report on 1007 patients from the Multi-institutional Collaborative RPS Working Group. *Ann Surg*. 2016;263(5):1002–1009. doi:10.1097/SLA.0000000000001447
36. Tan MC, Brennan MF, Kuk D, et al. Histology-based classification predicts pattern of recurrence and improves risk stratification in primary retroperitoneal sarcoma. *Ann Surg*. 2016;263(3):593–600. doi:10.1097/SLA.0000000000001149
37. Tseng WW, Madewell JE, Wei W, et al. Locoregional disease patterns in well-differentiated and dedifferentiated retroperitoneal liposarcoma: implications for the extent of resection? *Ann Surg Oncol*. 2014;21(7):2136–2143. doi:10.1245/s10434-014-3643-4
38. Anaya DA, Lahat G, Liu J, et al. Multifocality in retroperitoneal sarcoma: a prognostic factor critical to surgical decision-making. *Ann Surg*. 2009;249(1):137–142. doi:10.1097/SLA.0b013e3181928f2f
39. Gronchi A, Miceli R, Shurell E, et al. Outcome prediction in primary resected retroperitoneal soft tissue sarcoma: histology-specific overall survival and disease-free survival nomograms built on major sarcoma center data sets. *J Clin Oncol*. 2013;31(13):1649–1655. doi:10.1200/JCO.2012.44.3747
40. Nussbaum DP, Rushing CN, Lane WO, et al. Preoperative or postoperative radiotherapy versus surgery alone for retroperitoneal sarcoma: a case-control, propensity score-matched analysis of a nationwide clinical oncology database. *Lancet Oncol*. 2016;17(7):966–975. doi:10.1016/S1470-2045(16)30050-X
41. Baldini EH, Wang D, Haas RL, et al. Treatment guidelines for preoperative radiation therapy for retroperitoneal sarcoma: preliminary consensus of an International Expert Panel. *Int J Radiat Oncol Biol Phys*. 2015;92(3):602–612. doi:10.1016/j.ijrobp.2015.02.013
42. Catton CN, O'Sullivan B, Kotwall C, et al. Outcome and prognosis in retroperitoneal soft tissue sarcoma. *Int J Radiat Oncol Biol Phys*. 1994;29(5):1005–1010. doi:10.1016/0360-3016(94)90395-6
43. Kelly KJ, Yoon SS, Kuk D, et al. Comparison of perioperative radiation therapy and surgery versus surgery alone in 204 patients with primary retroperitoneal sarcoma: a retrospective 2-institution study. *Ann Surg*. 2015;262(1):156–162. doi:10.1097/SLA.0000000000001063
44. Haas RLM, Bonvalot S, Miceli R, et al. Radiotherapy for retroperitoneal liposarcoma: a report from the Transatlantic Retroperitoneal Sarcoma Working Group. *Cancer*. 2019;125(8):1290–1300. doi:10.1002/cncr.31927
45. Bonvalot S, Gronchi A, Le Pechoux C, et al. STRASS (EORTC 62092): a phase III randomized study of preopertative radiotherapy plus surgery versus surgery alone for patients with retroperitoneal sarcoma. *J Clin Oncol*. 2019;37(15 suppl):11001. doi:10.1200/JCO.2019.37.15_suppl.11001
46. Cassier PA, Kantor G, Bonvalot S, et al. Adjuvant radiotherapy for extremity and trunk wall atypical lipomatous tumor/well-differentiated LPS (ALT/WD-LPS): a French Sarcoma Group (GSF-GETO) study. *Ann Oncol*. 2014;25(9):1854–1860. doi:10.1093/annonc/mdu202
47. Zaidi MY, Canter R, Cardona K. Post-operative surveillance in retroperitoneal soft tissue sarcoma: the importance of tumor histology in guiding strategy. *J Surg Oncol*. 2018;117(1):99–104. doi:10.1002/jso.24927
48. Bagaria SP, Gabriel E, Mann GN. Multiply recurrent retroperitoneal liposarcoma. *J Surg Oncol*. 2018;117(1):62–68. doi:10.1002/jso.24929
49. Park JO, Qin LX, Prete FP, et al. Predicting outcome by growth rate of locally recurrent retroperitoneal liposarcoma: the one centimeter per month rule. *Ann Surg*. 2009;250(6):977–982. doi:10.1097/sla.0b013e3181b2468b
50. Ikoma N, Roland CL, Torres KE, et al. Salvage surgery for recurrent retroperitoneal well-differentiated liposarcoma: early reoperation may not provide benefit. *Ann Surg Oncol*. 2018;25(8):2193–2200. doi:10.1245/s10434-018-6417-6
51. Swallow CJ. Strategic delay: histology- and biology-driven decision-making in recurrent retroperitoneal sarcoma. *Ann Surg Oncol*. 2018;25(8):2117–2119. doi:10.1245/s10434-018-6472-z
52. Rhu J, Cho CW, Lee KW, et al. Optimal maximum duration for delaying salvage operation when recurrence of retroperitoneal liposarcoma is suspected: a single-center study. *Int J Clin Oncol*. 2019;24(5):583–589. doi:10.1007/s10147-018-01383-w
53. Honoré C, Faron M, Mir O, et al. Management of locoregional recurrence after radical resection of a primary nonmetastatic retroperitoneal soft tissue sarcoma: the Gustave Roussy experience. *J Surg Oncol*. 2018;118(8):1318–1325. doi:10.1002/jso.25291
54. Casadei L, Calore F, Creighton CJ, et al. Exosome-derived miR-25-3p and miR-92a-3p stimulate liposarcoma progression. *Cancer Res*. 2017;77(14):3846–3856. doi:10.1158/0008-5472.CAN-16-2984
55. Santoro A, Tursz T, Mouridsen H, et al. Doxorubicin versus CYVADIC versus doxorubicin plus ifosfamide in first-line treatment of advanced soft tissue sarcomas: a randomized study of the European Organization for Research and Treatment of Cancer Soft Tissue and Bone Sarcoma Group. *J Clin Oncol*. 1995;13(7):1537–1545. doi:10.1200/JCO.1995.13.7.1537

56. Judson I, Verweij J, Gelderblom H, et al. Doxorubicin alone versus intensified doxorubicin plus ifosfamide for first-line treatment of advanced or metastatic soft-tissue sarcoma: a randomised controlled phase 3 trial. *Lancet Oncol*. 2014;15:415–423. doi:10.1016/S1470-2045(14)70063-4
57. Jones RL, Fisher C, Al-Muderis O, et al. Differential sensitivity of liposarcoma subtypes to chemotherapy. *Eur J Cancer*. 2005;41:2853–2860. doi:10.1016/j.ejca.2005.07.023
58. Italiano A, Toulmonde M, Cioffi A, et al. Advanced well differentiated/dedifferentiated liposarcomas: role of chemotherapy and survival. *Ann Oncol*. 2012;23(6):1601. doi:10.1093/annonc/mdr485
59. Livingston JA, Bugano D, Barbo A, et al. Role of chemotherapy in dedifferentiated liposarcoma of the retroperitoneum: defining the benefit and challenges of the standard. *Sci Rep*. 2017;7(1):11836. doi:10.1038/s41598-017-12132-w
60. Casali PG, Sanfilippo R, D'Incalci M. Trabectedin therapy for sarcomas. *Curr Opin Oncol*. 2010;22(4):342–346. doi:10.1097/CCO.0b013e32833aaac1
61. Sanfilippo R, Bertulli R, Marrari A, et al. High-dose continuous-infusion ifosfamide in advanced well-differentiated/dedifferentiated liposarcoma. *Clin Sarcoma Res*. 2014;4(1):16. doi:10.1186/2045-3329-4-16
62. Elias A, Eder J, Shea T, et al. High-dose ifosfamide with mesna uroprotection. A phase I study. *J Clin Oncol*. 1990;8:170–178. doi:10.1200/JCO.1990.8.1.170
63. Le Cesne A, Antoine E, Spielmann M, et al. High-dose ifosfamide: circumvention of resistance to standard-dose ifosfamide in advanced soft tissue sarcomas. *J Clin Oncol*. 1995;13:1600–1608. doi:10.1200/JCO.1995.13.7.1600
64. Palumbo R, Palmeri S, AntimiM, et al. Phase II study of continuous infusion high-dose ifosfamide in advanced and/or metastatic pretreated soft tissue sarcomas. *Ann Oncol*. 1997;8:1159–1162. doi:10.1023/A:1008279426654
65. Schöffski P, Chawla S, Maki RG, et al. Eribulin versus dacarbazine in previously treated patients with advanced liposarcoma or leiomyosarcoma: a randomised, open-label, multicentre, phase 3 trial. *Lancet*. 2016;387:1629–1637. doi:10.1016/S0140-6736(15)01283-0
66. Chawla S, Schoffski P, Grignani G, et al. Subtype-specific activity in liposarcoma (LPS) patients (pts) from a phase 3, open-label, randomized study of eribulin (ERI) versus dacarbazine (DTIC) in pts with advanced LPS and leiomyosarcoma (LMS). *J Clin Oncol*. 2016;34(suppl):Abstr11037. doi:10.1200/JCO.2016.34.15_suppl.11037
67. Ray-Coquard I, Blay JY, Italiano A, et al. Effect of the MDM2 antagonist RG7112 on the P53 pathway in patients with MDM2-amplified, well-differentiated or dedifferentiated liposarcoma: an exploratory proof-of-mechanism study. *Lancet Oncol*. 2012;13(11):1133–1140. doi:10.1016/S1470-2045(12)70474-6
68. Dickson MA, Tap WD, Keohan ML, et al. Phase II trial of the CDK4 inhibitor PD0332991 in patients with advanced CDK4-amplified well-differentiated or dedifferentiated liposarcoma. *J Clin Oncol*. 2013;31(16):2024–2028. doi:10.1200/JCO.2012.46.5476
69. Gounder MM, Zer A, Tap WD, et al. Phase IB study of selinexor, a first-in-class inhibitor of nuclear export, in patients with advanced refractory bone or soft tissue sarcoma. *J Clin Oncol*. 2016;34(26):3166–3174. doi:10.1200/JCO.2016.67.6346
70. Tawbi HA, Burgess M, Bolejack V, et al. Pembrolizumab in advanced soft-tissue sarcoma and bone sarcoma (SARC028): a multicentre, two-cohort, single-arm, open-label, phase 2 trial. *Lancet Oncol*. 2017;18(11):1493–1501. doi:10.1016/S1470-2045(17)30624-1
71. Tseng WW, Demicco EG, Lazar AJ, et al. Lymphocyte composition and distribution in inflammatory, well-differentiated retroperitoneal liposarcoma: clues to a potential adaptive immune response and therapeutic implications. *Am J Surg Pathol*. 2012;36(6):941–944. doi:10.1097/PAS.0b013e31824f2594
72. Tseng WW, Malu S, Zhang M, et al. Analysis of the intratumoral adaptive immune response in well differentiated and dedifferentiated retroperitoneal liposarcoma. *Sarcoma*. 2015;2015:547460. doi:10.1155/2015/547460
73. Tseng WW, Chopra S, Engleman EG, Pollock RE. Hypothesis: the intratumoral immune response against a cancer progenitor cell impacts the development of well-differentiated versus dedifferentiated disease in liposarcoma. *Front Oncol*. 2016;6:134. doi:10.3389/fonc.2016.00134

10

Gastrointestinal Stromal Tumor

César Serrano and Suzanne George

INTRODUCTION

It was not until 1998 that gastrointestinal stromal tumors (GISTs) could be established as a distinctive tumor of mesenchymal origin due to the seminal discovery of the biologic and disease-defining role of *KIT* receptor tyrosine kinase (RTK) in this disease. Since then, GIST has emerged as a paradigm for clinically effective targeted inhibition of oncogenic driver mutations and a successful model to validate the preclinical concepts for drug response and drug resistance.

GIST is currently regarded as the most common malignant gastrointestinal (GI) mesenchymal neoplasm, and it is thought to arise from the interstitial cells of Cajal (ICC). GIST spans a wide clinical spectrum that ranges from lesions with essentially no metastatic potential to malignant and life-threatening metastatic tumors. Activating mutations of *KIT* and *PDGFRA* RTKs are early, and possibly initiating, oncogenic events in most GISTs, and they continue to be the crucial drivers of tumor development and maintenance once GISTs have undergone malignant transformation. Throughout, the acquisition of novel genomic events is critical for tumor progression, mainly boosting cell cycle dysregulation and metastases formation.

Over the past two decades, we have witnessed a spectacular increase in the overall survival (OS) of patients with this formerly untreatable disease. This is due to the exquisite addiction to oncogenic *KIT*/*PDGFRA*, which explains the profound effect of small-molecule *KIT* inhibitors on GIST cell viability and growth, both preclinically and clinically. However, even in patients with near-complete initial response to imatinib, there are invariably viable residual GIST cells, including imatinib-resistant subclones which harbor *KIT* secondary mutations, and subsequently manifest as clinical progression, typically in a median time of 20 to 24 months.

Secondary mutations in *KIT* constitute the main mechanism of failure to imatinib in 70% to 90% of GIST patients. These imatinib-resistant secondary mutations cluster in two hotspot regions of the *KIT* kinase domain: the adenosine triphosphate (ATP)-binding pocket (exons 13 and14) and the activation loop (exons 17 and 18). Treatment strategies after imatinib failure exploit this *KIT* dependence, and sunitinib and regorafenib, two tyrosine kinase inhibitors (TKIs) with broad *KIT* inhibitory activity, are approved, respectively, in the second and third line. However, the structural heterogeneity of different *KIT*-resistant oncoproteins complicates the design of drugs that could effectively bind to and specifically inhibit all mutants. Thus, *KIT* secondary subclones cannot be completely suppressed by any given currently approved *KIT* inhibitor, ultimately leading to clinical progression after a median of 4 to 6 months regardless of the TKI used post-imatinib. Therefore, imatinib-resistant disease is not only an unmet clinical need, but also a highly active and evolving area of preclinical and clinical research that will likely continue to shape the field both in the short and long term (Figure 10.1).

INCIDENCE AND DEMOGRAPHICS

GIST is the most common mesenchymal malignant neoplasm arising in the GI tract, although its estimated incidence is only 1% of all GI tumors. Epidemiologic studies estimate an annual incidence of GIST in the United States of approximately 4,000 to 6,000 new cases, which represents seven to 20 cases per million per year.

Recent European population-based, histologically confirmed studies establish the incidence rate of GIST between 1.2 and 1.5 cases per 100,000 per year. Notably, these studies also determined for the first time that GIST is the most frequent histological sarcoma subtype.

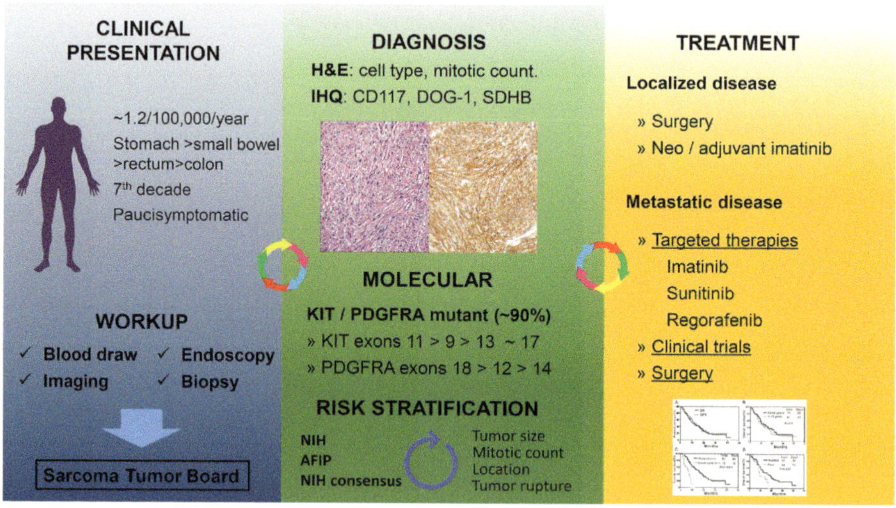

FIGURE 10.1 Work flow depicting clinical, diagnosis, and treatment management of GIST patients.

AFIP, Armed Forces Institute of Pathology; GIST, gastrointestinal stromal tumor; H&E, hematoxylin and eosin; IHQ, immunohistochemistry; NIH, National Institutes of Health.

GIST occurs predominantly in middle-aged and older individuals, with a peak of incidence in the seventh decade of life. GISTs are equally distributed across all geographic and racial groups, also without gender predilection. An exception to this is succinate dehydrogenase (SDH)-deficient GIST. SDH-deficient GISTs are an uncommon subgroup (see section "*KIT*/*PDGFRA* Wild-Type GIST"), demographically characterized by disease present in patients younger than 40 years—particularly in the second decade—and with female predominance.

CLINICAL PRESENTATION

As with many mesenchymal neoplasms, there are no specific confirmatory signs or symptoms of GIST diagnosis, and clinical manifestations depend on the tumor size, location of the primary tumor, and presence of metastatic disease. Thus, GISTs are asymptomatic or paucisymptomatic at an early stage of disease and patients may appear completely healthy on physical exam. A constellation of symptoms emerge as the tumor develops, usually associated with the GI portion of origin and involvement of adjacent structures.

GISTs may originate throughout the GI tract from the esophagus to the anus, and overt or occult GI bleeding at any point, together with the subsequent anemic syndrome, are the most common manifestations in up to two-thirds of patients. Abdominal mass, abdominal pain, and intestinal obstruction are present in 10% to 40% of the patients. Other symptoms are rather unspecific and may include hyporexia, postprandial fullness or early satiety, bloating, nausea, vomiting, dysphagia, constipation, weight loss, and fatigue. Constitutional symptoms are uncommon at early stages, even in patients with high tumor burden.

DIAGNOSTIC APPROACH: BIOPSY AND PATHOLOGIC EVALUATION

Tumor Biopsy

Imaging results and radiologic findings are commonly highly suggestive of GIST diagnosis, and therefore, the final decision to undertake an image-guided tumor biopsy should be discussed within a multidisciplinary team and based on the confidence of workup results. Tumor biopsy is mandatory to confirm the diagnosis of GIST and the mutational status prior to the initiation of neoadjuvant treatment, when indicated. Likewise, definitive diagnosis is made by tumor biopsy in the case of reasonable questions regarding the radiologic findings. In metastatic GIST patients, image-guided percutaneous core-needle tumor biopsy is appropriate at the time of presentation to establish the diagnosis before initiation of systemic treatment.

Pathologic Evaluation and Diagnosis

GIST shows a broad morphologic spectrum that ranges from spindle cell appearance (77%) to epithelioid (8%) or mixed (15%) histologic types. The epithelioid morphology is more frequently observed in the stomach. Nuclear atypia is relatively uncommon. Mitotic rate is currently obtained as the number of mitosis in an area of 5 mm^2, which equals 50 high-power fields (HPF) at a magnification of 40× in microscopes with traditional field size. Approximately two-thirds of GISTs at diagnosis have low or very low mitotic index (≤5 mitosis/5 mm^2).

Over 95% of GISTs stain for *CD117* (*KIT*), and thus, immunohistochemistry for *CD117* is routinely implemented for the diagnosis of GIST. *CD117* often shows a diffuse cytoplasmic pattern and, to a lesser extent, membranous or perinuclear expression. Although *DOG1* may be included in the initial panel, it is most useful in negative cases for *CD117*, in which *DOG1* is expressed in one-third of the tumors. Other commonly used stains and their percentage of positivity include CD34 (80%), actin (30%), S-100 (10%), and desmin (4%). These markers exclude different entities in the differential diagnosis, such as schwannomas, fibromatosis, leiomyosarcomas, or myofibroblastic inflammatory tumors.

Mutational analysis for *KIT* and *PDGFRA* mutations can confirm the diagnosis of GIST in challenging cases, particularly in GI mesenchymal neoplasms with a negative expression for *CD117* and *DOG1*. Regardless, for GIST diagnosis, it is strongly recommended to determine the molecular status of *KIT* and *PDGFRA*, because the type of mutation in patients with localized or metastatic GIST can be both prognostic and predictive of treatment response to TKIs.

SDH-deficient GISTs are characterized by epithelioid morphology, multinodularity, plexiform mural involvement, and low or very low mitotic index. Immunohistochemical staining for *SDHB* is widely used to confirm the diagnosis.

It is strongly recommended to evaluate GIST cases with complex or unusual histopathologic features in referral centers with expertise in sarcoma diagnosis.

RECOMMENDED IMAGING PROCEDURES AND CHARACTERISTIC FEATURES

Imaging Studies

Abdominopelvic CT scan is the initial procedure of choice for GIST workup. CT scans should be performed with both oral and intravenous contrast, which are critical to define the extent and location of the primary tumor and metastases, as well as other characteristics related to the clinical behavior (i.e., invasive components). GIST usually appears on CT scans as well-demarcated spherical masses that arise from the GI wall. They often project exophytically and/or intraluminally, and may have overlying mucosal ulceration. Central and extensive areas of necrosis and hemorrhage are commonly seen in larger GISTs owing to the outgrowth of vascular supplies.

Endoscopy and Endoscopy Ultrasound

GISTs appear at endoscopy as a submucosal mass protruding into the gastric lumen. Endoscopic ultrasound (EUS) exam further characterizes a gastric mass as suspicious for GIST, as GISTs are characteristically located in the fourth layer of the stomach, corresponding to the muscularis propria. Endoscopic biopsies using standard techniques often do not yield sufficient tissue for a definitive diagnosis; however, they can still be considered in certain cases.

MOLECULAR ABERRATIONS DRIVING GIST GROWTH AND SURVIVAL

KIT and *PDGFRA* Primary Mutations

Oncogenic activation of *KIT* or *PDGFRA* RTKs is central to GIST biology and is present in 85% to 90% of the patients. *KIT* is a transmembrane receptor that belongs to the type III RTK family, which also includes *KIT*-homologous receptor *PDGFRA*, among others. *KIT* and *PDGFRA* mutations are mutually exclusive and are likely the initiating event. Constitutive activation of *KIT* or *PDGFRA* triggers downstream cell signaling cascades that control critical cell functions, including survival, proliferation, and adhesion.

Oncogenic mutations in *KIT* are found in approximately 80% of GISTs. Two-thirds of GISTs harbor primary mutations in *KIT* juxtamembrane domain, encoded by exon 11 and distributed in the form of in-frame deletions, insertions, and substitutions, or combinations of these. Similar complexity is found, although less frequently, in other *KIT* regions distributed across the extracellular domain (exon 9), the ATP-binding pocket (exon 13), or the activation loop (exon 17). Primary mutations in *PDGFRA* (~10%) are found in homologous regions of the gene.

Cytogenetic Progression in GIST

Clinical and biologic progression of GIST represents a continuum that spans from micro-GISTs (<1 cm) to clinically aggressive and metastasizing GISTs. The crucial transforming and possibly initiating oncogenic event in most GISTs is the mutational activation of *KIT* or *PDGFRA*, which continues to be the essential driver of tumor development and maintenance, once the GISTs have undergone malignant transformation. However, *KIT* mutations alone are insufficient to induce malignant behavior, and additional genetic events are necessary to transform micro-GISTs into tumors with increasingly malignant potential. Thus, there is a well-established multistep cytogenetic progression involving typical chromosomic regions targeting genes not yet fully understood: *KIT*-activating mutation → 14q deletion (*MAX*) → 22q deletion → 1p deletion → 9p deletion (*CDKN2A*) → Xp deletion (*DMD*) (2–4). Deletion of *DMD* is almost universally present at a late stage in high-grade, lethal GIST, and conditions the metastatic spread.

KIT Secondary Mutations

Acquired resistance to first-line imatinib occurs in 70% to 90% of GIST patients through polyclonal expansion of heterogeneous subclones harboring different *KIT* secondary mutations that confer resistance to imatinib. Such mutations are not random and cluster in two regions of the *KIT* kinase domain: the ATP-binding pocket (encoded by exons 13 and 14) and the activation loop (encoded by exons 17 and 18). Other mechanisms, most likely involving *KIT*-independent activation of *KIT*-downstream signal intermediates (i.e., *RAS*; *PIK3CA*, *PTEN*), might have a potential role in imatinib resistance after several lines of treatment, although they are yet to be fully elucidated.

KIT/PDGFRA Wild-Type GIST

Wild-type (WT) GIST encompasses 10% to 15% of GISTs with heterogeneous molecular backgrounds sharing a lack of *KIT* or *PDGFRA* mutations.

SDH-deficient GISTs represent approximately 40% of WT GISTs, and comprise pediatric GIST, Carney tryad, Carney–Stratakis syndrome, and a small proportion of adult WT GISTs. Most SDH-deficient tumors present with the following features: appear at a young age (<40 years), female predominance, gastric origin, epithelioid morphology, multifocal nodular growth pattern, and frequent involvement of local lymph nodes. SDH-deficient WT GISTs normally follow a chronic and indolent course of disease. Loss of SDH function through inactivating mutations or epigenetic silencing triggers a recurrent DNA hypermethylation phenotype. Although the key driver genes and/or pathways remain unclear, hypoxia-inducible factor (HIF) and insulin growth factor receptor (IGFR) pathways have been found to be typically hyperactivated in these patients.

WT GISTs that are not SDH deficient may harbor a diversity of genetic events activating the *RAS*/mitogen-activated protein kinase (MAPK) pathway, uncommon fusions including *NTRK*, and unknown driver mechanisms.

COMMON LOCATION OF PRIMARY DISEASE

GISTs are the most common sarcomas of the GI tract and can arise virtually anywhere along the GI tract, although stomach and small intestine are the most common primary tumor locations in 60% and 30% of the patients, respectively. Duodenum and rectum are the less common primary sites (4% each), and more infrequent locations include esophagus, colon, appendix, and extra-GI GIST (i.e., omentum).

GENERAL THERAPEUTIC APPROACH FOR PRIMARY TUMOR

According to the National Comprehensive Cancer Network (NCCN) and European Society of Medical Oncology (ESMO) guidelines, management of GIST patients should be done in reference centers and/or within reference networks sharing multidisciplinary expertise and treating a high number of patients annually.

Surgery

All GISTs ≥2 cm in size should be resected because of their intrinsic metastatic potential. The standard and potentially curative therapy for localized GIST is surgical resection with the goal of complete removal with negative margins and an intact pseudocapsule. The extent of surgery usually involves a wedge resection of the stomach or bowel, as GIST, unlike epithelial GI tumors, commonly projects exophytically and/or intraluminally, and therefore, wide margins are not needed. Actually, the ideal margin of resection in GIST remains a matter of debate. Hence, while macroscopic incomplete resection is certainly associated with worse outcome, it seems that the presence of microscopically positive margins (R1) does not impact negatively on recurrence-free survival (RFS). Additionally, tumor rupture to the abdominal cavity during perioperative procedures is associated with a risk of recurrence close to 100%, and therefore, it should be avoided.

Routine lymphadenectomy is not recommended, given the virtual absence of nodal metastases in GIST, except in rare GIST subtypes such as SDH-deficient GIST. Abdomen and liver inspection should be performed in all cases with an aim to identify and remove any previously undetected peritoneal metastatic deposits.

There is no consensus on the management of small GISTs (<2 cm). On the one hand, incidental micro-GISTs (<1 cm) are present in up to one-third of the population and virtually never progress to clinically aggressive GIST. Thus, incidental lesions suggestive of micro-GIST might be initially followed to prove lack of increase in tumor size. By contrast, the clinical behavior of GISTs between 1 and 2 cm is unpredictable in the absence of pathologic evaluation. While surveillance might be considered in gastric GISTs between 1 and 2 cm, small bowel, colon, or rectal GISTs should be resected irrespective of the size, given the higher risk of recurrence and malignant potential.

Adjuvant and Neoadjuvant Imatinib

The success of imatinib in advanced disease prompted interest in its perioperative use with the final goal of preventing relapse after surgery. This includes both postoperative treatment for patients at high risk of recurrence after complete resection of a primary GIST and preoperative therapy for patients with unresectable disease or borderline resectable tumors. There are several well-defined criteria specifically created to identify the subset of GIST patients with the highest likelihood of relapse and who could obtain more benefit from adjuvant/neoadjuvant imatinib. According to the risk-stratification criteria, GIST patients are classified at low, intermediate, and high risk of recurrence after surgery (see section "Propensity to Metastasize: Risk Factor Stratification in GIST"), and high-risk patients benefit the most from perioperative treatment with imatinib.

Adjuvant Imatinib

Three years of adjuvant imatinib therapy is associated with reduced recurrence rates and improved OS in patients with high-risk primary GIST, and it is the current standard of care. This recommendation is the result of three randomized Phase 3 clinical trials that evaluated the role of imatinib 400 mg daily in the adjuvant setting: the American College of Surgeons Oncology Group (ACOSOG) trial Z9001[1], the Scandinavian Sarcoma Group (SSG) XVIII/Arbeitsgemeinschaft Internistische Onkologie (AIO) trial[2], and the European Organization for Research and Treatment of Cancer (EORTC) trial 62024[3].

In Z9001, resected GISTs ≥3 cm were randomly assigned to either imatinib or placebo for 1 year after surgery. One-year RFS was significantly improved from 83% in the placebo group to 98% in the imatinib group. No difference in OS was detected between both groups because of the crossover effect and because the trial was not powered to assess this difference. One of the main criticisms to this study was the inclusion of a wide range of GIST patients with different risks for relapse. Regardless, 1 year of treatment with adjuvant imatinib was accepted as the standard treatment after complete resection of GIST.

The SSG XVIII/AIO Phase 3 clinical trial subsequently investigated the differences between imatinib 400 mg daily for 1 year and the same regimen for 3 years. For this study, more stringent inclusion criteria were applied, and it only entered high-risk GIST patients based on the National Institutes of Health (NIH) consensus classification or those with tumor rupture. Patients assigned to the 3-year group had a 5-year RFS of 65.6% compared with 47.9% in the 1-year group. Although the trial was not powered to assess differences in OS, the analysis showed that 3-year treatment achieved a 5-year OS of 92% compared with 81.7% in the 1-year group. In view of these results, the NCCN and ESMO guidelines currently recommend 3 years of adjuvant treatment with imatinib in high-risk patients. The NCCN guidelines also recommend considering adjuvant imatinib in intermediate-risk patients on an individual basis. Adjuvant treatment for low-risk patients is not indicated.

The Phase 3 EORTC 62024 study randomized intermediate- and high-risk GIST patients to 2 years of imatinib or observation after surgical resection. Two years of adjuvant imatinib impacted positively on RFS, with a 3- and 5-year RFS rate in the experimental and placebo groups of 84% versus 66% and 69% versus 63%, respectively. OS did not differ between the treatment arms. Interestingly, this trial changed the primary endpoint to imatinib failure-free survival (IFFS) in order to capture the time when a different TKI was started in the advanced setting. No differences were observed regardless of the treatment group. This trial confirmed earlier studies in terms of RFS, but also observed that most of the benefit was lost after 1 to 3 years from the end of the adjuvant imatinib, thus suggesting that imatinib delayed the relapse. Therefore, this finding raises concerns about the mechanism of action of adjuvant imatinib in GIST, as it is not known whether recurrences are truly being prevented or just delayed.

Recently, the PERSIST-5 Phase 2, single-arm clinical trial[6] investigated whether longer duration of adjuvant imatinib 400 mg daily (5 years) had an impact on outcomes in completely resected intermediate- and high-risk GIST patients. Half of the patients discontinued the treatment owing to patient choice. Recurrence occurred within 2 years from imatinib discontinuation in those patients completing the 5 years on adjuvant treatment. The definitive answer to this question will come from the SSG XXII trial, which is currently evaluating 3 versus 5 years of adjuvant imatinib in locally resected GIST patients in an international Phase 3 study.

Other areas of uncertainty need to be addressed with prospective studies interrogating questions such as whether doses >400 mg should be used in the adjuvant setting and whether adjuvant imatinib might benefit uncommon GIST subgroups (i.e., SDH-deficient GIST).

Neoadjuvant Imatinib

Current evidence for the use of preoperative imatinib in localized GIST comes from retrospective series and a few prospective, single-arm Phase 2 trials. These studies[4,5] showed that most locally advanced GISTs shrink or stabilize in size after 6 to 12 months of preoperative imatinib, allowing subsequent surgery. Therefore, neoadjuvant treatment with imatinib is not a standard of care, and the decision must be made on an individual basis.

Several aspects need to be taken into account: first, based on the high rate of responses observed with imatinib in patients with metastatic GIST, preoperative use of imatinib aims to reduce tumor bulk to facilitate complete surgical resection. Thus, it can be considered in patients with rectal or duodenal GIST—to avoid resections that adversely impair the quality of life—and in patients with a large gastric GIST, which likely requires total or subtotal gastrectomy. Second, early assessment of response is required in order to minimize risks, because a delay could impede surgery if imatinib fails to shrink or stabilize the tumor size. Thus, tumor imaging by either PET/CT or CT at baseline and in the first 4 to 8 weeks on imatinib appears to be the most sensitive option, and it is our standard practice. Third, genotyping at baseline and identification of imatinib-nonresponsive mutations (e.g., *PDGFRA* D842V) are highly recommended. Finally, it should be noted that risk stratification in patients receiving neoadjuvant imatinib will likely be inaccurate, because both pretreatment biopsy and posttreatment specimens do not allow full evaluation of tumor mitotic rate. Thus, careful evaluation is needed for a correct indication for adjuvant imatinib.

RECOMMENDED FOLLOW-UP AFTER DEFINITIVE THERAPY

Abdominal CT scan is the usual procedure, given the abdominal location and the typical relapse in the peritoneum and liver. MRI is recommended to characterize the liver lesions, complex locations such as rectum, or allergic reactions to iodine contrast agent. PET is indicated when the previous studies are inconclusive.

There is a lack of studies assessing the effectiveness of duration, timing, and procedures for the follow-up of GIST patients undergoing treatment for localized disease with or without perioperative treatment with imatinib. In this absence of data, recent guidelines and recommendations advocate adjustments based on risk of recurrence and time after surgery.

Localized Disease

Annual CT Scan in Low-Risk Patients

For intermediate- and high-risk GIST, CT scan can be performed every 3 to 4 months during the first 2 years, every 6 months thereafter, and annually after 5 years of follow-up. It is important to note that once imatinib is withdrawn, recurrence mostly occurs during the following 12 to 24 months, and therefore, follow-up should be maintained during this period.

Advanced and Metastatic Disease

Follow-up should be conducted in GIST patients treated with TKIs approximately every 3 months, but can be prolonged to 4 to 6 months in patients with sustained response to a given TKI, particularly in the long-term responders (>5 years) to imatinib. RECIST (Response Evaluation Criteria in Solid Tumors) is the usual type of measurement in the follow-up, but Choi response criteria should be used to rule out pseudoprogression as a consequence of myxoid degeneration or intratumoral hemorrhage occurring in response to TKIs.

PROPENSITY TO METASTASIZE: RISK FACTOR STRATIFICATION IN GIST

According to some series, 40% to 50% of GIST patients may develop recurrent disease after surgery despite macroscopically complete resection. All GISTs >2 cm are at risk of recurrence, although their clinical behavior is highly variable. Several prognostic criteria are used among clinicians to estimate the risk of relapse after surgery and/or to predict the potential benefit of adjuvant treatment with imatinib.

Primary tumor size, mitotic count, and tumor location are the three main prognostic factors in GIST. Proliferation rate is assessed in GIST with the mitotic count using a total area of 5 mm^2 or 25 per HPF in modern microscopes. GISTs located outside the stomach have generally more unfavorable outcomes than GISTs arising in the stomach. Additionally, virtually all patients are considered at risk of relapse in the context of tumor rupture, either spontaneous or due to manipulation during the surgery.

Current risk-stratification systems include some or all of the aforementioned prognostic factors. The consensus criteria from the NIH, which is the oldest, stratifies risk based on tumor size and mitotic count. The Armed Forces Institute of Pathology (AFIP) risk criteria added tumor location as a prognostic factor, which improves differentiation between patients with moderate and intermediate risk. Finally, the revised NIH consensus criteria additionally incorporated tumor rupture. Despite these differences, these three methods are comparable and predict reasonably well. These risk-stratification systems are validated only in *KIT*-mutant GIST—other genotypes are underrepresented.

There is a well-established prognostic role of particular mutational status in GIST, although it is not included in any risk evaluation system. GISTs with *KIT* exon 11 deletions in codon 557 exhibit particularly aggressive behavior. This has been consistently shown in several studies and appears to be particularly helpful in gastric GIST with intermediate risk of relapse by the above-mentioned risk-stratification systems. These reports also agree that GISTs with primary mutations in *PDGFRA* exon 18 (D842V) are associated with a more favorable prognosis when localized and have a seemingly lower risk of recurrence and distant metastatic spread.

COMMON FEATURES OF METASTATIC DISEASE

GIST commonly spreads to the liver and/or the abdominal cavity (peritoneum, mesentery, omentum). At the time of diagnosis, approximately 50% of the cases are localized, 20% are locally advanced, and 25% are already present with metastatic disease.

THERAPEUTIC APPROACH FOR METASTATIC DISEASE

GIST has emerged as a paradigmatic and successful model for rational development of targeted agents against critical driver alterations in cancer. In the past 15 years, we have witnessed how the introduction of *KIT* inhibitors into the clinic has led to an extraordinary improvement of outcomes in this tumor, formerly deemed chemoresistant.

Targeted Therapy

Imatinib

Imatinib (Gleevec in the United States, Glivec elsewhere; Novartis Oncology, Basel, Switzerland), an orally available, small-molecule inhibitor with activity against *KIT*, *PDGFR*, and *ABL* kinases, was the first TKI that was granted the U.S. Food and Drug Administration (FDA) approval for the treatment of *KIT*-positive metastatic and/or unresectable GISTs, following the demonstration of sustained response to imatinib 400 mg daily in the landmark B2222 Phase 2 trial.[7] Approximately two-thirds of the patients achieved objective radiographic response to imatinib, 15% of patients had prolonged stable disease, and 10% to 15% exhibited primary resistance. Patients with stable disease had similar long-term benefit and favorable survival outcomes as those with objective responses. This study showed a median time to treatment progression (TTP) of 24 months and an estimated median OS of 57 months, with no differences between the doses of 400 and 600 mg daily. This benefit is particularly prolonged in a subset of GIST patients, with around one-third achieving progression-free survival (PFS) at 5 years and 5% to 10% achieving it for up to 10 years. Importantly, the *KIT* genotype predicted GIST outcomes, as *KIT* exon 11-mutant patients had a substantially greater likelihood of partial response and longer time to treatment failure compared with patients with either *KIT* exon 9 mutation or *KIT/PDGFRA* WT. Therapy is generally well tolerated, with diarrhea, edema, and fatigue being the most common treatment-related toxicities.

Two subsequent Phase 3 trials[8,9] supported these findings and further studied the efficacy of higher doses of imatinib (800 vs. 400 mg daily). Overall, a small but statistically significant PFS advantage was seen in GIST patients treated with imatinib 800 mg daily, with no difference in OS between the two arms, and patients on higher-dose therapy reported more side effects. The presence of *KIT* exon 9 mutation was the only significant predictive factor for benefit from higher doses.

Imatinib at a dose of 400 mg daily is the standard initial dose for the treatment of advanced or metastatic GIST patients. Dose escalation to 800 mg/d is a reasonable option for patients progressing on 400 mg/day—particularly in *KIT* exon 9 mutant—although there is no data or consensus favoring dose escalation versus initiation of second-line treatment. [10–12]

The main mechanism of resistance found in 70% to 90% of GIST patients entails the emergence of subpopulations with *KIT* secondary mutations impeding imatinib binding to the *KIT* receptor. Resistance involves substantial heterogeneity of secondary mutations between and within metastases from individual patients, which underscores the complexity of resistance as the main treatment challenge in patients with GIST after frontline imatinib treatment.

Sunitinib

Sunitinib (Sutent; Pfizer Inc., New York, NY, USA) is a multitargeted small-molecule TKI with potent activity against *KIT* and *PDGFRA*, among several other kinases, and is currently approved for the treatment of metastatic GIST in patients with imatinib resistance or intolerance. In a pivotal randomized, placebo-controlled Phase 3 trial[13] in patients with imatinib-refractory or -intolerant GISTs, 312 patients were enrolled and randomized to receive sunitinib or placebo. Sunitinib dose was 50 mg daily, 4 weeks on and 2 weeks off. Despite a low objective response rate in the sunitinib group (7% response rate), TTP, the primary endpoint, was fourfold longer in the sunitinib arm compared with placebo (27 vs. 6 weeks, respectively). Continuous dosing of sunitinib 37.5 mg daily is also active in the same setting, as shown in a nonrandomized Phase 2 clinical trial[14] that yielded a clinical benefit rate of 53% and a PFS of 34 weeks.

Regorafenib

Regorafenib (Stivarga; Bayer HealthCare Pharmaceuticals Inc., Montville, NJ, USA), an orally active multikinase inhibitor with activity against a variety of kinases including *KIT* and *PDGFRA*, obtained worldwide approval for the treatment of GIST after failure of imatinib and sunitinib. A pivotal Phase 3 trial[15] randomized GIST patients to regorafenib 160 mg once daily for the first 21 days of each 28-day cycle or placebo. Median PFS was also significantly longer in patients treated with regorafenib (4.8 months) compared to placebo (0.9 month). As observed with sunitinib, the overall response rate was low (4.5%), as most of the benefit was due to disease stabilization.

Other Therapies

There are currently no other therapies approved for the treatment of TKI-refractory GIST, and therefore, it remains an unmet clinical need. It is highly encouraged to treat these patients in clinical trials.

Resumption of imatinib with palliative purposes is a common practice, given the rapid progression and symptom worsening after TKI discontinuation, likely due to the rapid outgrowth of imatinib-sensitive disease. However, a Phase 3 randomized trial[16] showed no significant improvement in objective response or in OS compared to placebo in this setting. No improvement in quality of life measurements could be determined either, although other studies have demonstrated the positive impact of TKI maintenance on OS despite progression.

Pazopanib has recently proved to be effective in TKI-resistant GIST patients in a randomized Phase 2 trial,[17] achieving a significant improvement of median PFS (3.4 months) over placebo (2.4 months), again with <5% response rate, although these results have not been consistent across studies. The following TKIs with *KIT* inhibitory activity have been investigated in imatinib-resistant GIST, mostly in single-arm Phase 2 trials: sorafenib, ponatinib, nilotinib, dasatinib, and dovitinib. All of them share a similar activity profile, with a median PFS between 3 and 5 months and a response rate <10%, regardless of the line of treatment. Interestingly, small-molecule *KIT*-inhibitor monotherapies have a drug-specific activity profile against a subset of the *KIT* secondary mutational spectrum, which constitutes the molecular basis for the modest clinical benefit observed with successive lines of treatment in imatinib-resistant GIST.

Surgery

Resection of metastatic disease in GIST patients is not a standard procedure in all centers; however, in the absence of controlled trials, it can be considered on an individualized basis within multidisciplinary teams in sarcoma expert centers. Resection of metastatic disease aiming to achieve complete response may positively impact on outcomes in GIST patients either responding to TKIs or with focal progression. However, it is not recommended in patients experiencing generalized disease progression while receiving a TKI. Importantly, resection, even if complete, does not eliminate the need for continued treatment with TKI therapy.

SUMMARY

The molecular understanding of the biologic underpinnings of GIST has led and is currently leading to the rational development of therapeutic approaches successfully implemented into the clinic. All currently approved drugs for GIST are based on *KIT* inhibition, given the dominance of oncogenically active *KIT* signaling throughout all steps of GIST oncogenesis from micro-GIST to imatinib-resistant metastatic GIST. However, treatment of GISTs refractory to approved TKIs remains an unmet clinical need, as the heterogeneity of the resistant disease is a challenge. Thus, therapeutic strategies exploiting *KIT*, *KIT*-downstream pathways, or adaptive mechanisms to *KIT* inhibition through combination therapies or novel cross-cutting treatment strategies are being actively sought. Likewise, the high reliance of GIST on *KIT* or *PDGFRA* mutations, together with the relevance of *KIT* secondary genotype for response prediction to current TKIs make GIST an appealing model to validate circulating tumor DNA with the final goal of its implementation as a real-time biomarker for treatment selection. This approach remains under active investigation.

In the meantime, GIST patients, as in all rare diseases, should be consulted and/or referred to sarcoma expert centers for disease management and treatment. Patient tolerance of imatinib treatment facilitates its use in the community. However, there are several nuances and steps during the clinical course of the disease that need to be addressed by multidisciplinary teams. For instance, *KIT/PDGFRA* primary genotype is highly relevant for the indication of imatinib as a neoadjuvant/adjuvant treatment or in the setting of metastatic disease, and should be performed in all cases. Additionally, GIST genotype is increasingly important for the participation in clinical trials. On the other hand, unlike imatinib, the range of side effects of sunitinib and regorafenib is higher owing to the wider spectrum of target inhibition. Although the majority of them are manageable, prevention and timely dose/schedule adaptation are essential to avoid unnecessary definitive treatment withdrawals from potential effective treatments. Likewise, and as mentioned in the section "Surgery," surgery for metastatic disease potentially benefits a subset of GIST patients, and these opportunities should be evaluated in multidisciplinary sarcoma centers.

CASE STUDY

A 59-year-old female patient was referred to our institution with a suspected diagnosis of localized gastric GIST. Two weeks before, the patient was admitted at her home institution because of melena accompanied by anemic syndrome, without hemodynamic instability. The episode was spontaneously stabilized and it partially recovered after red blood cell (RBC) transfusion. The patient only had records for a 4-month history of mild asymptomatic microcytic anemia with normal colonoscopy. CT scan at the ED showed a 22-cm gastric mass protruding toward the abdominal cavity, with suggestive radiologic signs of microperforation. The lesion was highly suggestive of a gastric GIST. The rest of the examination was unremarkable. Blood draw at our institution showed grade 3 anemia despite prior transfusion, although without evidence for active bleeding. The patient remained hemodynamically stable.

The sarcoma board at our institution decided to perform surgery without neoadjuvant imatinib treatment, given the high risk of massive GI bleeding together with the suspicion of microperforation. During the surgical procedure, the surgeons identified multiple subcentimetric peritoneal metastases, with three of them being resected for pathologic evaluation. The gastric mass was resected through partial gastrectomy and it measured 21 cm. The microperforation was evidenced at the gross examination, together with extensive hemorrhagic and necrotic areas. The pathology report described a spindle cell–type GIST, 17 mitoses/5 mm^2, and diffuse stain for *CD117*. The molecular analysis identified a *KIT* exon 11 deletion (p.552_554del).

The patient was discharged 10 days after surgery and initiated with imatinib 400 mg daily for 3 weeks after the surgery. Tolerance was acceptable, with only mild transitory nausea reported within 1 hour of imatinib intake. Reevaluation visit was performed 10 weeks after imatinib initiation. At that time, the patient felt short of breath (grade 2 dyspnea), accompanied by occasional cough and pleuritic-like pain on deep inspiration in her right hemithorax. No other symptoms were described. The physical examination revealed semiology of pleural effusion that was confirmed in the upper images of the contrast-enhanced abdominopelvic CT scan. No peritoneal disease was radiologically visible. However, multiple subcentimetric hypodense liver lesions (>20) showed up in this first reevaluation. Overall, the case presentation was deemed pleural effusion due to imatinib toxicity and the response of previously undetectable subcentimetric liver lesions (Choi-like effect). PET/CT was performed, which was without fluorodeoxyglucose (FDG)-avid disease, further supporting the finding of pseudoprogression in this case. Imatinib was put on hold for 2 weeks and resumed at 200 mg daily together with a diuretic. Imatinib could be gradually escalated uneventfully to the standard dose of 400 mg daily within 2 months.

The patient remained on imatinib at 400 mg/day and underwent CT imaging every 3 months. Serial imaging demonstrated stability to the hepatic lesions, which became quite hypodense over time. She remains on imatinib with radiographically stable disease 2 years after imatinib initiation.

This case highlights the complexity of GIST management due to presenting symptoms and/or toxic effect, plus the relevance of a multidisciplinary tumor board with expertise in GIST. In addition, the subtle finding of "new liver lesions" interpreted as response rather than resistance allowed the patient to remain on an active therapy, imatinib, for at least 2 years.

REFERENCES

1. Dematteo RP, Ballman KV, Antonescu CR, et al. Adjuvant imatinib mesylate after resection of localised, primary gastrointestinal stromal tumour: a randomised, double-blind, placebo-controlled trial. *Lancet*. 2009;373(9669):1097–1104. doi:10.1016/S0140-6736(09)60500-6
2. Joensuu H, Eriksson M, Sundby Hall K, et al. One vs three years of adjuvant imatinib for operable gastrointestinal stromal tumor: a randomized trial. *JAMA*. 2012;307(12):1265–1272. doi:10.1001/jama.2012.347
3. Casali PG, Zalcberg J, Le Cesne A, et al. Ten-year progression-free and overall survival in patients with unresectable or metastatic GI stromal tumors: long-term analysis of the European Organisation for Research and Treatment of Cancer, Italian Sarcoma Group, and Australasian Gastrointestinal Trials Group Intergroup Phase III Randomized Trial on Imatinib at Two Dose Levels. *J Clin Oncol*. 2017;35(15):1713–1720. doi:10.1200/JCO.2016.71.0228
4. Eisenberg BL, Harris J, Blanke CD, et al. Phase II trial of neoadjuvant/adjuvant imatinib mesylate (IM) for advanced primary and metastatic/recurrent operable gastrointestinal stromal tumor (GIST): early results of RTOG 0132/ACRIN 6665. *J Surg Oncol*. 2009;99(1):42–47. doi:10.1002/jso.21160
5. McAuliffe JC, Hunt KK, Lazar AJ, et al. A randomized, phase II study of preoperative plus postoperative imatinib in GIST: evidence of rapid radiographic response and temporal induction of tumor cell apoptosis. *Ann Surg Oncol*. 2009;16:910–919.
6. Raut CP, Espat NJ, Maki RG, et al. Efficacy and tolerability of 5-year adjuvant imatinib treatment for patients with resected intermediate- or high-risk primary gastrointestinal stromal tumor: the PERSIST-5 clinical trial. *JAMA Oncol*. 2018;4(12):e184060. doi:10.1001/jamaoncol.2018.4060
7. Demetri GD, von Mehren M, Blanke CD, et al. Efficacy and safety of imatinib mesylate in advanced gastrointestinal stromal tumors. *N Engl J Med*. 2002;347(7):472–480. doi:10.1056/NEJMoa020461
8. Blanke CD, Rankin C, Demetri GD, et al. Phase III randomized, intergroup trial assessing imatinib mesylate at two dose levels in patients with unresectable or metastatic gastrointestinal stromal tumors expressing the kit receptor tyrosine kinase: S0033. *J Clin Oncol*. 2008;26:626–632. doi:10.1200/JCO.2007.13.4452

9. Verweij J, Casali PG, Zalcberg J, et al. Progression-free survival in gastrointestinal stromal tumours with high-dose imatinib: randomised trial. *Lancet*. 2004;364:1127–1134. doi:10.1016/S0140-6736(04)17098-0
10. Liegl B, Kepten I, Le C, et al. Heterogeneity of kinase inhibitor resistance mechanisms in GIST. *J Pathol*. 2008;216(1):64–74. doi:10.1002/path.2382
11. Corless CL, Barnett CM, Heinrich MC. Gastrointestinal stromal tumours: origin and molecular oncology. *Nat Rev Cancer*. 2011;11(12):865–878. doi:10.1038/nrc3143
12. Serrano C, Marino-Enriquez A, Tao DL, et al. Complementary activity of tyrosine kinase inhibitors against secondary kit mutations in imatinib-resistant gastrointestinal stromal tumours. *Br J Cancer*. 2019;120(6):612–620. doi:10.1038/s41416-019-0389-6
13. Demetri GD, van Oosterom AT, Garrett CR, et al. Efficacy and safety of sunitinib in patients with advanced gastrointestinal stromal tumour after failure of imatinib: a randomised controlled trial. *Lancet*. 2006;368:1329–1338. doi:10.1016/S0140-6736(06)69446-4
14. George S, Blay JY, Casali PG, et al. Clinical evaluation of continuous daily dosing of sunitinib malate in patients with advanced gastrointestinal stromal tumour after imatinib failure. *Eur J Cancer*. 2009;45:1959–1968. doi:10.1016/j.ejca.2009.02.011
15. Demetri GD, Reichardt P, Kang YK, et al. Efficacy and safety of regorafenib for advanced gastrointestinal stromal tumours after failure of imatinib and sunitinib (GRID): an international, multicentre, randomised, placebo-controlled, phase 3 trial. *Lancet*. 2013;381:295–302. doi:10.1016/S0140-6736(12)61857-1
16. Kang YK, Ryu MH, Yoo C, et al. Resumption of imatinib to control metastatic or unresectable gastrointestinal stromal tumours after failure of imatinib and sunitinib (RIGHT): a randomised, placebo-controlled, phase 3 trial. *Lancet Oncol*. 2013;14:1175–1182. doi:10.1016/S1470-2045(13)70453-4
17. Mir O, Cropet C, Toulmonde M, et al. Pazopanib plus best supportive care versus best supportive care alone in advanced gastrointestinal stromal tumours resistant to imatinib and sunitinib (PAZOGIST): a randomised, multicentre, open-label phase 2 trial. *Lancet Oncol*. 2016;17(5):632–641. doi:10.1016/S1470-2045(16)00075-9

11

Osteosarcoma

Matthew Chin and J. Andrew Livingston

INTRODUCTION

Osteosarcoma is the most common primary bone sarcoma, most often affecting adolescents and young adults or arising as a secondary osteosarcoma in older adults. Although osteosarcoma previously held a poor prognosis, overall survival improved dramatically after the adoption of multiagent chemotherapy, establishing multimodality treatment including surgery and chemotherapy as the standard of care. Since these advances over 30 years ago, overall treatment strategies for the primary treatment of osteosarcoma have not changed significantly, and therefore, overall survival has remained relatively stable. The mainstay of treatment involves neoadjuvant chemotherapy (most frequently, a combination of doxorubicin, cisplatin, high-dose methotrexate with or without ifosfamide), wide surgical resection with limb-sparing surgery if possible, followed by adjuvant chemotherapy. The treatment of metastatic disease remains a significant challenge. While patients with isolated pulmonary metastases may be cured with resection, unresectable disease portends a poor prognosis. Current approaches being developed include defining molecular subsets for targeted therapies and exploring the role of immunotherapy for the treatment of recurrent/metastatic disease.

INCIDENCE AND EPIDEMIOLOGY

Osteosarcoma follows a bimodal distribution, with a peak incidence in children and adolescents and a secondary peak in the elderly. According to the Surveillance, Epidemiology, and End Results Program (SEER) from the National Cancer Institute, the annual incidence in the United States is 4.4 per million for those 0 to 24 years of age, 1.7 for those 25 to 59 years of age, and 4.2 for adults older than 60 years.[1] Among adolescents and young adults, the majority of cases are conventional high-grade osteosarcoma (including osteoblastic, chondroblastic, and fibroblastic subtypes). Conversely, older adults have higher rates of osteosarcoma associated with Paget disease of bone or as a secondary cancer.[1] Overall, there is also a slight predominance in blacks and males, with an average male/female ratio of 1.22:1.[1]

Several studies have examined the prognostic factors and survival outcomes in the current treatment era of multimodality therapy. The recently completed European and American Osteosarcoma Study (EURAMOS-01), an international collaboration of the largest osteosarcoma trial performed to date, reported the 3- and 5-year overall survival rate from the date of diagnosis as 79% and 71%, respectively, in a cohort of patients aged ≤40 years with resectable high-grade osteosarcoma.[2] The 3- and 5-year event-free survival rates in this cohort were 59% and 54%, respectively. Factors associated with adverse outcome included both pulmonary and nonpulmonary metastases upon presentation, axial skeleton tumor site, and poor histologic response after chemotherapy (defined as ≥10% viable tumor), with poor histologic response being the most significant prognostic adverse factor.[2] Analysis across multiple cooperative group trials and registry-based studies have identified similar prognostic factors. The most important prognostic factor at the time of diagnosis is the presence of detectable metastatic disease. Survival outcomes for the 15% to 20% of patients who present with overt metastatic disease are poor, with a 10-year cause-specific survival rate of 24% as compared to 66% for patients with localized disease.[3] Male sex, axial tumor site, large tumor size, and older age at diagnosis have also been associated with inferior outcomes.[3,4] Following neoadjuvant chemotherapy, pathologic treatment response—with poor response often defined as <90% tumor necrosis in the primary tumor—correlates with both event-free and overall survival.[4,5] The prognosis for patients with secondary osteosarcomas, such as radiation-induced and pagetoid osteosarcoma, is poor, with overall survival rates at 5 years between

4% and 22%, likely due to a combination of chemoresistance, disease biology, and poor tolerance of standard chemotherapy in the elderly population.[6–8]

ETIOLOGY

The specific molecular pathogenesis of osteosarcoma remains unclear. Although the vast majority of cases occur sporadically, its occurrence has been classically linked to germline alterations in tumor suppressor genes implicated in several inherited familial cancer predisposition syndromes, such as germline mutations in the *RB1* gene in retinoblastoma, *TP53* gene in Li–Fraumeni syndrome, and *RECQL4* gene in Rothmand–Thomson syndrome.[9–11] A small, but clinically important subset of cases is caused by exposure to therapeutic radiation with an average latency period of >10 years between irradiation and the development of secondary osteosarcoma. In older adults, osteosarcoma is often associated with Paget disease of bone. However, the incidence of malignant transformation is <1%.

Unlike other sarcomas, osteosarcomas lack recurrent translocations or common driver mutations. Rather, osteosarcomas are characterized by complex karyotypes and genomic complexity attributed to mutations in the tumor suppressor genes *TP53* and *RB*. Initially thought to account for approximately half of osteosarcomas, now the vast majority (75%–95%) of all are estimated to harbor *TP53* alterations, frequently translocations in intron 1 of the *TP53* gene.[12] In addition to *TP53* mutations, chromosomal shattering, termed chromothripsis, is evident in 20% to 89%, contributing further to its genomic complexity.[13] More recent studies utilizing next-generation sequencing (whole-exome sequencing [WES] and whole-genome sequencing [WGS]) reveal a genomic landscape predominantly characterized by somatic copy number alterations (SCNAs) rather than somatic mutations. While the highest among pediatric solid tumors, the somatic mutation burden in osteosarcoma (0.79–1.3 per Mb) is modest in comparison to other adult-type solid tumors.[12,14]

PRESENTATION AND DIAGNOSTIC APPROACH

Patients most often present with deep-seated, constant pain and swelling in the affected location. As the most common locations are in the metaphysis of long bones, specifically the distal femur, proximal tibia, and proximal humerus, they will often endorse knee or shoulder pain or limited range of motion and attribute it to minor trauma, a sprain, or overuse injury. In some instances, patients may even present with pathologic fracture necessitating immobilization or provisional stabilization. Occasionally, patients may present with back or pelvic pain as well, as approximately 6% of cases occur in the axial skeleton.[4] Fortunately, these cases are uncommon, as they are typically the most challenging to resect surgically and often are not recognized until late in the disease course.

In addition to a detailed history and physical examination, the workup for osteosarcoma includes laboratory tests, radiographs, MRI of the entire bone to evaluate for skip lesions (i.e., discontinuous metastases in the primary bone site), technetium bone scan, and chest CT. Chest imaging is essential as the most common site of metastasis is the lungs. Although not universally accepted as the standard of care, whole body (i.e., head-to-toe) PET/CT is also often performed, which provides additional staging information and may aid in assessing treatment response. Favorable PET/CT responses are associated with improved progression-free survival (PFS), but this only partially correlates with the histologic response to chemotherapy.[15] Radiographic evaluation demonstrates an osteoblastic, osteolytic, or mixed lesion (Figure 11.1A–C) and also provides a measure by which treatment response may be evaluated. The classic appearance is a permeative, moth-eaten, or destructive lesion in bone with an associated ossified or "sunburst" appearance of calcification (Figure 11.2A and B). Codman triangle (Figure 11.2C), a periosteal calcification in the border of the tumor and healthy tissue that occurs as a reactive process to wall off the tumor, is also commonly seen on radiographs (Figure 11.3A and B). Secondary osteosarcomas can have a similar appearance with a calcified mass arising from Paget disease or within a prior radiation field (Figure 11.4A and B). MRI remains the best modality with which to evaluate soft tissue component, surrounding neurovascular structures, and intramedullary extension—features that can be valuable in surgical planning. While imaging guidelines for the workup, treatment, and follow-up of osteosarcoma patients differ slightly among the National Comprehensive Cancer Network (NCCN), European Society for Medical Oncology (ESMO), and the Children's Oncology Group (COG), the same imaging should be utilized during treatment and for posttreatment disease surveillance.

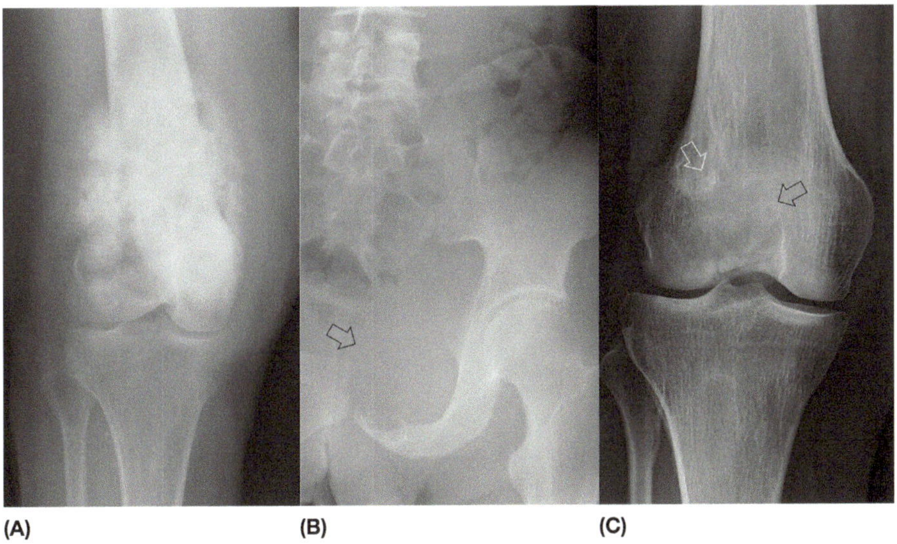

FIGURE 11.1 Variable appearance of osteosarcoma. (A) Typical blastic appearance. (B) Lytic appearance of small cell osteosarcoma. (C) Mixed lytic and blastic appearance.

Source: Used with permission from Behrang Amini, MD, Department of Diagnostic Radiology, The University of Texas MD Anderson Cancer Center.

Laboratory testing should include a complete blood count, electrolyte panel, blood urea nitrogen, creatinine, and liver function tests. Alkaline phosphatase and lactate dehydrogenase levels have also been described as a surrogate measure of tumor burden, with elevated levels correlating with poor prognosis,[16] but are not routinely followed as tumor markers. Pretreatment workup should also include echocardiogram and fertility counseling for patients with high-grade osteosarcoma who will go on to receive chemotherapy.

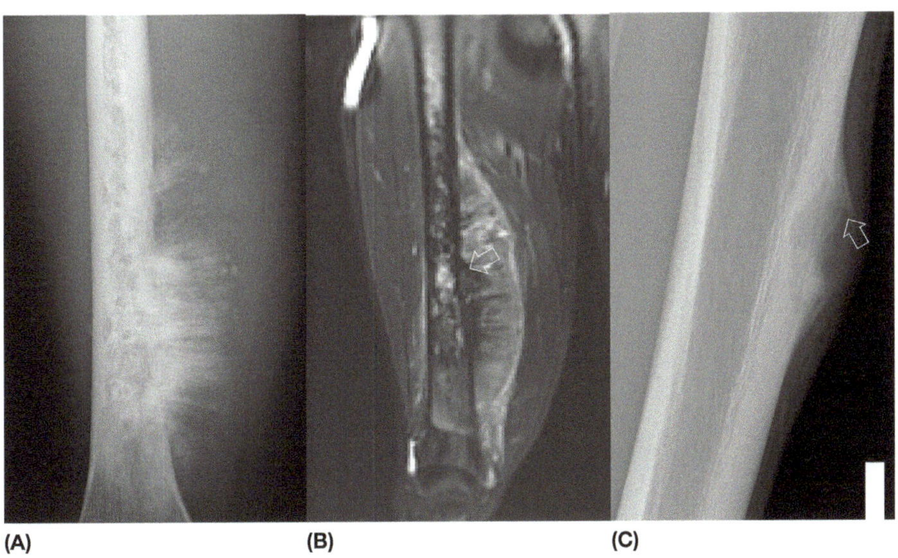

FIGURE 11.2 Periosteal reaction in osteosarcoma. (A) Sunburst appearance in conventional osteosarcoma on conventional radiography. (B) T2-weighted image showing calcification perpendicular to the cortex, lifting the periosteum (thin dark line, arrow). (C) Codman triangle (arrow) in a patient with periosteal osteosarcoma.

Source: Used with permission from Behrang Amini, MD, Department of Diagnostic Radiology, The University of Texas MD Anderson Cancer Center.

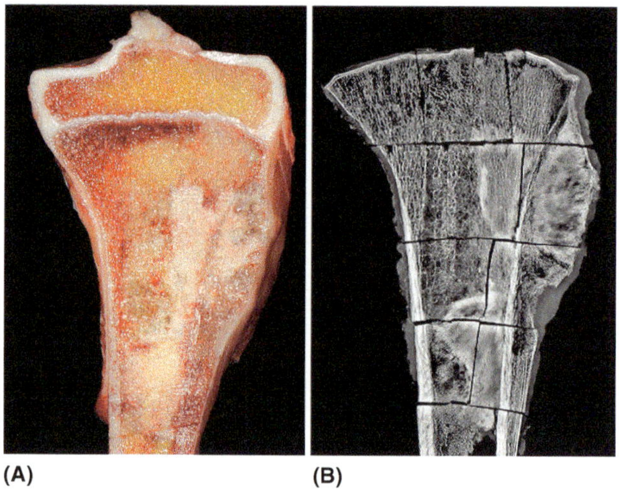

FIGURE 11.3 (A) Gross specimen of osteosarcoma involving metaphysis and diaphysis of tibia. Tumor is predominantly intramedullary and extends through cortex with prominent periosteal reaction. (B) The x-ray image of mapped cross section.

Source: Used with permission from Wei-Lien Wang, MD, Department of Pathology, The University of Texas MD Anderson Cancer Center.

In addition to radiographic evaluation and staging workup, the diagnosis must always be verified histologically with a biopsy. It is widely accepted and recommended that biopsies should be performed at specialized centers with experience treating sarcomas owing to their rarity, in order to ensure proper biopsy techniques and appropriate histologic examination and molecular testing when indicated. Core-needle biopsies are sufficient, but multiple samples should be obtained to improve diagnostic yield. With the increased accuracy of image-guided needle biopsies, the need for open biopsy has diminished, but it remains the gold standard for obtaining sufficient tissue for diagnosis. When necessary, open biopsies should be performed by experienced orthopedic oncologists. Placing the biopsy incision in line with the incision for definitive resection is essential because the biopsy tract must be excised as well.

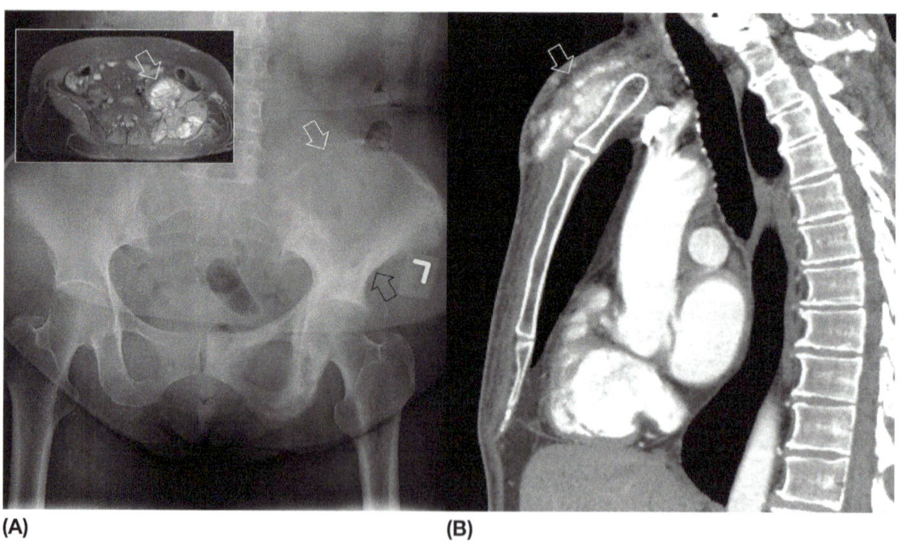

FIGURE 11.4 Secondary osteosarcoma. (A) Osteosarcoma (white arrow and inset) arising from Paget disease of the left ilium (black arrow). (B) Anterior chest wall osteosarcoma associated with radiation therapy for head and neck cancer.

Source: Used with permission from Behrang Amini, MD, Department of Diagnostic Radiology, The University of Texas MD Anderson Cancer Center.

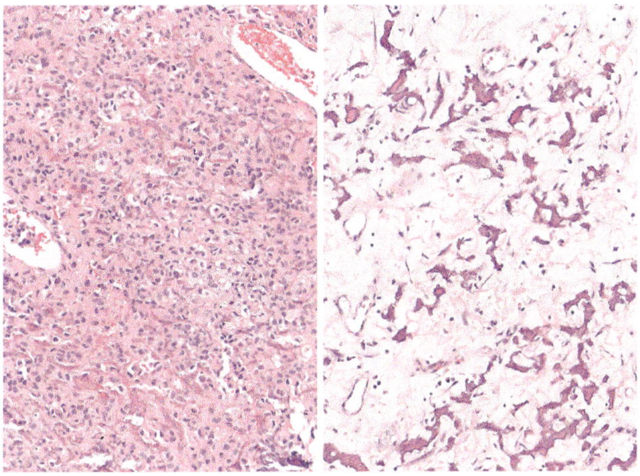

FIGURE 11.5 (A) Pretreatment biopsy. High-grade tumor composed of atypical epithelioid cells with osteoid matrix (H&E, 200×). (B) Posttreatment resection specimen. Treatment-related changes result in decreased cellularity and replacement by hyaline stroma. Osteoid matrix remains (H&E, 200×).

H&E, hematoxylin and eosin.

Source: Used with permission from Wei-Lien Wang, MD, Department of Pathology, The University of Texas MD Anderson Cancer Center.

The Musculoskeletal Tumor Society (MSTS) and the American Joint Committee on Cancer (AJCC) systems have been traditionally used for staging.[17,18] Most patients present with nonmetastatic conventional high-grade osteosarcoma with soft tissue component, or MSTS stage IIB disease. In the most recent eighth edition of the AJCC classification, which uses the traditional TNM (primary tumor, regional lymph nodes, and distant metastasis) staging of solid tumors, T stage is separated by the primary site, with spine and pelvis primary tumors classified separately from those arising in the appendicular skeleton, trunk, skull, or facial bones. Prognostic stage groups are defined for tumors arising in the appendicular skeleton, trunk, skull, or facial bones based upon T, N, M, and histologic grade. Clinically, neither staging system has been routinely incorporated into treatment planning; rather the presence or absence of overt metastatic disease remains the most significant prognostic factor. Histologic subtypes of osteosarcoma are described in the World Health Organization classification of bone-forming tumors.[19] All osteosarcoma subtypes are characterized by osteoid production in a malignant spindle cell stroma (Figure 11.5A and B). Conventional intramedullary osteosarcomas account for the largest subtype of osteosarcoma and are subdivided into osteoblastic, chondroblastic, and fibroblastic subtypes, named according to the predominant cellular component. Other intramedullary histologic subtypes are less common and include telangiectatic and small cell osteosarcoma. Variants such as surface osteosarcomas, which include parosteal, periosteal, and high-grade surface as well as osteosarcoma of the mandible, often differ in regard to natural history, prognosis, and treatment and are discussed in further detail in separate sections of this chapter. Extraskeletal osteosarcoma, a malignant mesenchymal tumor that arises in soft tissue (without bone involvement) and produces osteoid, is considered an entirely separate entity and is most often treated in line with other high-grade soft tissue sarcomas rather than conventional osteosarcoma.

GENERAL THERAPEUTIC APPROACH FOR PRIMARY TUMOR

The therapeutic approach for osteosarcoma is described in relation to treating conventional, high-grade osteosarcoma. Similar to biopsy principles, treatment is best completed in multidisciplinary referral centers with radiologists, pathologists, orthopedists, and medical oncologists experienced in treating bone sarcomas. Successful treatment requires both systemic chemotherapy and surgical resection. Osteosarcoma is not sensitive to radiation therapy at doses that would allow safe administration of systemic therapy, and therefore is reserved for select cases typically in a palliative setting for patients with incurable disease. Historically, metastatic disease recurrence was high and the long-term survival rate was low (<20%) in patients treated with surgery alone. Comparatively, 5-year overall survival rate is >60% for patients treated in the current era with chemotherapy and surgery and >70% for patients with localized osteosarcoma of the extremity.[20] These findings indicate the presence of micrometastatic disease in the majority who present with localized disease at the time of diagnosis and support the routine use of chemotherapy in addition to surgery.

The most active chemotherapeutic agents include high-dose methotrexate, doxorubicin, cisplatin, and ifosfamide.[21,22] While the specific combination or number of chemotherapeutic agents differs across protocols, most chemotherapy regimens use at least three of these four agents. Neoadjuvant chemotherapy is commonly administered as a three-drug combination of high-dose methotrexate, doxorubicin, and cisplatin (MAP). This regimen was agreed upon as the standard therapy for the pediatric EURAMOS-1 trial, based on a prospective, randomized trial performed by the COG.[2,23] Repeat imaging at the conclusion of neoadjuvant chemotherapy prior to resection is useful for surgical planning, but has limited utility in assessing treatment response. Histologic response to neoadjuvant chemotherapy measured as percent tumor necrosis (Figure 11.5B) has historically been considered the most significant prognostic factor for disease-free and overall survival. This has been confirmed in contemporary series as well.[2,4,24] Patients with <90% tumor necrosis after preoperative chemotherapy have more than double the risk of a subsequent event, whereas those with ≥90% tumor necrosis have a 5-year continuous disease-free survival rate of approximately 80%.[2,25]

For conventional osteosarcoma, limb-salvage surgery is feasible in >85% of patients without compromising overall survival when compared to amputation.[26] If preoperative imaging does not demonstrate extensive neurovascular involvement or a massive soft tissue component precluding safe resection, the limb may be spared and reconstructed using a variety of techniques, including endoprosthesis, allograft–prosthetic composite, or rotationplasty. Intra-articular resection can usually be performed if an MRI does not demonstrate invasion into the joint space or along cruciate or collateral ligaments. In spine and pelvic cases, en bloc spondylectomy or hemipelvectomy are the surgical options depending on the extent of invasion of the epidural space and dura, hip joint, and nearby neurovascular structures. Other surgical considerations include the presence of pathologic fracture, potential remaining skeletal growth in children and resultant limb length discrepancies, and functional demands after the procedure.

In order to ensure negative bone margins, frozen sections are taken from the marrow margins and grossly evaluated by the pathologist. Whenever possible, bone margins of 1 to 3 cm are recommended, although subcentimeter margins may be acceptable in epiphyseal-sparing resections when the tumor border is clearly delineated on MRI. The adequate soft tissue margin is more difficult to discern; some studies report local recurrences are significantly decreased using ≥2 mm as a cutoff.[27,28] Perhaps more important than an exact cutoff for an adequate margin is the response to chemotherapy, which may modulate aspects of the surgery performed and impact local control.

After resection of the primary tumor, patients typically resume adjuvant chemotherapy. While poor histologic response to neoadjuvant chemotherapy is a well-established prognostic factor, the role for modified postoperative chemotherapy for poor responders remains controversial. The concept of "tailoring" chemotherapy has been attempted since at least the 1970s, but early studies were difficult to interpret and relied upon neoadjuvant chemotherapy regimens that are no longer used.[29] In subsequent series, the addition of ifosfamide and etoposide (I/E) to postoperative MAP chemotherapy for poor responders resulted in an improvement in disease-free survival.[30] These and other studies showing the activity of I/E in osteosarcoma served as the basis for the trial design in EURAMOS-1 study in which patients with poor response to neoadjuvant MAP were randomized to either continue MAP alone or receive intensified postoperative chemotherapy with MAPIE. In this study, MAPIE failed to improve event-free survival among poor responders as compared to MAP and was associated with increased toxicity.[31]

The treatment of older adults with osteosarcoma warrants special consideration. In most series, older adults have a worse prognosis than children or young adults with osteosarcoma. However, curative intent treatment with combination chemotherapy and resection is warranted when feasible.[32] Older adults often have difficulty tolerating the dose and intensity of the pediatric MAP chemotherapy regimen. High-dose methotrexate, in particular, can be difficult to administer in older adults due to the slow clearance of methotrexate and overlapping toxicities of mucositis with doxorubicin and nephrotoxicity with cisplatin.[33] At several large sarcoma centers in the United States, adults are treated with neoadjuvant doxorubicin and cisplatin (AP) for up to four cycles, followed by resection and assessment of histologic treatment response. Patients with a favorable pathologic response go on to receive four cycles of adjuvant doxorubicin and ifosfamide (AI), omitting high-dose methotrexate. For patients with poor response, adjuvant chemotherapy consists of six cycles each of high-dose methotrexate and high-dose ifosfamide for up to 12 total cycles. This modified approach has been associated with improved disease-free survival among adults with poor response to neoadjuvant chemotherapy.[34]

FOLLOW-UP

Strict adherence to long-term follow-up is critical for successful treatment. The NCCN and the COG provide guidelines for general timing for follow-up and disease surveillance depending on the tumor grade and pathologic diagnosis.[35,36] Patients with high-grade osteosarcoma should be seen with post-treatment surveillance imaging every 3 months for the first 2 years after treatment, every 4 months in the third year, every 4 to 6 months in the fourth year, and every 6 months in the fifth year. Because late recurrence can be seen >10 years after the completion of treatment, consideration should be given to continuing disease surveillance every 12 months after 5 years. Surveillance imaging consists of radiographs and MRI of the primary bone, as well as chest imaging. Small subcentimeter nodules that are nonspecific are typically followed during surveillance with serial chest CT. Local recurrences are becoming less common with improved surgical technique and imaging, but have been reported in up to 10% of patients. They require wide local excision with negative margins, which sometimes can only be achieved with amputation in cases with extensive involvement.[37] After 10 years, the risk of recurrence or secondary malignancy is significantly decreased, but long-term follow-up is still recommended to monitor the status of orthopedic implants and late effects of chemotherapy. Endoprostheses are subject to high rates of wear over time and may eventually fail owing to aseptic loosening, polyethylene wear, hardware breakage, or instability necessitating revision. Allograft constructs may also exhibit nonunion, resorption, or degenerative joint disease requiring total joint arthroplasty. Amputees typically need lifelong follow-up with prosthetists to maintain and adjust their prostheses.

Long-term follow-up is also needed to evaluate and treat the frequent treatment-related late effects of chemotherapy. Among childhood cancer survivors, survivors of bone tumors face the highest of risk of developing severe or potentially life-threatening chronic health conditions including renal impairment, cardiomyopathy, hearing loss, and ongoing musculoskeletal problems.[38] Osteosarcoma survivors are at increased risk of doxorubicin-induced cardiac dysfunction and cardiomyopathy, which may require regular echocardiograms and evaluation of other cardiac risk factors. Renal impairment due to nephrotoxic chemotherapy such as ifosfamide and cisplatin may present many years after completion of therapy if potentiated by other nephrotoxic medications or other common causes of renal dysfunction such as hypertension, and therefore warrants ongoing monitoring of renal function, electrolytes, and blood pressure. Acute and long-term side effects from cisplatin include sensory neuropathy and ototoxicity; patients should undergo audiology evaluations prior to and during treatment and as clinically indicated. Secondary cancers including treatment-related myelodysplastic syndrome and acute myelogenous leukemia are infrequent but well described and have been specifically linked to alkylating agents and topoisomerase inhibitors.[39]

THERAPEUTIC APPROACH FOR METASTATIC DISEASE

The prognosis for patients with nonmetastatic conventional osteosarcoma has remained relatively constant since the introduction of chemotherapy, with a 5-year overall survival rate of roughly 65% to 75%.[2,4] Conventional high-grade osteosarcoma has a high propensity to metastasize, which is clearly evident prior to the introduction of chemotherapy, whereas low-grade variants such as well-differentiated intramedullary and parosteal osteosarcoma generally have low metastatic potential and are typically treated with surgery alone. Patients who present with metastatic disease have a significantly worse prognosis, with reported 5-year survival rates of 30% to 50%.[2,40] Approximately 10% to 20% of patients present with metastatic disease, which is most commonly in the lung, but can also manifest in the same bone as a skip lesion or other bones, and very rarely in lymph nodes. The initial preoperative treatment approach is the same as for patients with nonmetastatic disease, and the approach is with curative intent in those with resectable pulmonary metastases.

Relapse is seen in approximately 30% of patients with localized osteosarcoma and up to 80% of patients with primary metastatic disease. Importantly, a subset of patients with recurrent metastatic disease following the completion of primary therapy can achieve long-term remission or cure with surgery alone or in combination with additional chemotherapy. Prognosis in the recurrent metastatic setting depends upon the time to recurrence, location of disease, and the ability of achieving a second surgical remission. Among patients previously treated with neoadjuvant chemotherapy and surgery, the 5-year post-relapse survival rate is 35% for patients who relapsed >2 years from the initiation of treatment as compared to 14% for patients whose disease recurred in <2 years.[41] Pulmonary metastasectomy results in 5-year overall survival rate of 25% to 40%, even following second, third, or subsequent recurrences for patients who achieve surgical remission with no evidence of disease.[42,43] For patients with late disease recurrence, surgical resection alone is appropriate. For those patients with short-interval recurrence (i.e., <1 year from primary surgery), extensive, or borderline resectable disease, chemotherapy prior to or following surgery should be considered. While there are no well-controlled data demonstrating a survival benefit to adjuvant chemotherapy following pulmonary metastasectomy, this approach may prolong time to recurrence and potentially may cure. Neoadjuvant chemotherapy for oligometastatic disease has the added benefit of allowing for response assessment by imaging and tumor necrosis at the time of resection.

Chemotherapy is the treatment of choice for patients with recurrent unresectable disease where the prognosis remains exceedingly poor. A recent pooled analysis of seven negative Phase 2 trials from the COG and its predecessors demonstrated a 4-month event-free survival rate of only 12% in patients with unresectable disease.[44] In addition to retreatment with the standard agents (particularly for those with a long disease-free interval), second-line regimens for recurrent metastatic disease include high-dose ifosfamide with or without etoposide, the combination of gemcitabine and docetaxel, or more recently, tyrosine kinase inhibitors (TKIs).[21,45,46] The specific choice of second-line therapy depends upon the patient's prior treatment and comorbid conditions. While there are no predominant recurrent targetable alterations in osteosarcoma, multitargeted TKIs that target vascular endothelial growth factor receptor (VEGFR) have shown efficacy in the recurrent metastatic setting. Single-agent sorafenib, targeting VEGFR-1, -2, -3, Raf kinase, and platelet-derived growth factor receptor (PDGFR), has modest activity in osteosarcoma with a median PFS of 4-months and a 6-month PFS rate of 29%.[47] The addition of the mTOR (mammalian target of rapamycin) inhibitor everolimus to sorafenib also showed clinical activity (median PFS 5 months, 6-month PFS rate 45%), but failed to meet the study's primary efficacy endpoint targeting a 6-month PFS rate of 50%.[48] Regorafenib, an antiangiogenic TKI targeting VEGFRs as well as KIT, RET, RAF, BRAF, PDGFR, and fibroblast growth factor receptor (FGFR), has also shown activity in two recent placebo-controlled Phase 2 trials in metastatic osteosarcoma. In the French REGOBONE study, 17 of 26 (65%) patients treated with regorafenib were progression free at 8 weeks, as compared to zero of 12 patients receiving placebo.[49] Findings from the U.S.-led SARC024 study were comparable, with an improvement in median PFS with regorafenib (3.6 vs. 1.7 months).[50] Preliminary data for cabozantinib, which targets cMET, VEGFR2, AXL, and RET, also shows activity in patients with metastatic osteosarcoma.[51]

There has been a long-standing interest in the role of immune response and immunotherapy in osteosarcoma. Liposomal muramyl tripeptide-phosphatidylethanolamine (MTP-PE; also known as mifamurtide), a synthetic bacterial cell wall analog derived from bacille Calmette-Guerin (BCG) that activates macrophages and increases cytokines, was studied in a randomized trial. The addition of mifamurtide to standard MAP chemotherapy improved overall survival, but not event-free survival.[23] A subset analysis of patients with primary metastatic disease enrolled on the same study showed a trend toward improvement in overall survival and event-free survival with the addition of mifamurtide; however, these differences were not statistically significant.[52] These results led to its approval in Europe, Mexico, and several other countries, but not within the United States, and its role in the treatment of metastatic osteosarcoma remains controverted. As with other solid tumors, there has been a growing interest in the use of immune checkpoint inhibitors in osteosarcoma. In the SARC028 Phase 2 study of pembrolizumab, single-agent anti-PD-1 therapy demonstrated activity in specific soft tissue sarcoma cohorts, with 72% of advanced disease patients with undifferentiated pleomorphic sarcoma or liposarcoma achieving disease control (stable disease or partial response at 8 weeks). However, the response rate in osteosarcoma was low at 5% with disease control at 8 weeks seen in 32% (seven of 22 patients).[53] A second study evaluating nivolumab with or without ipilimumab demonstrated higher response rates with the combination among patients with soft tissue sarcomas, but no responses were seen in the two patients with osteosarcoma (one nivolumab alone, other one nivolumab + ipilimumab).[54] Based upon these initial clinical trials, further development of immune checkpoint inhibitors in bone sarcoma is focused on novel combinations.

LOW- AND INTERMEDIATE-GRADE OSTEOSARCOMA

Low-grade osteosarcoma may be intramedullary or parosteal, and is most commonly seen in the posterior aspect of the distal femur (Figure 11.6). Both forms are rare and may be difficult to distinguish from other ossified lesions such as heterotopic ossification, myositis ossificans, osteomyelitis, and other benign bone-forming lesions. Workup of other variants is the same as for conventional osteosarcoma, but treatment for low-grade lesions is wide local resection alone. Prognosis is excellent with reports of over 95%

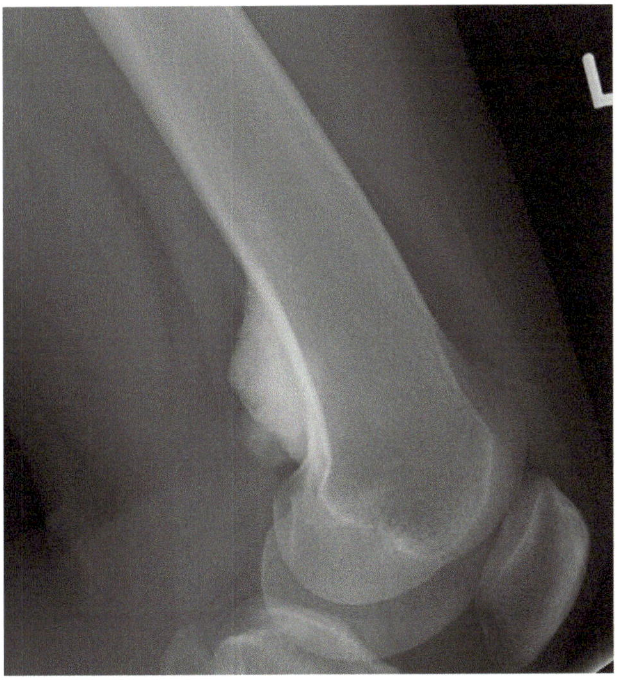

FIGURE 11.6 Parosteal osteosarcoma. Lateral radiograph showing well-defined osteoid lesion.

Source: Used with permission from Behrang Amini, MD, Department of Diagnostic Radiology, The University of Texas MD Anderson Cancer Center.

survival rate at 5 years, and local recurrence or metastasis is extremely rare, except in the setting of marginal or intralesional resection or areas of dedifferentiation.[55,56] Local recurrence is managed with repeat wide excision and close surveillance. Areas of even small foci of dedifferentiation warrant treatment similar to conventional high-grade osteosarcoma with preoperative and postoperative chemotherapy, as dedifferentiated parosteal osteosarcoma is associated with a high risk of metastatic disease recurrence. Limited data exist for the treatment of intermediate-grade osteosarcoma, but the use of conventional chemotherapy comparable to the treatment of high-grade osteosarcoma is generally favored.

CRANIOFACIAL OSTEOSARCOMA

Craniofacial osteosarcomas are a unique subset that deserves special mention, although only comprising about 10% of all osteosarcomas.[57] Though similar to conventional osteosarcoma histologically, they have a favorable natural history and low metastatic potential. Treatment involves wide surgical resection, with or without radiation. Combined modality treatment with radiation therapy and surgery is associated with improved local control and overall survival as compared to surgery alone.[58] The role of chemotherapy for craniofacial osteosarcoma remains controversial and is often reserved for patients with recurrent or unresectable disease. A recent meta-analysis concluded that chemotherapy improves survival in craniofacial osteosarcoma patients with adverse factors such as high-grade tumors, recurrent tumors, or those resected with positive margins.[59]

SUMMARY

Conventional osteosarcoma serves as the model for the diagnosis and management of high-grade bone sarcomas. Survival in patients with osteosarcoma dramatically improved with the addition of neoadjuvant and/or adjuvant chemotherapy to surgery >30 years ago and now remains the standard. For children and adults with conventional high-grade extremity osteosarcoma, treatment consists of neoadjuvant chemotherapy with a regimen containing cisplatin, doxorubicin, high-dose methotrexate, and/or ifosfamide; limb-sparing surgery; and adjuvant chemotherapy. Pathologic treatment response to neoadjuvant chemotherapy remains a significant prognostic factor; however, the role of modified postoperative chemotherapy in poor responders remains controversial and institution dependent. Following primary treatment, the lung is the most common site of metastatic disease recurrence. Resection of pulmonary metastasis should be pursued when complete resection is feasible. Using these treatment principles, a cure is attainable in the majority of patients with localized disease and a subset of patients with metastatic osteosarcoma. Unfortunately, in patients with recurrent unresectable disease, the prognosis remains poor and treatment options are limited. While VEGFR-targeted TKIs have shown clinical benefit, the use of immunotherapy including immune checkpoint inhibitors remains investigational and is the focus of ongoing clinical trials.

CASE STUDY

A 21-year-old male college student presents with a 2-month history of persistent left knee pain. Radiograph of the knee shows a mixed osteolytic and osteoblastic lesion of the distal left femur. Core biopsy reveals high-grade osteoblastic osteosarcoma. MRI of the left leg demonstrates a small soft tissue component. Results of routine laboratory studies are normal, except for serum alkaline phosphatase level of 250 IU/mL. Complete evaluation, including plain film and CT of the chest and radionuclide bone scan, reveals no evidence of metastatic disease. He is initiated on neoadjuvant chemotherapy including MAP. He then undergoes a limb-sparing procedure and placement of a femoral prosthesis. Pathology at resection demonstrates a favorable pathologic treatment response with 95% tumor necrosis. He goes on to complete additional adjuvant MAP chemotherapy, and his end of treatment studies including chest CT show no evidence of disease. He is followed with surveillance imaging every 3 months; at 2 years from the completion of primary therapy, he is found to have a solitary 2-cm left upper lobe calcified nodule. He undergoes thoracotomy and wedge resection with pathologic exam confirming metastatic osteosarcoma. Given the time to recurrence, he is dispositioned to surveillance and remains disease free at 10 years of follow-up.

REFERENCES

1. Mirabello L, Troisi RJ, Savage SA. Osteosarcoma incidence and survival rates from 1973 to 2004: data from the Surveillance, Epidemiology, and End Results Program. *Cancer*. 2009;115(7):1531–1543. doi:10.1002/cncr.24121
2. Smeland S, Bielack SS, Whelan J, et al. Survival and prognosis with osteosarcoma: outcomes in more than 2000 patients in the EURAMOS-1 (European and American Osteosarcoma Study) cohort. *Eur J Cancer*. 2019;109:36–50. doi:10.1016/j.ejca.2018.11.027
3. Duchman KR, Gao Y, Miller BJ. Prognostic factors for survival in patients with high-grade osteosarcoma using the Surveillance, Epidemiology, and End Results (SEER) Program database. *Cancer Epidemiol*. 2015;39(4):593–599. doi:10.1016/j.canep.2015.05.001
4. Bielack SS, Kempf-Bielack B, Delling G, et al. Prognostic factors in high-grade osteosarcoma of the extremities or trunk: an analysis of 1,702 patients treated on neoadjuvant cooperative osteosarcoma study group protocols. *J Clin Oncol*. 2002;20(3):776–790. doi:10.1200/JCO.2002.20.3.776
5. Bacci G, Longhi A, Versari M, et al. Prognostic factors for osteosarcoma of the extremity treated with neoadjuvant chemotherapy: 15-year experience in 789 patients treated at a single institution. *Cancer*. 2006;106(5):1154–1161. doi:10.1002/cncr.21724
6. Frassica FJ, Sim FH, Frassica DA, Wold LE. Survival and management considerations in postirradiation osteosarcoma and Paget's osteosarcoma. *Clin Orthop*. 1991;(270):120–127. doi:10.1097/00003086-199109000-00018
7. Shaylor PJ, Peake D, Grimer RJ, et al. Paget's osteosarcoma—no cure in sight. *Sarcoma*. 1999;3(3–4):191–192. doi:10.1080/13577149977631
8. Longhi A, Errani C, Gonzales-Arabio D, et al. Osteosarcoma in patients older than 65 years. *J Clin Oncol*. 2008;26(33):5368–5373. doi:10.1200/JCO.2007.14.9104
9. Friend SH, Bernards R, Rogelj S, et al. A human DNA segment with properties of the gene that predisposes to retinoblastoma and osteosarcoma. *Nature*. 1986;323(6089):643–646. doi:10.1038/323643a0
10. Malkin D, Li FP, Strong LC, et al. Germ line p53 mutations in a familial syndrome of breast cancer, sarcomas, and other neoplasms. *Science*. 1990;250(4985):1233–1238. doi:10.1126/science.1978757
11. Wang LL, Gannavarapu A, Kozinetz CA, et al. Association between osteosarcoma and deleterious mutations in the RECQL4 gene in Rothmund-Thomson syndrome. *J Natl Cancer Inst*. 2003;95(9):669–674. doi:10.1093/jnci/95.9.669

12. Chen X, Bahrami A, Pappo A, et al. Recurrent somatic structural variations contribute to tumorigenesis in pediatric osteosarcoma. *Cell Rep*. 2014;7(1):104–112. doi:10.1016/j.celrep.2014.03.003
13. Stephens PJ, Greenman CD, Fu B, et al. Massive genomic rearrangement acquired in a single catastrophic event during cancer development. *Cell*. 2011;144(1):27–40. doi:10.1016/j.cell.2010.11.055
14. Perry JA, Kiezun A, Tonzi P, et al. Complementary genomic approaches highlight the PI3K/mTOR pathway as a common vulnerability in osteosarcoma. *Proc Natl Acad Sci U S A*. 2014;111(51):E5564–5573. doi:10.1073/pnas.1419260111
15. Hawkins DS, Conrad EU, Butrynski JE, et al. [F-18]-fluorodeoxy-D-glucose-positron emission tomography response is associated with outcome for extremity osteosarcoma in children and young adults. *Cancer*. 2009;115(15):3519–3525. doi:10.1002/cncr.24421
16. Meyers PA, Heller G, Healey J, et al. Chemotherapy for nonmetastatic osteogenic sarcoma: the Memorial Sloan-Kettering experience. *J Clin Oncol*. 1992;10(1):5–15. doi:10.1200/JCO.1992.10.1.5
17. Enneking WF. A system of staging musculoskeletal neoplasms. *Clin Orthop*. 1986;(204):9–24. doi:10.1097/00003086-198603000-00003.
18. Kneisl JS, Rosenberg AE, Anderson PM. Bone. In: Amin MB, ed. *AJCC Cancer Staging Manual*. 8th ed. Chicago, IL: American College of Surgeons; 2017: 471–487.
19. Fletcher CD, Bridge JA, Hogendoorn PCW, Mertens F, eds. *WHO Classification of Tumours of Soft Tissue and Bone*. Lyon, France: IARC; 2003:305–310.
20. Allison DC, Carney SC, Ahlmann ER, et al. A meta-analysis of osteosarcoma outcomes in the modern medical era. *Sarcoma*. 2012;2012:704872. doi:10.1155/2012/704872
21. Patel SR, Vadhan-Raj S, Papadopolous N, et al. High-dose ifosfamide in bone and soft tissue sarcomas: results of phase II and pilot studies--dose-response and schedule dependence. *J Clin Oncol*. 1997;15(6):2378–2384. doi:10.1200/JCO.1997.15.6.2378
22. Isakoff MS, Bielack SS, Meltzer P, Gorlick R. Osteosarcoma: current treatment and a collaborative pathway to success. *J Clin Oncol*. 2015;33(27):3029–3035. doi:10.1200/JCO.2014.59.4895
23. Meyers PA, Schwartz CL, Krailo MD, et al. Osteosarcoma: the addition of muramyl tripeptide to chemotherapy improves overall survival—a report from the Children's Oncology Group. *J Clin Oncol*. 2008;26(4):633–638. doi:10.1200/JCO.2008.14.0095
24. Raymond AK, Chawla SP, Carrasco CH, et al. Osteosarcoma chemotherapy effect: a prognostic factor. *Semin Diagn Pathol*. 1987;4(3):212–236. PMID:3313606.
25. Jaffe N, Patel SR, Benjamin RS. Chemotherapy in osteosarcoma. Basis for application and antagonism to implementation; early controversies surrounding its implementation. *Hematol Oncol Clin North Am*. 1995;9(4):825–840. doi:10.1016/S0889-8588(18)30074-1
26. Rougraff BT, Simon MA, Kneisl JS, et al. Limb salvage compared with amputation for osteosarcoma of the distal end of the femur. A long-term oncological, functional, and quality-of-life study. *J Bone Joint Surg Am*. 1994;76(5):649–656. doi:10.2106/00004623-199405000-00004
27. Cates JMM. Reporting surgical resection margin status for osteosarcoma: comparison of the AJCC, MSTS, and margin distance methods. *Am J Surg Pathol*. 2017;41(5):633–642. doi:10.1097/PAS.0000000000000815
28. Bertrand TE, Cruz A, Binitie O, et al. Do surgical margins affect local recurrence and survival in extremity, nonmetastatic, high-grade osteosarcoma? *Clin Orthop*. 2016;474(3):677–683. doi:10.1007/s11999-015-4359-x
29. Rosen G, Caparros B, Huvos AG, et al. Preoperative chemotherapy for osteogenic sarcoma: selection of postoperative adjuvant chemotherapy based on the response of the primary tumor to preoperative chemotherapy. *Cancer*. 1982;49(6):1221–1230. doi:10.1002/1097-0142(19820315)49:6<1221::aid-cncr2820490625>3.0.co;2-e
30. Bacci G, Picci P, Ferrari S, et al. Primary chemotherapy and delayed surgery for nonmetastatic osteosarcoma of the extremities. Results in 164 patients preoperatively treated with high doses of methotrexate followed by cisplatin and doxorubicin. *Cancer*. 1993;72(11):3227–3238. doi:10.1002/1097-0142(19931201)72:11<3227::aid-cncr2820721116>3.0.co;2-c
31. Marina NM, Smeland S, Bielack SS, et al. Comparison of MAPIE versus MAP in patients with a poor response to preoperative chemotherapy for newly diagnosed high-grade osteosarcoma (EURAMOS-1): an open-label, international, randomised controlled trial. *Lancet Oncol*. 2016;17(10):1396–1408. doi:10.1016/S1470-2045(16)30214-5
32. Grimer RJ, Cannon SR, Taminiau AM, et al. Osteosarcoma over the age of forty. *Eur J Cancer*. 2003;39(2):157–163. doi:10.1016/s0959-8049(02)00478-1
33. Wagner MJ, Livingston JA, Patel SR, Benjamin RS. Chemotherapy for bone sarcoma in adults. *J Oncol Pract*. 2016;12(3):208–216. doi:10.1200/JOP.2015.009944
34. Livingston JA, Wagner MJ, Conley AP. Tailored post-operative therapy in adult osteosarcoma patients with poor necrosis: 30 years of treatment at MD Anderson Cancer Center. Presented at: Connective Tissue Oncology Society Annual Meeting; November 4, 2015; Salt Lake City, Utah.
35. Children's Oncology Group. Long-Term Follow-Up Guidelines for Survivors of Childhood, Adolescent, and Young Adult Cancers Version 5.0. Published October, 2018. http://www.survivorshipguidelines.org
36. Biermann JS, Chow W, Reed DR, et al. NCCN guidelines insights: bone cancer, version 2.2017. *J Natl Compr Cancer Netw*. 2017;15(2):155–167. doi:10.6004/jnccn.2017.0017
37. Takeuchi A, Lewis VO, Satcher RL, et al. What are the factors that affect survival and relapse after local recurrence of osteosarcoma? *Clin Orthop*. 2014;472(10):3188–3195. doi:10.1007/s11999-014-3759-7

38. Oeffinger KC, Mertens AC, Sklar CA, et al. Chronic health conditions in adult survivors of childhood cancer. *N Engl J Med*. 2006;355(15):1572–1582. doi:10.1056/NEJMsa060185
39. Bhatia S, Sklar C. Second cancers in survivors of childhood cancer. *Nat Rev Cancer*. 2002;2(2):124–132. doi:10.1038/nrc722
40. Bielack S, Jürgens H, Jundt G, et al. Osteosarcoma: the COSS experience. *Cancer Treat Res*. 2009;152:289–308. doi:10.1007/978-1-4419-0284-9_15
41. Gelderblom H, Jinks RC, Sydes M, et al. Survival after recurrent osteosarcoma: data from 3 European Osteosarcoma Intergroup (EOI) randomized controlled trials. *Eur J Cancer*. 2011;47(6):895–902. doi:10.1016/j.ejca.2010.11.036
42. Briccoli A, Rocca M, Salone M, et al. Resection of recurrent pulmonary metastases in patients with osteosarcoma. *Cancer*. 2005;104(8):1721–1725. doi:10.1002/cncr.21369
43. Bielack SS, Kempf-Bielack B, Branscheid D, et al. Second and subsequent recurrences of osteosarcoma: presentation, treatment, and outcomes of 249 consecutive cooperative osteosarcoma study group patients. *J Clin Oncol*. 2009;27(4):557–565. doi:10.1200/JCO.2008.16.2305
44. Lagmay JP, Krailo MD, Dang H, et al. Outcome of patients with recurrent osteosarcoma enrolled in seven phase II trials through Children's Cancer Group, Pediatric Oncology Group, and Children's Oncology Group: learning from the past to move forward. *J Clin Oncol*. 2016;34(25):3031-3038. doi:10.1200/JCO.2015.65.5381
45. Goorin AM, Harris MB, Bernstein M, et al. Phase II/III trial of etoposide and high-dose ifosfamide in newly diagnosed metastatic osteosarcoma: a pediatric oncology group trial. *J Clin Oncol*. 2002;20(2):426–433. doi:10.1200/JCO.2002.20.2.426
46. Palmerini E, Jones RL, Marchesi E, et al. Gemcitabine and docetaxel in relapsed and unresectable high-grade osteosarcoma and spindle cell sarcoma of bone. *BMC Cancer*. 2016;16:280. doi:10.1186/s12885-016-2312-3
47. Grignani G, Palmerini E, Dileo P, et al. A phase II trial of sorafenib in relapsed and unresectable high-grade osteosarcoma after failure of standard multimodal therapy: an Italian Sarcoma Group study. *Ann Oncol*. 2012;23(2):508–516. doi:10.1093/annonc/mdr151
48. Grignani G, Palmerini E, Ferraresi V, et al. Sorafenib and everolimus for patients with unresectable high-grade osteosarcoma progressing after standard treatment: a non-randomised phase 2 clinical trial. *Lancet Oncol*. 2015;16(1):98–107. doi:10.1016/S1470-2045(14)71136-2
49. Duffaud F, Mir O, Boudou-Rouquette P, et al. Efficacy and safety of regorafenib in adult patients with metastatic osteosarcoma: a non-comparative, randomised, double-blind, placebo-controlled, phase 2 study. *Lancet Oncol*. 2019;20(1):120–133. doi:10.1016/S1470-2045(18)30742-3
50. Davis LE, Bolejack V, Ryan CW, et al. Randomized double-blind phase II study of regorafenib in patients with metastatic osteosarcoma. *J Clin Oncol*. 2019;37(16):1424–1431. doi:10.1200/JCO.18.02374
51. Italiano A, Mir O, Mathoulin-Pelissier S, et al. Cabozantinib in patients with advanced Ewing sarcoma or osteosarcoma (CABONE): a multicentre, single-arm, phase 2 trial. *The Lancet Oncology*. 2020;21(3):446–455. doi:10.1016/S1470-2045(19)30825-3
52. Chou AJ, Kleinerman ES, Krailo MD, et al. Addition of muramyl tripeptide to chemotherapy for patients with newly diagnosed metastatic osteosarcoma: a report from the Children's Oncology Group. *Cancer*. 2009;115(22):5339–5348. doi:10.1002/cncr.24566
53. Tawbi HA, Burgess M, Bolejack V, et al. Pembrolizumab in advanced soft-tissue sarcoma and bone sarcoma (SARC028): a multicentre, two-cohort, single-arm, open-label, phase 2 trial. *Lancet Oncol*. 2017;18(11):1493–1501. doi:10.1016/S1470-2045(17)30624-1
54. D'Angelo SP, Mahoney MR, Van Tine BA, et al. Nivolumab with or without ipilimumab treatment for metastatic sarcoma (Alliance A091401): two open-label, non-comparative, randomised, phase 2 trials. *Lancet Oncol*. 2018;19(3):416–426. doi:10.1016/S1470-2045(18)30006-8
55. Okada K, Frassica FJ, Sim FH, et al. Parosteal osteosarcoma. A clinicopathological study. *J Bone Joint Surg Am*. 1994;76(3):366–378. doi:10.2106/00004623-199403000-00007
56. Hayashi K, Tsuchiya H, Yamamoto N, et al. Diagnosis and treatment of low-grade osteosarcoma: experience with nine cases. *Int J Clin Oncol*. 2014;19(4):731–738. doi:10.1007/s10147-013-0592-z
57. Mirabello L, Troisi RJ, Savage SA. International osteosarcoma incidence patterns in children and adolescents, middle ages and elderly persons. *Int J Cancer*. 2009;125(1):229–234. doi:10.1002/ijc.24320
58. Guadagnolo BA, Zagars GK, Raymond AK, et al. Osteosarcoma of the jaw/craniofacial region: outcomes after multimodality treatment. *Cancer*. 2009;115(14):3262–3270. doi:10.1002/cncr.24297
59. Liang L, Zhang T, You Y, et al. An individual patient data meta-analysis on the effect of chemotherapy on survival in patients with craniofacial osteosarcoma. *Head Neck*. 2019;41:2016–2023. doi:10.1002/hed.25668

12

Chondrosarcoma

Jonathan C. Trent and Luyuan Li

INTRODUCTION

Chondrosarcomas constitute a heterogeneous group of malignant cartilaginous matrix-producing bone neoplasms with diverse morphologic features and clinical behavior.[1] Following osteosarcoma, chondrosarcoma is the second most common primary bone tumor, accounting for 20% to 27% of primary bone malignancy.[2] The incidence of chondrosarcoma steadily increases with age, with a peak incidence in the fifth to seventh decades and a slight male predominance. The most commonly involved sites are the bones of the pelvis, followed by the femur, humerus, and ribs.[1] Most of the chondrosarcomas are sporadic, but they may develop from malignant transformation of two benign cartilaginous bone tumors, osteochondromas and enchondromas. Chondrosarcomas that arise de novo are called primary chondrosarcomas, while those superimposed on preexisting cartilaginous neoplasms such as enchondroma or osteochondroma are referred to as secondary chondrosarcomas.[3] The cornerstone of the management of localized chondrosarcomas is surgical resection. The majority of chondrosarcomas grow slowly and rarely metastasize, and they have an excellent prognosis after adequate surgery. However, chondrosarcomas tend to recur following the initial tumor resection and over 10% of recurrent chondrosarcomas are of a higher grade than the original neoplasm.[3] Many patients will eventually develop metastatic disease, which is nearly uniformly fatal in the absence of effective systemic therapy. The clinical challenge is to prevent recurrence and to find better treatment options for unresectable or metastatic disease. Here is a review of the classification, clinical characteristics, and therapeutic options of different subtypes of chondrosarcomas (Table 12.1), as well as the emerging novel therapeutic targets for this malignancy.

HISTOPATHOLOGIC FEATURES

Pathologic subgroups include conventional and nonconventional chondrosarcomas; 85% to 90% of chondrosarcomas are conventional type, which can be subdivided into the central, peripheral, and periosteal subgroups according to the osseous location in the bone. The vast majority (>85%) are central chondrosarcomas, which arise within the intramedullary space. Primary central chondrosarcoma typically affects patients older than 50 years. Pelvis, proximal femur, proximal humerus, distal femur, and ribs are the most frequently involved sites. Secondary central chondrosarcoma develops as malignant transformation of enchondroma (very rare) or enchondromatosis, such as Ollier disease or Maffucci syndrome. Patients with Ollier disease and Maffucci syndrome have a 25% to 30% risk of developing chondrosarcoma.[4] Peripheral chondrosarcoma (up to 15%) develops from the surface of bone, generally from the cartilage cap of preexisting osteochondromas. These are, therefore, referred to as secondary peripheral chondrosarcoma.[5] Osteochondromas are cartilaginous-capped bony projections and usually occur on the external surface of long bones, tibial, and femoral bone, around the knee. Malignant transformation occurs in 5% of cases of osteochondromas, either solitary or multiple form.[6] In addition, a minority (<1%) occur at the surface of bone, and are possibly of periosteal origin and designated as periosteal chondrosarcoma. This type tends to affect younger adults more often than other conventional types. The metaphyseal regions of long bones, especially the femur and the humerus, are most commonly affected.

Histologically, conventional chondrosarcoma is subdivided as grade I, II, and III (low, intermediate, and high grade) by hematoxylin and eosin (H&E) staining based on cellularity, matrix protein, and mitoses. Histopathologic grading is more related to tumor aggressiveness and disease prognosis. Grade I chondrosarcoma, now reclassified as an atypical cartilaginous tumor, shows low cellularity

TABLE 12.1 **Overview of Clinical Characteristics in Different Subtypes of Chondrosarcomas**

Characteristic	Conventional Central Chondrosarcoma	Conventional Secondary Peripheral Chondrosarcoma	Conventional Periosteal Chondrosarcoma	Dedifferentiated Chondrosarcoma	Mesenchymal Chondrosarcoma	Clear Cell Chondrosarcoma
Definition	Tumor arises within the intramedullary space	Tumor arises from the surface of bone, generally from the cartilage cap of preexisting osteochondromas	Tumor occurs at the surface of bone and is possibly of periosteal origin	Well-differentiated benign lesion or chondrosarcoma juxtaposed with a high-grade noncartilaginous component	Undifferentiated small round cell component admixed with islands of well-differentiated cartilage	Tumor cells with clear, empty cytoplasm
% in all chondrosarcomas	~75%	~10%	<1%	~10%	~3%	~2%
Age (years)	>50	40–60	20–30	Median age 59	10–20	20–30
Preferential location	Pelvis, proximal femur, proximal humerus, distal femur, ribs	Pelvis, shoulder girdle bones	Metaphyseal region of the long bones, especially the femur and the humerus	Pelvis and shoulder	Skeleton (jawbones, ribs, ilium, vertebrae); extraosseous (meninges)	Epiphysis of humeral or femoral head
Histologic grading	Grade I–III	Grade I/II	Grade I/II	High grade	High grade	Low grade
Prognosis	Good, with 5-year overall survival rates as follows: grade I, 89%; II and III, 57%[1]	Good, with 5-year overall survival rate ~90%[2]	Good, with 5-year overall survival rate ~83%[1]	Poor, with 5-year overall survival rates ranging from 7% to 24%[3]	Poor, with 10-year survival rate in the range of 27%–67%[4]	Good, with 5-year overall survival rate >80%[1]
Treatment	Surgical management (resistant to conventional chemotherapy and radiation therapy)			Surgery; possibly chemotherapy	Surgery; possibly chemotherapy and radiation therapy	Surgery

and is locally aggressive, but typically does not metastasize. Grade II and grade III conventional chondrosarcomas show increased cellularity with mitoses and reduced cartilaginous matrix, and a corresponding increase in metastasizing capacity alongside poor patient survival.[7] Approximately 90% of conventional chondrosarcomas are low to intermediate grade (grade I–II) and behave indolently and rarely metastasize. Only 5% to 10% of conventional chondrosarcomas are grade III and have high metastatic potential.[8] The main site of metastatic disease is lung, while the regional lymph nodes and liver are much less commonly involved.[2]

Nonconventional chondrosarcomas are some specialized types with distinctive microscopic and clinical features, including dedifferentiated, mesenchymal, clear cell, and myxoid chondrosarcoma. They together constitute 10% to 15% of all chondrosarcomas. Dedifferentiated chondrosarcoma is a highly malignant variant of chondrosarcoma and accounts for up to 10% of all chondrosarcomas. The age of presentation is a decade older than that for conventional chondrosarcoma. It is characterized by two distinct histopathologic components: a well-differentiated lesion or chondrosarcoma (usually low grade) sharply juxtaposed with a high-grade, noncartilaginous component, which most frequently exhibits features of osteosarcoma, fibrosarcoma, or undifferentiated pleomorphic sarcoma.[7,9] Mesenchymal chondrosarcoma is considered high-grade tumor type and accounts for approximately 3% of chondrosarcomas. It is characterized by a biphasic histologic pattern of undifferentiated small round cells admixed with islands of well-differentiated cartilage.[3,10] The small cell component shows positive staining for *SOX9* and negativity for FLI-1, which often helps in the differential diagnosis from Ewing sarcoma.[10] *HEY1–NCOA2* fusion gene has also been described in this subtype as a marker of diagnostic utility.[11] Clear cell chondrosarcoma is a variant of conventional chondrosarcoma behaving as low-grade malignant bone tumor and involves a younger population than the conventional type. It accounts for about 2% of all chondrosarcomas, demonstrating tumor cells with clear, empty cytoplasm in addition to hyaline cartilage.[7,8] Loss of p16 protein has been reported in patients with clear cell chondrosarcomas.[12] Extraskeletal myxoid chondrosarcoma is a slow-growing soft tissue tumor containing prominent myxoid material, but it is considered a misnomer because it lacks cartilaginous differentiation.[13]

CLINICAL PRESENTATION AND DIAGNOSTIC EVALUATION

Pain is nearly always present and is usually insidious, progressive, worse at night, and present for months to years prior to the patient seeking care. A palpable mass is frequently seen. Some patients present with pathologic fracture.[14] Tumors located in the skull base can cause neurologic symptoms. Plain radiography is used for initial evaluation, which allows the identification of the cartilaginous nature and aggressiveness of the lesion. CT and MRI are essential for the determination of the extent of the intraosseous and soft tissue involvement preoperatively. Tissue biopsy by an experienced surgeon or interventional radiologist is essential to diagnose and differentiate the lesion from another malignant bone tumor.

TREATMENT

The radiologic and histopathologic classifications in relation to the clinical symptoms, medical history, and performance status are important for treatment decisions. Surgical treatment is the only option for curative therapy. Low-grade chondrosarcoma confined to the bone can be managed by extensive intralesional curettage with local adjuvant treatment such as phenolization or cryosurgery, followed by filling the cavity with bone graft.[3,15,16] For intermediate- and high-grade chondrosarcoma, wide en bloc excision is the preferred surgical treatment.[3,17] Tumors with intra-articular or soft tissue involvement, larger tumors, and axial or pelvic tumors must be treated with wide excision. However, in the event of tumor location at a nonresectable site, such as in the skull or pelvis, or a metastatic disease, there is no curative treatment.

In general, chondrosarcoma is relatively resistant to conventional chemotherapy and radiation therapy, possibly because of the low mitotic fraction of cells and restricted drug penetration as a result of the abundant extracellular matrix and poor vascularity.[18] Chemotherapy is effective in mesenchymal chondrosarcoma[10] but has limited value in dedifferentiated chondrosarcoma. Patients with primary mesenchymal chondrosarcoma are treated with an adult, small cell sarcoma regimen (see Chapter 13, Rhabdomyosarcoma) such as vincristine 2 mg, doxorubicin 75 to 90 mg/m^2 (over 72-hour infusion or bolus with dexrazoxane), and ifosfamide 10 g/m^2 (divided over 4–5 days with mesna uroprotection) for six to eight cycles. On the other hand, primary dedifferentiated chondrosarcoma patients are generally approached like a poor-risk osteosarcoma (see Chapter 11, Osteosarcoma) using doxorubicin plus cisplatinum 90 to 120 mg/m^2 intra-arterially (or intravenously [IV]), followed by high-dose ifosfamide 14 g/m^2 for six cycles and high-dose methotrexate 12 g/m^2 for six cycles. These agents are active in the metastatic setting as well. Radiation therapy can be considered after incomplete resection or if resection is not feasible or would cause unacceptable morbidity. However, doses >60 Gy are needed in attempts to achieve local control after incomplete resection. Unfortunately, application of this high-dose radiation therapy with conventional photon therapy is often not feasible, especially in chondrosarcomas arising in the skull base and axial skeleton. Irradiation with protons or other charged particles seems beneficial in this situation.[3,19] Follow-up scans are extremely important for chondrosarcoma to make sure there has been no recurrence or metastasis.

PROGNOSIS

Prognosis highly depends on the histologic grade of malignancy. For conventional central chondrosarcoma, the 5-year survival rate by grade was 89% for patients with grade 1 and 57% for the combined group of patients with grades 2 and 3.[4] The prognosis for patients with conventional periosteal chondrosarcoma is favorable compared to that of central type. The overall 5-year metastasis-free survival rate is approximately 83%.[4] Most of the conventional peripheral chondrosarcomas are low grade and the overall prognosis is good, with long-term survival found in 70% to 90% of patients.[4] However, despite adequate wide surgical resection and adjuvant systemic therapy, the prognosis for patients with a primary dedifferentiated chondrosarcoma is poor, with the 5-year survival rate reported to be between 7% and 24%.[9] Mesenchymal chondrosarcoma shows a strong tendency toward late local and metastatic recurrences. Despite a potentially prolonged clinical course, the outcome for these patients ultimately appears to be poor, with reported 10-year survival rate in the range of 27% to 67%.[10]

NOVEL THERAPEUTIC APPROACHES

Novel therapeutic approaches for patients with unresectable or metastatic disease are urgently needed. Current research focuses on elucidating the molecular events underlying the pathogenesis of chondrosarcoma and aiming at the development of new molecularly targeted therapies. The emerging pharmaceutical targets in chondrosarcoma include *IDH* mutation, phosphatidylinositol 3-kinase (PI3K)/ protein kinase B (AKT)/mammalian target of rapamycin (mTOR), angiogenesis, and Hedgehog (HH) pathway.

Targeting *IDH* Mutations

Isocitrate dehydrogenases (IDHs) are enzymes involved in tricarboxylic acid cycle (TCA) that catalyze the oxidative decarboxylation of isocitrate into alpha-ketoglutarate (alpha-KG). Mutant IDHs lose the capacity to convert isocitrate to alpha-KG, and instead gain a new function of reducing alpha-KG to an oncometabolite, D-2-hydroxyglutarate (D-2HG). *IDH* mutations have been observed in a variety of tumors including cartilaginous tumors.[20] Intriguingly, these mutations are present in 87% of benign enchondromas, 38% to 70% of primary conventional central chondrosarcomas (central and periosteal), and 54% of dedifferentiated chondrosarcomas, but not in clear cell or mesenchymal chondrosarcomas.[20,21] Therefore, *IDH* mutation represents a new common genetic abnormality in chondrosarcomas, indicating a potential role of this mutation in the pathogenesis of chondrosarcomas. The exact mechanism by which *IDH* mutation and D-2HG causes tumor formation is unknown, although increasing evidence points toward epigenetic mechanisms. The emerging concept is that the accumulated D-2HG competitively inhibits the function of alpha-KG–dependent dioxygenases involved in DNA and histone demethylation, which leads to a hypermethylation status of genome that affects the gene expression required for cellular differentiation.[22] Inhibitors of mutant *IDH1*, *IDH2*, or both have been developed and evaluated in preclinical and clinical studies as single agents and in combination with other anticancer agents and have shown promising clinical benefits in some cancer types.[23,24] It has been reported that a mutant *IDH1* inhibitor showed antitumor activity in chondrosarcoma cell lines.[25] Mutant *IDH1* inhibitor AG-120 (NCT02073994), *IDH2* inhibitor AG-221 (NCT02273739), and pan-*IDH* inhibitor AG-881 (NCT02481154) are currently being evaluated in patients with advanced *IDH*-mutant solid tumors including chondrosarcoma (Table 12.2).

TABLE 12.2 **Ongoing Clinical Trials for Patients With Chondrosarcoma**

ClinicalTrial.gov Identifier	Drug	Mechanism	Condition	Phase	Status
Targeting *IDH* mutations					
NCT02073994	AG-120	Mutant IDH1 inhibitor	Advanced solid tumors, including chondrosarcoma, with an *IDH1* mutation	1	Active, not recruiting
NCT02273739	AG-221	Mutant IDH2 inhibitor	Advanced solid tumors, including chondrosarcoma, with an *IDH2* mutation	1/2	Completed
NCT02481154	AG-881	Pan-IDH mutant inhibitor	Advanced solid tumors, including chondrosarcoma, with an *IDH1* and/or *IDH2* mutation	1	Active, not recruiting
Targeting PI3K/AKT/mTOR pathway					
NCT02821507	Sirolimus Cyclophosphamide	mTOR inhibitor	Metastatic or unresectable myxoid liposarcoma and chondrosarcoma	2	Recruiting
NCT00401388	Perifosine	PI3K and AKT inhibitor	Chondrosarcoma, alveolar soft part sarcoma, and extraskeletal myxoid chondrosarcoma	2	Completed
NCT03190174	ABI-009 (nab-sirolimus)	mTOR inhibitor	Undifferentiated pleomorphic sarcoma, liposarcoma, chondrosarcoma, osteosarcoma, and Ewing sarcoma	1/2	Recruiting
NCT01560260	Linsitinib	IGF-1R inhibitor	Camey complex, chondrosarcoma, GIST, and paraganglioma	2	Completed
NCT00720174	Cixutumumab Doxorubicin	IGF-1R inhibitor	Unresectable, locally advanced, or metastatic soft tissue sarcoma	1	Completed
Targeting angiogenesis					
NCT01330966	Pazopanib	Selective multitargeted receptor tyrosine kinase inhibitor	Unresectable or metastatic chondrosarcoma	2	Completed
NCT02389244	Regorafenib	Multi-kinase inhibitor; targets angiogenic, stromal, and oncogenic receptor tyrosine kinase	High-grade osteosarcoma, Ewing sarcoma of bone, intermediate- or high-grade chondrosarcomas and chordomas	2	Recruiting
NCT01532687	Pazopanib, gemcitabine	Selective multitargeted receptor tyrosine kinase inhibitor	Refractory soft tissue sarcoma including extraskeletal myxoid chondrosarcoma	2	Recruiting
Targeting Hedgehog pathway					
NCT01310816	IPI-926	SMO inhibitor	Metastatic or unresectable chondrosarcoma	2	Completed
NCT01267955	Vismodegib	SMO inhibitor	Advanced chondrosarcomas	2	Active, not recruiting

GIST, gastrointestinal stromal tumor; IGF-1R, insulin-like growth factor 1 receptor; mTOR mammalian target of rapamycin; PI3K phosphatidylinositol 3-kinase; SMO, Smoothened.

Sources: Data from Kim MJ, Cho KJ, Ayala AG, Ro JY. Chondrosarcoma: with updates on molecular genetics. *Sarcoma*. 2011;2011:405437. doi:10.1155/2011/405437; Lin PP, Moussallem CD, Deavers MT. Secondary chondrosarcoma. *J Am Acad Orthop Surg*. 2010;18:608–615. doi:10.5435/00124635-201010000-00004; Strotman PK, Reif TJ, Kliethermes SA, et al. Dedifferentiated chondrosarcoma: a survival analysis of 159 cases from the SEER database (2001–2011). *J Surg Oncol*. 2017;116:252–257. doi:10.1002/jso.24650; Frezza AM, Cesari M, Baumhoer D, et al. Mesenchymal chondrosarcoma: prognostic factors and outcome in 113 patients. A European Musculoskeletal Oncology Society study. *Eur J Cancer*. 2015;51:374–381. doi:10.1016/j.ejca.2014.11.007.

Targeting PI3K/AKT/mTOR Pathway

The PI3K/AKT and the mTOR signaling pathways both contribute to a variety of cellular processes including nutrient uptake, anabolic reactions, cell growth, and survival.[26] They are so closely interconnected that, in a certain sense, they could be regarded as a single, unique pathway. This pathway is initiated by ligand activation of receptor tyrosine kinases (RTKs) such as insulin-like growth factor 1 receptor (IGF-1R) and platelet-derived growth factor receptor (PDGFR). Activation of this pathway results in a profound disturbance of control of cell growth and survival, which ultimately leads to a competitive growth advantage, metastatic competence, angiogenesis, and therapy resistance.[27] Targeting the components of this complex signaling pathway, such as IGF-1R, PI3K/AKT, or mTOR, has been taken into consideration as one of the most attractive targets for the development of anticancer agents. Several drugs such as the IGF-R inhibitor, linsitinib (NCT01560260), the PI3K/AKT inhibitor, perifosine (NCT00401388), and mTOR inhibitors, sirolimus (NCT02821507) and ABI-009 (nab-sirolimus) (NCT03190174), are currently being evaluated in chondrosarcoma patients (Table 12.2). Intriguingly, a combination of sirolimus and low-dose daily cyclophosphamide in patients with advanced conventional chondrosarcomas has shown meaningful clinical activity with a disease control rate of 70%.[28] A Phase 2 trial is further evaluating the efficacy of these two drugs in metastatic or unresectable myxoid liposarcoma and chondrosarcoma (NCT02821507; Table 12.2).

Targeting Angiogenesis

To support the high proliferative rate of cancer cells, tumors need to rapidly develop a new vascular network to meet the demand of nutrients and oxygen. Angiogenesis refers to the formation of new blood vessels from preexisting vasculature. It is a hallmark of cancer and plays a crucial role in tumor progression and metastasis.[29,30] Numerous inducers of angiogenesis have been identified, including the members of the vascular endothelial growth factor (VEGF) family, angiopoietins, transforming growth factors (TGFs), platelet-derived growth factor (PDGF), tumor necrosis factor-alpha (TGF-alpha), interleukins, and the members of the fibroblast growth factor (FGF) family.[31] Of these, VEGF was the first characterized vascular-specific growth factor and is one of the most critical drivers of tumor angiogenesis.[32] A few pharmacologic agents against angiogenesis that disrupt tumor vascular supply have been developed. Targeting VEGF and its cognate receptor (VEGFR) signaling seems to be the most effective in preclinical and clinical settings. A number of preclinical studies have shown clinical benefits of targeting angiogenesis in chondrosarcomas.[2] Pazopanib is a multitargeted tyrosine kinase inhibitor, with activity against VEGFR-1, -2, -3; PDGF receptors alpha and beta (PDGFR-alpha, -beta); and c-kit.[33] A Phase 2 trial recently reported pazopanib had clinically meaningful antitumor activity in patients with progressive and advanced extraskeletal myxoid chondrosarcoma and could be considered a suitable option after failure to respond to first-line chemotherapy in these patients.[34] It is currently being evaluated in patients with unresectable or metastatic chondrosarcoma (NCT01330966; Table 12.2). Regorafenib is a multi-kinase inhibitor that targets angiogenic, stromal, and oncogenic RTKs. Regorafenib shows antiangiogenic activity mainly due to its dual inhibition of VEGFR2 and tyrosine kinase with immunoglobulin and epidermal growth factor homology domain 2 (TIE2), an angiopoietin receptor.[35] This drug is currently being evaluated in a Phase 2 clinical trial on patients with advanced sarcoma including chondrosarcoma (NCT02389244; Table 12.2).

Targeting the HH Pathway

The HH pathway plays essential roles in the regulation of many fundamental processes in vertebrate embryonic development, including stem cell maintenance, cell differentiation, tissue polarity, and cell proliferation.[36] When the HH ligands bind to the canonical membrane protein Patched (Ptc), the suppression of Smoothened (Smo) by Ptc is relieved. Smo is then stabilized and mediates activation of the GLI transcription factor and consequent expression of HH-target genes to initiate a series of cellular responses.[37] Chondrogenesis is regulated by the Indian HH (IHH)/parathyroid hormone-related peptide (PTHrP) feedback loop. Aberrant activation of this pathway leads to constant signals from IHH, which induce chondrocyte proliferation and secretion of PTHrP that mediates inhibition of chondrocyte differentiation and apoptosis.[38] Tiet et al. reported that constitutive IHH signaling upregulates chondrosarcoma cell proliferation.[39] Therapeutic targeting of this pathway in chondrosarcoma with an SMO inhibitor vismodegib (GDC-0049) has been investigated in clinical trials, but results look discouraging.[40] A Phase 2 study of vismodegib in patients with advanced chondrosarcomas is still active, but not recruiting patients (NCT01267955; Table 12.2).

Other Targeted Treatments

In addition to the targets described above, other attractive therapeutic interventions include immunotherapy, histone deacetylase (HDAC) inhibitors, integrin-receptor antagonists, microRNAs (miRNAs), and so on. Kostine et al. reported the presence of PD-L1 expression in association with immune-infiltrating cells and HLA class I expression in nearly 50% of the dedifferentiated chondrosarcomas, which provides rationale for including these patients in clinical trials with immunotherapies.[41] Advanced chondrosarcomas are currently included in the following clinical trials of immunotherapeutic drugs: combination of a PD-1 inhibitor, nivolumab, and a CTLA4 inhibitor, ipilimumab (NCT02982486); autologous tumor-infiltrating lymphocyte LN-145, which is made by collecting and growing specialized white blood cells from the patient's tumor (NCT03449108), and recombinant humanized anti-PD-1 monoclonal antibody, toripalimab (NCT03474640). Moreover, as mediators of a wide spectrum of cancer cell activities, integrins represent an attractive target for cancer therapy. Our recent study showed that deregulation of integrin receptor-mediated processes contribute to the tumorigenicity of IDH1-mutant chondrosarcoma cells,[42] suggesting that integrin-receptor antagonists are appealing candidates for combinatorial regimens with mutant IDH inhibitors for chondrosarcomas that harbor IDH mutation.

SUMMARY

Chondrosarcomas are a heterogeneous group of tumors with highly diverse features and behavior patterns, ranging from indolent, nonmetastasizing lesions to highly aggressive metastasizing sarcomas. Prognosis highly depends on the histologic grade of malignancy. Chondrosarcoma is poorly treatable because it is highly resistant to chemotherapy and radiation therapy. Surgical resection remains the "gold standard" for the treatment of localized chondrosarcoma. Owing to lack of effective treatment, the clinical management of advanced chondrosarcomas is exceptionally challenging. The past few years' research that focused on elucidating the molecular events underlying the pathogenesis of chondrosarcoma has led to the identification of several new potential therapeutic targets such as *IDH* mutation, PI3k/AKT/mTOR, angiogenesis, HH pathway, and immunotherapy. Future studies should further explore the utility of these candidate molecular targeted therapies in advanced chondrosarcoma patients.

CASE STUDY

A 45-year old woman develops a painful right hip that interferes with her ability to ride her bicycle and requires daily analgesics. She is evaluated by her primary care physician, who orders a plain x-ray exam that reveals a lytic lesion. She is referred to an orthopedic surgeon, who evaluates the x-ray and obtains an MRI of the right hip with and without contrast. These studies show a mass occupying the ischium and surrounding the right acetabulum, but no extraosseous extension. The patient is then referred to an orthopedic oncologist who reviews her case and performs a biopsy of the pelvic mass that is subsequently reviewed by a sarcoma pathologist who determines the lesion is most consistent with a conventional chondrosarcoma. The patient has a follow-up appointment with the orthopedic oncologist to discuss the results and treatment options. Unfortunately, the only oncologic resection possible is an external hemipelvectomy with amputation of the right leg. The patient decides to seek a second opinion at a sarcoma center.

Upon evaluation by a sarcoma medical oncologist, the patient is considered for clinical trials because there is no standard chemotherapy that is effective against conventional chondrosarcoma. A recently opened clinical trial of an inhibitor of mutant *IDH* is available for the patient, but requires the presence of mutant *IDH*. Internal molecular testing identifies the presence of mutant *IDH-1* that is targetable by the clinical trial agent. Once enrolled in the clinical trial, the patient reports no adverse events as well as the disappearance of pain and ability to ride her bicycle without discomfort. The patient continues this therapy for >2 years, with MRI showing decrease in tumor volume by 80% over this time interval.

REFERENCES

1. Speetjens FM, de Jong Y, Gelderblom H, Bovee JVMG. Molecular oncogenesis of chondrosarcoma: impact for targeted treatment. *Curr Opin Oncol*. 2016;28:314–322. doi:10.1097/CCO.0000000000000300
2. Polychronidou G, Karavasilis V, Pollack SM, et al. Novel therapeutic approaches in chondrosarcoma. *Future Oncol*. 2017;13:637–648. doi:10.2217/fon-2016-0226

3. Gelderblom H, Hogendoorn PC, Dijkstra SD, et al. The clinical approach towards chondrosarcoma. *Oncologist*. 2008;13:320–329. doi:10.1634/theoncologist.2007-0237
4. Kim MJ, Cho KJ, Ayala AG, Ro JY. Chondrosarcoma: with updates on molecular genetics. *Sarcoma*. 2011;2011:405437. doi:10.1155/2011/405437
5. Doyle LA. Sarcoma classification: an update based on the 2013 World Health Organization Classification of Tumors of Soft Tissue and Bone. *Cancer*. 2014;120:1763–1774. doi:10.1002/cncr.28657
6. Nazeri E, Gouran Savadkoohi M, Majidzadeh AK, Esmaeili R. Chondrosarcoma: an overview of clinical behavior, molecular mechanisms mediated drug resistance and potential therapeutic targets. *Crit Rev Oncol Hematol*. 2018;131:102–109. doi:10.1016/j.critrevonc.2018.09.001
7. van Oosterwijk JG, Anninga JK, Gelderblom H, et al. Update on targets and novel treatment options for high-grade osteosarcoma and chondrosarcoma. *Hematol Oncol Clin North Am*. 2013;27:1021–1048. doi:10.1016/j.hoc.2013.07.012
8. Chow WA. Chondrosarcoma: biology, genetics, and epigenetics. *F1000Res*. 2018;7. doi:10.12688/f1000research.15953.1
9. Strotman PK, Reif TJ, Kliethermes SA, et al. Dedifferentiated chondrosarcoma: a survival analysis of 159 cases from the SEER database (2001-2011). *J Surg Oncol*. 2017;116:252–257. doi:10.1002/jso.24650
10. Frezza AM, Cesari M, Baumhoer D, et al. Mesenchymal chondrosarcoma: prognostic factors and outcome in 113 patients. A European Musculoskeletal Oncology Society study. *Eur J Cancer*. 2015;51:374–381. doi:10.1016/j.ejca.2014.11.007
11. Wang L, Motoi T, Khanin R, et al. Identification of a novel, recurrent HEY1-NCOA2 fusion in mesenchymal chondrosarcoma based on a genome-wide screen of exon-level expression data. *Gene Chromosome Cancer*. 2012;51:127–139. doi:10.1002/gcc.20937
12. Meijer D, de Jong D, Pansuriya TC, et al. Genetic characterization of mesenchymal, clear cell, and dedifferentiated chondrosarcoma. *Gene Chromosome Cancer*. 2012;51:899–909. doi:10.1002/gcc.21974
13. Goh YW, Spagnolo DV, Platten M, et al. Extraskeletal myxoid chondrosarcoma: a light microscopic, immunohistochemical, ultrastructural and immuno-ultrastructural study indicating neuroendocrine differentiation. *Histopathology*. 2001;39:514–524. doi:10.1046/j.1365-2559.2001.01277.x
14. Flemming DJ, Murphey MD. Enchondroma and chondrosarcoma. *Semin Musculoskelet Radiol*. 2000;4:59–71. doi:10.1055/s-2000-6855
15. Veth R, Schreuder B, van Beem H, et al. Cryosurgery in aggressive, benign, and low-grade malignant bone tumours. *Lancet Oncol*. 2005;6:25–34. doi:10.1016/S1470-2045(05)70023-1
16. Leerapun T, Hugate RR, Inwards CY, et al. Surgical management of conventional grade I chondrosarcoma of long bones. *Clin Orthop Relat Res*. 2007;463:166–172. doi:10.1097/BLO.0b013e318146830f
17. Fiorenza F, Abudu A, Grimer RJ, et al. Risk factors for survival and local control in chondrosarcoma of bone. *J Bone Joint Surg Br*. 2002;84:93–99. doi:10.1302/0301-620X.84B1.0840093
18. Bovee JV, Cleton-Jansen AM, Taminiau AH, Hogendoorn PC. Emerging pathways in the development of chondrosarcoma of bone and implications for targeted treatment. *Lancet Oncol*. 2005;6:599–607. doi:10.1016/S1470-2045(05)70282-5
19. Mavrogenis AF, Gambarotti M, Angelini A, et al. Chondrosarcomas revisited. *Orthopedics*. 2012;35:e379–e390. doi:10.3928/01477447-20120222-30
20. Amary MF, Bacsi K, Maggiani F, et al. IDH1 and IDH2 mutations are frequent events in central chondrosarcoma and central and periosteal chondromas but not in other mesenchymal tumours. *J Pathol*. 2011;224:334–343. doi:10.1002/path.2913
21. Pansuriya TC, van Eijk R, d'Adamo P, et al. Somatic mosaic IDH1 and IDH2 mutations are associated with enchondroma and spindle cell hemangioma in Ollier disease and Maffucci syndrome. *Nat Genet*. 2011;43(12):1256–1261. doi:10.1038/ng.1004
22. Schaap FG, French PJ, Bovée JVMG. Mutations in the isocitrate dehydrogenase genes IDH1 and IDH2 in tumors. *Adv Anat Pathol*. 2013;20(1):32–38. doi:10.1097/PAP.0b013e31827b654d
23. Tommasini-Ghelfi S, Murnan K, Kouri F M, et al. Cancer-associated mutation and beyond: the emerging biology of isocitrate dehydrogenases in human disease. *Sci Adv*. 2019;5:eaaw4543. doi:10.1126/sciadv.aaw4543
24. Li L, Eid JE, Paz AC, Trent JC. Metabolic enzymes in sarcomagenesis: progress toward biology and therapy. *BioDrugs*. 2017;31(5):379–392. doi:10.1007/s40259-017-0237-2
25. Li L, Paz A C, Wilky B A, et al. Treatment with a small molecule mutant IDH1 inhibitor suppresses tumorigenic activity and decreases production of the oncometabolite 2-hydroxyglutarate in human chondrosarcoma cells. *PLoS One*. 2015;10:e0133813. doi:10.1371/journal.pone.0133813
26. Luo J, Manning BD, Cantley LC. Targeting the PI3K-Akt pathway in human cancer: rationale and promise. *Cancer Cell*. 2003;4(4):257–262. doi:10.1016/s1535-6108(03)00248-4
27. Porta C, Paglino C, Mosca A. Targeting PI3K/Akt/mTOR signaling in cancer. *Front Oncol*. 2014;4:64. doi:10.3389/fonc.2014.00064
28. Bernstein-Molho R, Kollender Y, Issakov J, et al. Clinical activity of mTOR inhibition in combination with cyclophosphamide in the treatment of recurrent unresectable chondrosarcomas. *Cancer Chemother Pharmacol*. 2012;70(6):855–860. doi:10.1007/s00280-012-1968-x
29. Hanahan D, Weinberg RA. Hallmarks of cancer: the next generation. *Cell*. 2011;144(5):646–674. doi:10.1016/j.cell.2011.02.013

30. Albini A, Tosetti F, Li VW, et al. Cancer prevention by targeting angiogenesis. *Nat Rev Clin Oncol*. 2012;9(9):498–509. doi:10.1038/nrclinonc.2012.120
31. Otrock ZK, Mahfouz RAR, Makarm JA, Shamseddine AI. Understanding the biology of angiogenesis: review of the most important molecular mechanisms. *Blood Cell Mol Dis*. 2007;39:212–220. doi:10.1016/j.bcmd.2007.04.001
32. Ferrara N. Vascular endothelial growth factor as a target for anticancer therapy. *Oncologist*. 2004;9(suppl 1):2–10. doi:10.1634/theoncologist.9-suppl_1-2
33. Sonpavde G, Hutson TE. Pazopanib: a novel multitargeted tyrosine kinase inhibitor. *Curr Oncol Rep*. 2007;9(2):115–119. doi:10.1007/s11912-007-0007-2
34. Stacchiotti S, Ferrari S, Redondo A, et al. Pazopanib for treatment of advanced extraskeletal myxoid chondrosarcoma: a multicentre, single-arm, phase 2 trial. *Lancet Oncol*. 2019;20(9):1252–1262. doi:10.1016/S1470-2045(19)30319-5
35. Wilhelm SM, Dumas J, Adnane L, et al. Regorafenib (BAY 73-4506): a new oral multikinase inhibitor of angiogenic, stromal and oncogenic receptor tyrosine kinases with potent preclinical antitumor activity. *Int J Cancer*. 2011;129(1):245–255. doi:10.1002/ijc.25864
36. Gupta S, Takebe N, Lorusso P. Targeting the Hedgehog pathway in cancer. *Ther Adv Med Oncol*. 2010;2(4):237–250. doi:10.1177/1758834010366430
37. Wu F, Zhang Y, Sun B, et al. Hedgehog signaling: from basic biology to cancer therapy. *Cell Chem Biol*. 2017;24(3):252–280. doi:10.1016/j.chembiol.2017.02.010
38. Rubin LL, de Sauvage FJ. Targeting the Hedgehog pathway in cancer. *Nat Rev Drug Discov*. 2006;5(12):1026–1033. doi:10.1038/nrd2086
39. Tiet TD, Hopyan S, Nadesan P, et al. Constitutive hedgehog signaling in chondrosarcoma up-regulates tumor cell proliferation. *Am J Pathol*. 2006;168(1):321–330. doi:10.2353/ajpath.2006.050001
40. Italiano A, Le Cesne A, Bellera C, et al. GDC-0449 in patients with advanced chondrosarcomas: a French Sarcoma Group/US and French National Cancer Institute Single-Arm Phase II Collaborative Study. *Ann Oncol*. 2013;24(11):2922–2926. doi:10.1093/annonc/mdt391
41. Kostine M, Cleven AH, de Miranda NFCC, et al. Analysis of PD-L1, T-cell infiltrate and HLA expression in chondrosarcoma indicates potential for response to immunotherapy specifically in the dedifferentiated subtype. *Mod Pathol*. 2016;29(9):1028–1037. doi:10.1038/modpathol.2016.108
42. Li L, Hu X, Eid JE, et al. Mutant IDH1 depletion downregulates integrins and impairs chondrosarcoma growth. *Cancers*. 2020;12(1):141. doi:10.3390/cancers12010141

13

Rhabdomyosarcoma

Pamela Abdayem and Sarah Dumont

INTRODUCTION

Rhabdomyosarcoma (RMS) is a soft tissue sarcoma composed of small round cells and spindle cells of unknown origin mimicking the striated aspect of skeletal muscle, thus the Greek prefix "rhabdo" meaning rod shape. RMS is traditionally classified into embryonal, alveolar, and pleomorphic subtypes. The spindle/sclerosing subtype, once considered a variant of embryonal subtype, is now a distinct fourth subtype according to the 2015 World Health Organization (WHO) classification. Being the most common soft tissue sarcoma and the third most common extracranial solid tumor after neuroblastoma and Wilms tumor in children, RMS is generally considered a pediatric tumor.[1] With the combined use of chemotherapy, radiation therapy (RT), and surgery, 80% of patients with localized disease remain alive at 5 years. Conversely, the 5-year overall survival (OS) rates seldom exceed 30% in patients with metastatic disease.[2] On the other hand, 40% of RMS cases occur in adults. Management of adult RMS is still extrapolated from pediatric protocols, despite several studies showing distinct biologic and clinical disease patterns. More studies are needed in this specific patient population in order to improve the outcomes of this rare and heterogeneous disease.

EPIDEMIOLOGY

Incidence

RMS is a rare tumor that accounts for 4% of childhood malignancies and about 3% of all adult soft tissue sarcomas in the United States. According to the Surveillance, Epidemiology, and End Results (SEER) database, 350 new cases are diagnosed each year in the United States and the annual incidence of RMS in children and adults younger than 20 years of age is around 4.3 cases per 1 million. The French Sarcoma Group published one of the largest prospective cohorts performed in a multicenter setting at a national level for adult RMS. The estimated incidence of adult RMS was around 0.9 case per million per year.[3]

Half the cases occur in children under the age of 10, while 40% of them affect adults. Incidence of pediatric RMS is highest between the ages of 2 and 6 years, and 10 and 18 years. Adult RMS usually occurs between the third and seventh decades of life. Embryonal RMS (E-RMS) affects approximately four cases per 1 million children younger than 4 years of age. It is less frequent in adolescents and very rare in adults. Incidence of alveolar RMS (A-RMS) is around one per 1 million children and adolescents. Pleomorphic RMS (P-RMS) occurs in <2% of children, but is the second most frequent entity in the adult population (19%).

There is a slight male predominance in children with a male to female ratio between 1.3:1 and 1.5:1 that varies according to the histologic subtype (E-RMS being more common in males, while A-RMS is gender independent) and tumor location (predominance of genitourinary [GU] tract and orbital tumors in males and females, respectively). On the other hand, the incidence of RMS is equivalent between male and female adults.

In addition to being gender dependent, tumor location also varies with age. Children more often present with GU tract, orbital, and head and neck tumors that are almost always of the embryonal type. Adolescents and adults experience more extremity, truncal, and paratesticular tumors that are frequently of the alveolar type.

Incidence of RMS is slightly higher in black patients between 15 and 19 years of age, compared to white patients. It is lowest in the Asian population.[4] No geographic distribution has been reported.

Risk Factors

There is a lack of solid data concerning risk factors. Some studies suggested a higher incidence of RMS in patients previously exposed to alkylating agents or to radiation in utero, those with accelerated in utero growth, children from families with a low socioeconomic status, those who received antibiotics soon after birth, and those whose parents used recreational drugs (marijuana or cocaine) during pregnancy.[5–7] Other studies suggest a protective role for higher birth order, immunizations, and immune-related factors (allergies, atopy, day-care attendance, breastfeeding for 12 or more months).[8–10]

Inherited Syndromes

Most cases of RMS are sporadic; however, Zhang et al. identified germline pathogenic or probably pathogenic mutations by next-generation sequencing in 7% of children with RMS.[11] In another study by Ruymann et al., congenital abnormalities were found in 37 of 115 (32%) children and adolescents autopsied with RMS. These patients also had an increased incidence of congenital malformations affecting the central nervous system (CNS) or GU, cardiovascular (CV), and gastrointestinal (GI) systems.[12] The following hereditary syndromes have a higher incidence of RMS:

- Li–Fraumeni syndrome: Inactivating germline mutations of the *p53* tumor suppressor genes predispose patients to a spectrum of cancers, including soft tissue sarcomas.[13] Incidence of RMS in this setting may be greatest among children under 3 years of age, who should therefore be screened for germline *p53* mutations.[14] In addition, patients with Li–Fraumeni syndrome usually develop anaplastic forms of RMS.[15]
- Beckwith–Wiedemann syndrome: This hereditary disease shares the same chromosomal abnormalities (11p15, the locus for the *IGF-2* gene) with certain pediatric tumors such as RMS, hepatoblastoma, Wilms tumor, and adrenocortical carcinoma.[16]
- Costello syndrome: In addition to postnatal growth retardation, macrocephaly, coarse facies, loose skin, nonprogressive cardiomyopathy, developmental delay, and papillomas, the presence of a mutation in the *HRAS* proto-oncogene predisposes patients to several tumors including RMS, epithelioma, bladder carcinoma, and vestibular schwannoma.[17–22]
- Neurofibromatosis: Incidence of RMS is 20 times higher compared with the general population.[23]
- *DICER1* syndrome: In this autosomal dominant, pleiotropic, tumor-predisposition disorder resulting from a germline *DICER1* gene mutation, there is an increased risk for GU E-RMS.[24,25]
- Rubinstein–Taybi syndrome: predisposes to neural and developmental tumors including nasopharyngeal RMS.[26,27]
- Gorlin basal cell nevus syndrome: There are several case reports of RMS associated with this syndrome, a rare autosomal dominant, inherited disorder that is characterized by development of basal cell carcinomas from a young age.[28,29]

CLINICAL PRESENTATION

RMS presents with variable signs and symptoms according to tumor location, patient age, and presence or absence of metastases. While a painless enlarging mass is easily palpated in the head and neck or the limbs, diagnosis of parameningeal or retroperitoneal RMS can be challenging.

Head and Neck Primary RMS

This is the most frequent primary tumor site (35%–40% of cases). Tumors can arise in the orbit (25%) resulting in proptosis or diplopia, in parameningeal sites (middle ear, nasal cavity, paranasal sinuses, nasopharynx, and infratemporal fossa; 50%) resulting in nasal obstruction or cranial nerve palsies, as well as in other head and neck locations (25%).[30] E-RMS predominates and lymph node (LN) involvement is infrequent.[31]

GU Tract

Twenty-five percent of RMS occurs in the GU tract. Embryonal subtype is predominant with specific occurrence of the botryoid variant. Bladder tumors cause hematuria and urinary obstruction. Prostate tumors present as large pelvic masses resulting in obstructive and irritative urinary symptoms, as well as constipation and bowel obstruction. Vaginal tumors may produce a mucosanguineous discharge in young girls, along with a protruding polypoid mass. Older girls present with cervical and uterine tumors. A painless scrotal or inguinal mass may be reported in boys with paratesticular RMS.[32] More than half of these boys older than 10 years of age have nodal involvement.[33]

Extremities

Twenty percent of RMS cases present as a bulging, nontraumatic, nontender mass in the extremities, with or without skin erythema. They mainly occur in adolescents, spread to LNs (50%) and along fascial planes, and are of the alveolar subtype (50%–75%).

Metastatic Disease

Metastatic disease is identified in <25% of patients at diagnosis. The most frequent metastatic site is the lung (50%). Patients with metastatic disease to the bones (30%) may present with skeletal-related events. Bone marrow involvement occurs in 30% of cases and results in cytopenias leading to a false diagnosis of leukemia. Other metastatic sites include the omentum (16%) and the pleura (13%). Visceral and brain metastases are rare.[34–37]

DIAGNOSTIC APPROACH

Biopsy

In patients with a suspicious mass, an open or core-needle biopsy is needed to establish the diagnosis. Whenever there is a suspicion for sarcoma, the patient should be referred to an expert center and the case displayed at the multidisciplinary tumor board. A surgical biopsy should be performed by an experienced sarcoma surgeon to prevent dissemination of tumor cells. An alternative to this method is a 14-gauge core-needle biopsy performed by an experienced interventional radiologist. The diagnostic material should be reviewed by a pathologist with an expertise in this domain, which ensures proper tissue processing and allows for special cytogenetic and molecular studies necessary for diagnosis and classification.

Imaging Workup

Imaging of the primary tumor site varies according to the tumor location and may include the following:

- Plain x-ray studies to identify calcifications and bone involvement of the primary tumor
- CT scan to serve as a baseline for future evaluations and to assess for bone erosions
- MRI, which evaluates local extension more accurately than CT scan in orbital, paraspinal, and parameningeal locations

Once the pathologic diagnosis of RMS is established, the following imaging exams should be performed to rule out metastatic disease:

- CT scan of the chest to identify secondary lung lesions
- CT scan or ultrasound of the liver in patients with abdominal and pelvic primary tumors
- ^{99}Tc bone scan to identify bone metastases
- Spinal and pelvic MRI to search for bone marrow involvement and guide subsequent biopsies
- 18-Fluorodeoxyglucose (18-FDG) PET-CT scan to search for regional nodal involvement as well as metastatic disease, especially to the bone; also to assess early response to chemotherapy
- Brain MRI in patients with neurologic symptoms

Laboratory Workup

Laboratory studies may reveal abnormalities in favor of metastatic diseases and are necessary to assess the patient's condition before starting treatment. They include the following:

- Complete blood count (CBC) to search for inflammatory anemia or other cytopenia
- Renal and liver function exams
- Albumin: to evaluate the nutritional status
- Urinalysis: to detect hematuria in RMS of the GU tract

Other Diagnostic Exams

Cooperative group studies often require a full metastatic workup, namely a CT of the chest, a bone scan, and bilateral bone marrow aspiration and biopsy to rule out marrow involvement. However, because the overall incidence of metastatic disease is low, a risk-oriented rather than disease-oriented staging strategy is currently being adopted. In fact, the most important factors that predict metastatic disease are nodal involvement, tumor invasiveness (>5 cm), and tumor histology (fusion-positive [FP] disease),

Weiss et al., from the Children's Oncology Group (COG) soft tissue sarcoma committee, showed that the risk of bone and bone marrow metastases is <1% in a retrospective analysis of 955 fusion-negative (FN) RMS patients without nodal or lung involvement.[38] Therefore, in selected children (tumors <5 cm, FN RMS, no evidence of nodal disease), omission of bone marrow biopsy is acceptable.

On the other hand, lumbar puncture and cerebrospinal fluid analysis could be solely performed in parameningeal disease.

Despite the data mentioned above, lumbar puncture for cerebrospinal fluid cytology in parameningeal tumors and bone marrow aspiration and biopsy remain "mandatory" in pediatric RMS. However, this is not the case in adult patients. These explorations are limited to symptomatic adult patients with suspicion of CNS or marrow involvement.

Cardiac ultrasound or nuclear medicine test is recommended before initiating chemotherapy with anthracyclines in order to establish a baseline ejection fraction.

Genetic counseling should be considered in younger patients with anaplastic features at diagnosis or in those with a family history of malignant disease.

PATHOLOGY

Morphologic analysis of fixed, paraffin-embedded biopsy tissue samples establishes the diagnosis of RMS which is characterized by the presence of muscle differentiation features. The latter is further classified into embryonal, alveolar, and pleomorphic subtypes. Cytologic material is generally insufficient to confirm diagnosis.[39] Immunohistochemistry (IHC) confirms the diagnosis by using specific antibodies that detect antigens involved in myogenic differentiation. Molecular biology using fluorescent in situ hybridization (FISH) as well as reverse transcriptase-polymerase chain reaction (RT-PCR) assays when FISH is unavailable or uninformative is a complementary diagnostic tool whenever morphologic diagnosis is difficult to obtain. In addition, it may detect chromosomal and molecular abnormalities with prognostic implications. Currently, FISH, next-generation sequencing, or RT-PCR for *FOXO1* rearrangement is performed on all RMS tumors, regardless of the histology.

Morphology

RMS is composed of small round blue cells that resemble other pediatric tumors such as lymphoma, small cell osteosarcoma, mesenchymal chondrosarcoma, and Ewing sarcoma. Identification of rhabdomyoblasts or cross striations that are characteristic of skeletal muscle on light microscopy is necessary to classify a tumor as RMS. Tumor architecture helps determine the histologic subtype: while small round cells grow in cohesive sheets in E-RMS, they are typically detached in A-RMS. In the botryoid variant of E-RMS, there is a typical cambium layer composed of dense subepithelial rhabdomyoblast aggregates. A-RMS cells line up along thin membranes similar to the lung alveoli. In addition, P-RMS encompasses malignant large spindle cells oriented in fascicles (Figures 13.1–13.3).

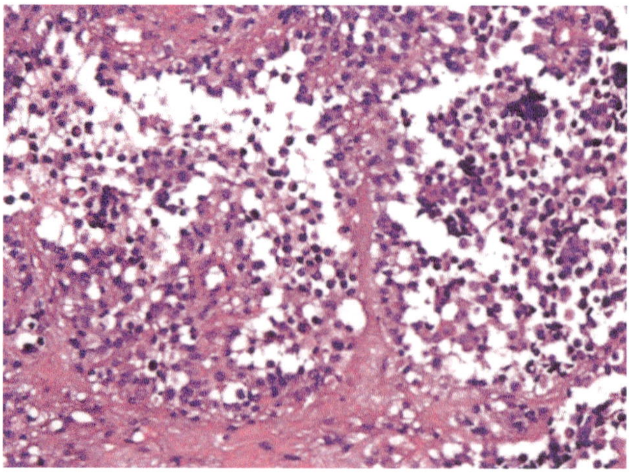

FIGURE 13.1 Embryonal rhabdomyosarcoma with tight sheets of small round cells.

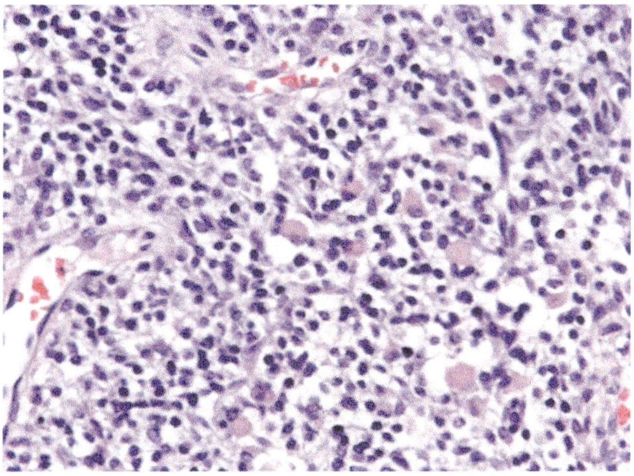

FIGURE 13.2 Alveolar rhabdomyosarcoma with loose aggregates of small round cells.

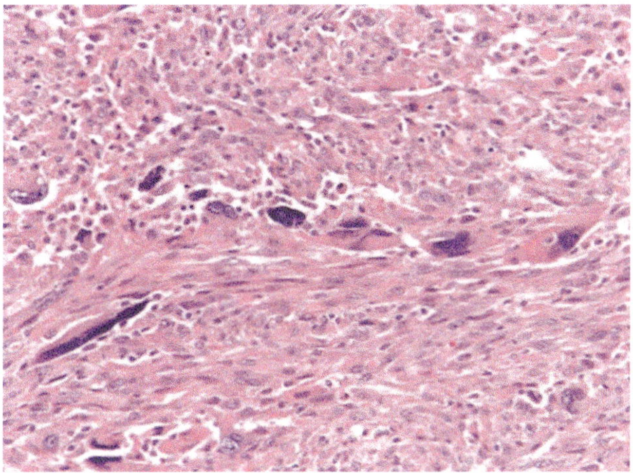

FIGURE 13.3 Pleomorphic rhabdomyosarcoma with fascicles of large spindle cells.

Immunohistochemistry

Muscle-specific proteins such as actin (95% of RMS), myosin, polyclonal desmin (99% of RMS), myoglobin (78% of RMS), Z-band protein, and myogenic differentiation 1 (MyoD1) can be identified by IHC.[40,41] Myogenin, present in 95% of tumors, is more often expressed in A-RMS and is an independent marker of poor survival in the pediatric setting.[42,43]

Cytogenetics and Molecular Biology

Molecular studies such as RT-PCR and FISH identify characteristic fusion proteins in ambiguous cases, especially in A-RMS where FISH for *FOXO1* rearrangement became a necessary test to confirm diagnosis based on the recommendations of the Soft Tissue Sarcoma Committee of the COG. Nowadays, FISH or RT-PCR for *FOXO1* rearrangement is performed on all RMS tumors.

This detailed diagnostic approach is summarized in Exhibit 13.1, taken from a 2018 report from the COG Soft Tissue Sarcoma Committee.[44]

RMS SUBTYPES: CLINICAL, PATHOLOGIC, GENETIC, AND MOLECULAR FEATURES

The International Classification of Rhabdomyosarcoma was derived from detailed pathologic study of patients who were enrolled in the first four Intergroup Rhabdomyosarcoma Study Group (IRSG)

EXHIBIT 13.1 Rhabdomyosarcoma Diagnostic and Staging Workup

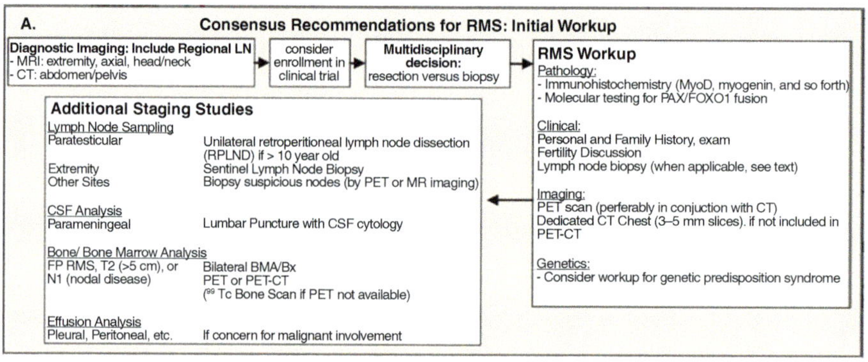

BMA/Bx, bone marrow aspiration and biopsy; CSF, cerebrospinal fluid; FP RMS, fusion-positive RMS; LN, lymph node; MyoD, myogenic differentiation; RMS, rhabdomyosarcoma; RPLND, retroperitoneal lymph node dissection.

Source: Reproduced with permission from Borinstein SC, Steppan D, Hayashi M, et al. Consensus and controversies regarding the treatment of rhabdomyosarcoma. *Pediatr Blood Cancer*. 2018;65(2):e26809. doi:10.1002/pbc.26809

therapeutic trials (IRS-I to -IV).[31,40] According to the 2015 WHO classification of skeletal muscle tumors in pediatric RMS, four major histologic subtypes with characteristic treatment strategies and prognostic implications were described.[45]

Embryonal RMS

As mentioned in the section "Incidence," E-RMS affects young children and is mostly found in the head, neck, and GU sites. This entity accounts for 59% of all RMS cases. Eighty-four percent of E-RMS cases are of the classic subtype. The botryoid variant is diagnosed in 10% of cases. Typical rhabdomyoblasts have a moderate to deeply eosinophilic cytoplasm representing poorly formed myofilaments, and are arranged in sheets and large nests, with infrequent intermixed fusiform cells (Figure 13.1). E-RMS lacks specific translocations, but usually has loss of heterozygosity (LOH) at the 11p15 locus, the site of insulin-like growth factor 2 (*IGF-2*), an imprinted gene. This results in upregulation of *IGF-2* expression in tumor cells, which in turn stimulates tumor growth.[46–49] Other genetic and epigenetic aberrations in E-RMS include the following:

- Alteration of genes at 11p15.5 locus (in addition to *IGF-2*): *H19*, *CDKN1C*, and *HOTS*
- *ALK* copy gain
- Mutations in *pRb*, *TP53*, *GLI*, *CDKN2A*, *CDKN2B*, *RAS*, *FGFR4*, *PIK3CA*, *CTNNB1* (beta-catenin), and *MyoD1*
- Deletion in *NF1* gene
- DNA methylation aberrations

Botryoid Variant

Sarcoma botryoid has a grape-like gross appearance. It only affects infants and typically arises from the wall of the bladder or the vagina.

Spindle Cell/Sclerosing RMS

Spindle cell/sclerosing RMS (S-RMS) has been recently identified as a new subtype. However, patients are still stratified based on more established risk factors while awaiting new data on treatment modalities. These forms are more prevalent in males. Poor prognostic features include adult age, parameningeal tumors, and the presence of *MYOD1* mutations.[50,51]

The spindle variant occurs in infants younger than 1 year of age. When needed, IHC for desmin, myogenin, and MyoD1 should be performed to distinguish this tumor from congenital/infantile fibrosarcoma. Unique translocations with rearrangements of *VGLL2* and *NCOA2* facilitate diagnosis. Infants <1 year of age with this particular histology usually have a favorable outcome.

The sclerosing variant is an aggressive, poor prognostic form occurring in children older than 1 year of age as well as in adults. Mutations in *MyoD1* and/or *PI3KCA* genes are characteristic.

Alveolar RMS

A-RMS typically affects the trunk or the extremities in children. It has a poorer prognosis than E-RMS with 5-year survival rates barely reaching 50%. Similar to pulmonary alveoli, the morphology of A-RMS consists of pseudoalveolar spaces separated by fibrovascular septa that are lined with round, loosely adherent rhabdomyoblasts. The latter frequently shed into these spaces.

A-RMS is characterized by a specific translocation t(2;13)(q35; q14) between the following:

- The long arm of chromosome 2 that includes the *PAX3* gene, a transcription regulator during early neuromuscular development and
- The long arm of chromosome 13 that harbors the *FOXO1* gene, a transcription factor[52,53]

Several cases have been reported with a variant t(1;13)(p36;q14) translocation, resulting in a fusion between *PAX7* and *FOXO1* genes.[54] *PAX3* and *PAX7* encode related DNA-binding domains; the resulting fusion transcript promotes the development of a transformed phenotype through mechanisms that are yet to be determined.[55] FISH test using a *FOXO1* probe and/or RT-PCR assays that detect the presence of either of these fusion genes are both rapid and accurate tests for identifying these translocations. Of 78 children with A-RMS, Sorensen et al. detected *PAX3* and *PAX7* fusion transcripts in 55% and 22% of cases, respectively. Twenty-three percent were fusion negative. They also demonstrated a higher risk of failure ($p = .025$), death ($p = .019$), and increased bone marrow involvement in metastatic tumors harboring a *PAX3–FOXO1* translocation.[56,57] Conversely, the *PAX7–FOXO1* translocation occurs in younger patients, affects the extremities, and has better outcomes.

According to the Soft Tissue Sarcoma Committee of the COG, the diagnosis of A-RMS requires the presence of a typical architectural pattern in >50% of the tumor as well as the presence of a *FOXO1* rearrangement, t(1;13) or t(2;13), by FISH or RT-PCR (when cytogenetic testing is unavailable). The latter is also beneficial for risk stratification as well as confirmation of diagnosis in the ambiguous cases.

Other genetic/epigenetic abnormalities include the following:

- *PAX3/FOXO4*, *PAX3/NCOA1*, *PAX3/NCOA2*, and *FOXO1/FGFR1* translocations
- *CDK4* amplification
- *TP53*, *CDKN2A*, *CDKN2B* mutations
- *FGFR4* and *ALK* copy gains
- *RASSF*, *HIC1*, *CASP8* tumor suppressor mutations
- DNA methylation: Compared to E-RMS, A-RMS has a distinct DNA methylation pattern and is enriched in DNA hypermethylation of polycomb target genes

Up to 45% of RMS with alveolar morphology lack *FOXO1* (or *FKHR*) rearrangement or other known genetic abnormalities and often behave like E-RMS with a more favorable outcome.[58,59] This suggests that fusion gene status regardless of histology is an essential factor in risk stratification of RMS. Adult patients with FN RMS have a better prognosis compared to FP RMS. Unlike in children, no significant difference in prognosis between *PAX3/FOXO1* and *PAX7/FOXO1* fusions was detected. In consequence, nonpleomorphic RMS could be classified into two major subgroups: FN RMS and FP RMS.

Pleomorphic RMS

P-RMS is the subtype that mainly affects adults. The risk factors, biology, and genetics remain unclear because of the low incidence of this disease and the lack of corresponding studies in adults. Tumor architecture consists of large spindle cells that may resemble other types of spindle cell sarcomas (pleomorphic myogenic soft tissue sarcoma). This subtype is extremely genetically heterogeneous.

Noujaim et al. published a series of 45 adult patients with P-RMS. Median age at diagnosis was 71.5 years. Median OS was 12.8 and 7.1 months in localized and metastatic disease, respectively. Response rates to pediatric chemotherapy protocols were low and relapse rate was high (53.8%).[60]

STAGING

Two major staging systems are used in newly diagnosed pediatric RMS: Clinical Group (CG) and TNM.[61] Conversely, traditional soft tissue sarcoma staging systems are still used in adults.

CG Classification

Developed by the IRSG in 1972, this widely used surgical pathologic staging system (Table 13.1) includes four disease categories with different prognoses.[62,63] It evaluates the quality of the surgical

TABLE 13.1 Clinical Group and Description

Clinical Group I	Localized disease, completely resected, regional nodes not involved. This includes both gross inspection and microscopic confirmation of complete resection
Clinical Group II	Total gross resection with evidence of regional spread a. Grossly resected tumor with microscopic residual disease (tumor at margin) b. Regional involved nodes, completely resected with no microscopic residual disease c. Regional involved nodes and microscopic residual disease
Clinical Group III	Incomplete resection or biopsy with gross residual disease
Clinical Group IV	Distant metastatic disease present at onset

resection based on the presence of residual disease and microscopic LN involvement. While it helps define treatment strategies, this classification does not consider other prognostic factors such as age, primary site, histology, cytogenetics, tumor size, and nodal involvement.

TNM Classification

This classification (Table 13.2) was developed and incorporated into the fourth IRSG protocol (IRS-IV).[64] Patients are assigned to one of four stages according to the site and size of the primary tumor, regional node involvement, and the absence or presence of distant metastases. Favorable disease sites include the orbit and eyelid, other nonparameningeal head and neck locations, and nonbladder, nonprostate GU tumors (e.g., paratesticular tumors), while unfavorable sites include the extremities, bladder and prostate, cranial parameningeal sites, trunk, and retroperitoneum.

TABLE 13.2 TNM Staging System of Rhabdomyosarcoma

Stage	Sites	T	Size	N	M
1	Orbit	T1 or T2	a or b	N0 or N1 or Nx	M0
	Head and neck (excluding parameningeal)				
	GU—nonbladder/nonprostate				
	Biliary tract/liver				
2	Bladder/prostate	T1 or T2	a	N0 or Nx	M0
	Extremity, cranial				
	Parameningeal, other (includes trunk, retroperitoneum, etc.)				
	Except biliary tract/liver				
3	Bladder/prostate	T1 or T2	a	N1	M0
	Extremity cranial		b	N0 or N1 or Nx	M0
	Parameningeal, other (includes the trunk, retroperitoneum, etc.)				
	Except biliary tract/liver				
4	All	T1 or T2	a or b	N0 or N1	M1

T: Tumor

T1(site) confined to anatomic site of origin

T2(site) extension and/or fixative to surrounding tissue

(a) ≤5 cm in diameter

(b) >5 cm in diameter

N: Regional nodes

N_0 regional nodes not clinically involved

N1: regional nodes clinically involved by neoplasm defined as (a) >1 cm by CT or MRI or (b) 18F-FDG avid

N_x clinical status of regional nodes unknown (especially the sites that preclude lymph node evaluation)

M: Metastasis

M_0 no distant metastasis

M_1 metastasis present

FDG, fluorodeoxyglucose.

The TNM and CG staging systems complement each other, and both of them are used to assess prognosis and select treatment for individual patients with RMS.

PROGNOSTIC FACTORS

According to the SEER program, mortality of RMS patients is predominantly related to age, tumor site, histology, and disease extension.

Age

In the past decades, mortality rate from cancer in children has been cut by half. However, these favorable results are yet to be achieved in adolescents and adults. The 5-year OS rate of RMS is 67% in children, 51% in adolescents, and 27% in adults. The most favorable age group is between 1 and 9 years with a 5-year survival rate of 87% according to the IRSG trials. Infants younger than 1 year of age and children older than 9 years have a 5-year survival rate of 76%. Among the adult population, the 5-year OS is inversely proportional to age and reaches 36%, 29%, and 11% in young adult, middle-aged, and elderly patients, respectively. According to the SEER database of the National Cancer Institute (NCI), adults tend to have unfavorable histologic subtypes (pleomorphic subtype) at unfavorable sites (65% vs. 55%, $p < .0001$). They also have overall worse survival than children for similar subtypes, especially in the nonmetastatic setting (5-year survival rate 47% vs. 82%).[65]

Tumor Site

Prognosis is linked to the primary tumor site, but not always to the possibility of resection. In fact, orbital and GU tumors have a better prognosis than those occurring in the extremities, retroperitoneum, or trunk.

Histology

Classically, E-RMS is correlated with a better prognosis than either A-RMS or P-RMS. A-RMS is more often diagnosed in unfavorable age groups or locations (<1 year of age or older patients, extremities, metastatic sites). Adult P-RMS is a particularly aggressive undifferentiated tumor, with a behavior similar to undifferentiated pleomorphic soft tissue sarcoma. It is treated suboptimally with pediatric protocols, hence the dismal prognosis (Figure 13.4).

Molecular Biology

PAX3/PAX7–FOXO1 fusion is observed in A-RMS. FN A-RMS tends to have a better outcome, more consistent with E-RMS, and is often reclassified as such. FP tumors involving *PAX7* may have a better outcome than those with *PAX3* fusions (Figure 13.4).

Disease Extension

Patients presenting with metastatic disease have a worse prognosis than those with localized disease. Moreover, patients with metastatic disease lacking other poor risk factors known as the Oberlin criteria, such as unfavorable sites, more than three sites, bone marrow involvement, and age younger than 1 year or older than 10 years, have a higher event-free survival (EFS) than those with three to four adverse features (50% vs. 10%).[66]

Prognostic Models: the IRSG Model

Risk-based algorithms help select treatment in pediatric RMS. There are currently no risk-based models for adults.

The IRSG, now known as the Soft Tissue Sarcoma Committee of the COG, developed a recurrence risk-based model to refine therapy in children. Favorable prognostic factors include absence of metastases; orbital, nonparameningeal head/neck, and GU nonbladder/non-prostate primary sites; grossly complete surgical removal of localized tumor at the time of diagnosis; embryonal/botryoid histology; tumor size ≤5 cm; and age younger than 10 years at diagnosis[67] (Table 13.3). Other classifications exist such as the one used in European RMS studies that define subgroups from A to H.[68] More recent COG protocols (ARST0431 and ARST1431) have a distinct risk-based classification with intermediate- and high-risk groups that were adapted to each protocol.

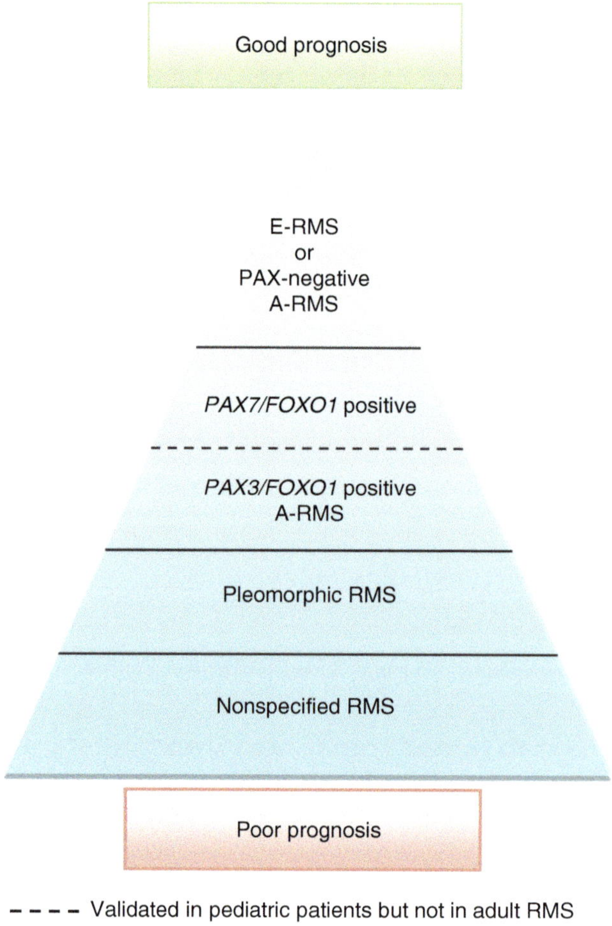

FIGURE 13.4 Prognosis of rhabdomyosarcoma according to histology and molecular biology.

A-RMS, alveolar RMS; E-RMS, embryonal RMS; RMS, rhabdomyosarcoma.

TREATMENT OF PEDIATRIC AND ADULT RMS

Common Treatment Strategies in Children and Adults

All patients diagnosed with RMS should be treated in experienced centers. The treatment strategy (type of treatment, timing, intensity) should be elaborated by a multidisciplinary sarcoma board that includes an experienced pathologist, a surgeon, a radiation oncologist, and a medical oncologist. Decisions should also be discussed directly with the patient. They often involve a multimodal approach that combines surgery, chemotherapy, and RT. Short- and long-term toxicities should be taken into consideration. All patients should be encouraged to participate in clinical trials.

Pediatric RMS

Micrometastatic disease is often present at diagnosis of RMS. The addition of chemotherapy and RT to surgery increased cures rates in children from 20% to 70%. Nowadays, treatment of pediatric RMS is based on chemotherapy in the neoadjuvant and adjuvant settings, surgery if possible, and RT to improve local control. Large cooperative international groups such as the COG in the United States and the more recently founded European Pediatric Soft Tissue Sarcoma Study Group (EpSSG) in Europe developed several multimodality treatment protocols based on the estimated risk of disease recurrence. Risk-adapted therapy uses prognostic tables such as the IRSG risk classification table (Table 13.3) to decide treatment strategy.[2,62,69]

TABLE 13.3 Rhabdomyosarcoma Prognostic Classification in Children According to the Intergroup Rhabdomyosarcoma Study Group Experience

Prognosis	Stage	Clinical Group	Site	Size	Age (Years)	Histology	Metastasis	Nodes
Excellent (>85%) Low-risk subset A	1	I	Favorable	a or b	<21	Fusion negative	M0	N0
	1	II	Favorable	a or b	<21	Fusion negative	M0	N0
	1	III	Orbit only	a or b	<21	Fusion negative	M0	N0
	2	I	Unfavorable	a	<21	Fusion negative	M0	N0 or Nx
	1	II	Favorable	a or b	<21	Fusion negative	M0	N1
Very good (70%–85%) Low-risk subset B	1	III	Orbit only	a or b	<21	Fusion negative	M0	N1
	1	III	Favorable, excluding orbit	a or b	<21	Fusion negative	M0	N0 or N1 or Nx
	2	II	Unfavorable	a	<21	Fusion negative	M0	N0 or Nx
	3	I or II	Unfavorable	a	<21	Fusion negative	M0	N1
	3	I or II	Unfavorable	b	<21	Fusion negative	M0	N0 or N1 or Nx
Good (50%–70%) Intermediate risk	2	III	Unfavorable	a	<21	Fusion negative	M0	N0 or Nx
	3	III	Unfavorable	a	<21	Fusion negative	M0	N1
	3	III	Unfavorable	b	<21	Fusion negative	M0	N0 or N1 or Nx
	1, 2, 3	I, II, III	Favorable or unfavorable	a or b	<21	Fusion positive	M0	N0 or N1 or Nx
	4	IV	Favorable or unfavorable	a or b	<10	Fusion negative	M1	N0 or N1 or Nx
Poor (<30%) High risk	4	IV	Favorable or unfavorable	a or b	≥10	Fusion negative	M1	N0 or N1 or Nx
	4	IV	Favorable or unfavorable	a or b	<21	Fusion positive	M1	N0 or N1 or Nx

Note: a, tumor size 5 cm in diameter; b, tumor size >5 cm in diameter; favorable site, orbit/eyelid, head and neck (excluding parameningeal), genitourinary (not bladder or prostate), and biliary tract; M0, no distant metastases; M1, distant metastases present; N0, regional nodes clinically not involved; N2, regional nodes clinically involved; Nx, node status unknown; unfavorable site, bladder, prostate, extremity, parameningeal, trunk, retroperitoneal, pelvis, other.

Source: Adapted with permission from Raney RB, Anderson JR, Barr FG, et al. Rhabdomyosarcoma and undifferentiated sarcoma in the first two decades of life: a selective review of intergroup Rhabdomyosarcoma Study Group Experience and rationale for Intergroup Rhabdomyosarcoma Study V. *J Pediatr Hematol Oncol*. 2001;23:215–220. doi:10.1097/00043426-200105000-00008. Copyright ©2001 Lippincott Williams & Wilkins.

Surgery

Patient outcomes depend on the extent of surgical resection, which should be complete in localized disease if functional and cosmetic results are acceptable. If a resection with negative margins is not possible or if RMS involves the orbit, biliary tract, or the GU tract (except for paratesticular RMS), neoadjuvant chemotherapy should be administered.

Clinically and radiographically suspicious LNs should be excised. Given the low risk of LN involvement, routine cervical sampling is not mandatory in head and neck tumors (except orbital tumors). On the other hand, up to 47% of adolescents with radiographically negative retroperitoneal LNs have pathologic documentation of LN metastasis. Therefore, all boys after the age of 10 with paratesticular

RMS should undergo ipsilateral nerve-sparing retroperitoneal LN dissection along with radical inguinal orchiectomy. Moreover, patients with positive nodes usually receive additional RT and cyclophosphamide, while those with negative nodes are only given a two-drug regimen (vincristine dactinomycin [VA]).[33,70] Sentinel LN biopsy is recommended in patients with extremity RMS.[71]

Re-excision should be considered in case of positive resection margins. Second-look surgery to document the histopathologic response to chemotherapy did not demonstrate any survival benefit. However, it may be considered in children with CG III disease to identify those who may benefit from reduced-dose RT.[72]

Survival advantage from resection of distant metastases has not been proved yet. The decision to perform metastasectomy should be thoroughly discussed at the tumor board on a case-by-case basis.

Radiation Therapy

RT is recommended for local control in all patients with RMS, except those who have embryonal/FN (any site) CG I disease. Three-dimensional (3D) conformal RT along with intensity-modulated RT should be privileged to minimize toxicities. Proton beam RT significantly reduces late toxicities in orbit and parameningeal tumors.[73] Tumor volume should include at least a 1-cm margin of normal tissue as well as involved LNs. Although no studies have shown a benefit for specific timing, radiation is usually initiated after four cycles of chemotherapy, even in patients with cranial nerve palsy or skull base erosion from parameningeal RMS.[74] Radiation doses are adapted according to the CG and the LN involvement. Several attempts to decrease RT doses to limit long-term toxicities in various tumor locations have been made, some with encouraging results. Craniospinal RT is indicated when tumor cells are found in the cerebrospinal fluid. Whole-brain RT should be delivered in case of several brain metastases and a negative CSF cytology. Brachytherapy should be considered for small critically located tumors (GU, head and neck).[75,76] In addition, RT may be used in metastatic disease to control both the primary and metastatic sites. Some protocols even recommend whole-lung RT (generally up to 14.4 Gy) for patients with multiple lung lesions.

Chemotherapy

All patients with RMS should receive chemotherapy along with local treatment. Chemotherapy may be administered both in the neoadjuvant setting (induction treatment) to facilitate subsequent surgery and to test for tumor chemosensitivity. It can also be given in the postoperative setting to eradicate micrometastases and prevent recurrence. A classic chemotherapy regimen in pediatric RMS includes an alkylating agent (cyclophosphamide or ifosfamide), vincristine, and dactinomycin. None of the trials performed since the 1970s has been able to identify a chemotherapy protocol more effective than vincristine, dactinomycin, and cyclophosphamide (VAC) or ifosfamide, vincristine, and dactinomycin (IVA).

Based on the COG studies, the VAC regimen is considered standard of care in North America. Intensification of VAC by adding other agents such as etoposide, ifosfamide, topotecan, melphalan, and doxorubicin failed to improve outcomes compared with VAC.[77,78] The ARST0531 trial compared the alternation of VAC and VI (vincristine and irinotecan) to standard VAC in patients with intermediate-risk disease (patients with nonmetastatic alveolar tumors and patients with stage 2 or 3, group III embryonal tumors). OS and EFS were similar between the two arms; however, the VAC/VI arm was associated with less hematologic toxicity and lower cumulative cyclophosphamide doses.[79]

On the other hand, the EpSSG replaces cyclophosphamide with ifosfamide because of the lower gonadal toxicity rates with the former. IVA is the European standard of care in pediatric RMS. The EpSSG RMS 2005 trial is the first multicenter, randomized controlled, open-label Phase 3 study that investigated the benefit of adding doxorubicin 30 mg/m^2 given as a 4-hour infusion on days 1 and 2 to a standard IVA regimen, as well as the benefit of a maintenance treatment in patients with high-risk localized disease. Unfortunately, no survival benefit was found and toxicity was worse in the IVA plus doxorubicin group (IVAdo).

Table 13.4 features the most commonly used regimens for pediatric RMS.

Treatment strategies according to risk group (North American experience) are discussed in the following sections (Exhibit 13.2). In all the risk groups, RT, when indicated, is usually started at week 13 of chemotherapy. Dose reductions are necessary for children younger than 3 years of age. Dactinomycin administration should be held during RT and resumed thereafter.

Low Risk

Subset A

This category includes embryonal and alveolar FN, stage 1/2, CG I/II tumors, as well as stage 1, CG III orbital tumors. Three-year failure-free survival (FFS) rate exceeds 85%.[80] Fifteen to sixteen cycles of

TABLE 13.4 Most Frequently Used Chemotherapy Regimens in Pediatric Rhabdomyosarcoma

Regimen	Drug and Dose	Schedule
VA (15 cycles, 45 weeks)[a]	• Vincristine 1.5 mg/m² (max 2 mg) • Dactinomycin 0.045 mg/kg (max 2.5 mg)	• Weekly during weeks 0 to 8, 12 to 20, 24 to 32, 36 to 44 • Every 3 weeks during weeks 0 through 45
VAC/VA (eight cycles, 24 weeks)[b]	• Vincristine 1.5 mg/m² (max 2 mg) • Dactinomycin 0.045 mg/kg (max 2.5 mg) • Cyclophosphamide 1,200 mg/m² with mesna and as needed hematopoietic growth factor support	• Weekly during weeks 1 to 9, 13 to 21 • Every 3 weeks during weeks 1 through 22 • Every 3 weeks during weeks 1 to 10 for a total of four doses
VAC (14 cycles, 40 weeks)[c]	• Vincristine 1.5 mg/m² (max 2 mg) • Dactinomycin 0.045 mg/kg (max 2.5 mg) • Cyclophosphamide 1,200 mg/m² with mesna and as needed hematopoietic growth factor support	• Weekly during weeks 1 to 13, 19 to 25, 31 to 37, 40 • Every 3 weeks during weeks 1 through 40 • Every 3 weeks during weeks 1 through 40
VAC/VI (14 cycles, 40 weeks)[d]	• Vincristine 1.5 mg/m² (max 2 mg) • Dactinomycin 0.045 mg/kg (max 2.5 mg) • Cyclophosphamide 1,200 mg/m² with mesna and as needed hematopoietic growth factor support • Irinotecan 50 mg/m² days 1 to 5	• On weeks 1 to 13, 16, 17, 19, 20, 22 to 26, 28, 31 to 34, 37, 38, 40 • On weeks 1, 7, 13, 22, 28, 34, 40 • On weeks 1, 7, 13, 22, 28, 34, 40 • On weeks 4, 10, 16, 19, 25, 31, 37
IVA (nine cycles, 27 weeks)[e]	• Ifosfamide 3 g/m², with mesna 3 g/m² • Vincristine 1.5 mg/m² • Dactinomycin 1.5 mg/m²	• 3-hour intravenous infusion on days 1 and 2 every 21 days • Weekly during the first 7 weeks then only on day 1 of each cycle • On day 1

[a]The IRSG D9602 protocol (1997–2004) objectives were to decrease toxicity in similar patients by RT doses and eliminate cyclophosphamide for the lowest-risk patients. Raney RB, Walterhouse DO, Meza JL, et al. Results of the Intergroup Rhabdomyosarcoma Study Group D9602 protocol, using vincristine and dactinomycin with or without cyclophosphamide and radiation therapy, for newly diagnosed patients with low-risk embryonal rhabdomyosarcoma: a report from the Soft Tissue Sarcoma Committee of the Children's Oncology Group. *J Clin Oncol.* 2011;29:1312–1318. doi:10.1200/JCO.2010.30.4469.

[b]Walterhouse DO, Pappo AS, Meza JL, et al. Shorter-duration therapy using vincristine, dactinomycin, and lower-dose cyclophosphamide with or without radiotherapy for patients with newly diagnosed low-risk rhabdomyosarcoma: a report from the Soft Tissue Sarcoma Committee of the Children's Oncology Group. *J Clin Oncol.* 2014;32:3547–3552. doi:10.1200/JCO.2014.55.6787.

[c]VAC doses and schedule are modified from the most recent COG protocol for intermediate-risk disease, ARST0531 Regimen A. Hawkins DS, Chi YY, Anderson JR, et al. Addition of vincristine and irinotecan to vincristine, dactinomycin, and cyclophosphamide does not improve outcome for intermediate-risk rhabdomyosarcoma: a report from the Children's Oncology Group. *J Clin Oncol.* 2018;36:2770–2777. doi:10.1200/JCO.2018.77.9694.

[d]VAC/VI doses and schedule are based on the COG protocol ARST1431. Hawkins DS, Chi YY, Anderson JR, et al. Addition of vincristine and irinotecan to vincristine, dactinomycin, and cyclophosphamide does not improve outcome for intermediate-risk rhabdomyosarcoma: a report from the Children's Oncology Group. *J Clin Oncol.* 2018;36:2770–2777. doi:10.1200/JCO.2018.77.9694.

[e]Bisogno G, Jenney M, Bergeron C, et al. Addition of dose-intensified doxorubicin to standard chemotherapy for rhabdomyosarcoma (EpSSG RMS 2005): a multicentre, open-label, randomised controlled, phase 3 trial. *Lancet Oncol.* 2018;19:1061–1071. doi:10.1016/S1470-2045(18)30337-1.

COG, Children's Oncology Group; IRSG, Intergroup Rhabdomyosarcoma Study Group; IVA, ifosfamide, vincristine, and dactinomycin; RT, radiation therapy; VA, vincristine dactinomycin; VAC, vincristine, dactinomycin, and cyclophosphamide; VI, vincristine and irinotecan.

VA (as per regimen D9602)[81] or four short cycles of VAC followed by four cycles of VA (as per regimen ARST0331)[82] could be administered.

Subset B

This subset includes nonorbit stage 1, CGIII or stage 3, CG I/II embryonal and alveolar FN tumors. Three-year FFS rate is around 70%.[83] Fourteen cycles of VAC as per ARST0531 regimen A are recommended.[79]

Intermediate Risk

This category includes the following:

- Stage 2, 3, CG III embryonal and alveolar FN tumors;
- Metastatic embryonal and alveolar FN tumors in children <10 years of age; and
- Alveolar FP tumors, CG I to III.

EXHIBIT 13.2 Rhabdomyosarcoma Consensus Treatment Algorithm Created by a Panel of Pediatric and Adolescent and Young Adult Sarcoma Experts

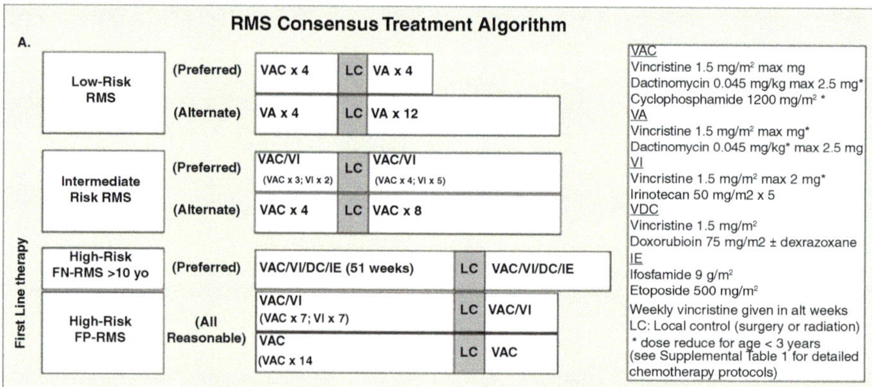

Up-Front Resection Radiation Recommendations

Surgical Group	Margin	Node	XRT (Gy)
I (FN-RMS)	Neg	N0	0
IIA (FP-RMS)	Neg	N0	36
IIA (N0)	Pos	N0	36
IIA (N1)	Neg	N1	36
IIC (N1)	Pos	N1	41.4
III (any)	N/A	Nx	50.4
III (orbit)	N/A	Nx	45 – 50.4

Delayed Resection Radiation Recommendations

Resection Margin	Node	XRT (Gy)
Neg.	N0	36
Microscopic	N0	41.4
	N1	41.4
No Resection or Gross residual*	Any	50.4

* Orbital RMS = 45 Gy and complete response to induction chemotherapy, otherwise 50.4 Gy

Note: N0, no evidence of nodal disease; N1, evidence of nodal disease; Nx, nodal disease status unknown.

FN, fusion negative; FP, fusion positive; IVA, ifosfamide, vincristine, and dactinomycin; RMS, rhabdomyosarcoma; RT, radiation therapy; SOC, standard of care therapy; VA, vincristine dactinomycin; VAC, vincristine, dactinomycin, and cyclophosphamide; VI, vincristine and irinotecan.

Source: Reproduced with permission from Borinstein SC, Steppan D, Hayashi M, et al. Consensus and controversies regarding the treatment of rhabdomyosarcoma. *Pediatr Blood Cancer*. 2018;65(2):e26809. doi:10.1002/pbc.26809.

Three-year EFS rate is between 50% and 70%. Also, 12 to 14 cycles of VAC or VAC/VI could be administered. There are not adequate data to conclude that VAC/VI is as effective. However, it is associated with less hematologic toxicity and fewer hospitalizations.[79] Tumors that have an alveolar histology but are FN should be treated with the VAC-only regimen.

Temsirolimus is currently being tested in combination with chemotherapy in a randomized Phase 3 study in patients with intermediate-risk RMS (Trial NCT02567435).

Maintenance chemotherapy using weekly intravenous vinorelbine plus daily oral cyclophosphamide resulted in a borderline significant improvement in 3-year EFS when compared to induction/adjuvant chemotherapy alone (78.4% vs. 72.3%, hazard ratio [HR]: 0.68, 95% confidence interval [95% CI]: 0.45–1.02, $p = .06$), but significantly better 3-year OS rate (86.5% vs. 73.7%, HR: 0.52, 95% CI: 0.32–0.86).[84] However, the latter results come from the EpSSG and cannot be extrapolated into the standard regimen for patients treated as per the COG guidelines.

High Risk

This category includes the following:

- Metastatic embryonal and alveolar FN tumors in patients older than 10 years of age
- Metastatic alveolar FP tumors

Five-year EFS rate is around 30% with standard therapy.[67] Fourteen cycles of VAC according to regimen A of the ARST0531 is the standard of care when patients cannot be included in clinical trials.

According to the results of two meta-analyses, high-dose chemotherapy followed by stem cell rescue failed to demonstrate survival advantage over conventional chemotherapy and had a greater risk of grade 3 and 4 adverse events.[85,86] It should not be administered outside the setting of a clinical trial.

Evaluation of Response

In the EpSSG protocols, response is usually assessed with appropriate imaging after three courses of chemotherapy. It is classified as follows:

- Complete response: absence of measurable tumor
- Good response: tumor volume reduction of more than two-thirds in relation to the initial volume

EXHIBIT 13.3 Treatment Response: Rhabdomyosarcoma Consensus Treatment Algorithm Created by a Panel of Pediatric and Adolescent and Young Adult Sarcoma Experts

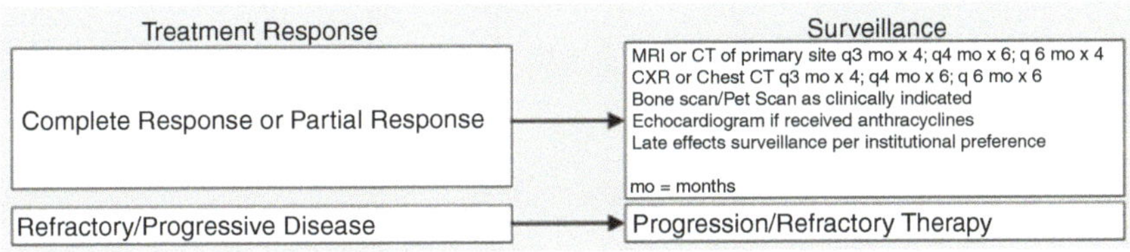

Source: Reproduced with permission from Borinstein SC, Steppan D, Hayashi M, et al. Consensus and controversies regarding the treatment of rhabdomyosarcoma. *Pediatr Blood Cancer*. 2018;65(2):e26809. doi:10.1002/pbc.26809.

- Poor response: volume reduction of more than one-third and less than two-thirds in relation to the initial volume
- Objective response: volume reduction of more than one-third in relation to the initial volume
- Progressive disease: volume increase of more than one-third or development of new lesions

Exhibit 13.3 suggests a surveillance plan after achieving complete or partial response. When volume reduction is less than 50%, chemotherapy intensification is considered.

On the other hand, interim imaging is not necessary in the COG protocols. Response rates are not correlated with outcomes and are not used for treatment intensification. In addition, complete response by cross-sectional imaging is seldom obtained, though PET scans show no signs of hypermetabolism. Management of residual hypermetabolic masses remains controversial; biopsy/resection of PET-avid masses in high-risk patients should be thoroughly discussed at the tumor board.

Treatment of Recurrent Disease

In most cases, RMS recurs within 2 years following diagnosis. Late relapses are rare (9%), and are especially frequent in patients with both advanced disease (Group III/IV) and large primary tumors at diagnosis (>5 cm).[87] Metastatic disease at relapse, previous use of alkylating agents and RT, alveolar histology, shorter time to relapse (within 18 months of diagnosis), and higher stage and CG at diagnosis were associated with a poor prognosis.[88,89] Exhibit 13.4 features a consensus treatment algorithm for relapsed RMS. Local therapy should always be considered. Less toxic regimens (cyclophosphamide, vinorelbine) should be administered in case of very advanced incurable relapses. The following treatments may be used in second-line setting (see Exhibit 13.4):

- Full VAC or VAC/VI regimen in patients who received VA or short course VAC in first line
- Doxorubicin, ifosfamide, and etoposide[90]
- Doxorubicin, ifosfamide, and dacarbazine (MAID)[91]
- Cyclophosphamide and topotecan[92]
- Cyclophosphamide, vinorelbine, and temsirolimus[93]

EXHIBIT 13.4 Relapsed rhabdomyosarcoma consensus treatment algorithm created by a panel of pediatric and adolescent and young adult sarcoma experts.

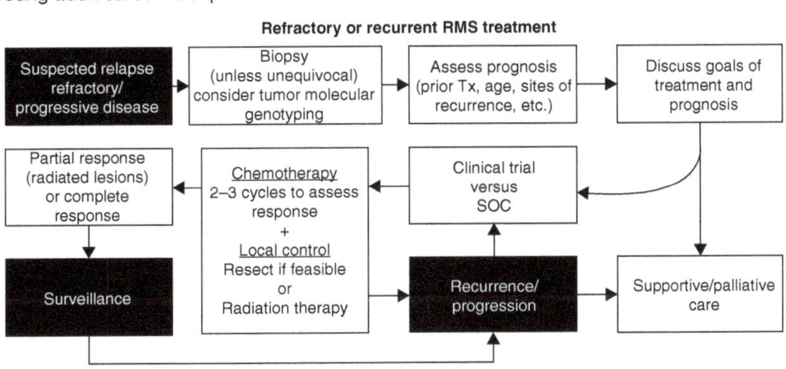

RMS, rhabdomyosarcoma; SOC, standard of care; Tx, treatment.

Source: Reproduced with permission from Borinstein SC, Steppan D, Hayashi M, et al. Consensus and controversies regarding the treatment of rhabdomyosarcoma. *Pediatr Blood Cancer*. 2018;65(2):e26809. doi:10.1002/pbc.26809.

Long-Term Complications

Long-term sequelae are common after multimodality treatment and require careful follow-up:

- Bowel and bladder complications: incontinence, frequency, hemorrhagic cystitis, primary hypogonadism
- Dentofacial abnormalities: bony hypoplasia/facial asymmetry, trismus, tooth/root agenesis, microdontia, enamel defects, and osteonecrosis
- Cardiac dysfunction: anthracyclines, high-dose cyclophosphamide
- Secondary tumors: leukemias, radiation-induced bone sarcomas
- Hypopituitarism following RT to the hypothalamic–pituitary area
- Cataracts and orbital hypoplasia in patients with orbital tumors

Adult RMS

In general, the same pediatric principles are adopted in the treatment of adult patients with RMS. Higher radiation doses are permitted in contrast to children who might develop late growth-related radiation sequelae. Selecting the optimal treatment sequence is yet to be determined. In a study by the French Sarcoma Group (FSG), patients older than 25 years of age received less chemotherapy and numerous treatments. While the 5-year survival in pediatric A/E-RMS has improved with time, the benefit did not extend to adult patients with A/E-RMS. The inferior results in adults could be due to advanced age and differences in clinical presentation or in intensity and duration of treatment. In addition, a molecular and genetic comparison between the two age groups might help explain this difference.

Surgery

R0 surgery remains the cornerstone of treatment in localized adult sarcoma, regardless of histology.[94–96] Univariate and multivariate analyses showed that the absence of surgery as well as incomplete resection were associated with worse outcomes, whereas adjuvant RT and the use of pediatric protocols were beneficial.[3] Furthermore, in the studies conducted by the FSG, MD Anderson Cancer Center, and the French Pediatric Society, local surgery showed survival benefit in advanced disease.[3,97,98] OS is also improved with RT in both localized and metastatic settings. These data suggest that local treatment strategies should always be debated even in the metastatic setting. However, patients often present with large-volume disease in "delicate" locations such as the head and neck, where R0 surgery and, in some cases, radiation are very complicated to perform and might result in devastating long-term sequelae.

Chemotherapy

Overall, RMS is a chemosensitive disease. Doxorubicin, vincristine, and ifosfamide remain the most potent chemotherapy agents. Other options, mainly for relapsed disease, include etoposide, dactinomycin, cyclophosphamide, irinotecan, melphalan, and temozolomide. Pediatric protocols have a positive impact on OS in patients with E-RMS and A-RMS.[3,98,99] In a retrospective analysis of 171 adult patients, results were similar to what has been reported in pediatric series when physicians adhered to the current guidelines for treatment of children.[100] However, P-RMS is not as sensitive to chemotherapy as A-RMS and E-RMS. In a small study, Bompas et al. failed to show a survival advantage of chemotherapy in localized P-RMS.[3] Wide surgical resection along with neoadjuvant/adjuvant RT is the pillar of therapy for localized pleomorphic disease. Unfortunately, outcomes with this approach result in high recurrence rates. Although not widely accepted, consideration should be given to neoadjuvant/adjuvant chemotherapy with vincristine 2 mg fixed dose, doxorubicin 75 to 90 mg/m^2 (72-hour infusion or bolus with dexrazoxane), and ifosfamide 10 g/m^2 (divided over 4–5 days with mesna uroprotection) for six cycles for patients with tumors >5 cm. Furthermore, unlike A-RMS and E-RMS and owing to the absence of positive survival data as well as the reduced tolerance to treatment in adults, pediatric regimens are not the treatment of choice in adult P-RMS. Doxorubicin alone or in combination with ifosfamide, as outlined above, remains the standard while awaiting new recommendations. Moreover, there is no current standard of care in older (>50 years of age) patients with A/E-RMS who will likely not tolerate pediatric protocols.

Neoadjuvant/Adjuvant Chemotherapy

Neoadjuvant chemotherapy recently achieved a survival benefit in high-risk patients with soft tissue sarcoma and is currently discussed at tumor boards before surgery.[101] Although found to result in disease-free survival and OS benefit, adjuvant chemotherapy is still a matter of debate at some centers.[102] Moreover, P-RMS is still regarded as refractory to standard chemotherapy; combination of surgery and RT for localized disease is the standard.

TABLE 13.5 **Chemotherapy Regimens Reported by the FSG Study**

Regimen*	Number of Patients (%) Total = 127	Agents
Adult protocols	**70 (55)**	
A	9 (13)	Adriamycin
MAI	23 (33)	Adriamycin ifosfamide
MAID	20 (28)	Adriamycin ifosfamide dacarbazine
MAIDO	1 (1.4)	Adriamycin ifosfamide dacarbazine vincristine
API	4 (6)	Adriamycin cisplatin ifosfamide
TNF-melphalan	1 (1.4)	TNF-melphalan
CYVADIC	4 (6)	Cyclophosphamide vincristine Adriamycin dacarbazine
AD	3 (4)	Adriamycin dacarbazine
EP	1 (1.4)	Etoposide cisplatin
IV	1 (1.4)	Ifosfamide vincristine
Trofosfamide	1 (1.4)	Trophosphamid
DECAV	1 (1.4)	Ifosfamide Adriamycin dacarbazine vindesine cisplatin
	1 (1.4)	Adriamycin vindesine ifosfamide cisplatin
Pediatric protocols	**52 (41)**	
IVA	9 (1.1)	Ifosfamide vincristine Adriamycin
VAC	14 (27)	Ifosfamide vincristine actinomycin
IVA/IVADo	6 (11.5)	Ifosfamide vincristine actinomycin doxorubicin
MAIDO/IVA/CEV	2 (3.8)	Ifosfamide vincristine actinomycin Adriamycin
IVAD	8 (15.3)	Ifosfamide vincristine Adriamycin dacarbazine
VIDE	2 (3.8)	Vincristine ifosfamide doxorubicin etoposide
IVA/IVE/CEV	3 (5.7)	Ifosfamide vincristine actinomycin etoposide carboplatin epirubicin
Protocol SIOP/MMT	6 (11.5)	
IVA/CEV	2 (3.8)	Ifosfamide vincristine actinomycin carboplatin epirubicin
NA	**5 (3)**	

*Drugs within these protocols are listed under Agents in this table.

FSG, French Sarcoma Group; TNF, tumor necrosis factor.

Source: From Bompas E, Campion L, Italiano A, et al. Outcome of 449 adult patients with rhabdomyosarcoma: an observational ambispective nationwide study. *Cancer Med*. 2018;7(8):4023–4035. doi:10.1002/cam4.1374.

Table 13.5 lists both adult and pediatric chemotherapy regimens used to treat adult RMS in France. Table 13.6 shows the most important studies about adult RMS. The majority of these studies are retrospective; survival results should therefore be interpreted with caution.[103–106]

RELAPSED DISEASE

According to the results of the FSG study, the relapse rate after multimodality treatment is between 33% and 57%. Metastatic disease is detected in 48% to 68% of relapsed cases. It mostly occurs during the first year, leading to death in 6 to 12 months with a median survival of 9, 8, and 7 months for patients with local relapse, metastatic relapse, and both, respectively. The dismal outcomes confirm the poor prognosis of adult RMS.[3] There is no current standard of care in second line. Few studies test the efficacy of chemotherapy agents and targeted therapies used in soft tissue sarcomas, such as gemcitabine, docetaxel, and pazopanib.[107,108]

TREATMENT OF ADULT RMS AT OUR INSTITUTION

All cases are discussed at the weekly sarcoma board, sometimes at the pediatric tumor board often in the presence of the patient. Patients are encouraged to enroll in clinical trials whenever possible. Owing

TABLE 13.6 Studies Conducted in Adult Rhabdomyosarcoma

Author (Year)[a]	Number of Patients	Age (Median)	Tumor Characteristics	Surgery	Chemotherapy	Radiation	Response Rate	EFS/PFS/OS
Sultan et al. (2009)[65]	1,071 adults	Age >19	Unfavorable site category: 65% M+: E-RMS: 20.4% A-RMS: 14.5% P-RMS: 19% Spindle cell: 1% NOS subtype: 43%	NA	NA	NA	NA	OS @ 5 y: 27%
Bompas et al. (2018)[3]	157 (retrospective cohort) Treated between 2010 and 2014	37	M+: 29% E-RMS: 21% A-RMS: 35% P-RMS: 44% EXT: 48% H&N: 25% GU: 9%	Surgery of primary: 69% (80% of M– patients and 41% of M+ patients)	81% Neoadjuvant 31% Adjuvant 23% Both 8%, palliative 18% PP: 53% of patients with A-RMS who received CT, 69% of E-RMS, and 12% of P-RMS	Retrospective: 68%	CR: 59% CR M–: 72% CR M+: 28%	@ 8.5 y: mOS 49 mo if CR+ mOS 9 mo if CR– ($p < .0001$) mOS 40 mo in M– mOS 13 mo in M+
Bompas et al. (2018)[3]	292 (prospective cohort) Treated between 2010 and 2014	55	M+: 70% E-RMS: 17% A-RMS: 18% P-RMS: 65% EXT: 38% H&N: 22%	NA	NA	NA	NA	mOS: A-RMS: 35 mo P-RMS: 37 mo E-RMS: not reached mPFS: A-RMS: 19 mo P-RMS: 11 mo E-RMS: 27 mo OS @ 5 y 30%
Hawkins et al. (2001)[103]	84 (1982–1999)	23	M+: 44% E-RMS: 51% A-RMS: 30% P-RMS: 17%	75%	92% Vincristine, dactinomycin, cyclophosphamide, ifosfamide, etoposide	63% EBRT: 49% Brachytherapy: 12%	NA	mDFS: 22 months OS 35% @ 5 y

Dumont et al. (2013)[98]	239 117 older than 20 (49%) (1957–2003)	19	M+: 32% E-RMS: 38% A-RMS: 23% P-RMS: 10% H&N: 44%	NA	100% Dactinomycin: 17% Ifosfamide: 26% Doxorubicin: 70%	NA	NA	mOS M–: 3.8 y mOS M+: 1.4 y OS @ 15 y: 14.4% in M+ disease + bimodality tx OS @ 14 y: 37.5% in M+ disease + trimodality tx mPFS 0.9 y
Esnaola et al. (2001)[104]	39 (1973–1996)	26	33% M+ E-RMS: 18% A-RMS: 56% P-RMS: 13% H&N: 33% EXT: 31%	54% Complete resection: 18%	95% VAC: 46% MAID: 35% Other ifosfamide-based regimen: 8% Other doxorubicin-based regimen: 11%	69% Median dose 55 Gy (range 30–66) Brachytherapy 5%	CR to chemo: 41% PR: 32% RR: 73%	OS @ 5 y: 31% OS @ 10 y: 27% M–: OS @ 5 y: 44% M+: OS @ 5 y: 0%
Little et al. (2002)[105]	82 (1960–1998)	27	M+: 10% E-RMS: 34% A-RMS: 23% P-RMS: 43% H&N: 52%	55%	71%	66%	ORR to chemo: 75%	DFS @ 10 y: 41% OS @ 10 y: 40% MFS @ 15 y: 53%
Ferrari (2003)[100,b]	171 (1975–2001)	27	M+: 17% E-RMS: 33% A-RMS: 34% P-RMS: 21% NOS: 12% H&N: 29% EXT: 27%	NA	72.5% 58% multidrug regimen containing cyclophosphamide or ifosfamide, in addition to doxorubicin, epirubicin, or dactinomycin; most regimens also included vincristine	61%	ORR to chemo 85%	EFS @ 5 y: 28% OS @ 5 y: 40%

(continued)

TABLE 13.6 **Studies Conducted in Adult Rhabdomyosarcoma** (*continued*)

Author (year)	Number of patients	Age (median)	Tumor characteristics	Surgery	Chemotherapy	Radiation	Response rate	EFS/PFS/OS
Gerber (2013)[99]	148 (1990–2011)	28	M+: 32% E-RMS: 54%, A-RMS: 33%, P-RMS: 12%, NOS RMS: 2% Parameningeal: 25% GU nonbladder non-prostate: 22%	NA	91% Cyclophosphamide, doxorubicin, vincristine: 58% VAC: 26% Others: AI, MAID	73%	NA	OS @ 5 y: 45% in M– OS @ 5 y for all cohort: 34%
Noujaim et al. (2015)[60]	45 (1995–2014)	71.5	M+ 28.9% P-RMS: 51.1%	81.3% of localized diseases	31.1% First-line palliative Multi-agent PP: 6.6% Ifosfamide–doxorubicin: 8.8% Single-agent doxorubicin: 15.5%	NA	NA	mOS M–: 12.8 mo mOS M+: 7.1 mo Relapse rate 53.8%[a] mPFS: 2.3 mo
Liu et al. (2019)[106]	20 (2004–2015)	34	M+ 20% H&N and paramenin-geal: 60% E-RMS: 15% A-RMS: 40% P-RMS: 45%	-	95% VAC-based chemotherapy in the majority of patients	65%	-	OS @ 3 y: 56.25% M– 0% M+

[a]Some patients also received dacarbazine, cisplatin, carboplatin, or etoposide, in addition to cyclophosphamide/ifosfamide and anthracyclines. Five patients received intrathecal methotrexate for parameningeal RMS, and four patients with metastases received high-dose chemotherapy. In 20 cases, chemotherapy did not include cyclophosphamide or ifosfamide (i.e., single-agent chemotherapy with doxorubicin or a two-agent regimen involving doxorubicin plus dacarbazine was used; both treatments were based on regimens used to treat adults with soft tissue sarcomas).

AP, adult protocol; A-RMS, alveolar RMS; CR, complete response; DFS, disease-free survival; EBRT, external beam radiation therapy; EFS, event-free survival; E-RMS, embryonal RMS; EXT, extremities; GU, genitourinary; H&N, head and neck; M+, metastatic disease; M–, nonmetastatic disease; MAID, Mesna, doxorubicin, ifosfamide, dacarbazine; mDFS, median DFS; MFS, metastasis-free survival; mOS, median overall survival; mPFS, median progression-free survival; NA, data not available; NOS, not otherwise specified; ORR, objective response rate; OS, overall survival; PFS, progression-free survival; PP, pediatric protocol; PR, partial response; P-RMS, pleomorphic RMS; RMS, rhabdomyosarcoma; RR, response rate; tx, treatment; VAC, vincristine, dactinomycin, cyclophosphamide.

to the postoperative sequelae that could be devastating, we have adopted a more conservative treatment approach. RT is almost always considered. The utility of induction chemotherapy is discussed at the tumor board in case of extensive surgery or risk of R2 disease. Neoadjuvant chemotherapy may improve local control and allow lowering of RT doses, which in turn reduces long-term complications. Embryonal and alveolar subtypes in fit adolescents and young adults are treated with pediatric regimens such as VAC or IVA. P-RMS or RMS in older adults is managed similarly to other soft tissue sarcomas. Adriamycin 60 mg/m^2 combined with ifosfamide 3 g/m^2 on days 1, 2, and 3 (Neo AI protocol) is the treatment of choice at our institution. Chest CT as well as adequate imaging of the primary location of the disease is performed every two to three cycles. Patients are regularly assessed for potential R0 surgery. Isolated limb perfusion, palliative and stereotactic RT, as well as interventional radiology procedures (radiofrequency, cryoablation) are often used to treat symptomatic or critical sites in both oligometastatic and widespread disease.

SUMMARY

RMS is a rare, complex disease with poor outcomes, especially in adults and relapsed cases. Studies are scarce and mostly retrospective. Multidisciplinary management at a sarcoma center and participation in clinical trials are crucial to improve survival and quality of life. Pediatric and adult patients should be referred to expert sarcoma centers and enrolled in clinical trials whenever possible.

Overall, there are four subtypes of RMS: embryonic, alveolar, spindle cell/sclerosing, and pleomorphic. Adult patients achieve worse outcomes due to several factors: increased prevalence of the more aggressive pleomorphic subtype (up to 43% of cases), delayed disease presentation and access to care in expert centers, poor adherence to aggressive treatment regimens, potential pharmacokinetic differences, and limited accrual on clinical trials. Furthermore, all patients with RMS should undergo molecular testing for *PAX/FOXO1* fusions, which are present in 75% of A-RMS and are associated with worse outcomes. Note that A-RMS with absence of *FOXO1* translocation behaves more like E-RMS. Nonpleomorphic RMS should rather be classified as FP or FN disease.

The most common metastatic locations are the LNs, lungs, cortical bone, and bone marrow. A risk-specific rather than a disease-specific approach to staging should be considered. Surgery is essential to the optimal management of RMS in all stages and risk groups. Induction chemotherapy is required when complete resection of the primary is impossible or results in significant morbidity. Adjuvant RT is recommended for all patients, except those with margin-negative E-RMS/FN A-RMS. Resection quality, *FOXO1* fusion status, nodal disease, and tumor site and size help determine radiation doses.

Standard chemotherapy regimens include VAC/IVA in pediatric patients and in adults with nonpleomorphic RMS. Although no formal trials have tested the efficacy of chemotherapy regimens in adult RMS patients, some sarcoma centers utilize the combination vincristine, doxorubicin, and ifosfamide. Because P-RMS behaves similarly to adult soft tissue sarcomas, chemotherapy with an anthracycline and alkylating agents (±vincristine) is usually administered (neo VAI). Relapsed/refractory disease is most often fatal. Standard of care is still lacking.

CASE STUDY

A 29-year-old man with no significant past medical history presented to ear, nose, and throat clinic with right hemifacial swelling, headaches, blurry vision, and enlarged cervical LNs. MRI of the face showed a right ethmoidal mass extending into the frontal and right maxillary sinuses. CT scan of the head, neck, chest, abdomen, and pelvis additionally showed right cervical and supraclavicular lymphadenopathies along with two lung nodules located in the middle and left lower lobes (Figure 13.5). An ultrasound-guided core-needle biopsy of a right submandibular LN revealed poorly differentiated small, round tumor cells with positive expression of desmin and myogenin on IHC. The pathologic aspect was in favor of grade II A-RMS. 18-FDG PET-CT scan did not show any distant hypermetabolic lesions. The case was discussed at the weekly sarcoma board. Given the rapidly progressive symptoms, chemotherapy combining doxorubicin (60 mg/m^2 on day 2) and ifosfamide (3 g/m^2 on days 2, 3, and 4) was decided and initiated rapidly, while awaiting molecular confirmation of diagnosis (neo AI regimen). A significant reduction

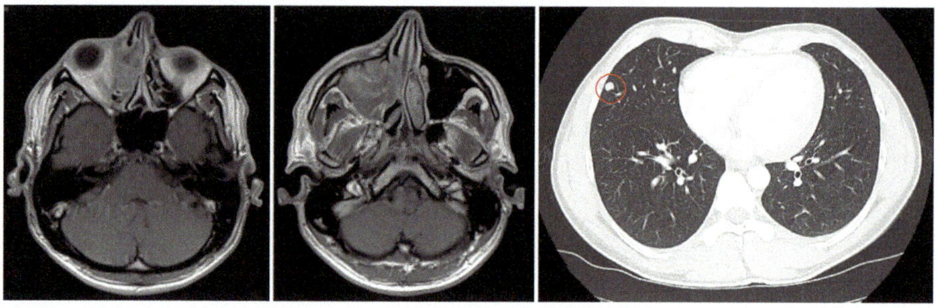

(A) (B) (C)

FIGURE 13.5 Right ethmoidal mass (A and B) with right middle lobe nodule (C).

of facial swelling and shrinking of cervical nodes were observed after the first cycle. The diagnosis of locally advanced A-RMS was later confirmed when RT-PCR revealed the presence of a *PAX3–FOXO1* fusion. The chemotherapy regimen was therefore switched from neo AI to IVAdo (ifosfamide 3 g/m^2 on days 1 and 2, dactinomycin 1.5 mg/m^2 on day 1, doxorubicin 30 mg/m^2 on days 1 and 2, and vincristine 1.5 mg/m^2 on days 1, 8, and 15). The patient received two cycles of neo AI followed by four cycles of IVAdo. The last cycle was administered without doxorubicin because of an altered left ventricular ejection fraction. A very good local partial response was obtained both clinically and radiologically. However, the lung nodules remained unchanged. After discussion at the sarcoma, head and neck, and pediatric tumor boards, a radical surgical treatment was abandoned, given the probability of metastatic disease in the lungs. The patient was instead treated with RT to the head and neck regions (70 Gy ethmoidal residue, 60 Gy tumor and LN, 33 fractions). He also received three cycles of ifosfamide, two of which were given concomitantly with RT (vincristine discontinued owing to grade 3 peripheral neuropathy, dactinomycin discontinued owing to the risk of toxicity when given with RT). After that, he underwent a wedge resection by video thoracoscopic surgery of the right middle lobe pulmonary nodule. Histologic analysis revealed a 0.8-cm hamartochondroma and no signs of malignancy. Maintenance treatment with oral vinorelbine and cyclophosphamide was given for 12 months. The patient was last seen 4 months after the end of oral chemotherapy. He was in a very good clinical condition, and imaging exams showed no signs of local or metastatic progression.

Commentary: In this case, you can see that RMS management slightly differed from the recommendations we stated in this chapter. However, the main elements are present, that is, multidisciplinary decision-making, induction chemotherapy, and evaluation for a local treatment upon response to initial chemotherapy.

REFERENCES

1. Pastore G, Peris-Bonet R, Carli M, et al. Childhood soft tissue sarcomas incidence and survival in European children (1978–1997): report from the Automated Childhood Cancer Information System project. *Eur J Cancer*. 2006;42:2136–2149. doi:10.1016/j.ejca.2006.05.016
2. Punyko JA, Mertens AC, Baker KS, et al. Long-term survival probabilities for childhood rhabdomyosarcoma. A population-based evaluation. *Cancer*. 2005;103(7):1475–1483. doi:10.1002/cncr.20929
3. Bompas E, Campion L, Italiano A, et al. Outcome of 449 adult patients with rhabdomyosarcoma: an observational ambispective nationwide study. *Cancer Med*. 2018;7(8):4023–4035. doi:10.1002/cam4.1374
4. Stiller CA, McKinney PA, Bunch KJ, et al. Childhood cancer and ethnic group in Britain: a United Kingdom Children's Cancer Study Group (UKCCSG) study. *Br J Cancer*. 1991;64(3):543–548. doi:10.1038/bjc.1991.347
5. Grufferman S, Schwartz AG, Ruymann FB, Maurer HM. Parents' use of cocaine and marijuana and increased risk of rhabdomyosarcoma in their children. *Cancer Causes Control*. 1993;4(3):217–224. doi:10.1007/bf00051316
6. Grufferman S, Wang HH, DeLong ER, et al. Environmental factors in the etiology of rhabdomyosarcoma in childhood. *J Natl Cancer Inst*. 1982;68(1):107–113. doi:10.1093/jnci/68.1.107
7. Magnani C, Pastore G, Luzzatto L, et al. Risk factors for soft tissue sarcomas in childhood: a case-control study. *Tumori*. 1989;75(4):396–400. doi:10.1177/030089168907500418
8. Lupo PJ, Zhou R, Skapek SX, et al. Allergies, atopy, immune-related factors and childhood rhabdomyosarcoma: a report from the Children's Oncology Group. *Int J Cancer*. 2014;134(2):431–436. doi:10.1002/ijc.28363

9. Sankaran H, Danysh HE, Scheurer ME, et al. The role of childhood infections and immunizations on childhood rhabdomyosarcoma: a report from the Children's Oncology Group. *Pediatr Blood Cancer*. 2016;63(9):1557–1562. doi:10.1002/pbc.26065
10. Von Behren J, Spector LG, Mueller BA, et al. Birth order and risk of childhood cancer: a pooled analysis from five US states. *Int J Cancer*. 2011;128(11):2709–2716. doi:10.1002/ijc.25593
11. Zhang J, Nichols KE, Downing JR. Germline mutations in predisposition genes in pediatric cancer. *N Engl J Med*. 2016;374:1391. doi:10.1056/NEJMc1600338
12. Ruymann FB, Maddux HR, Ragab A, et al. Congenital anomalies associated with rhabdomyosarcoma: an autopsy study of 115 cases. A report from the Intergroup Rhabdomyosarcoma Study Committee (representing the Children's Cancer Study Group, the Pediatric Oncology Group, the United Kingdom Children's Cancer Study Group, and the Pediatric Intergroup Statistical Center). *Med Pediatr Oncol*. 1988;16(1):33–39. doi:10.1002/mpo.2950160109
13. Malkin D, Li FP, Strong LC, et al. Germ line p53 mutations in a familial syndrome of breast cancer, sarcomas, and other neoplasms. *Science*. 1990;250(4985):1233–1238. doi:10.1126/science.1978757
14. Diller L, Sexsmith E, Gottlieb A, et al. Germline p53 mutations are frequently detected in young children with rhabdomyosarcoma. *J Clin Invest*. 1995;95(4):1606–1611. doi:10.1172/JCI117834
15. Hettmer S, Archer NM, Somers GR, et al. Anaplastic rhabdomyosarcoma in TP53 germline mutation carriers. *Cancer*. 2014;120(7):1068–1075. doi:10.1002/cncr.28507
16. Steenman M, Westerveld A, Mannens M. Genetics of Beckwith-Wiedemann syndrome-associated tumors: common genetic pathways. *Genes Chromosomes Cancer*. 2000;28(1):1–13. doi:10.1002/(sici)1098-2264(200005)28:1<1::aid-gcc1>3.0.co;2-#
17. Aoki Y, Niihori T, Kawame H, et al. Germline mutations in HRAS proto-oncogene cause Costello syndrome. *Nat Genet*. 2005;37(10):1038–1040. doi:10.1038/ng1641
18. Feingold M. Costello syndrome and rhabdomyosarcoma. *J Med Genet*. 1999;36(7):582–583. https://jmg.bmj.com/content/36/7/582
19. Franceschini P, Licata D, Di Cara G, et al. Bladder carcinoma in Costello syndrome: report on a patient born to consanguineous parents and review. *Am J Med Genet*. 1999;86(2):174–179. doi:10.1002/(SICI)1096-8628(19990910)86:2<174::AID-AJMG17>3.0.CO;2-Y
20. Gripp KW, Scott CI Jr, Nicholson L, et al. Five additional Costello syndrome patients with rhabdomyosarcoma: proposal for a tumor screening protocol. *Am J Med Genet*. 2002;108(1):80–87. doi:10.1002/ajmg.10241
21. Menke J, Pauli S, Sigler M, et al. Uniparental trisomy of a mutated HRAS proto-oncogene in embryonal rhabdomyosarcoma of a patient with Costello syndrome. *J Clin Oncol*. 2015;33:e62–e65. doi:10.1200/JCO.2013.49.6539
22. Quezada E, Gripp KW. Costello syndrome and related disorders. *Curr Opin Pediatr*. 2007;19(6):636–644. doi:10.1097/MOP.0b013e3282f161dc
23. Sung L, Anderson JR, Arndt C, et al. Neurofibromatosis in children with rhabdomyosarcoma: a report from the Intergroup Rhabdomyosarcoma study IV. *J Pediatr*. 2004;144:666–668. doi:10.1016/j.jpeds.2004.02.026
24. Doros L, Yang J, Dehner L, et al. DICER1 mutations in embryonal rhabdomyosarcomas from children with and without familial PPB-tumor predisposition syndrome. *Pediatr Blood Cancer*. 2012;59(3):558–560. doi:10.1002/pbc.24020
25. Stewart DR, Best AF, Williams GM, et al. Neoplasm risk among individuals with a pathogenic germline variant in DICER1. *J Clin Oncol*. 2019;37:668–676. doi:10.1200/JCO.2018.78.4678
26. Miller RW, Rubinstein JH. Tumors in Rubinstein-Taybi syndrome. *Am J Med Genet*. 1995;56(1):112–115. doi:10.1002/ajmg.1320560125
27. Sobel RA, Woerner S. Rubinstein-Taybi syndrome and nasopharyngeal rhabdomyosarcoma. *J Pediatr*. 1981;99(6):1000–1001. doi:10.1016/s0022-3476(81)80043-1
28. Beddis IR, Mott MG, Bullimore J. Case report: nasopharyngeal rhabdomyosarcoma and Gorlin's naevoid basal cell carcinoma syndrome. *Med Pediatr Oncol*. 1983;11(3):178–179.
29. Bresler SC, Padwa BL, Granter SR. Nevoid basal cell carcinoma syndrome (Gorlin syndrome). *Head Neck Pathol*. 2016;10(2):119–124.
30. Months SR, Raney RB. Rhabdomyosarcoma of the head and neck in children: the experience at the Children's Hospital of Philadelphia. *Med Pediatr Oncol*. 1986;14(5):288–292. doi:10.1002/mpo.2950140508
31. Hicks J, Flaitz C. Rhabdomyosarcoma of the head and neck in children. *Oral Oncol*. 2002;38(5):450–459. doi:10.1016/s1368-8375(01)00105-1
32. Shapiro E, Strother D. Pediatric genitourinary rhabdomyosarcoma. *J Urol*. 1992;148(6):1761–1768. doi:10.1016/s0022-5347(17)37023-4
33. Wiener ES, Anderson JR, Ojimba JI, et al. Controversies in the management of paratesticular rhabdomyosarcoma: is staging retroperitoneal lymph node dissection necessary for adolescents with resected paratesticular rhabdomyosarcoma? *Semin Pediatr Surg*. 2001;10:146–152. doi:10.1053/spsu.2001.24695
34. Breneman JC, Lyden E, Pappo AS, et al. Prognostic factors and clinical outcomes in children and adolescents with metastatic rhabdomyosarcoma—a report from the Intergroup Rhabdomyosarcoma Study IV. *J Clin Oncol*. 2003;21:78–84. doi:10.1200/JCO.2003.06.129
35. Koscielniak E, Rodary C, Flamant F, et al. Metastatic rhabdomyosarcoma and histologically similar tumors in childhood: a retrospective European multi-center analysis. *Med Pediatr Oncol*. 1992;20(3):209–214. doi:10.1002/mpo.2950200305

36. Raney RB Jr, Tefft M, Maurer HM, et al. Disease patterns and survival rate in children with metastatic soft-tissue sarcoma. A report from the Intergroup Rhabdomyosarcoma Study (IRS)-I. *Cancer*. 1988;62(7):1257–1266. doi:10.1002/1097-0142(19881001)62:7<1257::aid-cncr2820620703>3.0.co;2-k
37. Ruymann FB, Newton WA Jr, Ragab AH, et al. Bone marrow metastases at diagnosis in children and adolescents with rhabdomyosarcoma. A report from the intergroup rhabdomyosarcoma study. *Cancer*. 1984;53(2):368–373. doi:10.1002/1097-0142(19840115)53:2<368::aid-cncr2820530233>3.0.co;2-3
38. Weiss AR, Lyden ER, Anderson JR, et al. Histologic and clinical characteristics can guide staging evaluations for children and adolescents with rhabdomyosarcoma: a report from the Children's Oncology Group Soft Tissue Sarcoma Committee. *J Clin Oncol*. 2013;31:3226–3232. doi:10.1200/JCO.2012.44.6476
39. Pohar-Marinsek Z. Difficulties in diagnosing small round cell tumours of childhood from fine needle aspiration cytology samples. *Cytopathology*. 2008;19:67–79. doi:10.1111/j.1365-2303.2008.00555.x
40. Qualman SJ, Coffin CM, Newton WA, et al. Intergroup Rhabdomyosarcoma Study: update for pathologists. *Pediatr Dev Pathol*. 1998;1:550–561. doi:10.1007/s100249900076
41. Wachtel M, Runge T, Leuschner I, et al. Subtype and prognostic classification of rhabdomyosarcoma by immunohistochemistry. *J Clin Oncol*. 2006;24:816–822. doi:10.1200/JCO.2005.03.4934
42. Dias P, Chen B, Dilday B, et al. Strong immunostaining for myogenin in rhabdomyosarcoma is significantly associated with tumors of the alveolar subclass. *Am J Pathol*. 2000;156(2):399–408. doi:10.1016/S0002.-9440(10)64743-8
43. Heerema-McKenney A, Wijnaendts LCD, Pulliam JF, et al. Diffuse myogenin expression by immunohistochemistry is an independent marker of poor survival in pediatric rhabdomyosarcoma: a tissue microarray study of 71 primary tumors including correlation with molecular phenotype. *Am J Surg Pathol*. 2008;32(10):1513–1522. doi:10.1097/PAS.0b013e31817a909a
44. Borinstein SC, Steppan D, Hayashi M, et al. Consensus and controversies regarding the treatment of rhabdomyosarcoma. *Pediatr Blood Cancer*. 2018;65(2):e26809. doi:10.1002/pbc.26809
45. Rudzinski ER, Anderson JR, Hawkins DS, et al. The World Health Organization classification of skeletal muscle tumors in pediatric rhabdomyosarcoma: a report from the Children's Oncology Group. *Arch Pathol Lab Med*. 2015;139(10):1281–1287. doi:10.5858/arpa.2014-0475-OA
46. El-Badry OM, Minniti C, Kohn EC, et al. Insulin-like growth factor II acts as an autocrine growth and motility factor in human rhabdomyosarcoma tumors. *Cell Growth Differ*. 1990;1:325–331. http://cgd.aacrjournals.org/cgi/reprint/1/7/325
47. Kalebic T, Tsokos M, Helman LJ. *In vivo* treatment with antibody against IGF-1 receptor suppresses growth of human rhabdomyosarcoma and down-regulates $p34^{cdc2}$. *Cancer Res*. 1994;54(21):5531–5534. https://cancerres.aacrjournals.org/content/54/21/5531.full-text.pdf
48. Scrable H, Witte D, Shimada H, et al. Molecular differential pathology of rhabdomyosarcoma. *Genes Chromosomes Cancer*. 1989;1(1):23–35. doi:10.1002/gcc.2870010106
49. Scrable HJ, Witte DP, Lampkin BC, Cavenee WK. Chromosomal localization of the human rhabdomyosarcoma locus by mitotic recombination mapping. *Nature*. 1987;329:645–647. doi:10.1038/329645a0
50. Agaram NP, Chen CL, Zhang L, et al. Recurrent MYOD1 mutations in pediatric and adult sclerosing and spindle cell rhabdomyosarcomas: evidence for a common pathogenesis. *Genes Chromosomes Cancer*. 2014;53(9):779–787. doi:10.1002/gcc.22187
51. Alaggio R, Zhang L, Sung YS, et al. A molecular study of pediatric spindle and sclerosing rhabdomyosarcoma: identification of novel and recurrent VGLL2-related fusions in infantile cases. *Am J Surg Pathol*. 2016;40(2):224–235. doi:10.1097/PAS.0000000000000538
52. Galili N, Davis RJ, Fredericks WJ, et al. Fusion of a fork head domain gene to PAX3 in the solid tumour alveolar rhabdomyosarcoma. *Nat Genet*. 1993;5(3):230–235. doi:10.1038/ng1193-230
53. Shapiro DN, Sublett JE, Li B, et al. Fusion of PAX3 to a member of the forkhead family of transcription factors in human alveolar rhabdomyosarcoma. *Cancer Res*. 1993;53(21):5108–5112. https://cancerres.aacrjournals.org/content/53/21/5108.full-text.pdf
54. Davis RJ, D'Cruz CM, Lovell MA, et al. Fusion of *PAX7* to *FKHR* by the variant t(1;13)(p36;q14) translocation in alveolar rhabdomyosarcoma. *Cancer Res*. 1994;54(11):2869–2872. https://cancerres.aacrjournals.org/content/54/11/2869.full-text.pdf
55. Kephart JJG, Tiller RGJ, Crose LES, et al. Secreted Frizzled-Related Protein 3 (SFRP3) is required for tumorigenesis of PAX3-FOXO1-positive alveolar rhabdomyosarcoma. *Clin Cancer Res*. 2015;21:4868–4880. doi:10.1158/1078-0432.CCR-14-1797
56. Skapek SX, Anderson J, Barr FG, et al. PAX-FOXO1 fusion status drives unfavorable outcome for children with rhabdomyosarcoma: a children's oncology group report. *Pediatr Blood Cancer*. 2013;60(9):1411–1417. doi:10.1002/pbc.24532
57. Sorensen PHB, Lynch JC, Qualman SJ, et al. PAX3-FKHR and PAX7-FKHR gene fusions are prognostic indicators in alveolar rhabdomyosarcoma: a report from the children's oncology group. *J Clin Oncol*. 2002;20:2672–2679. doi:10.1200/JCO.2002.03.137
58. Parham DM, Qualman SJ, Teot L, et al. Correlation between histology and PAX/FKHR fusion status in alveolar rhabdomyosarcoma: a report from the Children's Oncology Group. *Am J Surg Pathol*. 2007;31(6):895–901. doi:10.1097/01.pas.0000213436.99492.51

59. Williamson D, Missiaglia E, Reyniès A, et al. Fusion gene-negative alveolar rhabdomyosarcoma is clinically and molecularly indistinguishable from embryonal rhabdomyosarcoma. *J Clin Oncol*. 2010;28:2151–2158. doi:10.1200/JCO.2009.26.3814
60. Noujaim J, Thway K, Jones RL, et al. Adult pleomorphic rhabdomyosarcoma: a multicentre retrospective study. *Anticancer Res*. 2015;35(11):6213–6217. http://ar.iiarjournals.org/content/35/11/6213.full
61. Lawrence W, Anderson JR, Gehan EA, Maurer H. Pretreatment TNM staging of childhood rhabdomyosarcoma: a report of the Intergroup Rhabdomyosarcoma Study Group. *Cancer*. 1997;80:1165–1170. doi:10.1002/(sici)1097-0142(19970915)80:6<1165::aid-cncr21>3.0.co;2-5
62. Crist W, Gehan EA, Ragab AH, et al. The third intergroup rhabdomyosarcoma study. *J Clin Oncol*. 1995;13:610–630. doi:10.1200/JCO.1995.13.3.610
63. Crist WM, Garnsey L, Beltangady MS, et al. Prognosis in children with rhabdomyosarcoma: a report of the intergroup rhabdomyosarcoma studies I and II. Intergroup Rhabdomyosarcoma Committee. *J Clin Oncol*. 1990;8:443–452. doi:10.1200/JCO.1990.8.3.443
64. Crist WM, Anderson JR, Meza JL, et al. Intergroup rhabdomyosarcoma study-IV: results for patients with nonmetastatic disease. *J Clin Oncol*. 2001;19:3091–3102. doi:10.1200/JCO.2001.19.12.3091
65. Sultan I, Qaddoumi I, Yaser S, et al. Comparing adult and pediatric rhabdomyosarcoma in the surveillance, epidemiology and end results program, 1973 to 2005: an analysis of 2,600 patients. *J Clin Oncol*. 2009;27:3391–3397. doi:10.1200/JCO.2008.19.7483
66. Oberlin O, Rey A, Lyden E, et al. Prognostic factors in metastatic rhabdomyosarcomas: results of a pooled analysis from United States and European cooperative groups. *J Clin Oncol*. 2008;26:2384–2389. doi:10.1200/JCO.2007.14.7207
67. Raney RB, Anderson JR, Barr FG, et al. Rhabdomyosarcoma and undifferentiated sarcoma in the first two decades of life: a selective review of intergroup Rhabdomyosarcoma Study Group experience and rationale for Intergroup Rhabdomyosarcoma Study V. *J Pediatr Hematol Oncol*. 2001;23(4):215–220. doi:10.1097/00043426-200105000-00008
68. Sultan I, Ferrari A. Selecting multimodal therapy for rhabdomyosarcoma. *Expert Rev Anticancer Ther*. 2010;10(8):1285–1301. doi:10.1586/era.10.96
69. Sutow WW, Sullivan MP, Ried HL, et al. Prognosis in childhood rhabdomyosarcoma. *Cancer*. 1970;25(6):1384–1390. doi:10.1002/1097-0142(197006)25:6<1384::aid-cncr2820250617>3.0.co;2-t
70. Walterhouse DO, Barkauskas DA, Hall D, et al. Demographic and treatment variables influencing outcome for localized paratesticular rhabdomyosarcoma: results from a pooled analysis of North American and European Cooperative Groups. *J Clin Oncol*. 2018;36:JCO2018789388. doi:10.1200/JCO.2018.78.9388
71. McMulkin HM, Yanchar NL, Fernandez CV, Giacomantonio C. Sentinel lymph node mapping and biopsy: a potentially valuable tool in the management of childhood extremity rhabdomyosarcoma. *Pediatr Surg Int*. 2003;19:453–456. doi:10.1007/s00383-003-0956-y
72. Rodeberg DA, Wharam MD, Lyden ER, et al. Delayed primary excision with subsequent modification of radiotherapy dose for intermediate-risk rhabdomyosarcoma: a report from the Children's Oncology Group Soft Tissue Sarcoma Committee. *Int J Cancer*. 2015;137:204–211. doi:10.1002/ijc.29351
73. Ladra MM, Szymonifka JD, Mahajan A, et al. Preliminary results of a phase II trial of proton radiotherapy for pediatric rhabdomyosarcoma. *J Clin Oncol*. 2014;32:3762–3770. doi:10.1200/JCO.2014.56.1548
74. Spalding AC, Hawkins DS, Donaldson SS, et al. The effect of radiation timing on patients with high-risk features of parameningeal rhabdomyosarcoma: an analysis of IRS-IV and D9803. *Int J Radiat Oncol Biol Phys*. 2013;87:512–516. doi:10.1016/j.ijrobp.2013.07.003
75. Magné N, Oberlin O, Martelli H, et al. Vulval and vaginal rhabdomyosarcoma in children: update and reappraisal of Institut Gustave Roussy brachytherapy experience. *Int J Radiat Oncol Biol Phys*. 2008;72:878–883. doi:10.1016/j.ijrobp.2008.01.034
76. Nag S, Cano ER, Demanes DJ, et al. The American Brachytherapy Society recommendations for high-dose-rate brachytherapy for head-and-neck carcinoma. *Int J Radiat Oncol Biol Phys*. 2001;50:1190–1198. doi:10.1016/s0360-3016(01)01567-x
77. Arndt CAS, Stoner JA, Hawkins DS, et al. Vincristine, actinomycin, and cyclophosphamide compared with vincristine, actinomycin, and cyclophosphamide alternating with vincristine, topotecan, and cyclophosphamide for intermediate-risk rhabdomyosarcoma: children's oncology group study D9803. *J Clin Oncol*. 2009;27:5182–5188. doi:10.1200/JCO.2009.22.3768
78. Sandler E, Lyden E, Ruymann F, et al. Efficacy of ifosfamide and doxorubicin given as a phase II "window" in children with newly diagnosed metastatic rhabdomyosarcoma: a report from the Intergroup Rhabdomyosarcoma Study Group. *Med Pediatr Oncol*. 2001;37:442–448. doi:10.1002/mpo.1227
79. Hawkins DS, Chi YY, Anderson JR, et al. Addition of vincristine and irinotecan to vincristine, dactinomycin, and cyclophosphamide does not improve outcome for intermediate-risk rhabdomyosarcoma: a report from the Children's Oncology Group. *J Clin Oncol*. 2018;36:2770–2777. doi:10.1200/JCO.2018.77.9694
80. Ferrer FA, Isakoff M, Koyle MA. Bladder/prostate rhabdomyosarcoma: past, present and future. *J Urol*. 2006;176:1283–1291. doi:10.1016/j.juro.2006.06.019
81. Raney RB, Walterhouse DO, Meza JL, et al. Results of the Intergroup Rhabdomyosarcoma Study Group D9602 protocol, using vincristine and dactinomycin with or without cyclophosphamide and radiation therapy, for newly diagnosed patients with low-risk embryonal rhabdomyosarcoma: a report from the Soft Tissue Sarcoma Committee of the Children's Oncology Group. *J Clin Oncol*. 2011;29:1312–1318. doi:10.1200/JCO.2010.30.4469

82. Walterhouse DO, Pappo AS, Meza JL, et al. Shorter-duration therapy using vincristine, dactinomycin, and lower-dose cyclophosphamide with or without radiotherapy for patients with newly diagnosed low-risk rhabdomyosarcoma: a report from the Soft Tissue Sarcoma Committee of the Children's Oncology Group. *J Clin Oncol*. 2014;32:3547–3552. doi:10.1200/JCO.2014.55.6787
83. Walterhouse DO, Pappo AS, Meza JL, et al. Reduction of cyclophosphamide dose for patients with subset 2 low-risk rhabdomyosarcoma is associated with an increased risk of recurrence: a report from the Soft Tissue Sarcoma Committee of the Children's Oncology Group. *Cancer*. 2017;123:2368–2375. doi:10.1002/cncr.30613
84. Bisogno G, De Salvo GL, Bergeron C, et al. Maintenance low-dose chemotherapy in patients with high-risk (HR) rhabdomyosarcoma (RMS): a report from the European Paediatric Soft Tissue Sarcoma Study Group (EpSSG). *J. Clin Oncol*. 2018;36:LBA2. doi:10.1200/JCO.2018.36.18_suppl.LBA2
85. Admiraal R, Paardt M, Kobes J, et al. High-dose chemotherapy for children and young adults with stage IV rhabdomyosarcoma. *Cochrane Database Syst Rev*. 2010;12:CD006669. doi:10.1002/14651858.CD006669.pub2
86. Peinemann F, Kröger N, Bartel C, et al. High-dose chemotherapy followed by autologous stem cell transplantation for metastatic rhabdomyosarcoma—a systematic review. *PloS One*. 2011;6:e17127. doi:10.1371/journal.pone.0017127
87. Sung L, Anderson JR, Donaldson SS, et al. Late events occurring five years or more after successful therapy for childhood rhabdomyosarcoma: a report from the Soft Tissue Sarcoma Committee of the Children's Oncology Group. *Eur J Cancer*. 2004;40:1878–1885. doi:10.1016/j.ejca.2004.04.005
88. Chisholm JC, Marandet J, Rey A, et al. Prognostic factors after relapse in nonmetastatic rhabdomyosarcoma: a nomogram to better define patients who can be salvaged with further therapy. *J Clin Oncol*. 2011;29:1319–1325. doi:10.1200/JCO.2010.32.1984
89. Pappo AS, Anderson JR, Crist WM, et al. Survival after relapse in children and adolescents with rhabdomyosarcoma: a report from the Intergroup Rhabdomyosarcoma Study Group. *J Clin Oncol*. 1999;17:3487–3493. doi:10.1200/JCO.1999.17.11.3487
90. Miser JS, Kinsella TJ, Triche TJ, et al. Ifosfamide with mesna uroprotection and etoposide: an effective regimen in the treatment of recurrent sarcomas and other tumors of children and young adults. *J Clin Oncol*. 1987;5:1191–1198. doi:10.1200/JCO.1987.5.8.1191
91. Antman K, Crowley J, Balcerzak SP, et al. A Southwest Oncology Group and Cancer and Leukemia Group B phase II study of doxorubicin, dacarbazine, ifosfamide, and mesna in adults with advanced osteosarcoma, Ewing's sarcoma, and rhabdomyosarcoma. *Cancer*. 1998;82(7):1288–1295. doi:10.1002/(SICI)1097-0142(19980401)82:7<1288::AID-CNCR11>3.0.CO;2-2
92. Saylors RL, Stine KC, Sullivan J, et al. Cyclophosphamide plus topotecan in children with recurrent or refractory solid tumors: a Pediatric Oncology Group phase II study. *J Clin Oncol*. 2001;19:3463–3469. doi:10.1200/JCO.2001.19.15.3463
93. Mascarenhas L, Meyer WH, Lyden E, et al. Randomized phase II trial of bevacizumab and temsirolimus in combination with vinorelbine (V) and cyclophosphamide (C) for first relapse/disease progression of rhabdomyosarcoma (RMS): a report from the Children's Oncology Group (COG). *J Clin Oncol*. 2014;32:10003–10003. doi:10.1200/jco.2014.32.15_suppl.10003
94. Bonvalot S, Raut CP, Pollock RE, et al. Technical considerations in surgery for retroperitoneal sarcomas: position paper from E-Surge, a master class in sarcoma surgery, and EORTC-STBSG. *Ann Surg Oncol*. 2012;19(9):2981–2991. doi:10.1245/s10434-012-2342-2
95. Ray-Coquard I, Thiesse P, Ranchère-Vince D, et al. Conformity to clinical practice guidelines, multidisciplinary management and outcome of treatment for soft tissue sarcomas. *Ann Oncol*. 2004;15:307–315. doi:10.1093/annonc/mdh058
96. Stoeckle E, Gardet H, Coindre JM, et al. Prospective evaluation of quality of surgery in soft tissue sarcoma. *Eur J Surg Oncol*. 2006;32:1242–1248. doi:10.1016/j.ejso.2006.05.005
97. Ben Arush M, Minard-Colin V, Mosseri V, et al. Does aggressive local treatment have an impact on survival in children with metastatic rhabdomyosarcoma? *Eur J Cancer*. 2015;51:193–201. doi:10.1016/j.ejca.2014.11.009
98. Dumont SN, Araujo DM, Munsell MF, et al. Management and outcome of 239 adolescent and adult rhabdomyosarcoma patients. *Cancer Med*. 2013;2(4):553–563. doi:10.1002/cam4.92
99. Gerber NK, Wexler LH, Singer S, et al. Adult rhabdomyosarcoma survival improved with treatment on multimodality protocols. *Int J Radiat Oncol Biol Phys*. 2013;86(1):58–63. doi:10.1016/j.ijrobp.2012.12.016
100. Ferrari A, Dileo P, Casanova M, et al. Rhabdomyosarcoma in adults. A retrospective analysis of 171 patients treated at a single institution. *Cancer*. 2003;98(3):571–580. doi:10.1002/cncr.11550
101. Casali PG, Abecassis N, Aro HT, et al. Soft tissue and visceral sarcomas: ESMO-EURACAN Clinical Practice Guidelines for diagnosis, treatment and follow-up. *Ann Oncol*. 2018;29:iv268–iv269. doi:10.1093/annonc/mdy321
102. Pervaiz N, Colterjohn N, Farrokhyar F, et al. A systematic meta-analysis of randomized controlled trials of adjuvant chemotherapy for localized resectable soft-tissue sarcoma. *Cancer*. 2008;113:573–581. doi:10.1002/cncr.23592
103. Hawkins WG, Hoos A, Antonescu CR, et al. Clinicopathologic analysis of patients with adult rhabdomyosarcoma. *Cancer*. 2001;91:794–803. doi:10.1002/1097-0142(20010215)91:4<794::AID-CNCR1066>3.0.CO;2-Q
104. Esnaola NF, Rubin BP, Baldini EH, et al. Response to chemotherapy and predictors of survival in adult rhabdomyosarcoma. *Ann Surg*. 2001;234:215–223. doi:10.1097/00000658-200108000-00012

105. Little DJ, Ballo MT, Zagars GK, et al. Adult rhabdomyosarcoma: outcome following multimodality treatment. *Cancer*. 2002;95:377–388. doi:10.1002/cncr.10669
106. Liu YT, Wang CW, Hong RL, Kuo SH. Prognostic factors and treatment outcomes of adult patients with rhabdomyosarcoma after multimodality treatment. *Anticancer Res*. 2019;39:1355–1364. doi:10.21873/anticanres.13249
107. Bay JO, Ray-Coquard I, Fayette J, et al. Docetaxel and gemcitabine combination in 133 advanced soft-tissue sarcomas: a retrospective analysis. *Int J Cancer*. 2006;119:706–711. doi:10.1002/ijc.21867
108. Subbiah V, Meyer C, Zinner R, et al. Phase Ib/II study of the safety and efficacy of combination therapy with multikinase VEGF inhibitor pazopanib and MEK inhibitor trametinib In advanced soft tissue sarcoma. *Clin Cancer Res*. 2017;23:4027–4034. doi:10.1158/1078-0432.CCR-17-0272

14

Ewing Sarcoma

Warren Alperstein and Matteo Trucco

INTRODUCTION

The Ewing sarcoma (EWS) family of tumors is a group of tumors consisting of typical EWS, extraosseous EWS, atypical EWS, primitive neuroectodermal tumor (PNET), and Askin tumor. The unifying feature of these tumors is the specific chromosomal translocation fusing the *EWS* gene to a subset of ETS transcription factor family members, most commonly the *FLI1* gene (less frequently, *ERG*, *ETV1*, *E1A-F*, or *FEV*). The peak incidence of EWS is during adolescence. Treatment of these tumors requires a multidisciplinary approach. The ideal team consists of experienced oncologists, orthopedists, radiation oncologists, radiologists, pathologists, and supportive care members. Despite extensive research leading to the finding of the disease-defining translocations, our understanding of the biology and its clinical correlation is still limited and there has been little progress in our ability to cure this disease in the past 30 years. Given the lack of recent clinical progress, optimal management of these patients by experienced teams is of particular importance. There have not been major advances in survival in patients with metastatic disease since standard use of adjuvant chemotherapy was adopted in the 1970s. Therefore, it is imperative to continue developing clinical trials and encouraging enrollment into these studies. This chapter will discuss the current approach to diagnosis and management for those with the EWS family of tumors.

EPIDEMIOLOGY

EWS is the second most common primary bone malignancy of childhood and young adulthood. About 80% of EWS occurs in patients younger than 20 years at the time of diagnosis.[1] The annual incidence of EWS in this population is approximately 2.9 cases per million.[2] The incidence is slightly higher in males than females at a ratio of 1.2:1. The most striking epidemiologic feature of EWS is the difference in racial distribution. It occurs more frequently in Caucasians, with a lower occurrence rate in people of Asian and African American (AA) descent.[1,2] Worch et al. looked at the National Cancer Institute (NCI) Surveillance, Epidemiology, and End Results (SEER) database from 1973 to 2005 and found that the racial distribution of EWS was 78.6% white non-Hispanic, 14% Hispanic, 4.9% Asian, and 2.5% AA.[3] This indicates lower occurrence in people of AA descent, as this group makes up about 13% of the population. This racial difference is seen at every age, and the explanation has yet to be fully elucidated. Beck et al., looking at the different length polymorphisms of the *NR0B1* and *CAV1* GGAA microsatellite in both European and African populations, were able to demonstrate that the number of GGAA microsatellite repeats is considerably higher in African populations, as a possible explanation.[4] Additional research is needed to look into these racial differences and the correlation of the GGAA microsatellite repeats.

CLINICAL PRESENTATION

The presenting symptoms for EWS depend on the location of the tumor. When presenting in the bone, pain is a common presenting symptom, though a painless mass is not uncommon. When the initial site is in the soft tissue, the patient will often present with a mass, which may or may not be painful. Given that the primary incidence is in adolescence, pain is often mistaken for so-called "growing pains." It is not uncommon for it to take weeks to months from the onset of symptoms for a diagnosis of EWS. EWS most often arises in the bones (85%), with the remaining 15% occurring in soft tissues.[2] Additional presenting symptoms may include local swelling, pathologic fractures, and systemic symptoms such as fever and weight loss. EWS can be found in almost any bone or soft tissue. Approximately 38% of EWS appears at the diaphysis of the long bone in the extremities. EWS can present at the flat bones of the axial skeleton, such as the ribs and pelvis, at about 27%.[2] Although extremity lesions are still more common, central lesions are seen in EWS more frequently. EWS that arises from the bone can also have a relatively large soft tissue component, especially when compared to osteosarcoma.

There are no specific laboratory findings or tumor markers associated with EWS. Nonspecific findings such as an elevated serum lactate dehydrogenase (LDH) and alkaline phosphatase are seen with increased tumor burden, cell turnover, and bone destruction. Van Maldegem et al. completed a meta-analysis looking at possible biomarkers as prognostic factors.[10] It was thought that LDH was a prognostic marker, but has been shadowed by the prognostic impact of metastatic disease, which clearly has the most impact on overall survival (OS). Decreases in white blood cells, hemoglobin, and platelets are not typically seen in EWS, unless there is significant bone marrow involvement.

DIAGNOSTIC APPROACH

Tissue diagnosis by an experienced pathologist is essential. Upfront resection of these tumors is not typically attempted in preference of biopsy, whether by percutaneous core-needle biopsy or via an open surgical procedure (Figure 14.1). The most common approach is to defer complete surgical

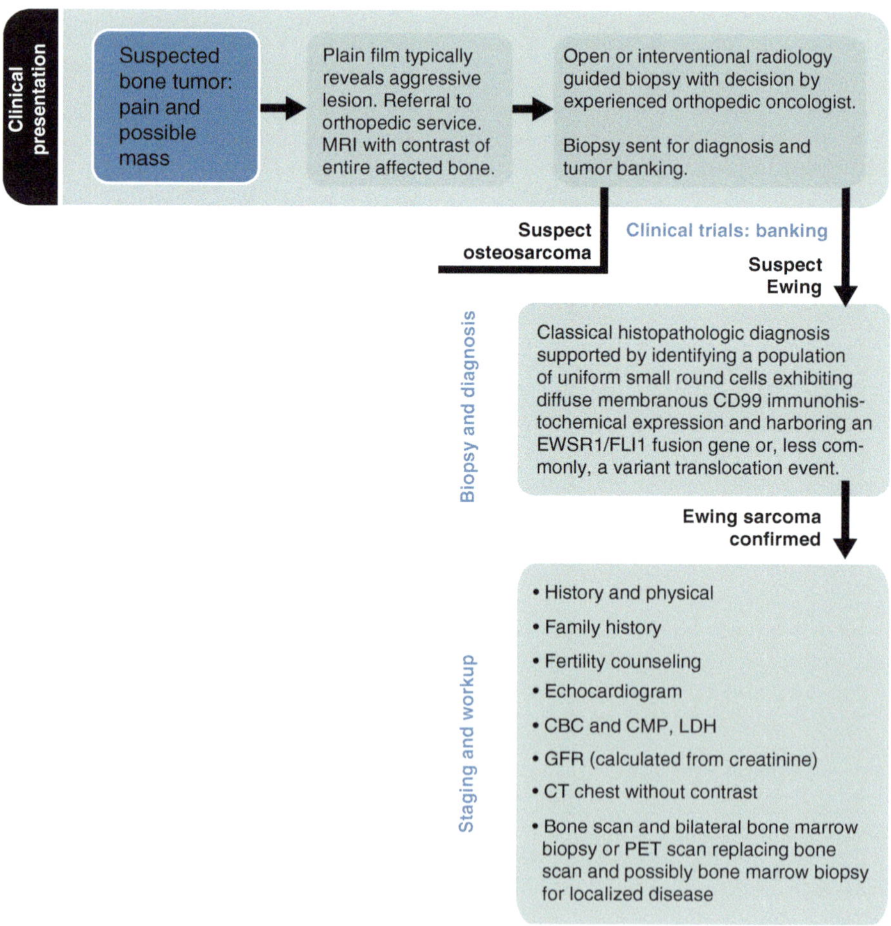

FIGURE 14.1 Workup for newly suspected bone sarcoma.

CBC, complete blood count; CMP, complete metabolic panel; GFR, glomerular filtration rate; LDH, lactate dehydrogenase.

Source: With permission from Reed DR, Hayashi M, Wagner L, et al. Treatment pathway of bone sarcoma in children, adolescents, and young adults. *Cancer*. 2017;123(12):2206–2218. doi: 10.1002/cncr.30589.

resection until after the patient has received neoadjuvant chemotherapy. This has multiple benefits including allowing time for preparation for the surgery and obtaining custom prostheses if needed. Neoadjuvant chemotherapy typically also reduces the size of the tumor, which may facilitate surgical resection. Finally, neoadjuvant chemotherapy allows for immediate systemic therapy to treat/prevent the development of macroscopic and microscopic metastases.

Core-needle biopsy with image guidance can provide sufficient samples for diagnosis and, being less invasive, is the preferred initial biopsy technique.[2] In rare cases, a core-needle biopsy does not provide enough tissue for diagnosis and a repeat or open biopsy must be attempted. It is imperative to minimize the tissue contamination from needle or open biopsy. The biopsy tract should be excised at the time of definitive surgery; hence, discussion with an experienced orthopedic oncologist on biopsy location is critical. If possible, the same surgical team performing the definitive surgery should obtain the biopsy or be consulted about the optimal image-guided core biopsy approach.

Radiographic Features (Prior to Biopsy)

At the time of diagnosis, a plain radiograph of the affected bone is done in addition to cross-sectional imaging, such as MRI or CT. In EWS, there will typically be x-ray findings in the diaphysis of the long bones that extend toward the metaphysis. The classic "onion skin" appearance of EWS is a lamellated periosteal reaction. It is seen in about 23% of presentations.[1] More common nonspecific features seen on x-ray image include lytic lesions (75%), soft tissue extension (64%), and reactive bone formation (25%).[1] Less common findings include radiating spicules, a.k.a. "sunburst appearance" (20%); periosteal thickening (19%); sclerosis (16%); and fracture (13%). The aforementioned sunburst appearance is more classically associated with osteosarcoma; however, it can be seen in both. The major difference between images of osteosarcoma and EWS is the location, which is typically at the metaphysis for osteosarcoma and diaphysis for EWS.[1] Those with soft tissue EWS may have normal x-ray imaging, unless there is bony erosion or the soft tissue mass is large enough to be radiopaque. Once the initial x-ray study is completed, additional imaging is mandated as part of the workup. More detailed imaging of the primary site is needed using MRI with gadolinium contrast agent. This provides the resolution needed for proper surgical mapping prior to the biopsy and definitive surgery. In addition, a CT scan of the chest is required to assess for metastatic disease to the lungs, as it is the most common site for metastasis. Typically, a CT scan of the chest without intravenous (IV) contrast is sufficient, as the air provides the "contrast" needed when looking for metastatic tissue in the lungs; however, contrast may be needed if assessing the soft tissue component of an EWS involving the chest. Historically, technetium bone scan was used to assess for local and metastatic bone disease. The advantage to the bone scan is that it is cheaper and involves less radiation. However, more recently, there has been a shift to the fluorodeoxyglucose (FDG) positron emission tomography/computed tomography (PET/CT) as it is more sensitive for metastatic disease in EWS and can help assess nonskeletal lesions.[2,5]

MOLECULAR BIOLOGY

The pathognomonic molecular finding in EWS family tumors is a reciprocal chromosomal translocation, most commonly occurring between the chromosomes 11 and 22. More specifically, t(11;22)(q24;q12) occurs in about 85% of cases. The gene name for the chromosome 22 translocation partner is *EWSR1*, and the gene name for the chromosome 11 partner is *FLI1*. The presence of this fusion protein correlates with a high expression of cell surface sialoglycoprotein CD99.[2] Of the 15% of EWSs that do not harbor the *EWSR1–FLI1* translocation, these tumors typically have evidence for gene rearrangements for *EWSR1* to a different fusion partner, the most common being *ERG* on chromosome 21q22, which is seen in about 10% of EWS family tumors. Other less frequent fusion partners seen in less than 1% of cases include *ETV1* on chromosome 7p22, *ETV4* on chromosome 17q12, and *FEV* on chromosome 2q33. In addition to *EWSR1*-associated translocations, other chromosomal changes can also be simultaneously present. Trisomy 8 and 12 are observed in 50% and 33% of cases, respectively.[2] Structural changes at chromosomes 1 and 16 are observed in about 20% of cases, typically leading to the gain of 1q, a loss of 16q, or the formation of a derivative chromosome der(1;16). There have been some reports describing fusions between *FUS* and either *ERG* or *FEV* in EWS. The FUS protein is highly related to *EWS*. The clinical significance of these various translocation partners to *EWSR1*, along with the other structural chromosomal changes, is unknown at this time. Additional research is needed to determine their significance.

It is believed that a second mutational event is needed to immortalize these *EWS–FLI1*-expressing cells. It was initially thought that p53 pathway was involved, but aberrations in p53 are relatively rare in EWS, occurring in less than 15% of tumors. Some preclinical data suggest that NOTCH signaling or insulin-like growth factor 1 receptor (IGF1R) circuit is involved.[2]

There is no conclusive evidence that any of these varying aberrations, such as the varying translocation partners with *EWSR1*, such as *FLI1*, *ERG*, *ETV1*, *E1A-F*, or *FEV* gene, play a role in a clinically meaningful way in regard to prognosis. Currently, the main prognostic factor remains the presence or absence of metastatic disease. It is important to acknowledge that in Europe, they also look at the response to neoadjuvant chemotherapy, which at the time of writing this chapter had not yet been incorporated in North American protocols.

THERAPEUTIC APPROACH

EWS requires a multidisciplinary team approach to treatment, including orthopedic oncology, interventional radiology, radiation oncology, radiology, and medical/pediatric oncology (see Figure 14.2). A specialized orthopedic oncologist can take care of the biopsy and the surgical resection of the primary tumor. The biopsy could also be completed by interventional radiology with consultation of the primary surgical team to identify the proper approach to ensure removal of the biopsy tract when the patient undergoes definitive surgical resection of the primary tumor. Radiation oncology is involved to provide radiation for local control of the primary tumor site when needed if complete surgical resection is not possible, the patient is not a surgical candidate, the patient declines surgery, or there are positive margins after surgical resection. A pediatric or medical oncologist is involved to administer systemic chemotherapy. When available, patients should be encouraged to participate in clinical trials to further advance our treatment strategies and potentially receive improved treatment. Neoadjuvant chemotherapy should be initiated quickly after completing histologic confirmation of the diagnosis, metastatic workup, and baseline assessment.

The use of chemotherapy to treat EWS started only in the 1960s. It was Sutow and Sullivan who, in 1962, published a report on cyclophosphamide to treat EWS.[11] In 1974, Rosen et al. from Memorial Sloan Kettering first started treating EWS with multiple agents together, as is currently done.[12] Their initial regimen consisted of vincristine, cyclophosphamide, actinomycin D, and doxorubicin (VACD). Chemotherapy greatly improved the outcomes of patients with EWS. The first cooperative study by Intergroup Ewing's Sarcoma Study (IESS) from 1973 to 1978 showed that the addition of doxorubicin to VAC had a 5-year OS rate of about 60%, which was compared to 24% with VAC alone.[6] The American Intergroup Ewing's trial (INT-0091/POG-8850/CCG7881) determined that the addition of ifosfamide and etoposide (IE) to VACD improved the event-free survival (EFS) rate to 69% in those with localized disease.[6] There was, however, no benefit in metastatic disease.

The combination of cooperative groups in North America has allowed for increased enrollment of patients with this rare tumor into therapeutic clinical trials. The Children's Oncology Group (COG) is one of the leading cooperative groups in pediatric oncology in North America. The COG trial AEWS0031 demonstrated improved survival in EWS patients with localized disease when treated with an interval-compressed version of VDC/IE given every 2 weeks instead of every 3 weeks. In Europe, a different standard regimen of VIDE is used, which consists of vincristine, ifosfamide, doxorubicin, and etoposide.[5] The Euro-E.W.I.N.G. 99 clinical trial looked at the safety of treating with VIDE, compared to earlier standard of vincristine, actinomycin D, and cyclophosphamide (VAC) or vincristine, actinomycin D, and ifosfamide (VAI) in Europe. It demonstrated tolerance and efficacy, and thus, the Europeans now treat with VIDE (vincristine 1.5 mg/m^2 × 1 day, ifosfamide 3 g/m^2 × 3 days, doxorubicin 20 mg/m^2 × 3 days, and etoposide 150 mg/m^2 × 3 days). Currently, an ongoing Euro-Ewing 12 study (EudraCT number 2012-002107-17) is being conducted which looks at a direct comparison of VIDE and VDC/IE. Historically, the outcomes have been comparable between regimens; however, only now are they being compared head to head.

The therapeutic regimen used in North America consists of vincristine (1.5 mg/m^2, on day 1), doxorubicin (75 mg/m^2 on days 1 and 2), cyclophosphamide (1,200 mg/m^2 on day 1) alternating every 2 weeks with ifosfamide (1,800 mg/m^2 on days 1–5) and etoposide (100 mg/m^2 on days 1–5). This is referred to as VDC/IE and is considered the current standard of care for a pediatric oncologist in North America. It currently consists of 12 weeks of neoadjuvant chemotherapy, followed by local control with surgery and/or radiation and then an additional 16 weeks of adjuvant chemotherapy for a total of 28 weeks of therapy.

While most pediatric oncologists follow the COG regimen described above, adult medical oncologists treat with different protocols. As demonstrated in the National Comprehensive Cancer Network (NCCN) Guidelines Version 1.2019, the possible regimens medical oncologists use to treat localized EWS are: VDC/IE (same as pediatrics), VDI (vincristine 2 mg/m^2, doxorubicin 75 mg/m^2, and

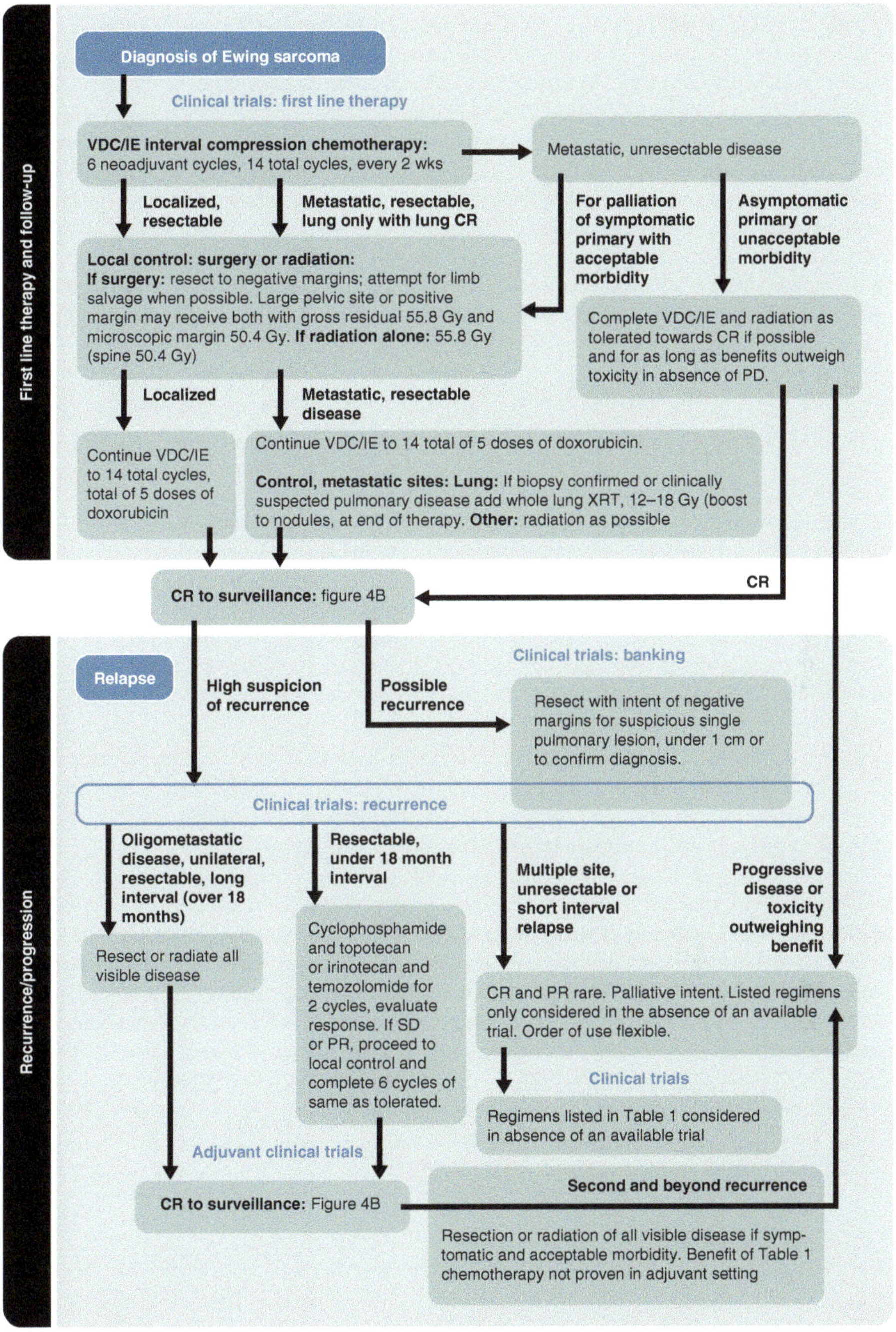

FIGURE 14.2 Pathway for treating newly diagnosed and relapsed Ewing sarcoma.

CR, complete response; IE, ifosfamide and etoposide; PD, progressive disease; PR, partial response; SD, stable disease; VDC, vincristine, doxorubicin, and cyclophosphamide; XRT, x-ray therapy.

Source: Used with permission from Reed DR, Hayashi M, Wagner L, et al. Treatment pathway of bone sarcoma in children, adolescents, and young adults. *Cancer*. 2017;123(12):2206–2218. doi:10.1002/cncr.30589.

ifosfamide 10 g/m^2), and VIDE. When treating metastatic disease, they use the same three regimens plus the additional option of VDC alone.

The choice of local control is dependent on the location of the tumor and the ability to obtain negative surgical margins. Surgical resection is preferred if negative margins are obtainable and the associated morbidity is not extreme. The use of radiation can provide an acceptable alternative to surgery for local control when negative margins are not obtainable and surgical morbidity is great.

Debulking operations that leave gross residual tumor are never indicated as they will just delay chemotherapy and the patient would require full-dose radiation therapy (RT) to treat gross residual disease, the same as if the surgery did not occur. A 2015 COG report by DuBois et al. showed that the choice of local control, between surgery and radiation, did not have a significant impact on OS.[13] However, the risk of local failure was greater in those who received radiation rather than surgery, with a statistically significant hazard ratio of 2.41, although the anatomic sites treated with surgery (i.e., extremity, rib) are generally different from those treated with radiation (i.e., spine, sacrum, pelvis); so, these patient cohorts are often quite different. Nevertheless, radiation does have additional long-term effects, such as the risk of secondary malignancies.[5] Surgical advances have continued to improve to allow for about 90% of extremity surgeries to be limb sparing, avoiding amputation as much as possible. Postoperative radiation is typically employed only if surgical margins are positive. For those patients receiving radiation as local control, it should be administered concurrently with consolidation therapy, specifically with the ifosfamide/etoposide portion. In addition, doxorubicin is held while radiation is being administered.[7] If clinicians are treating according to the COG trial regimen, the week 13 doxorubicin dose is given just prior to the initiation of radiation and then followed by back-to-back cycles of ifosfamide/etoposide to avoid enhancement of normal tissue radiation toxicity expected with concurrent doxorubicin (Adriamycin).

The total radiation fractions and dose (measured in Gy) depend on the location of the primary site, on whether there was a resection with positive margins, or if there was metastatic disease. For example, the total recommended dose for gross disease is 55.8 Gy. However, if resected with microscopic residual (unable to obtain clean margins), then 50.4 Gy is used. In addition, for nonosseous lesions with complete response to chemotherapy, 50.4 Gy is used as well. Dose-escalated RT to limited fields may be beneficial for high-risk tumors and may reduce local recurrence rates. A single-institutional Phase 2 trial employed focal limited-margin RT using conformal or intensity-modulated techniques.[8] Unresected tumors <8 cm at diagnosis received a standard dose of 55.8 Gy, and tumors >8 cm received an escalated dose of 64.8 Gy. Radiation is typically administered at a maximum of 1.5 to 1.8 Gy per fraction, given over an estimated 25 to 30 fractions. Given the variability in doses and fractions, the young age of the patients, and the need to integrate radiation with chemotherapy and possibly surgery, it is important to have a radiation oncologist well versed in treating EWS.

If a patient has metastatic disease at the time of diagnosis, the same systemic chemotherapy regimen is used. However, it is important to note that the five-drug regimen of VDC/IE was never shown to be more beneficial than VDC alone in treating metastatic disease. Also, the clinical trial demonstrating the superiority of administering chemotherapy every 2 versus 3 weeks did not include patients with metastatic disease; hence, the benefit of giving chemotherapy every 2 weeks has not yet been proved for metastatic disease. However, most oncologists will treat patients with metastatic disease with the same regimen used for localized disease, as most are reluctant to treat metastatic disease less aggressively than localized. The additional variability lies in local control, not only of the primary site but also of the sites of metastatic disease. It is dependent on where the metastatic disease is and if it can be surgically removed. Local control with radiation is also involved and the dose depends on the location site. For additional details of radiation in metastatic disease, refer to Chapter 4, Radiation Oncology.

METASTATIC DISEASE

About 25% to 30% of patients present with metastatic disease at the time of diagnosis. The incidence of metastatic disease at diagnosis correlates to the location of the primary tumor. Those with a central primary tumor, such as the pelvis, have the highest incidence of metastases at about 40%. Those with a proximal primary site have a 30% incidence of metastases. Also, those with a distal primary tumor have the lowest rate of incidence at about 15%.[1]

EWS metastasizes most commonly to three specific locations: lung, bone, and bone marrow. Their incidence is about 38%, 31%, and <10%, respectively.[1] Metastatic disease can also appear in the brain, liver, and soft tissue; however, these sites are much rarer. Given the high rate of metastatic disease at diagnosis, it is imperative to get a chest CT and an FDG PET/CT for all patients at the time of initial diagnosis and staging. Chest CT is needed in addition to PET/CT as the PET is not of high-enough resolution to properly evaluate for pulmonary metastasis. Historically, bilateral bone marrow biopsies were done routinely at the time of diagnosis. However, the yield of bone marrow biopsy is extremely low and it is no longer performed by many practitioners unless required for clinical trials.[5] Metastases to the bone marrow are not homogeneous, and therefore require a bilateral biopsy. Given the lack of homogeneity of metastatic disease to the bone marrow, sampling error resulting in false negative can be a problem. In addition, if the FDG PET/CT is negative, the likelihood for finding metastatic disease in the bone marrow is extremely low. In general, bone marrow involvement can often be seen on PET/CT, thus calling into question the value of a bone marrow biopsy. Once a positive PET/CT is obtained and it is determined to be metastatic disease, a bone marrow biopsy will not impact the treatment plan. For these reasons, the bone marrow biopsy is falling out of favor as a diagnostic requirement.

Therapeutic Approach for Metastatic Disease

Despite advances in survival for localized EWS, metastatic disease in EWS continues to have an unacceptably poor prognosis outcome with <30% survival.[5] Survival differs if metastases are limited to the lung only or have spread to the bone or bone marrow. When limited to lung metastases, the 5-year survival rate is slightly better than 30%, while if the disease has spread to other sites, survival rate is only 15% to 30%. Given this continued poor survival, treatment for metastatic disease should be encouraged to be given on clinical trials. At this time, the standard of care for metastatic disease at diagnosis consists of the same systemic regimen of interval-compressed VDC/IE used in North America, with other reasonable regimens being VDC, VAI, and VIDE. There are more options for metastatic disease because interval-compressed VDC/IE has not been shown to improve survival in metastatic disease. However, the standard of care remains the same, as most physicians do not feel comfortable treating metastatic disease less aggressively then localized disease. However, more aggressive systemic therapy with myeloablative chemotherapy with an autologous stem cell rescue has not been demonstrated as advantageous when given as induction therapy. Nevertheless, at relapse, some studies have demonstrated increased survival in chemotherapy-sensitive disease with an autologous stem cell rescue after high-dose chemotherapy, with the 5-year survival rate approaching 40% to 50%.[9] Given the poor outcome to standard chemotherapy, one should encourage patients to enroll in clinical trials when available, which offer the potential for improved outcomes.

The current COG Phase 3 clinical trial for metastatic EWS is AEWS1221. This trial explores the addition of ganitumab to the current standard of care of VDC/IE. Ganitumab is a monoclonal antibody directed against IGF1R. It prevents the binding of the natural ligand IGF-1, and therefore prevents activation of the signaling pathway PI3K/AKT. Inhibition of this survival signal is thought to inhibit tumor cell proliferation and cause an induction of tumor cell apoptosis. This is an excellent frontline therapeutic option for metastatic disease. Additionally, this COG trial looks at the effectiveness of compressed intervals (from 3 to 2 weeks) in metastatic disease, as it has been shown to be effective in localized disease but not previously tested in metastatic disease. For those patients with pulmonary metastases, it is recommended to administer whole lung radiation (at a dose of 12–15 Gy) after the completion of systemic therapy.

Relapse disease typically occurs within the first 2 years after the initial diagnosis, most often in either the lungs or the bones. Three factors that give patients the highest risk for relapsed disease are metastatic disease at the time of diagnosis, a primary lesion in the pelvis, or a poor histologic response to neoadjuvant chemotherapy.[5] Recurrent EWS has an estimated 5-year OS rate of <15%. However, those who have local relapsed disease or later relapsed disease do still have a potential for cure. Researchers Rodriguez-Galindo et al. at St. Jude Children's Research Hospital reviewed their data of relapsed EWS patients. The 5-year relapse-free survival rate was 18%. However, those who relapsed >2 years from diagnosis had a 5-year relapse-free survival rate of 35%. In addition, those with isolated local relapse only had a slightly higher 5-year relapse-free survival rate of 22% versus the general 18%.[14]

In relapsed disease, enrollment into a clinical trial should also be strongly considered. However, if trials are not available, the patient does not qualify, or the patient declines, a few different therapeutic regimens exist.[5] The two more commonly used regimens that give about 25% response rate are cyclophosphamide with topotecan and temozolomide with irinotecan plus vincristine. Another two options that have been used, with a lower response rate, are high-dose ifosfamide or gemcitabine plus docetaxel. The consensus opinion among experts in the field is to use the combination of temozolomide with irinotecan as the first option.[5] It is intriguing that if an irinotecan-containing regimen fails, a patient would still be able to use a topotecan-containing regimen; despite being in the same family of drugs, they have different patterns of resistance. It is important to note that the response rates to the cyclophosphamide/topotecan regimen were correlated with the relapse interval. Those who had disease progression while receiving therapy did not respond to this regimen. However, if >2 years had passed since the completion of therapy, then there was about a 50% response rate to this regimen.[5]

Cure is difficult to achieve in those patients with relapsed disease; patients who do receive therapy typically have a temporary response, with the median postrecurrence survival ranging from 9 to 17 months.[5] From a quality of life perspective, it is important to note that those with painful lesions will typically respond to palliative radiation. There is insufficient data to support the use of high-dose chemotherapy with autologous stem cell rescue in these patients with relapsed disease at this time. A recent review by Tenneti et al.[9] looked at the role of high-dose chemotherapy and autologous hematopoietic stem cell rescue (HSCT). It appears that giving high-dose chemotherapy followed by autologous HSCT after consolidation chemotherapy improved survival for some patients with EWS. In most of these studies, those who had high-dose chemotherapy followed by HSCT had an OS rate of 20% to 60% at 1 to 2 years and those who received consolidation chemotherapy had an OS rate of 20% to 25% at 5 years. The EFS rate for those with relapsed disease was 25% at 1 to 2 years for those with consolidation chemotherapy alone compared to 42% to 47% in those who had HSCT.[9] Those that received high-dose chemotherapy followed by HSCT in induction did not demonstrate a survival benefit. However, the heterogeneity of the studies reviewed was so significant that no conclusive statement could be made. A prospective randomized controlled study is needed for these patients.

FOLLOW-UP

Once a patient has completed therapy and is in remission, there is a consensus that surveillance follow-up should be conducted for every patient. Surveillance consists of primary site imaging, lung imaging, and lab tests at various intervals: the first year it should be every 3 months, the second year every 3 to 4 months, the third year every 4 to 6 months, and then yearly during the fourth and fifth years after treatment. The primary site should have an x-ray exam and/or MRI with contrast. The MRI is necessary for those with a soft tissue primary lesion, as it will not be seen on x-ray. The lung surveillance consists of a non-contrast CT in the first and second years, followed by x-ray studies. Some patients will need follow-up nuclear medicine imaging, depending on if the PET/CT or bone scan at diagnosis was positive. However, if at diagnosis the nuclear medicine scan was negative, then no follow-up scans are needed. Given the cumulative dose of anthracyclines given during EWS treatment, an echocardiogram is recommended every 1 to 2 years, as is a complete blood count with differential.

SUMMARY

Though EWS is the second most common primary bone malignancy of childhood and young adulthood, it is a rare tumor. While most oncology practices will likely encounter some patients with EWS, only high-volume sarcoma centers see enough patients to truly develop expertise with this family of tumors. While the chemotherapy used is familiar to most oncologists, and general approach to treatment is relatively straightforward, the care of these patients is nuanced and can easily become exceedingly complex. At the very minimum, consultation with a high-volume sarcoma center, including involvement of properly trained and experienced orthopedic, medical/pediatric, and radiation oncologists, along with radiologists and pathologists, is essential for assuring the best outcome for these patients. Additionally, support services, including physical therapy, psychosocial services, and fertility preservation experts, are extremely valuable. These tumors require a multidisciplinary team approach, with excellent communication between the various members of the care team. Metastatic disease, the potentially significant side effects of the treatment regimens, and/or relapsed disease raise the complexity of the care of these patients exponentially and underscore the importance of expert involvement.

Biologically, EWS is one of the genetically "quietest malignancies," driven by the defining translocation of *EWSR1–FLI1*. Despite this, much work is still needed to understand the underpinnings and heterogeneity within this family of tumors. Innovative treatments are currently being tested in clinical trials, with more to come. Sarcoma centers are propelling these advances in research and therapy, and should coordinate and collaborate with other centers and community practitioners to optimize the care for patients affected by this challenging malignancy.

CASE STUDY

Among the magnitude of cases that could be used to illustrate the complexity of EWS, this case was selected to demonstrate the importance of seeking treatment from teams with extensive experience in treating sarcomas, such as those that can be found at the sarcoma centers. This patient was a 20-year-old woman who initially presented with right-sided chest pain. The pain continued to worsen to the point that she sought medical care. Of note, at this time, the patient lived with her family outside the United States. The primary team initially did an ultrasound exam and chest radiograph to assess the area, and a bone mass was revealed arising from the right tenth rib. The patient was then referred to a surgical team. The surgical team attempted a complete resection of the mass and the right tenth rib at the time of diagnosis. The pathology returned as EWS, as fluorescence in situ hybridization (FISH) was positive for *EWSR1–FLI1* translocation. Unfortunately, for the patient, the correct surgical approach was not taken. In EWS of the chest wall/ribs, the standard approach is to remove the ribs above and below the lesion. Additionally, upfront surgery is not recommended for EWS, and instead, local therapy is typically to be done only after 12 weeks of chemotherapy. This approach increases the likelihood of negative margins, thus decreasing the risk for relapse. In contrast, this patient's surgery was done in her country of origin prior to any neoadjuvant chemotherapy. The patient then presented to pediatric oncology about 2 months after surgery. A repeat comprehensive staging workup was completed, including imaging of the primary site, chest CT, and a PET/CT. At this time, she was found to have metastatic disease with pulmonary nodules on the chest CT, which were not present initially at the time of her diagnosis. There were about six small pulmonary nodules of 2 to 3 mm in different areas of the left lower lobe of lung. In addition, the PET/CT was positive at the site of the initial lesion. Postsurgical changes could be seen; but given the time since surgery (about 2 months), the PET/CT was concerning for active disease. She was offered clinical trials, but did not enroll. She was then treated with interval-compressed VDC/IE. After 12 weeks of therapy, radiation was used for local control. She received right flank radiation at a dose of 50.4 Gy in 28 fractions. She then continued with consolidation therapy for 16 additional weeks. At the conclusion of her systemic therapy, she received whole lung radiation of 15 Gy in 10 fractions. Fourteen months after completion of therapy, she remains disease free, though still at high risk for recurrence. This case demonstrates two very important components of optimal care for EWS patients: the multidisciplinary approach with each team member (surgeon, medical/pediatric oncologist, radiation oncologist, pathologist, diagnostic radiologist) having a full understanding of the disease and how it is best treated and the need for comprehensive staging workup at diagnosis and relapse. Adherence to the recommended treatment guidelines could have altered the patient's outcome. To date, the patient remains disease free, but concern remains that the inappropriate surgical approach upfront has negatively impacted her prognosis. Another important feature of this case is that patients with EWS should be seen without delay by an experienced multidisciplinary team because of the risk of developing metastatic spread if systemic therapy is delayed. In this case, the patient may have been spared the addition of RT to both the chest wall and lungs, which places the patient at risk for future lung fibrosis and other secondary complications.

REFERENCES

1. Lanzkowsky P. *Lanzkowsky's Manual of Pediatric Hematology and Oncology*. 6th ed. San Diego, CA: Elsevier Science; 2016:533–543.
2. Pizzo PA, Poplack DG. *Principles and Practice of Pediatric Oncology*. 7th ed. Philadelphia, PA: Wolters Kluwer Health; 2015.
3. Worch J, Matthay KK, Neuhaus J, et al. Ethnic and racial differences in patients with Ewing sarcoma. *Cancer*. 2010;116(4):983–988. doi:10.1002/cncr.24865
4. Beck R, Monument MJ, Watkins WS, et al. EWS/FLI-responsive GGAA microsatellites exhibit polymorphic differences between European and African populations. *Cancer Genet*. 2012;205(6):304–312.
5. Reed DR, Hayashi M, Wagner L, et al. Treatment pathway of bone sarcoma in children, adolescents, and young adults. *Cancer*. 2017;123(12):2206–2218. doi:10.1002/cncr.30589

6. Jain S, Kapoor G. Chemotherapy in Ewing's sarcoma. *Indian J Orthop*. 2010;44(4):369–377. doi:10.4103/0019-5413.69305
7. Children's Oncology Group AEWS1221. Randomized Phase 3 Trial Evaluating the Addition of the IGF-1R Monoclonal Antibody Ganitumab (AMG 479, NSC# 750008, IND# 120449) to Multiagent Chemotherapy for Patients with Newly Diagnosed Metastatic Ewing Sarcoma. An Intergroup NCTN Phase 3 Study. December 2014.
8. Talleur AC, Navid F, Spunt SL, et al. Limited margin radiation therapy for children and young adults with ewing sarcoma achieves high rates of local tumor control. *Int J Radiat Oncol Biol Phys*. 2016;96:119.
9. Tenneti P, Zahid U, Iftikhar A, et al. Role of high-dose chemotherapy and autologous hematopoietic cell transplantation for children and young adults with relapsed Ewing's sarcoma: a systematic review. *Sarcoma*. 2018;2018:2640674. doi:10.1155/2018/2640674
10. van Maldegem AM, Hogendoorn PCW, Hassan AB. The clinical use of biomarkers as prognostic factors in Ewing sarcoma. *Clin Sarcoma Res*. 2012;2:7. doi:10.1186/2045-3329-2-7
11. Sutow WW, Sullivan MP. Cyclophosphamide therapy in children with Ewing's sarcoma. *Cancer Chemother Rep*. 1962;23:55–60. PMID:13979408
12. Rosen G, Wollner N, Tan C, et al. Proceedings: disease-free survival in children with Ewing's sarcoma treated with radiation therapy and adjuvant four-drug sequential chemotherapy. *Cancer*. 1974;33(2)384–393. doi:10.1002/1097-0142(197402)33:2<384::aid-cncr2820330213>3.0.co;2-t
13. DuBois SG, Krailo MD, Gebhardt MC, et al. Comparative evaluation of local control strategies in localized Ewing sarcoma of bone: a report from the Children's Oncology Group. *Cancer*. 2105;123(3):467–475. doi:10.1002/cncr.29065
14. Rodriguez-Galindo C, Billups CA, Kun LE, et al. Survival after recurrence of Ewing tumors: the St. Jude Children's Research Hospital experience, 1979–1999. *Cancer*. 2002;94:561–569. doi:10.1002/cncr.10192

15

Alveolar Soft Part Sarcoma

Emily E. Jonczak and Breelyn A. Wilky

Alveolar soft-part sarcoma [is] a type of soft-part sarcoma quite unlike any well-documented tumor of which we are aware. . . . Even though one cannot classify a tumor, it is desirable to recognize it as something one does not fully understand, for only through such recognition can one offer opinions as to probable behavior.

—William M. Christopherson, et al., 1952[1]

INTRODUCTION

Alveolar soft part sarcoma (ASPS) is a rare, translocation-driven soft tissue sarcoma (STS) classically affecting adolescents and young adults. The disease was first formally described in 1952 by Christopherson et al., who coined the term "alveolar soft part sarcoma" based on its unique histologic features, which included the presence of an organoid to pseudoalveolar pattern and large eosinophilic tumor cells.[1] Further description of ASPS is credited to Dr. Pierre Masson, who first described the intracytoplasmic crystalline structures in his 1956 text, *Tumeurs Humaines: Histologie, Diagnostics et Techniques*.[2] With advances in technology and our improved understanding of molecular genetics, we further elucidated that ASPS is defined not only by its characteristic histologic features but also by a conserved unbalanced translocation t(X;17)(p11;q25), which leads to a chimeric ASPL–transcription factor E3 (TFE3) fusion protein that leads to aberrant transcription.[3,4]

Clinically, ASPS is known for its indolent behavior, propensity to metastasize early, and its inherent resistance to conventional doxorubicin-based chemotherapy typically employed in the management of STS. Given the rarity of ASPS, the majority of our understanding of the disease comes from small case series, retrospective analysis, and clinical experience. The discovery of the *ASPL–TFE3* fusion protein and identification of angiogenic factors as critical mediators of ASPS pathophysiology has opened new doors to the exploration of novel treatment options including the use of tyrosine kinase inhibitors (TKIs) and most recently, modern immunotherapy including immune checkpoint inhibitors (ICIs). In this chapter, we review the epidemiology, clinical presentation, diagnostic approach, molecular drivers, and treatment options for ASPS.

EPIDEMIOLOGY

While STSs are a rare and heterogeneous group of cancers with an estimated 13,040 new cases diagnosed in 2018 representing only 0.8% of all new cancer diagnosis, ASPS accounts for <1% of newly diagnosed STS cases.[5] Based on data from the Surveillance, Epidemiology, and End Results (SEER) database, a mere 267 new cases were diagnosed in the United States between 1973 and 2014.[6] Most commonly, ASPS presents in young adults between the ages of 15 and 35. Diagnosis before age 30 has been shown to have a female-to-male predominance, with reversal of this ratio in patients older than 30 at the time of diagnosis.[4,7] No links to particular ethnicity or race have been reported.

CLINICAL PRESENTATION AND NATURAL HISTORY

ASPS frequently presents as a slow-growing mass in the deep tissues of the extremities, typically in the buttock and thighs. This is the primary disease site in approximately 60% of adult patients. Alternatively, unusual primary disease sites have been described, including the gastrointestinal tract, female genital tract, mediastinum, breast, urinary bladder, bone, and lung. Children with ASPS commonly present with tumors in the orbits or head and neck region. Given the indolent nature of the tumor, patients often do not develop functional impairment and describe a history of a slow-growing mass over years. Most commonly, patients present once the mass has become symptomatic or with signs and symptoms of metastatic disease. Gastrointestinal bleeding, vaginal bleeding, and proptosis have been reported as the presenting symptoms in patients with unusual disease sites. On physical exam, the clinician may appreciate a pulsatile mass and bruit on auscultation, as these tend to be highly vascular tumors (Figure 15.1A).[4,8]

A recent case series of 69 patients diagnosed with ASPS retrospectively reviewed from four major institutions reported that the median age at diagnosis was 17 years and 64% of patients were female.[8] The primary sites of disease included limbs (58%), trunk/retroperitoneum/pelvis (16%), and less commonly, tongue/pharynx (9%) and orbits (3%). All the 26 patients tested for *ASPL–TFE3* translocation were positive. Thirty-one patients presented with localized disease with Intergroup Rhabdomysarcoma Study (IRS) staging I, II, and III being 28%, 10%, and 7%, respectively. Thirty-eight (55%) of the patients had stage IV disease at the time of diagnosis. The sites of metastatic disease included lung (97%), bone (26%), and brain (4%). In the 31 patients presenting with localized disease, the 5-year event-free survival (EFS) rate was 80% and overall survival (OS) rate was 87%; alternatively, in those presenting with stage IV disease, the EFS and OS rates were 7% and 61%, respectively.[8]

In another relatively large series of 70 patients over 39 years from MD Anderson Cancer Center (MDACC), the population was slightly older with a median age of 26 years.[9] Overall, 51% of patients in this series were female; however, in patients over the age of 30, 58% of the patients were male. Metastatic disease at diagnosis was detected in 65% of patients.[9] At a median follow-up of 9 years, two of 22 patients who initially presented with localized disease developed local recurrence and three of 22 patients developed metastatic disease to the lungs. Five-year disease-free survival (DFS) rate of patients with localized disease was 71% and OS rate was 88%. In contrast, the median survival of patients with metastatic disease was 40 months, with a 5-year survival rate of 20%. Importantly, this series revealed an even higher proportion of patients with brain metastases. In contrast to other subtypes of STS, where brain involvement is rare, nine of 48 patients (19%) who presented with metastatic ASPS were noted to have brain lesions, which were always found in the presence of metastases to other sites as well. No patients with isolated brain lesions as the sole site of metastasis were identified, suggesting that routine intracranial imaging is unlikely to benefit patients without evidence of other metastatic disease.

Despite the historically dire prognosis of metastatic disease, it is critical to recognize that not all patients will experience rapid disease progression. Like other indolent STSs, such as epithelioid hemangioendothelioma, some patients may have relatively low-burden metastatic disease in the lungs that can remain stable and controlled without progression for months to years. In the MDACC series, two patients were noted to be alive with disease for 11 and 28 years, respectively, after the diagnosis of metastatic ASPS. Because of this observation, many providers will opt for close monitoring for newly diagnosed metastatic patients to identify patients with indolent biologic behavior and to reserve treatment for radiographic or symptomatic disease progression.

DIAGNOSTIC APPROACH

Given the rarity of this tumor, high clinical suspicion is required for accurate diagnosis. Like any soft tissue mass, early evaluation with gadolinium-enhanced MRI is critical to identify features suggestive of a malignant process. Referral to a multidisciplinary sarcoma center for initial management, including biopsy, pathologic review, and surgical resection for localized disease, is paramount for the best outcomes.[10] Initial staging should include a high-quality contrast-enhanced CT scan of the lungs, as well as abdomen, pelvis, and bone scan. PET/CT scan may be useful to identify occult lesions particularly in advanced disease, but early lung metastases are often subcentimeter in size and below the threshold of PET detection. Additionally, PET avidity is variable, particularly given the indolent nature of some ASPS. MRI of the brain should be performed at diagnosis and periodically in patients with metastatic disease in other sites.

Radiographic Features

ASPS tumors appear highly vascular on angiography and MRI with evidence of torturous, dilated veins (Figure 15.1B and C). On MRI, it is typical to see signs of prominent venous vasculature and high signal intensity on T1- and T2-weighted images. Cui et al. performed a retrospective analysis of

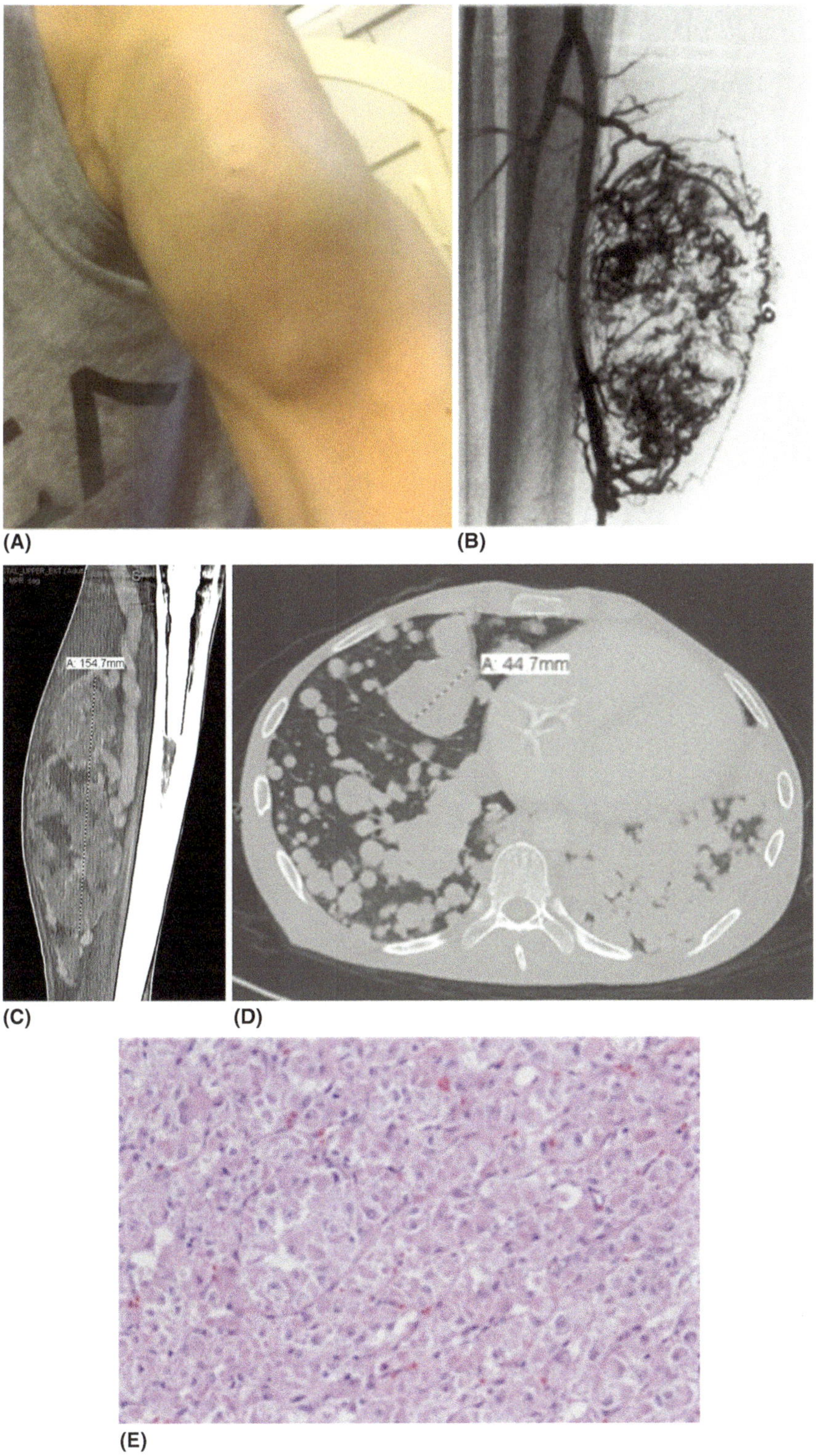

FIGURE 15.1 **Clinical, radiographic, and pathologic features of ASPS.** (A) Clinical image of large soft tissue mass of the left upper arm. (B) Angiogram of right lower extremity showing marked vascularity of the ASPS tumor with large tortuous arteries and veins and arteriovenous shunting. (C) MRI showing sagittal view of large lower extremity tumor. (D) CT of the chest showing substantial burden of metastatic disease common in ASPS. (E) Biopsy stained with hematoxylin and eosin, low-power view, showing the organoid and pseudoalveolar appearance of the tumor with central clearing and thin-walled vascular spaces.

ASPS, alveolar soft part sarcoma.

Source: Figure 15.1B reproduced with permission from Temple HT, Scully SP, O'Keefe RJ, et al. Clinical presentation of alveolar soft-part sarcoma. *Clin Orthop Relat Res*. 1994:300: Figure 5, p. 216. PMID:8131338.

MRI features in a case series of 12 patients with ASPS confirmed by pathology. They concluded that low signals or radiating flow voids accompanied by high signals of slow blood flow or blood sinuses in the center part of the tumor have high significance for the diagnosis of ASPS.[11] Ultrasound can also reveal vascular flow through ASPS lesions, which can sometimes be mistaken for large hemangiomas. In metastatic disease, virtually all patients will have innumerable lung metastases, and remarkably most patients can tolerate substantial burden of disease with mild clinical symptoms such as cough or decreased exercise tolerance (Figure 15.1D).[12]

Histopathologic Features

ASPS has a distinctive appearance microscopically and interestingly varies little from case to case; however, the differentiation and cell origin remain ambiguous. Uniform organoid nests of polygonal tumor cells, separated by fibrovascular septa, and delicate capillary-sized vascular channels define the histologic appearance (Figure 15.1E). The "alveolar" component of the name is due to the pseudoalveolar pattern, which appears to be due to necrosis of centrally located cells in the nests. Intravascular extension is present at the periphery in nearly all cases and may contribute to the high rate of metastatic disease. The cells often contain an abundant eosinophilic cytoplasm with a central nucleus and prominent nucleolus and intracytoplasmic crystals.[3]

The role of immunohistochemistry has historically been limited for the diagnosis for ASPS. Typically, these tumors are negative for epithelial markers including cytokeratins and epithelial membrane antigen, negative for neuroendocrine markers such as chromogranin A and synaptophysin, and negative for melanocytic markers including HMB-45 and Melan-A. Nonspecific markers including desmin and antibodies to actins in pan, smooth, and skeletal muscle have been reported to be positive in nearly 50% of patients. This has been an area of interest, given the controversy over cell of origin and possible myogenous differentiation.[3]

MOLECULAR AND BIOLOGIC DRIVERS

ASPS is defined by a tumor-specific translocation, t(X;17)(p11;q25).[13] This translocation results in a fusion of the transcription factor *TFE3* located on Xp11.22 with a novel gene at 17q25 named *ASPL*, also known as *ASPSCR1*. Detection of this translocation can be achieved through polymerase chain reaction (PCR) or identification of *TFE3* rearrangements by fluorescence in situ hybridization (FISH). Historically, a small subset of ASPS has been thought to be fusion negative; however, with modern whole-genome sequencing, the fusion is generally detected in these patients, likely with an alternative breakpoint that is missed by FISH probes. The recognition of this translocation provides an important diagnostic tool in differentiating ASPS from other tumor types based on histology alone, including renal cell carcinoma, hepatocellular carcinoma, paraganglioma, granular cell tumor, melanoma, and adrenal cortical carcinoma. It is important to note that some renal cell carcinomas have also been shown to be driven by related *TFE3* translocations.[14]

The *ASPS1–TFE3* fusion protein acts through altered regulation of activity of *TFE3*, a member of the microphthalmia transcription factor (MITF) transcription factor family, which drives ASPS biology through aberrant transcription and upregulation of several key pathways. First, a *TFE3*-binding site is located in the promoter of the proto-oncogene *MET*, which encodes the tyrosine kinase receptor c-MET, and multiple studies have identified increased functional protein production of c-MET and its ligand hepatocyte growth factor (HGF) in the setting of *ASPS1–TFE3* activity.[15–17] Downstream effects include upregulation of MAPK (mitogen-activated protein kinases)/ERK (extracellular signal-regulated kinases) and AKT (protein kinase B) pathways, key oncogenic regulators in other types of cancer. Additionally, numerous proangiogenic factors including vascular endothelial growth factor (VEGF), midkine, angiogenin, hypoxia-inducible factor 1 alpha (HIF-1alpha), and transforming growth factor beta (TGF-beta) have been shown to be highly expressed in ASPS, with subsequent chromatin immunoprecipitation analysis confirming direct binding of the fusion protein to the promoters of some targets such as angiopoietin-like 2 protein.[18] However, the majority of upregulated angiogenesis genes have not been shown to be direct transcriptional targets.

Emerging evidence suggests that ASPS biology, including the dependence on angiogenesis, may be highly impacted by the tumor, stromal, and immune microenvironmental factors. In a mouse model of ASPS, with conditional and inducible expression of the *ASPSCR1–TFE3* fusion gene transcript, lactate critically affected tumor cell metabolism, induced HIF-1alpha stabilization, and enhanced proliferation and angiogenesis.[19] Additionally, a different ex vivo mouse model of ASPS demonstrated that the tumor-associated vasculature permitted intravasation of tumor cells surrounded by nonmalignant hemangiopericytes, a phenomenon observed in human ASPS as well.[20] The authors postulated that hemangiopericytic encapsulation might protect tumor cells from attack by the immune system and facilitate metastatic spread.

The natural history of ASPS, with a prolonged indolent state followed by rapid tumor growth and metastasis, suggests that the human immune system may be capable of suppressing the growth of ASPS at least initially. The cancer immunoediting hypothesis describes an initial period of equilibrium, where the immune system is capable of suppressing tumor cell growth and proliferation; but with acquisition of additional immune evasion mechanisms, immunoedited resistant clones gradually take over and escape, leading to clinically apparent tumors.[21] A few case reports have described spontaneous regression of ASPS metastatic lesions, particularly after resection of the primary tumor.[22] Patients undergoing metastasectomy in the setting of limited disease generally show improved OS, which can also be seen in other types of STS. Features consistent with an immunosuppressive microenvironment in ASPS tumors include robust stroma and angiogenic networks, expression of genes like TGF-β, a potential immunosuppressive cytokine, as well as reports of expression of the immune checkpoint protein programmed-death ligand 1 (PD-L1).

Another potential mechanism in which *ASPL–TFE3* may play a role in tumorigenesis and promote an immunosuppressive microenvironment was investigated by Ishiguro et al., who demonstrated that in vitro models with ectopic expression of *ASPS1–TFE3* resulted in cell cycle arrest and increased levels of protein and mRNA of p21 (p21WAF1/CIP1). When *ASPL–TFE3* was expressed in human bone marrow mesenchymal stem cells, they observed upregulation of p21 and induction of senescence-associated galactosidase activity. When p21 was suppressed, they observed significant decrease in the induction of ASPL–TFE3-mediated cellular senescence. Furthermore, the expression of *ASPL–TFE3* was shown to induce proinflammatory cytokines including interleukin (IL)-1, IL-6, and IL-8 with senescence-associated secretory phenotype (SAPS), which further promote an immunosuppressive tumor microenvironment.[23] Finally, faulty metabolism within tumor sites, including lactate dependence, has been recently shown to greatly impact the activity and functionality of tumor-infiltrating lymphocytes, which could be a critical factor in ASPS.[24] Overall, further exploration and characterization of the immune microenvironment in ASPS are critical, particularly given the early activity observed with immunotherapy.

TREATMENT CONSIDERATIONS

Management of the Primary Tumor

The definitive treatment for ASPS with localized disease is complete surgical resection upfront. In a recent SEER analysis of 251 patients with ASPS from 1973 to 2012, 67% of patients had locoregional disease at presentation and 43% had distant metastasis. The 5-year OS rate for patients was 56%; but for those with localized disease, it was 82% and for those with distant metastasis at presentation, it was only 27%. The analysis identified that older age at diagnosis, tumor size >10 cm, distant metastasis, and truncal primary site were independent risk factors predicting worse OS. For the patients with localized disease, the analysis found that patients treated with surgery plus radiation had improved OS in comparison to surgery alone (p = .014); however, even for patients with distant metastasis, surgery of the primary site significantly improved OS (p < .001).[25]

The surgical margins postoperatively and/or the presence of metastatic disease have largely guided the clinician's decision to treat with chemotherapy and/or radiation in the adjuvant setting. It is largely accepted that ASPS is resistant to typical sarcoma doxorubicin-based chemotherapy regimens. Based on one European review of the literature of 68 patients who received upfront chemotherapy with anthracycline- or ifosfamide-containing regimens, only 4% achieved complete remission (CR), 3% had partial response (PR), 41% had stable disease, and 51% had progression of disease.[26] In another prospective European study in the pediatric population, 22 patients with a diagnosis of ASPS were evaluated. The patients were risk stratified postoperatively based on the completeness of the resection, IRS staging, and the size and grade of the tumor. Chemotherapy with doxorubicin and ifosfamide was offered to patients in IRS group III (local tumor that has not metastasized, but cannot be completely resected) and radiation was performed in patients in IRS groups II and III (II: resected with positive margins) and/or with tumor grades 2 and 3. The majority of patients (20) had localized disease and 19 had upfront surgical resection. Of the four patients who received conventional chemotherapy, none had a response. Three of 20 patients with localized disease later developed metastasis; all patients were alive at median follow-up of 61.7 months from diagnosis and the 5-year EFS rate was 91.7% and the OS rate was 100%. Of the three patients who developed metastasis, two had IRS I and small tumors <5 cm at the time of diagnosis and were treated with resection alone, developing metastatic relapse at 10 years and 4 months, respectively. The third patient was IRS III and was initially treated with two cycles of doxorubicin and ifosfamide followed by surgery and radiation; the patient developed metastatic relapse after 85.8 months.[27]

Overall, primary ASPS lesions should undergo complete resection when possible without significant morbidity, even in the setting of low-burden metastatic disease, and remains the best strategy for cure. Unfortunately, metastasis is common even in tumors <5 cm and recurrence can occur after a much longer disease-free interval than in other STSs, even a decade beyond the primary tumor diagnosis.[28,29] Therefore, these patients should be followed closely with serial imaging of the initial primary site with MRI or ultrasound and long-term chest imaging with CT scans while weighing the risks of radiation exposure from imaging versus early detection of metastatic disease. At the time of development of metastatic disease, like in other STSs, selected patients may benefit from metastasectomy, although the overall effect that surgical resection has on survival in these patients is unclear.[30]

Management of Metastatic Disease

Anti-VEGF Receptor TKIs

As discussed in the section "Molecular and Biologic Drivers," upregulation of angiogenesis-related transcripts has been identified in ASPS, prompting clinical investigation of antiangiogenic TKIs. Although none of these drugs are approved by the U.S. Food and Drug Administration (FDA) specifically for this indication, overall, anti-VEGF receptor TKIs have proved the most effective therapies for ASPS to date. Most of the data support the activity of cediranib, based on two completed clinical trials in the United States and Europe. The international CASPS trial compared cediranib versus placebo in patients with metastatic ASPS in a Phase 2, 2:1 double-blind randomized trial. Patients were unblinded at 24 weeks or sooner if the disease had progressed, and those in the placebo arm were allowed to crossover to cediranib if they had progressed. The primary endpoint was a percentage change in the sum of target marker lesions, with progression-free survival (PFS) and RECIST (Response Evaluation Criteria in Solid Tumors) response rate being the secondary endpoints. Forty-four evaluable patients were recruited between 2011 and 2016 from 12 centers in the United Kingdom, Australia, and Spain. Median change in target lesions was −8% in cediranib versus 13% in placebo ($p = .0013$). Best response at 24 weeks was RECIST partial response seen in six of 28 patients on cediranib versus zero of 16 receiving placebo. Median PFS on cediranib was 10.8 months versus 3.7 months in the placebo arm. CAPS is the largest randomized trial to date and confirms the activity by reduction in tumor burden and improvement in PFS.[31] Kummar et al. also observed substantial single-agent activity of cediranib in treatment of metastatic ASPS in a Phase 2 trial of cediranib 30 mg daily. They enrolled 46 patients and 43 were evaluable at the time of analysis. The primary endpoint of objective response rate (ORR) was 35%, with 15 of 43 patients achieving a partial response. Twenty-six patients (60%) had stable disease at 24 weeks. The disease control rate (partial response or stable disease) was 84% at 24 weeks. These results led to an ongoing open-label, multicenter, randomized Phase 2 trial for patients with metastatic ASPS comparing cediranib with another VEGF receptor inhibitor, sunitinib (ClinicalTrials.gov Identifier: NCT01391962).[32]

Anlotinib is a similar pan-VEGF receptor TKI with remarkable activity in ASPS. In a report of the Phase 2B trial conducted in China, out of 56 patients with ASPS, the median PFS was 18.23 months with anlotinib versus 3 months with placebo.[33] An ongoing Phase III trial in the United States includes an ASPS arm with open-label dosing of anlotinib, with intent for registration (ClinicalTrials.gov Identifier: NCT03016819). Activities of multiple other anti-VEGF receptor TKIs have been reported in the literature, including a small Phase 2 trial with pazopanib, which is FDA approved for other types of STS. Out of six patients, one achieved partial response and five showed stable disease with a median follow-up of 33 months. PFS was 5.5 months and OS was not reached.[34] Sunitinib has also been used regularly in the off-label setting, with one study of 15 ASPS patients reporting six patients with partial response, eight with stable disease, and one with progressive disease. The median PFS was 19 months, median OS was 56 months, and 5-year OS was 49%.[35] Several other therapies targeting VEGF have been reported in case studies and small clinical trials, including dasatinib, bevacizumab, and apatinib. A Phase 2 trial of dasatinib was conducted in patients with ASPS, chondrosarcoma, chondroma, epithelioid sarcoma, or solitary fibrous tumor. Twelve of the 109 patients had ASPS. The 6-month PFS, 2-year OS, and 5-year OS rates for patients with ASPS were 62%, 50%, and 30%, respectively.[36] A case report of single-agent bevacizumab, a monoclonal antibody against VEGF, showed marked improvement in symptoms and prolonged PR of lung metastasis of 16 months in an elderly patient who had previously failed sunitinib.[37] A case report showed a single patient with metastatic ASPS at diagnosis to the lungs which was treated with surgical resection of the primary mass and chemotherapy with gemcitabine–docetaxel with progression after two cycles. The patient was subsequently placed on apatinib 500 mg/day, a VEGFR-2 inhibitor, and achieved partial response at 1 month of therapy and remained progression free till the date of publication.[38] In general, these drugs are reasonably well tolerated, with common toxicities including neutropenia, thrombocytopenia, hypothyroidism, hypertension, and hand–foot syndrome.[35] These numerous examples suggest that blockade of VEGF receptors exhibits promising therapeutic advancement in the treatment of metastatic ASPS.

Targeting c-MET

With c-MET identified as a direct target of the fusion protein, the selective MET inhibitor tivantinib was also evaluated in a clinical trial including ASPS patients. Tivantinib appears to work through a different mechanism of action to block angiogenesis by impairing MET activity and likely having downstream effects on VEGF receptor activity. A multicenter, single-arm Phase 2 clinical trial was conducted on patients with advanced MITF-associated tumors. This is a rare group of tumors, which includes ASPS, clear cell sarcoma, and translocation-associated renal cell carcinoma, in which dysregulated expression of oncogenic MITF family transcription factors is found. The *MET* receptor tyrosine kinase gene is transcriptionally activated by MITF proteins, including TFE3. The study enrolled 47 patients with a median age of 25 years, of whom 27 had ASPS. They received tivantinib 120 mg orally twice daily and then 360 mg twice daily as per the protocol. The primary endpoint was overall response rate and the secondary endpoints included safety and PFS. There were no responses observed; however, stable disease was seen in 28 patients (60%), and median PFS was 5.5 months in the ASPS arm.[39]

Of notable interest, two patients with ASPS were long-term responders to tivantinib. The first was a 15-year-old girl diagnosed with ASPS on the left thigh with widely metastatic disease in the lungs at the time of diagnosis in 2007. She was previously treated with resection of the primary mass, radiation to the surgical bed, and resection of a tumor nodule in her lung. She was started on sorafenib, but was discontinued after 4 months because of progression of disease in the lungs. She was enrolled on the clinical trial, at which time she had several pulmonary nodules, which have been stable since last reported in a case series in January 2013. The second excellent responder was a 12-year-old boy with ASPS on the left thigh again with numerous lung lesions at the time of diagnosis in 2007. He was treated with preoperative radiation followed by resection of the primary mass. He was started on imatinib 600 mg daily for 4 months, but had progression of disease in the lungs. He was enrolled on the study and two target lesions in lungs have been closely followed. He was maintained on tivantinib for 199 weeks with stable disease as of January 2013. The prolonged stability of disease observed in these patients suggests this agent may show benefit in combination with another TKI or immunotherapy in the future.[40]

Overall, while the use of VEGF-receptor and MET TKIs has proved ability to stabilize ASPS, with some patients remaining on these agents for years prior to progression, complete responses are rare and these therapies are not curative.

Immunotherapy for ASPS

In the past decade, we have seen a revolution in cancer therapy with the development of modern immunotherapy, including ICIs. Monoclonal antibodies to the immune checkpoints CTLA-4 and the programmed death 1 (PD-1)/PD-L1 axis block suppression of T-cell activation and cytotoxicity, and have shown remarkable activity in numerous chemotherapy-refractory solid and hematologic malignancies. In sarcomas, the first trials of checkpoint inhibitors have shown meaningful and durable responses in a small subset of patients, with response rates of just under 20% with anti-PD-1 antibody pembrolizumab monotherapy and combination CTLA-4/PD-1 blockade with ipilimumab and nivolumab.[41,42] Unlike other cancers such as non-small cell lung cancer and urothelial cancer, in most cases, PD-1/PD-L1 expression has not been a reliable biomarker for the response to ICI in sarcomas, and additional biomarkers for patients likely to respond are still under investigation. However, early evidence of remarkable efficacy has been observed in patients with ASPS with checkpoint inhibitor therapy.

In a review of 50 patients enrolled in immunotherapy trials at MDACC with 14 different subtypes of sarcoma, four patients with metastatic ASPS who had received multiple prior lines of therapy were included. Two of the ASPS patients who received anti-PD-L1 therapy had partial responses nearing complete responses lasting 8 to 12 months and the other two achieved stable disease.[43] Recently presented preliminary data from a study of the PD-L1 inhibitor atezolizumab for ASPS revealed eight out of 19 patients achieving partial response (42%), nine having stable disease, and one having progressive disease. The median time to first response was five cycles, and the median time on treatment was 11 cycles.[44] In an ongoing study of tremelimumab/durvalumab, three of six patients with ASPS[45] had achieved partial response at the time of presentation. One partial response was reported in the Alliance study of ipilimumab/nivolumab in an ASPS patient receiving nivolumab monotherapy.[41]

Tumor angiogenesis has been shown to be a major contributor to the immunosuppressive tumor microenvironment, with cytokines such as HIF-1α and VEGF promoting accumulation of suppressive phenotypes of macrophages, dendritic cells, myeloid-derived suppressor cells, and T cells.[46] In melanoma and renal cell carcinoma, combinations of VEGF receptor inhibitors with immune checkpoint blockade have led to improved immune cell infiltration and tumor responses relative to either drug alone.[47,48] In an early trial of granulocyte–macrophage colony stimulating factor (GM-CSF) secreting vaccines with autologous tumor lysates in patients with ASPS and clear cell sarcoma, investigators noted postvaccine induction of serum antibodies to downstream VEGF-mediated factors including tissue-type plasminogen activator and angiopoietins-1/2. PD-1 and PD-L1 were also expressed on cytotoxic T cells and tumor cells in posttreatment tumor biopsies.[49] While no responses were seen, this was further evidence of a link between tumor angiogenesis and antitumor immunity in ASPS.

Given the importance of angiogenesis in the biology of ASPS, and the activity of anti-VEGF receptor TKIs in many types of STS, we conducted a Phase 2 trial of the anti-VEGF receptor TKI axitinib plus the anti-PD-1 checkpoint inhibitor pembrolizumab in patients with progressing, advanced, or metastatic ASPS and other STSs (ClinicalTrials.gov Identifier: NCT02301039). Out of 11 evaluable ASPS patients, six patients achieved partial response (54.5%, 95% confidence interval [CI]: 24.6–81.9) and two additional patients achieved stable disease for a clinical benefit rate of 72.7% (95% CI: 32.3–92.7). The median duration of response for ASPS patients was 29 weeks, with one patient maintaining partial response for 85 weeks before developing progressive disease and one patient who continues with a near-complete response for 94 weeks.[50] All ASPS tumor biopsies were positive for PD-L1 expression on tumor cells with robust immune cell infiltrates, suggesting that ASPS likely displays an inflamed phenotype, which is correlated with the response to ICI in other types of cancer. However, further evaluation of escape mechanisms is critical, given that most patients still ultimately develop resistance to immunotherapy.

SUMMARY

ASPS is an exceedingly rare and unique subset of STS. Despite the initial indolent nature, the early tendency of ASPS to metastasize has historically made this an incurable and ultimately fatal disease in all patients, many of whom are young. With anti-VEGF receptor TKIs, outcomes have clearly improved over the past several years; however, despite prolonging the disease course, ASPS remains incurable in nearly all cases. The early activity of ICIs against PD-1/PD-L1 represents significant hope for these patients, and with better understanding of the biology and development of counteractive combinations to resistance mechanisms, cure may be achievable one day.

CASE STUDY

A 30-year-old woman with ASPS was originally diagnosed with a primary lesion of the tongue at the age of 3 years in February 1991. At the time of diagnosis, she underwent an initial resection of the lesion in February 1991 followed by re-resection in March 1991 with no residual disease appreciated. She was treated with adjuvant chemotherapy on protocol POG 8653 from March 1991 to February 1992 with vincristine, D-actinomycin, and cyclophosphamide. She did well until the age of 6 (September 1994), at which time she had a recurrence in the chest and underwent right lower lobe thoracotomy and wedge resection. Remarkably, she was disease free until the age of 17 (2005) when she again incidentally was found to have a chest wall mass. Between 2005 and 2009, she required three wedge resections for recurrent masses in the lungs. No additional chemotherapy or radiation was given for these events.

She remained disease free between 2009 and 2012. Her next recurrence was identified during pregnancy when she was noted to have a left ventricular cardiac mass. She underwent an early cesarean section. After safe delivery, the mass regressed slightly and she was managed conservatively with observation until progression of the tumor in 2015. She was placed on sunitinib 37.5 mg orally daily in May 2015. By February 2016, her CT scans showed widespread metastatic disease with lesions in the liver, spleen, and soft tissue, including lesions in the infraspinatus muscle and the right intercostals. In March 2016, routine imaging prior to clinical trial enrollment identified multifocal brain metastasis requiring whole brain radiation. In May 2016, she was enrolled on a clinical trial combining a VEGF receptor inhibitor axitinib and the anti-PD-1 ICI pembrolizumab (ClinicalTrials.gov Identifier: NCT02301039). She achieved a durable partial response, with a decrease of >80% of her target tumor lesions. She remained on study for 20 months before developing autoimmune oligoarthritis related to pembrolizumab that required study treatment discontinuation. She is now 9 months off all treatments with stable, minimal residual disease. This case presentation highlights the unique biologic behavior of ASPS as an indolent tumor with high propensity to metastasize many years after the initial diagnosis, and highlights the complex, multidisciplinary approaches required including novel treatment modalities.

REFERENCES

1. Christopherson WM, Foote FW Jr, Stewart F W. Alveolar soft-part sarcomas; structurally characteristic tumors of uncertain histogenesis. *Cancer*. 1952;5(1):100–111. doi:10.1002/1097-0142(195201)5:1<100::aid-cncr2820050112>3.0.co;2-k
2. Masson P. *Tumeurs Humaines: Histologie, Diagnostics et Techniques*. 2nd ed. Paris, France: Libraire Maloine; 1956
3. Folpe AL, Deyrup AT. Alveolar soft-part sarcoma: a review and update. *J Clin Pathol*. 2006;59(11):1127–1132. doi:10.1136/jcp.2005.031120
4. Paoluzzi L, Ghesani M. Extraskeletal myxoid chondrosarcoma with massive pulmonary metastases. *Clin Sarcoma Res*. 2018;8:20. doi:10.1186/s13569-018-0108-8
5. Siegel RL, Miller KD, Jemal A. Cancer statistics, 2018. *CA Cancer J Clin*. 2018;68(1):7–30. doi:10.3322/caac.21442
6. Amer KM, Amer R, Sumrein N, et al. Epidemiology, incidence and survival of aveolar soft-part sarcoma: SEER database analysis. Presented at: Connective Tissue Oncology Society (CTOS) 2017 Annual Meeting; November 8–11, 2017; Maui, Hawaii.
7. Fletcher CB, Eakin EL, Rothman PE. Fetal ascites—liver giant-cell transformation. Report of a case with recovery. *Am J Dis Child*. 1964;108:554–558. https://www.ncbi.nlm.nih.gov/pubmed/14209692. PMID:14209692.
8. Flores RJ, Harrison DJ, Federman NC, et al. Alveolar soft part sarcoma in children and young adults: a report of 69 cases. *Pediatr Blood Cancer*. 2018;65(5):e26953. doi:10.1002/pbc.26953
9. Portera CA Jr, Ho V, Patel SR, et al. Alveolar soft part sarcoma: clinical course and patterns of metastasis in 70 patients treated at a single institution. *Cancer*. 2001;91(3):585–591. doi:10.1002/1097-0142(20010201)91:3<585::aid-cncr1038>3.0.co;2-0
10. Abarca T, Gao Y, Monga V, et al. Improved survival for extremity soft tissue sarcoma treated in high-117 facilities. *J Surg Oncol*. 2018;117(7):1479–1486. doi:10.1002/jso.25052
11. Cui JF, Chen HS, Hao DP, et al. Magnetic resonance features and characteristic vascular pattern of alveolar soft-part sarcoma. *Oncol Res Treat*. 2017;40(10):580–585. doi:10.1159/000477443
12. Temple HT, Scully SP, O'Keefe RJ, et al. Clinical presentation of alveolar soft-part sarcoma. *Clin Orthop Relat Res*. 1994;300:213–218. PMID:8131338
13. Ladanyi M, Lui MY, Antonescu CR, et al. The der(17)t(X;17)(p11;q25) of human alveolar soft part sarcoma fuses the TFE3 transcription factor gene to ASPL, a novel gene at 17q25. *Oncogene*. 2001;20(1):48–57. doi:10.1038/sj.onc.1204074
14. Zhong M, De Angelo P, Osborne L, et al. Translocation renal cell carcinomas in adults: a single-institution experience. *Am J Surg Pathol*. 2012;36(5):654–662. doi:10.1097/PAS.0b013e31824f24a6
15. Lazar AJ, Lahat G, Myers SE, et al. Validation of potential therapeutic targets in alveolar soft part sarcoma: an immunohistochemical study utilizing tissue microarray. *Histopathology*. 2009;55(6):750–755. doi:10.1111/j.1365-2559.2009.03436.x
16. Tsuda M, Davis IJ, Argani P, et al. TFE3 fusions activate MET signaling by transcriptional up-regulation, defining another class of tumors as candidates for therapeutic MET inhibition. *Cancer Res*. 2007;67(3):919–929. doi:10.1158/0008-5472.CAN-06-2855
17. Jun HJ, Lee J, Lim DH, et al. Expression of MET in alveolar soft part sarcoma. *Med Oncol*. 2010;27(2):459–465. doi:10.1007/s12032-009-9234-8
18. Kobos R, Nagai M, Tsuda M, et al. Combining integrated genomics and functional genomics to dissect the biology of a cancer-associated, aberrant transcription factor, the ASPSCR1-TFE3 fusion oncoprotein. *J Pathol*. 2013;229(5):743–754. doi:10.1002/path.4158
19. Goodwin ML, Jin H, Straessler K, et al. Modeling alveolar soft part sarcomagenesis in the mouse: a role for lactate in the tumor microenvironment. *Cancer Cell*. 2014;26(6):851–862. doi:10.1016/j.ccell.2014.10.003
20. Tanaka M, Homme M, Yamazaki Y, et al. Modeling alveolar soft part sarcoma unveils novel mechanisms of metastasis. *Cancer Res*. 2017;77(4):897–907. doi:10.1158/0008-5472.CAN-16-2486

21. Schreiber RD, Old LJ, Smyth MJ. Cancer immunoediting: integrating immunity's roles in cancer suppression and promotion. *Science*. 2011;331(6024):1565–1570. doi:10.1126/science.1203486
22. BaniHani MN, Al Manasra AR. Spontaneous regression in alveolar soft part sarcoma: case report and literature review. *World J Surg Oncol*. 2009;7:53. doi:10.1186/1477-7819-7-53
23. Ishiguro N, Yoshida H. ASPL-TFE3 oncoprotein regulates cell cycle progression and induces cellular senescence by up-regulating p21. *Neoplasia*. 2016;18(10):626–635. doi:10.1016/j.neo.2016.08.001
24. Buck MD, Sowell RT, Kaech SM, Pearce EL. Metabolic instruction of immunity. *Cell*. 2017;169(4):570–586. doi:10.1016/j.cell.2017.04.004
25. Wang H, Jacobson A, Harmon DC, et al. Prognostic factors in alveolar soft part sarcoma: a SEER analysis. *J Surg Oncol*. 2016;113(5):581–586. doi:10.1002/jso.24183
26. Reichardt P, Lindner T, Pink D, et al. Chemotherapy in alveolar soft part sarcomas. What do we know? *Eur J Cancer*. 2003;39(11):1511–1516. doi:10.1016/s0959-8049(03)00264-8
27. Brennan B, Zanetti I, Orbach D, et al. Alveolar soft part sarcoma in children and adolescents: the European Paediatric Soft Tissue Sarcoma study group prospective trial (EpSSG NRSTS 2005). *Pediatr Blood Cancer*. 2018;65(4):e26942. doi:10.1002/pbc.26942
28. Pappo AS, Parham DM, Cain A, et al. Alveolar soft part sarcoma in children and adolescents: clinical features and outcome of 11 patients. *Med Pediatr Oncol*. 1996;26(2):81–84. doi:10.1002/(SICI)1096-911X(199602)26:2<81::AID-MPO2>3.0.CO;2-Q
29. van Ruth S, van Coevorden F, Peterse JL, Kroon BBR. Alveolar soft part sarcoma. A report of 15 cases. *Eur J Cancer*. 2002;38(10):1324–1328. doi:10.1016/s0959-8049(02)00032-1
30. Billingsley KG, Burt ME, Jara E, et al. Pulmonary metastases from soft tissue sarcoma: analysis of patterns of diseases and postmetastasis survival. *Ann Surg*. 1999;229(5):602–610; discussion 610–612. doi:10.1097/00000658-199905000-00002
31. Judson IR, Morden JP, Leahy MG, et al. Activity of cediranib in alveolar soft part sarcoma (ASPS) confirmed by CASPS (cediranib in ASPS), and international, randomised phase II trial (C2130/A12118). *J Clin Oncol*. 2017;35(15):11004. doi:10.1200/JCO.2017.35.15
32. Kummar S, Allen D, Monks A, et al. Cediranib for metastatic alveolar soft part sarcoma. *J Clin Oncol*. 2013;31(18):2296–2302. doi:10.1200/JCO.2012.47.4288
33. Chi Y, Sun Y, Cai J, et al. Phase II study of anlotinib for treatment of advanced soft tissue sarcomas. *J Clin Oncol*. 2017;34(15 suppl):11005. https://ascopubs.org/doi/10.1200/JCO.2016.34.15_suppl.11005
34. Kim M, Kim TM, Keam B, et al. A Phase II trial of pazopanib in patients with metastatic alveolar soft part sarcoma. *Oncologist*. 2019;24(1):e20–e29. doi:10.1634/theoncologist.2018-0464
35. Jagodzińska-Mucha P, Świtaj T, Kozak K, et al. Long-term results of therapy with sunitinib in metastatic alveolar soft part sarcoma. *Tumori*. 2017;103(3):231–235. doi:10.5301/tj.5000617
36. Schuetze SM, Bolejack V, Choy E, et al. Phase 2 study of dasatinib in patients with alveolar soft part sarcoma, chondrosarcoma, chordoma, epithelioid sarcoma, or solitary fibrous tumor. *Cancer*. 2017;123(1):90–97. doi:10.1002/cncr.30379
37. Mir O, Boudou-Rouquette P, Larousserie F, et al. Durable clinical activity of single-agent bevacizumab in a nonagenarian patient with metastatic alveolar soft part sarcoma. *Anticancer Drugs*. 2012;23(7):745–748. doi:10.1097/CAD.0b013e3283514b8c
38. Zhou Y, Tang F, Wang Y, et al. Advanced alveolar soft part sarcoma responds to apatinib. *Oncotarget*. 2017;8(30):50314–50322. doi:10.18632/oncotarget.18599
39. Wagner AJ, Goldberg JM, Dubois SG, et al. Tivantinib (ARQ 197), a selective inhibitor of MET, in patients with microphthalmia transcription factor-associated tumors: results of a multicenter phase 2 trial. *Cancer*. 2012;118(23):5894–5902. doi:10.1002/cncr.27582
40. Goldberg JM, Gavcovich T, Saigal G, et al. Extended progression-free survival in two patients with alveolar soft part sarcoma exposed to tivantinib. *J Clin Oncol*. 2014;32(34):e114–e116. doi:10.1200/JCO.2013.48.7462
41. D'Angelo SP, Mahoney MR, Van Tine BA, et al. Nivolumab with or without ipilimumab treatment for metastatic sarcoma (Alliance A091401): two open-label, non-comparative, randomised, phase 2 trials. *Lancet Oncol*. 2018;19(3):416–426. doi:10.1016/S1470-2045(18)30006-8
42. Tawbi HA, Burgess M, Bolejack V, et al. Pembrolizumab in advanced soft-tissue sarcoma and bone sarcoma (SARC028): a multicentre, two-cohort, single-arm, open-label, phase 2 trial. *Lancet Oncol*. 2017;18(11):1493–1501. doi:10.1016/S1470-2045(17)30624-1
43. Groisberg R, Hong DS, Behrang A, et al. Characteristics and outcomes of patients with advanced sarcoma enrolled in early phase immunotherapy trials. *J Immunother Cancer*. 2017;5(1):100. doi:10.1186/s40425-017-0301-y
44. Coyne GO, Sharon E, Moore N, et al. Phase II study of atezolizumab in patients with alveolar soft part sarcoma. Presented at: Connective Tissue Oncology Society (CTOS) Meeting; November 14–17, 2018; Rome, Italy.
45. Somaiah N, Conley A, Lin H, et al. A phase II multi-arm study to test the efficacy of durvalumab and tremelimumab in multiple sarcoma subtypes. Presented at: Connective Tissue Oncology Society CTOS Meeting; November 8–11, 2017; Maui, Hawaii.
46. Kwilas AR, Donahue RN, Tsang KY, Hodge JW. Immune consequences of tyrosine kinase inhibitors that synergize with cancer immunotherapy. *Cancer Cell Microenviron*. 2015;2(1):e677. doi:10.14800/ccm.677
47. Hodi FS, Lawrence D, Lezcano C, et al. Bevacizumab plus ipilimumab in patients with metastatic melanoma. *Cancer Immunol Res*. 2014;2(7):632–642. doi:10.1158/2326-6066.CIR-14-0053

48. Atkins MB, Plimack ER, Puzanov I, et al. Axitinib in combination with pembrolizumab in patients with advanced renal cell cancer: a non-randomised, open-label, dose-finding, and dose-expansion phase 1b trial. *Lancet Oncol*. 2018;19(3):405–415. doi:10.1016/S1470-2045(18)30081-0
49. Goldberg JM, Fisher DE, Demetri GD, et al. Biologic activity of autologous, granulocyte-macrophage colony-stimulating factor secreting alveolar soft-part sarcoma and clear cell sarcoma vaccines. *Clin Cancer Res*. 2015;21(14):3178–3186. doi:10.1158/1078-0432.CCR-14-2932
50. Wilky BA, Trucco MM, Kolonias D, et al. A phase II trial of axitinib plus pembrolizumab for patients with advanced alveolar soft part sarcoma (ASPS) and other soft tissue sarcomas (STS). *J Clin Oncol*. 2018;36:(15 suppl):11547–11547. doi:10.1200/jco.2018.36.15_suppl.11547

16

Tenosynovial Giant Cell Tumor/Pigmented Villonodular Synovitis

Edward Y. Cheng, Christian M. Ogilvie, and Paari Murugan

INTRODUCTION

A mass-like growth arising from the synovial tissue was described by several early authors,[1–3] but it was not until 1941 that Jaffe and Lichenstein[4] coined the term pigmented villonodular synovitis (PVNS), based upon the gross appearance of xanthomatous nodular densities arising in a synovial joint. This term continues to be used in modern parlance. Masses that arise from extra-articular synovial tissue of the tendon sheaths were also recognized, but it was unclear if these were neoplastic or reactive in etiology and the terms giant cell tumor of tendon sheath (GCT-TS) and nodular tenosynovitis were used to describe these entities. More recently, the 2013 World Health Organization soft tissue classification schema categorized the origin of all of these entities as a "so-called fibrohistiocytic origin tumor," termed tenosynovial giant cell tumor (TGCT)[5] with the older traditional terms considered different forms of TGCT (Figure 16.1).

The clinical spectrum of diseases caused by TGCT is broad, ranging from benign, small nodular growths in the tendon sheaths of the digits (giant cell tumor of tendon sheath, GCT-TS) to intra-articular soft tissue masses (PVNS), either focal or involving diffuse synovitis, with or without extra-articular extension, to a rarely found, but nonetheless described, malignant tumor with fatal metastases. This tumor usually occurs in middle-aged adults.[6,7] Nearly always, clinicians encounter the benign nodular growth form in the tenosynovial tissues of the hand/wrist/foot or the intra-articular mass form in a synovial joint, most often the knee. When a nodular or solitary focal mass only is identified, the disease is considered *localized*. When multiple focal masses or extensive synovitis is present in a synovial joint, the disease is considered *diffuse*. The disease is usually monoarticular, with occasional polyarticular involvement when locally spread to a nearby, adjacent joint occurs, for example in the carpal joints of the wrist or the tibiotalar and subtalar joints of the hindfoot and ankle. Differentiation between a localized versus diffuse form of disease can be problematic when a focal intra-articular mass has some degree of reactive synovitis or changes from hemarthrosis present, but not sufficient to make a diagnosis of neoplastic involvement of the synovium.

Despite the plethora of names and clinical presentation, the histologic findings (Figure 16.2) are the same for each of these entities, with the exception of the malignant type.[5]

For many years, the management of this disease has been focused on the local control of the disease, which could be slowly destructive to local tissues resulting in debilitating arthritis, or relatively indolent with minor symptoms that cause minimal disability for patients. More recently, research findings have clearly identified the clonal, neoplastic growth of this disease and molecular insights into the genetic background of the tumor have opened the door to targeted therapies that are under investigation.

ESTIMATED INCIDENCE PER YEAR, GENDER, AND RACE

Incidence

TGCT is an uncommon benign tumor and according to cancer agencies, it is rare by any definition (National Cancer Institute: incidence <15 per 100,000 population; European Union: incidence <50 per 100,000). The true incidence of TGCT is not known exactly; however, three prior studies have provided some insight. From 1960 to 1976, Myers et al. performed a pathology review survey of 12 Tennessee hospitals finding 166 new cases of TGCT. When broken down by type, the incidence of GCT-TS was 9.2 cases per million population and for PVNS (localized and diffuse) 1.8 cases per million population.[8]

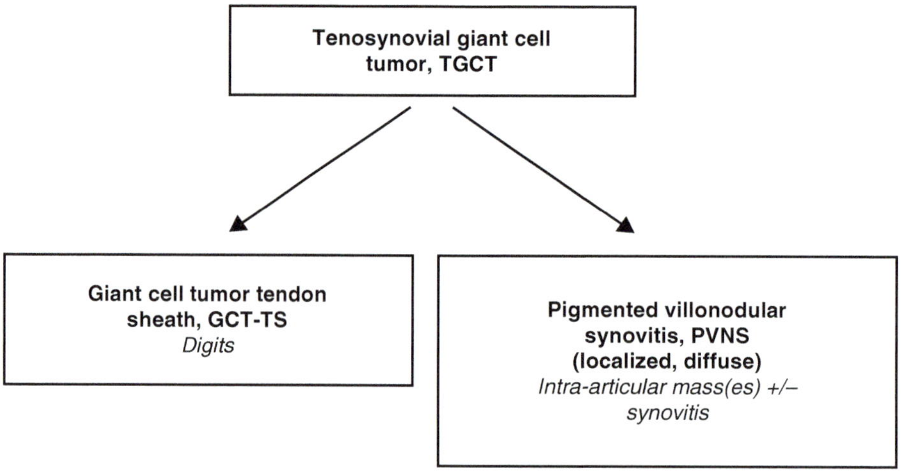

FIGURE 16.1 Types of tenosynovial giant cell tumor and nomenclature commonly used.

From 1990 to 1997, a study from Edinburgh of localized type PVNS revealed an incidence of 20 cases per million.[7] From 2009 to 2013, Mastboom et al. completed a survey of Dutch hospitals and found 2,815 cases involving digits and 1,323 cases involving nondigits. The incidences found were GCT-TS, 34 per million person-years; PVNS localized extremity, 11 per million; and PVNS diffuse, 5 per million.[6] When adjusted for worldwide population data, the estimated incidences were GCT-TS, 29 per million; PVNS localized extremity, 10 per million; and PVNS diffuse, 4 per million.[6]

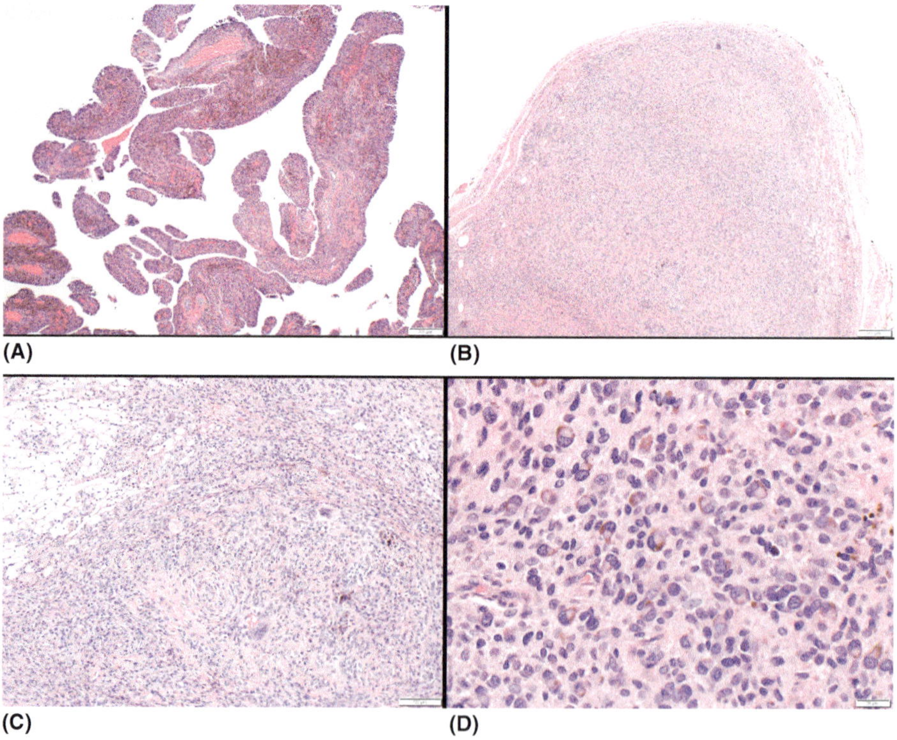

FIGURE 16.2 Diffuse-type tenosynovial giant cell tumor (pigmented villonodular synovitis): Hematoxylin and eosin-stained sections demonstrate a synovium-based hemosiderin pigment-laden neoplasm with papillovillous (A) and nodular architecture (B) (H&E ×100). Higher magnification reveals a diffuse proliferation of mononuclear cells in a background of multinucleate giant cells, histiocytes, and lymphocytes (C) (H&E ×200). The neoplastic mononuclear cells are large, epithelioid with eccentrically placed nuclei and a wreath-like deposition of hemosiderin ("ladybug" cells) (D) (H&E ×400).

H&E, hematoxylin and eosin.

Gender

A slight predilection for females is present in all epidemiologic studies of TGCT. The Tennessee study found a female/male ratio of 1.25:1 ($p < .01$).[8] The Dutch study had a similar sex distribution of female to male, 1.5:1.[6] The Edinburgh study of localized PVNS had a female/male ratio of 1.6:1.[7]

Race

No studies have found any racial differences among black versus white versus other populations.

MOST COMMON PRESENTING SYMPTOMS

The clinical presentation for TGCT varies depending upon the anatomic site and disease type. For hand and foot localized disease, presentation was painless swelling (93%) in the Edinburgh study.[7] Among the patients in the Tennessee study, GCT-TS patients most often presented with a mass (99%), of which 76% were asymptomatic. Among the PVNS patients, joint swelling (75%), pain (79%), or other dysfunction (37%) were much more common than a mass (10%).

Symptoms usually develop over a long period of time. When a synovial joint is involved, patients notice the intermittent joint effusions, probably related to hemarthroses, and also complain of mechanical symptoms of locking and catching. Trauma is unlikely to be etiologic, given the rarity of disease, yet minor trauma, even from daily activities, may herald the onset of symptoms, especially if hemarthroses develop. The initiation of prospective clinical trials for targeted therapy agents has resulted in the collection of patient-reported outcomes measures. In a Phase 1 trial of pexidartinib for diffuse (19) and localized (3) PVNS, the most common symptoms cited by patients were pain (82%), swelling (86%), stiffness (73%), reduced range of motion (64%), and joint instability (64%).[9]

DIAGNOSTIC APPROACH

The workup and subsequent diagnosis of TGCT is based upon clinical suspicion, after ruling out other more common intra-articular pathology, by performing a history and physical examination, MRI, and eventual tissue biopsy confirmation. Biopsy in the most common clinical scenarios will differ, depending upon the type of disease suspected and the anatomic site. For example, for GCT-TS involving either the digits, wrist, or other extra-articular sites, the size of the lesion is usually small, for example, <5 cm, and simple excisional biopsy is not only diagnostic but also adequate treatment for the disease. For the uncommon larger extra-articular lesions, concerns about a possible sarcoma are prudent and therefore incisional biopsy, or a core-needle biopsy, is warranted to preserve surgical options for a wide excision, should that become necessary. For intra-articular masses or joint synovitis, an arthroscopic biopsy is satisfactory, provided a sufficient amount of tissue is sampled. If the diagnosis can be made upon frozen section, then proceeding with surgical excision, as appropriate, under the same anesthetic can be undertaken. However, if a frozen section is equivocal, then it is optimal to delay any definitive procedure until the diagnosis is confirmed.

RADIOGRAPHIC FEATURES AND RECOMMENDED IMAGING

While plain radiographs are appropriate to look for either destructive joint changes or calcifications, which might suggest alternate diagnoses, the optimal imaging of TGCT is MRI (Figure 16.3).[10–12] A gradient echo sequence is most diagnostic with the key finding being the blooming artifact that occurs from the presence of metal (iron) in the hemosiderin-laden tissue often present[13] (Figure 16.3A). Other types of proprietary and nonproprietary gradient echo type sequences, for example, a fast field echo sequence, are acceptable as well.[14] Both clinicians and imaging review centers for clinical trials use MRI for assessing both treatment response and surveillance for relapse.[12,15] Metrics for measuring treatment response are lacking, however, as the Response Evaluation Criteria in Solid Tumors (RECIST)[16] and Choi criteria[17] have not been validated for this disease. Given the intra-articular and synovitic nature of some of the tumors, volumetric assessment using multiple MRI slices is likely to be the most accurate as opposed to measuring joint effusion or other parameters.

TGCT demonstrates hypermetabolic activity on PET, which is therefore a modality that is sensitive for detecting TGCT, either primary or recurrent; however, hypermetabolic regions must be differentiated from either metastatic or other primary sarcomas by either other techniques or clinical correlation as PET is not specific enough to make this distinction.[18–20]

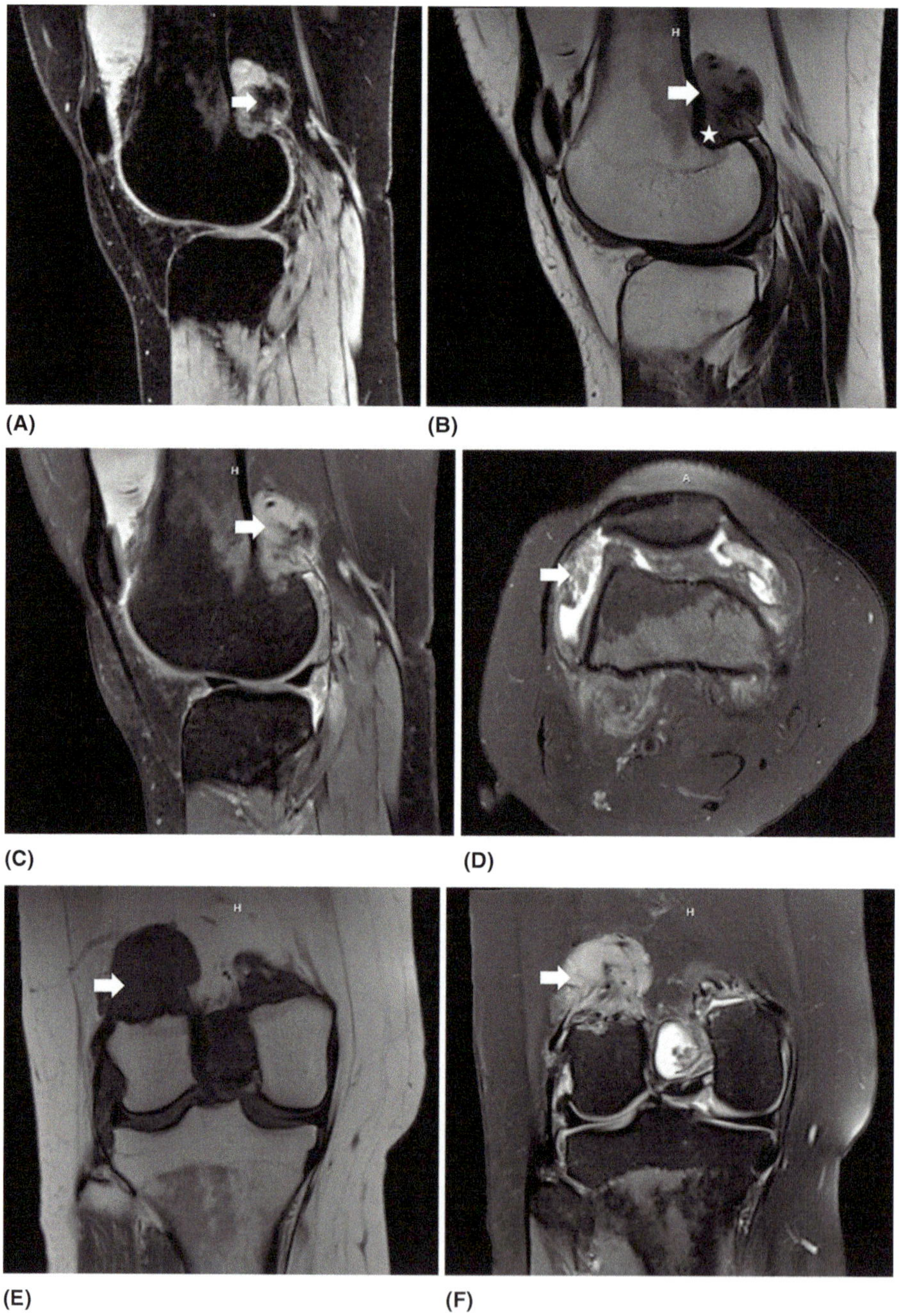

FIGURE 16.3 MRI of the right knee of a 26-year-old woman with several months of gradually increasing and intermittent knee swelling followed by 3 months of persistent knee swelling, decreased range of motion, and discomfort. (A) Sagittal gradient echo sequence demonstrating a dark signal void (blooming) of pigmented villonodular synovitis (arrow). (B) Sagittal T2 sequence demonstrating low to intermediate signal characteristic of pigmented villonodular synovitis (arrow) and periarticular bone erosion just proximal to the femoral condyle (star). (C) Sagittal fat-saturated proton density sequence also demonstrating low to intermediate signal of pigmented villonodular synovitis (arrow) and additional pigmented villonodular synovitis signal behind the posterior horn of the meniscus. (D) Axial fat-saturated T2 sequence showing pigmented villonodular synovitis in the lateral gutter (arrow). (E) Coronal T1 sequence shows low signal (arrow). (F) Coronal fat-saturated proton density sequence with pigmented villonodular synovitis next to femoral condyle (arrow).

MOLECULAR ABERRATION DRIVING THE TUMOR

TGCT is a clonal neoplasm that is typically characterized by rearrangements, involving the short arm of chromosome 1 (1p11–13) besides chromosome 5 and 7 trisomies.[21,22] The majority of the cases show rearrangements of the macrophage colony stimulating factor-1 (*CSF1*) gene located at the 1p13 locus.[23] Although the most common translocation partner is *COL6A3* at 2q37 [t(1;2)(p13;q37)],[24,25] multiple other fusions, including a novel *CSF1-S100A10* fusion gene and *CSF1* transcript have also been documented.[21,22,25,26] These aberrations can be detected by cytogenetic analyses, such as karyotyping and in situ hybridization as well as by reverse transcription polymerase chain reaction (RT-PCR) and RNA sequencing techniques. The neoplastic cells harboring the *CSF1* fusion transcripts that induce overexpression of the protein constitute only a minority of the tumor mass, the bulk of which is made up of *CSF1R* (*CSF1* receptor) containing reactive cells of the monocyte–macrophage lineage. This suggests the neoplastic cells create a tumor landscape that results in autocrine proliferation as well as the recruitment and induction of nonneoplastic macrophages and osteoclast-like giant cells.[27] The overexpression of *CSF1* and *CSF1R* is also seen in cases of TGCT that do not harbor translocations, suggesting alternative mechanisms of *CSF1* upregulation.[23,27] In addition to *CSF1* overexpression, Huang et al.[28] have shown alterations of cyclin A, P53, and 15q region in a cohort of malignant TCGT cases. The latter events may represent mechanisms leading to the rarely encountered malignant transformation in these tumors. From a management perspective, especially in cases that are recurrent or locally advanced, the abundance of *CSF1R* transmembrane tyrosine kinase receptors in these tumors offers a promising therapeutic target.

The differential diagnosis of TCGT includes other neoplasms and reactive synovitides, such as hemosiderotic synovitis, detritic synovitis, rheumatoid arthritis, crystal associated arthropathies, and chronic nonspecific synovitis that may result in synovial proliferation, inflammation, and hemosiderin deposition. However, these disorders do not exhibit a diffuse proliferation of mononuclear epithelioid cells in the typical heterogeneous background of multinucleate giant cells, histiocytes, and lymphocytes as seen in TCGT (Figure 16.2). In addition, although *CSF1* may be overexpressed in the lining cells of some of the reactive entities,[27] the characteristic molecular findings found in TCGT are not present in other diseases.

COMMON ANATOMIC LOCATIONS

Excluding the digits, the knee is by far the most common anatomic site for both localized and diffuse PVNS (46% and 64%, respectively).[6] Other common sites for localized disease are the hand/foot (30%) and the wrist and ankle (17%), while for the diffuse form, the ankle (10%) and hip (9%) are more common, and the hand and foot are less common (6%).

GENERAL THERAPEUTIC APPROACH

Giant Cell Tumor–Tendon Sheath

As this usually occurs in the digits of the hand and foot or around the wrist and is localized, surgical excision is the mainstay of treatment (Table 16.1). Most clinical presentations involve a differential diagnosis of other types of tenosynovitis. Prior steroid injections may have been administered. Upon surgical exposure, either a xanthomatous type nodule or hypertrophic synovium is usually evident. Complete, gross total excision, *en bloc* as possible, results in successful local control of the disease in 85% to 90% of cases.[29–32]

Localized Pigmented Villonodular Synovitis

The clinical presentation of this type of disease is usually an intra-articular focal mass associated with mechanical symptoms of joint dysfunction. In many cases, the MRI alone, with appropriate gradient echo sequences, is sufficient to have a high index of suspicion for the disease. Usually the differential diagnosis includes other intra-articular masses, such as synovial chondromatosis, lipoma arborescens, rheumatoid arthritis, gout, or amyloid associated arthropathy. Intra-articular masses are almost always benign, although cases of intra-articular sarcomas have been reported. More often, an extra-articular sarcoma has grown through and invaginated the synovial membrane, appearing as an intra-articular mass.

TABLE 16.1 Summary Table of Management Recommendations

TGCT Type	Anatomic Sites	Recurrence Risk	Management
GCT-TS	Digits, hand, foot, wrist	Low	Surgical excision
Localized PVNS	Intra-articular; knee, hip, hand/foot, wrist/ankle	Low	Surgical excision, *en bloc*, possibly arthroscopic
Diffuse PVNS	Intra-articular and extra-articular; knee, ankle, hip	High	1. Complete, gross total excision with synovectomy, anterior and posterior 2. Recurrence a. Imatinib or other tyrosine kinase inhibitor b. CSF1/CSF1R targeted agent, as available c. Radiation synovectomy, external beam radiation, for recurrent disease in elderly patients 3. Total joint arthroplasty, if joint destruction present, age and site dependent

CSF1, colony stimulating factor 1; CSF1R, CSF1 receptor; GCT-TS, giant cell tumor of tendon sheath; PVNS, pigmented villonodular synovitis; TGCT, tenosynovial giant cell tumor.

Optimal management is surgical resection of the mass.[33–36] While this usually can be accomplished technically with arthroscopic techniques, this is only advisable as long as morselization is not required and the mass can be removed *en bloc*. If morselization is needed, the consequent intra-articular contamination will increase the risk of local relapse, and therefore, an open technique enabling an *en bloc* excision is preferable.

Diffuse Pigmented Villonodular Synovitis

The clinical presentation again is similar to the localized form of the disease, yet recurrent hemarthroses and effusions are more common. The disease is locally aggressive but nonmetastasizing. Extra-articular soft tissue extension is common, and a diligent search for disease in the posterior intercondylar notch, the popliteus muscle, and behind the gastrocnemius muscle origin along the posterior femoral condyles is paramount to accurately assess the extent of disease. If surgical excision is undertaken, all diseased tissue must be excised to attain a gross total excision if durable local control is to be achieved. Traditionally, the mainstay of treatment is surgical excision with the goal of gross total excision as noted. The local recurrence-free survival is dependent upon the completeness of tumor excision.[37,38] Often, an extensile posterior approach to the posterior capsule of the knee, detaching the gastrocnemius muscle heads, is needed to adequately visualize the full extent of disease in the posterior knee[39] (Figure 16.3B).

Controversy exists regarding an arthroscopic versus open approach to surgical resection and synovectomy. Clearly, arthroscopic techniques are associated with less morbidity, yet the risk of recurrence has been reported to be higher owing to incomplete excision and inability to resect extra-articular disease.[33,40–42]

Regardless of the surgical approach, it is clear that the local recurrence risk is higher in the diffuse form of PVNS with a 5-year local recurrence-free survival rate of 50% or less.[38]

Attempts to improve local control and limit morbidity have included radiosynovectomy with yttrium-90 or phosphorus-32, either combined with surgery[43–45] or alone.[46] Other isotopes such as rhenium-186 sulfide colloid have been described.[47] External beam radiation has been used for treatment of PVNS; however, incurring the toxicity of radiation for treating a benign disease limits the enthusiasm for this treatment modality.[48–50]

With the knowledge that macrophage colony stimulating factor (M-CSF), also known as CSF-1, and CSF-1R are overexpressed in PVNS, tyrosine kinase inhibitors were studied for efficacy in PVNS.[51] A case report of a complete response to imatinib[52] demonstrated proof of concept in disrupting the CSF-1:CSR-1R paracrine loop. Further investigation revealed some efficacy in PVNS with RECIST defined responses in 19% of cases[53] as well as two cases of nilotinib-resistant disease.[15] Nilotinib has been investigated in inoperable or relapsing PVNS in a European trial, which revealed a partial response rate of 6% (3/51 patients).[54]

More recently, specific novel agents targeting both *CSF1* and *CSF1R* have been developed. A humanized monoclonal anti-M-CSF antibody that blocks phosphorylation of the CSF-1R (Novartis MCS110),[55] a small molecule inhibitor of *CSF1R* (Daiichi Sankyo, Pexidartinib, PLX-3397), and a humanized monoclonal anti-*CSF1R* antibody (Daiichi Sankyo, Emactuzumab, RG7155)[56] have been studied in clinical trials for PVNS.[57,58] For MCS110, a Phase 1/2 trial revealed a 40% reduction in tumor volume with tolerable side effects (periorbital edema).[55] For pexidartinib, a Phase 3 trial revealed a 55% reduction in tumor volume; however, serious liver toxicity was noted.[57] This study led to the Food and Drug Administration (FDA) approval in the United States in 2019 and is considered standard therapy for patients who are not candidates for definitive surgical resection. Many questions remain to be answered including the optimal dosages, frequency, and duration of treatment.

Malignant Pigmented Villonodular Synovitis

A malignant form of PVNS has been described in several case reports.[59,60] However, it is extremely rare, with less than 20 cases reported in the medical literature.[61] Six cases, all with pulmonary metastases, were treated with a combination of either doxorubicin or gemcitabine/docetaxel, at times with a tyrosine kinase inhibitor.[62] All six patients died of their disease at a median of 22 months after diagnosis.

RECOMMENDED FOLLOW-UP AFTER DEFINITIVE THERAPY

Monitoring for relapse after treatment for TGCT is important, yet scant evidence is available to guide recommendations. The likelihood of relapse is much greater for the diffuse type of PVNS as opposed to the localized type or GCT-TS of the digits. In addition, patients who relapse with either the localized form or digital GCT-TS are likely to either have symptoms or will notice a recurrent mass. Patient education and self-examination should be sufficient in these patients. Therefore, surveillance with imaging can be limited to only patients with the diffuse form of PVNS. MRI is the best imaging modality for detecting recurrent disease. While fluorodeoxyglucose (FDG)-PET might be considered, the limited specificity and higher cost argue against using this modality. How frequent to image and for what duration are determined by both a physician's judgment and patient's tolerance for evaluations; nonetheless, relapses have been reported at over 5 years after treatment.[50]

SUMMARY

The management of TGCT is changing as our understanding of the chromosomal translocations involving the *CSF1* and *CSF1R* pathway driving the development of this tumor are further elucidated. While surgical excision continues to be the initial treatment for both GCT-TS and localized PVNS, the management of diffuse PVNS is likely to evolve as other effective, nonsurgical therapies become available. With the efficacy of pexidartinib demonstrated, the challenge will be in determining the optimal role for this targeted agent. Possible roles are in the neoadjuvant setting to facilitate surgical excision, the adjuvant setting to lower the risk of local relapse, or as the primary sole treatment of PVNS, eliminating the need for surgical resection. Given the efficacy and toxicity profiles demonstrated to date, however, it is unlikely that surgery will be relegated to a historical treatment. Nonetheless, these new agents are the most exciting development in many decades regarding the treatment of TGCT.

CASE STUDY

A 15-year-old male had diffuse PVNS and underwent multiple local excisions, but continued to have recurrent disease and then underwent intra-articular dysprosium radiation synovectomy at age 17. Relapses continued despite two open posterior synovectomies, and he was treated with external beam radiation at age 29. The relapses still continued and two recurrent nodules were excised in the following 3 years. He was then disease free for 18 years, but developed degenerative knee disease resulting in a knee arthroplasty at age 37. Eleven years later, another anterior and posterior synovectomy was completed; however, 2 years afterward a mass developed in his quadriceps muscle and PVNS was confirmed with a core needle biopsy. Imatinib 400 mg per day was given for 1 year with partial response. He still had a palpable extra-articular mass and was symptomatic. Therefore, he enrolled in a clinical trial using an anti-M-CSF antibody (Novartis MCS-110) and was given four infusions resulting in a dramatic response as demonstrated both clinically (size reduction) and by reduction in SUVmax on FDG-PET (Figure 16.4). He has been disease free since the last treatment 5 years ago.

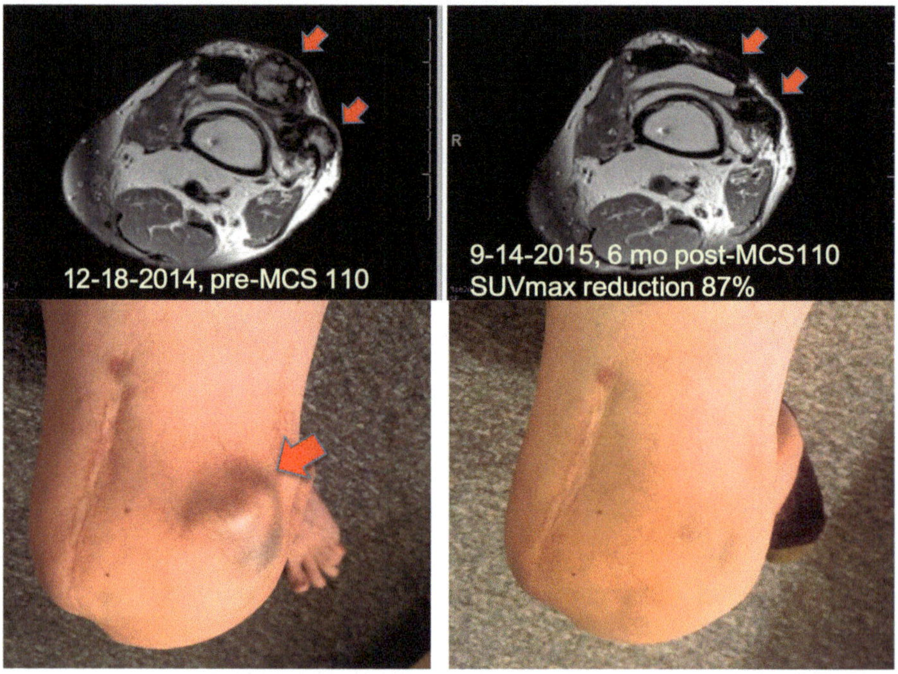

FIGURE 16.4 Magnetic resonance axial T1 image demonstrating recurrent, extra-articular pigmented villonodular synovitis proximal to patella in vastus lateralis muscle before (top left) and after (top right) treatment with MCS110. Clinical photographs (anteroposterior view of knee flexed to 90 degrees) of the patient's knee demonstrating the visual appearance of the palpable, extra-articular pigmented villonodular synovitis soft tissue mass before (bottom left) and after (bottom right) treatment with MCS110.

REFERENCES

1. Chassaignac M. Cancer de la gaine des tendons. *Gaz Hosp Civ Milit*. 1852;47:185–186.
2. Moser E. Primäres sarkom der fussgelenklapsel. Extirpation. Dauerheiung. *Dtsch Z Chir*. 1909;98(2–3):306–310.
3. Simon G. Extirpation einer sehr grossen, mit dickem stiele angewachsenen kniegelenkmaus mit glucklichem erfolge. *Arch Klinn Chir*. 1864;6:573–576.
4. Jaffe HL, Lichtenstein L, Sutro CJ. Pigmented villonodular synovitis, bursitis, and tenosynovitis: a discussion of the synovial and bursal equivalents of the tenosynovial lesions commonly denoted as xanthoma xanthogranuloma, giant cell tumor, or myeloplaxoma of the tendon sheath, with some consideration for the tendon sheath lesion itself. *Arch Pathol*. 1941;31:731–765.
5. de St. Aubain Somerhausen N, van de Rijn M. Tenosynovial giant cell tumor, localized type/diffuse type. In: Fletcher CDS, Bridge JA, Hogendoorn PC, Mertens F, eds. *WHO Classification of Tumors of Soft Tissue and Bone*. Lyon, France: IARC Press; 2013:100–103.
6. Mastboom MJL, Verspoor FGM, Verschoor AJ, et al. Higher incidence rates than previously known in tenosynovial giant cell tumors. *Acta Orthop*. 2017;88(6):688–694. doi:10.1080/17453674.2017.1361126
7. Monaghan H, Salter DM, Al-Nafussi A. Giant cell tumour of tendon sheath (localised nodular tenosynovitis): clinicopathological features of 71 cases. *J Clin Pathol*. 2001;54(5):404–407. doi:10.1136/jcp.54.5.404
8. Myers BW, Masi AT. Pigmented villonodular synovitis and tenosynovitis: a clinical epidemiologic study of 166 cases and literature review. *Medicine (Baltimore)*. 1980;59(3):223–238. https://journals.lww.com/md-journal/Citation/1980/05000/Pigmented_Villonodular_Synovitis_and.4.aspx
9. Gelhorn HL, Tong S, McQuarrie K, et al. Patient-reported symptoms of tenosynovial giant cell tumors. *Clin Ther*. 2016;38(4):778–793. doi:10.1016/j.clinthera.2016.03.008
10. Bhimani MA, Wenz JF, Frassica FJ. Pigmented villonodular synovitis: keys to early diagnosis. *Clin Orthop Relat Res*. 2001;386:197–202. doi:10.1097/00003086-200105000-00025
11. Muscolo DL, Makino A, Costa-Paz M, Ayerza M. Magnetic resonance imaging evaluation and arthroscopic resection of localized pigmented villonodular synovitis of the knee. *Orthopedics*. 2000;23(4):367–369. https://www.ncbi.nlm.nih.gov/pubmed/10791586

12. Poletti SC, Gates HS 3rd, Martinez SM, Richardson WJ. The use of magnetic resonance imaging in the diagnosis of pigmented villonodular synovitis. *Orthopedics*. 1990;13(2):185–190. https://www.healio.com/orthopedics/journals/ortho/1990-2-13-2/%7Ba2ffd1fa-06f0-4259-94c2-52de28045d6a%7D/the-use-of-magnetic-resonance-imaging-in-the-diagnosis-of-pigmented-villonodular-synovitis
13. Murphey MD, Rhee JH, Lewis RB, et al. Pigmented villonodular synovitis: radiologic-pathologic correlation. *Radiographics*. 2008;28(5):1493–1518. doi:10.1148/rg.285085134
14. Cheng XG, You YH, Liu W, et al. MRI features of pigmented villonodular synovitis (PVNS). *Clin Rheumatol*. 2004;23(1):31–34. doi:10.1007/s10067-003-0827-x
15. Stacchiotti S, Crippa F, Messina A, et al. Response to imatinib in villonodular pigmented synovitis (PVNS) resistant to nilotinib. *Clin Sarcoma Res*. 2013;3(1):8. doi:10.1186/2045-3329-3-8
16. Michaelis LC, Ratain MJ. Measuring response in a post-RECIST world: from black and white to shades of grey. *Nat Rev Cancer*. 2006;6(5):409–414. doi:10.1038/nrc1883
17. Choi H, Charnsangavej C, de Castro Faria S, et al. CT evaluation of the response of gastrointestinal stromal tumors after imatinib mesylate treatment: a quantitative analysis correlated with FDG PET findings. *AJR Am J Roentgenol*. 2004;183(6):1619–1628. doi:10.2214/ajr.183.6.01831619
18. Chang KJ, Byun BH, Moon HS, et al. Tenosynovial giant cell tumor of diffuse type mimicking bony metastasis detected on F-18 FDG PET/CT. *Nucl Med Mol Imaging*. 2014;48(3):230–232. doi:10.1007/s13139-014-0275-3
19. Cohen-Levy WB, Pretell-Mazzini J, Singer AD, et al. Significance of incidental intra-articular and peri-articular FDG avid foci on PET/CT. *Acta Radiol*. 2019;60(1):78–84. doi:10.1177/0284185118770901
20. Takeuchi A, Yamamoto N, Hayashi K, et al. Tenosynovial giant cell tumors in unusual locations detected by positron emission tomography imaging confused with malignant tumors: report of two cases. *BMC Musculoskelet Disord*. 2016;17:180. doi:10.1186/s12891-016-1050-7
21. Nilsson M, Höglund M, Panagopoulos I, et al. Molecular cytogenetic mapping of recurrent chromosomal breakpoints in tenosynovial giant cell tumors. *Virchows Arch*. 2002;441(5):475–480. doi:10.1007/s00428-002-0640-y
22. Sciot R, Rosai J, Dal CP, et al. Analysis of 35 cases of localized and diffuse tenosynovial giant cell tumor: a report from the Chromosomes and Morphology (CHAMP) study group. *Mod Pathol*. 1999;12(6):576–579. https://www.ncbi.nlm.nih.gov/pubmed/10392632
23. West RB, Rubin BP, Miller MA, et al. A landscape effect in tenosynovial giant-cell tumor from activation of CSF1 expression by a translocation in a minority of tumor cells. *Proc Natl Acad Sci U S A*. 2006;103(3):690–695. doi:10.1073/pnas.0507321103
24. Möller E, Mandahl N, Mertens F, Panagopoulos I. Molecular identification of COL6A3-CSF1 fusion transcripts in tenosynovial giant cell tumors. *Genes Chromosomes Cancer*. 2008;47(1):21–25. doi:10.1002/gcc.20501
25. Nishio J, Kamachi Y, Iwasaki H, Naito M. Diffuse-type tenosynovial giant cell tumor with t(1;17)(p13;p13) and trisomy 5. *In Vivo*. 2014;28(5):949–952. http://iv.iiarjournals.org/content/28/5/949.full
26. Panagopoulos I, Brandal P, Gorunova L, et al. Novel CSF1-S100A10 fusion gene and CSF1 transcript identified by RNA sequencing in tenosynovial giant cell tumors. *Int J Oncol*. 2014;44(5):1425–1432. doi:10.3892/ijo.2014.2326
27. Cupp JS, Miller MA, Montgomery KD, et al. Translocation and expression of CSF1 in pigmented villonodular synovitis, tenosynovial giant cell tumor, rheumatoid arthritis and other reactive synovitides. *Am J Surg Pathol*. 2007;31(6):970–976. doi:10.1097/PAS.0b013e31802b86f8
28. Huang HY, West RB, Tzeng CC, et al. Immunohistochemical and biogenetic features of diffuse-type tenosynovial giant cell tumors: the potential roles of cyclin A, P53, and deletion of 15q in sarcomatous transformation. *Clin Cancer Res*. 2008;14(19):6023–6032. doi:10.1158/1078-0432.CCR-08-0252
29. Gibbons CLMH, Khwaja HA, Cole AS, et al. Giant-cell tumour of the tendon sheath in the foot and ankle. *J Bone Joint Surg Br*. 2002;84(7):1000–1003. doi:10.1302/0301-620x.84b7.13115
30. Koutserimpas C, Kastanis G, Ioannidis A, et al. Giant cell tumors of the tendon sheath of the hand: an 11-year retrospective study. *J BUON*. 2018;23(5):1546–1551. https://jbuon.com/archive/23-5-1546.pdf
31. Suresh SS, Zaki H. Giant cell tumor of tendon sheath: case series and review of literature. *J Hand Microsurg*. 2010;2(2):67–71. doi:10.1007/s12593-010-0020-9
32. Williams J, Hodari A, Janevski P, Siddiqui A. Recurrence of giant cell tumors in the hand: a prospective study. *J Hand Surg Am*. 2010;35(3):451–456. doi:10.1016/j.jhsa.2009.12.004
33. De Ponti A, Sansone V, Malchere M. Result of arthroscopic treatment of pigmented villonodular synovitis of the knee. *Arthroscopy*. 2003;19(6):602–607. doi:10.1016/s0749-8063(03)00127-0
34. Dines JS, DeBerardino TM, Wells JL, et al. Long-term follow-up of surgically treated localized pigmented villonodular synovitis of the knee. *Arthroscopy*. 2007;23(9):930–937. doi:10.1016/j.arthro.2007.03.012
35. Kim SJ, Shin SJ, Choi NH, Choo ET. Arthroscopic treatment for localized pigmented villonodular synovitis of the knee. *Clin Orthop Relat Res*. 2000;379:224–230. doi:10.1097/00003086-200010000-00026
36. Zvijac JE, Lau AC, Hechtman KS, et al. Arthroscopic treatment of pigmented villonodular synovitis of the knee. *Arthroscopy*. 1999;15(6):613–617. doi:10.1053/ar.1999.v15.015061
37. Chin KR, Barr SJ, Winalski C, et al. Treatment of advanced primary and recurrent diffuse pigmented villonodular synovitis of the knee. *J Bone Joint Surg Am*. 2002;84-A(12):2192–2202. doi:10.2106/00004623-200212000-00011
38. Sharma V, Cheng EY. Outcomes after excision of pigmented villonodular synovitis of the knee. *Clin Orthop Relat Res*. 2009;467(11):2852–2858. doi:10.1007/s11999-009-0922-7
39. Cheng EY, Sharma V. Synovectomy for pigmented villonodular synovitis. In: Jackson DW, ed. *Reconstructive Knee Surgery*. 3rd ed. Philadelphia, PA: Lippincott Williams & Wilkins; 2008:499–514.

40. Chiari C, Pirich C, Brannath W, et al. What affects the recurrence and clinical outcome of pigmented villonodular synovitis? *Clin Orthop Relat Res*. 2006;450:172–178. doi:10.1097/01.blo.0000224051.01873.fb
41. Chin KR, Brick GW. Extraarticular pigmented villonodular synovitis: a cause for failed knee arthroscopy. *Clin Orthop Relat Res*. 2002;404:330–338. PMID:12439277
42. Ogilvie-Harris DJ, McLean J, Zarnett ME. Pigmented villonodular synovitis of the knee. The results of total arthroscopic synovectomy, partial, arthroscopic synovectomy, and arthroscopic local excision. *J Bone Joint Surg Am*. 1992;74(1):119–123. https://jbjs.org/reader.php?id=89927&rsuite_id=564932&native=1&source=The_Journal_of_Bone_and_Joint_Surgery/74/1/119/abstract&topics=kn#info
43. Shabat S, Kollender Y, Merimsky O, et al. The use of surgery and yttrium 90 in the management of extensive and diffuse pigmented villonodular synovitis of large joints. *Rheumatology (Oxford)*. 2002;41(10):1113–1118. doi:10.1093/rheumatology/41.10.1113
44. Kat S, Kutz R, Elbracht T, et al. Radiosynovectomy in pigmented villonodular synovitis. *Nuklearmedizin*. 2000;39(7):209–213. https://www.ncbi.nlm.nih.gov/pubmed/11127050
45. Ward WG Sr, Boles CA, Ball JD, Cline MT. Diffuse pigmented villonodular synovitis: preliminary results with intralesional resection and p32 synoviorthesis. *Clin Orthop Relat Res*. 2007;454:186–191. doi:10.1097/01.blo.0000229345.57092.a2
46. Kamaleshwaran KK, Rajan D, Krishnan B, et al. Use of yttrium-90 hydroxyapatite radiosynovectomy as a primary modality of treatment in diffuse pigmented villonodular synovitis of the knee joint: a first case report. *Indian J Nucl Med*. 2015;30(1):47–50. doi:10.4103/0972-3919.147539
47. Koca G, Ozsoy H, Atilgan HI, et al. Application of rhenium-186 radiosynovectomy in elbow diffuse pigmented villonodular synovitis. A case report with multiple joint involvement. *Nucl Med Mol Imaging*. 2012;46(3):215–217. doi:10.1007/s13139-012-0152-x
48. Berger B, Ganswindt U, Bamberg M, Hehr T. External beam radiotherapy as postoperative treatment of diffuse pigmented villonodular synovitis. *Int J Radiat Oncol Biol Phys*. 2007;67(4):1130–1134. doi:10.1016/j.ijrobp.2006.10.016
49. Mazonakis M, Tzedakis A, Lyraraki E, Damilakis J. Organ-specific radiation-induced cancer risk estimates due to radiotherapy for benign pigmented villonodular synovitis. *Phys Med Biol*. 2016;61(17):6400–6412. doi:10.1088/0031-9155/61/17/6400
50. Park G, Kim YS, Kim JH, et al. Low-dose external beam radiotherapy as a postoperative treatment for patients with diffuse pigmented villonodular synovitis of the knee: 4 recurrences in 23 patients followed for mean 9 years. *Acta Orthop*. 2012;83(3):256–260. doi:10.3109/17453674.2012.678803
51. Brahmi M, Vinceneux A, Cassier PA. Current systemic treatment options for tenosynovial giant cell tumor/pigmented villonodular synovitis: targeting the CSF1/CSF1R axis. *Curr Treat Options Oncol*. 2016;17(2):10. doi:10.1007/s11864-015-0385-x
52. Blay JY, El Sayadi H, Thiesse P, et al. Complete response to imatinib in relapsing pigmented villonodular synovitis/tenosynovial giant cell tumor (PVNS/TGCT). *Ann Oncol*. 2008;19(4):821–822. doi:10.1093/annonc/mdn033
53. Cassier PA, Gelderblom H, Stacchiotti S, et al. Efficacy of imatinib mesylate for the treatment of locally advanced and/or metastatic tenosynovial giant cell tumor/pigmented villonodular synovitis. *Cancer*. 2012;118(6):1649–1655. doi:10.1002/cncr.26409
54. Gelderblom H, Cropet C, Chevreau C, et al. Nilotinib in locally advanced pigmented villonodular synovitis: a multicentre, open-label, single-arm, phase 2 trial. *Lancet Oncol*. 2018;19(5):639–648. doi:10.1016/S1470-2045(18)30143-8
55. Cheng EY, Anna KA, Block JA, et al. *MCS110, an anti-CSF-1 antibody, for the treatment of pigmented villonodular synovitis*. Presented at: International Society of Limb Salvage and Musculoskeletal Tumor Society Meeting; October 6–10, 2015; Orlando, FL.
56. Cassier PA, Italiano A, Gomez-Roca CA, et al. CSF1R inhibition with emactuzumab in locally advanced diffuse-type tenosynovial giant cell tumours of the soft tissue: a dose-escalation and dose-expansion phase 1 study. *Lancet Oncol*. 2015;16:949–956. doi:10.1016/S1470-2045(15)00132-1
57. Tap WD, Gelderblom W, Stacchiotti S, et al. *Final results of ENLIVEN: A global, double-blind, randomized, placebo-controlled, phase 3 study of pexidartinib in advanced tenosynovial giant cell tumor (TGCT)*. Presented at: American Society of Clinical Oncology; June 1–5, 2018; Chicago, IL.
58. Tap WD, Wainberg ZA, Anthony SP, et al. Structure-guided blockade of CSF1R kinase in tenosynovial giant-cell tumor. *N Engl J Med*. 2015;373(5):428–437. doi:10.1056/NEJMoa1411366
59. Imakiire N, Fujino T, Morii T, et al. Malignant pigmented villonodular synovitis in the knee—report of a case with rapid clinical progression. *Open Orthop J*. 2011;5:13–16. doi:10.2174/1874325001105010013
60. Yoon HJ, Cho YA, Lee JI, et al. Malignant pigmented villonodular synovitis of the temporomandibular joint with lung metastasis: a case report and review of the literature. *Oral Surg Oral Med Oral Pathol Oral Radiol Endod*. 2011;111(5):e30–e36. doi:10.1016/j.tripleo.2010.11.031
61. Sistla R, Vidyasagar JVS, Afroz T. Malignant pigmented villonodular synovitis—a rare entity. *J Orthop Case Rep*. 2014;4(4):9–11. doi:10.13107/jocr.2250-0685.214
62. Nakayama R, Jagannathan JP, Ramaiya N, et al. Clinical characteristics and treatment outcomes in six cases of malignant tenosynovial giant cell tumor: initial experience of molecularly targeted therapy. *BMC Cancer*. 2018;18(1):1296. doi:10.1186/s12885-018-5188-6

17

Epithelioid Sarcoma

Andrea P. Espejo-Freire and Jonathan C. Trent

INTRODUCTION

Epithelioid sarcoma (ES) is an aggressive malignant soft tissue sarcoma (STS) that mainly affects young adults. It is often multifocal at presentation, with propensity for local recurrence and distant metastasis.[1] It was first described as a unique entity in 1970 by Franz Enzinger in a series of 62 cases. Enzinger identified cases of soft tissue neoplasia with particular clinical and histologic behavior. These cases were previously misdiagnosed as multiple benign and malignant conditions, including chronic inflammatory process, necrotizing granulomas, synovial sarcoma, and squamous cell carcinoma.[2] There are two variants of this disease. One is classic ES, which usually presents as a subcutaneous or deep dermal mass in the distal extremities of young patients. The other is proximal ES, which has a predisposition for limb girdles and trunk, and a slightly later onset of presentation. Each variant has distinctive histologic features. However, both are associated with the loss of SMARCCB1/INI1 protein expression.[3] Given the rarity of ES, the majority of our ES understanding derives from small retrospective case series and subset analysis of prospective (STS) trials. This chapter reviews the epidemiology, clinical presentation, diagnostic approach, molecular drivers, and treatment options for ES.

EPIDEMIOLOGY

ES is a rare STS that accounts for only 0.6% to 1.0% of sarcomas, with an estimated annual incidence of 0.041 per 100,000 population.[4,5] It usually presents in young adults between 20 and 40 years of age and rarely is seen in young children and older people. In children and adolescents, it is estimated to represent 5% to 8% of childhood nonrhabdomyosarcomatous STSs.[6] Two variants have been described: classical type, which characteristically involves the distal extremities and affects adolescents and young adults between ages 10 and 40 (median age 33 years); and the proximal type with predilection for proximal limbs, limb girdles, and midtrunk, which presents slightly later in life, between ages 20 and 65 (median age 38 years).[1,2,4,7,8] A male predisposition is noted in numerous series, with a male-to-female ratio of 1.6:1 to 1.9:1.[4,8] Additionally, Caucasian race is predominant in the series. In a cohort of 441 patients from the Surveillance, Epidemiology, and End Results (SEER) database in 2008, 80% of patients were white, 12% black, and 8% reported as other. According to ethnicity, 9% were identified as Hispanic and 91% as non-Hispanic. These data are concordant with Enzinger's original case series, in which the majority of cases were Caucasian and only a few were black.[2,5,8]

CLINICAL PRESENTATION AND NATURAL HISTORY

ES habitually develops as indolent slow-growing lesions in the dermis, subcutaneous tissues, and deeper along the superficial fascia and tendons. Majority of tumors present as indolent firm, hard palpable masses, which are often multifocal. When located within the dermis, they present as superficial nodules that may become ulcerated 2 to 3 months after the primary lesion is noted. Ulceration ensues in about 12% of cases. These lesions are often misdiagnosed as indurated abscesses, infected ulcers, or infected sinus tracts that fail to heal despite intensive treatment. Subcutaneous lesions, on the other hand, present as small nodules described as lumps or warts that grow slowly and steady, and are not associated with limitation of function. Deep lesions occur along fascial planes, aponeurosis, and tendons, felt as multinodular or irregular masses that may move along with limb motion. Usually, deeper lesions are larger at presentation, and in about 25% of cases, are associated with low-grade pain. Only a minority of patients present with severe pain, motion limitation, and sensory abnormalities, which is more common in deeper lesions. Because of the absence of symptoms other than the palpated mass, patients often delay care for several months. The mean duration of symptoms prior to definitive diagnosis is around 10.5 months (range 9–30 months), and up to 30% have symptoms for more than 2 years prior to diagnosis.[2,8,9] The most frequent location is the distal upper extremity (hand and forearm), which is involved in over 50% of cases. Next in frequency is the distal lower extremity, followed by proximal lower extremities, proximal upper extremity, trunk, and head and neck. Uncommon locations include the scalp, perineum, and vulva.[2,5,8,9]

Unlike other sarcoma, ES spreads mainly by the lymphatic system and has a tenacious propensity for local recurrence.[5] Up to 70% of patients develop local recurrence, at a median length of 9.5 months after wide local excision (range 3–56 months), and over 40% of patients will have metastasis to regional lymph nodes and distant sites, most frequently to lungs. At initial diagnosis, around 47% of patients have localized disease, 28% local lymph node involvement, and 25% distant metastasis.[10]

Overall, patients with localized disease have substantial better prognosis than patients with regional or metastatic disease. Five-year survival rate for local disease is around 75%, for regional involvement it is 49%, and none of the patients who presented with metastatic disease were alive at 5 years. One-year survival rate for metastatic disease is around 46%. Median overall survival (OS) is about 88 months from the time of diagnosis and 5-year survival rate is about 66%.[5,9,10]

DIAGNOSTIC APPROACH

Given the rarity of this tumor, high clinical suspicion is required for accurate diagnosis. Like any soft tissue mass, early evaluation with gadolinium-enhanced MRI is mandatory to identify features suggestive of a malignant process and the extent of tissue involvement. Referral to a multidisciplinary sarcoma center for initial management including biopsy, pathologic review, and surgical resection for localized disease is critical to improve outcomes. Initial staging should include a high-quality contrast-enhanced CT scan of the lungs, abdomen, and pelvis. PET/CT scan may be useful to identify occult lesions, particularly in advanced disease.

Radiographic Features

Multiple small series and case reports of radiographic characteristics are reported in the literature and support the diversity of features encountered in this tumor. On MRI, the majority of cases are of infiltrative masses. In the majority of cases, they may extend, lacking well-defined margins, and may present as multifocal lesions. In the classical subtype, some cases are seen as mainly intramuscular, while more superficial tumors have a creeping infiltrative manner extending from dermis or subcutaneous tissues deep into tendons and ligaments. Encasement of neurovascular structures and direct invasion to bone are seen in extensive tumors.[11] On T1-weighted images, the majority are isointense with muscle. However, heterogeneous enhancement with areas of increased uptake are seen, corresponding to foci of hemorrhagic necrosis. Areas of central hypointensity are present in tumors with extensive necrosis. In general, necrosis is seen in up to 70% of cases and its extent correlates with tumor size, local lymph node involvement, and distant metastasis. Furthermore, necrotic nodes were seen in all patients with node involvement, but some false positives were reported. Some cases also showed areas of punctuated hyperintensity on T1-weighted images that were consistent with macrocalcifications. Similarly, T2-weighted images varied from case to case. While some tumors showed heterogeneous enhancement, others were homogeneous with different intensities compared to fat. Mild to moderate T2-weighted peritumoral edema is seen as a feathery radial pattern of nonselective high signaling on T2-weighted or STIR (short-tau inversion recovery) series.[11,12] Figure 17.1 shows the radiographic findings of a patient with proximal type ES at the time of local presentation and upon progression with metastatic disease.

A case report of ES showed a honeycombing pattern of fat that simulated lymphedema. Cortical necrosis was also present, exemplifying the highly heterogeneous radiologic features of this tumor.[13] In the case of proximal type ES, lesions are commonly located in the chest wall, inguinal region, thigh, and perineum. By CT or MRI, these tumors were mononodular or multinodular masses with irregular indistinct borders. Calcifications were seen only in one patient of this series and were located in the periphery. It is worth mentioning that in Enzinger's series in 1970 and subsequently in 1985, the only identified radiologic feature was the occasional presence of calcifications by x-ray exam.[2,8] Low central attenuation consistent with necrosis was also common in the proximal type.[14]

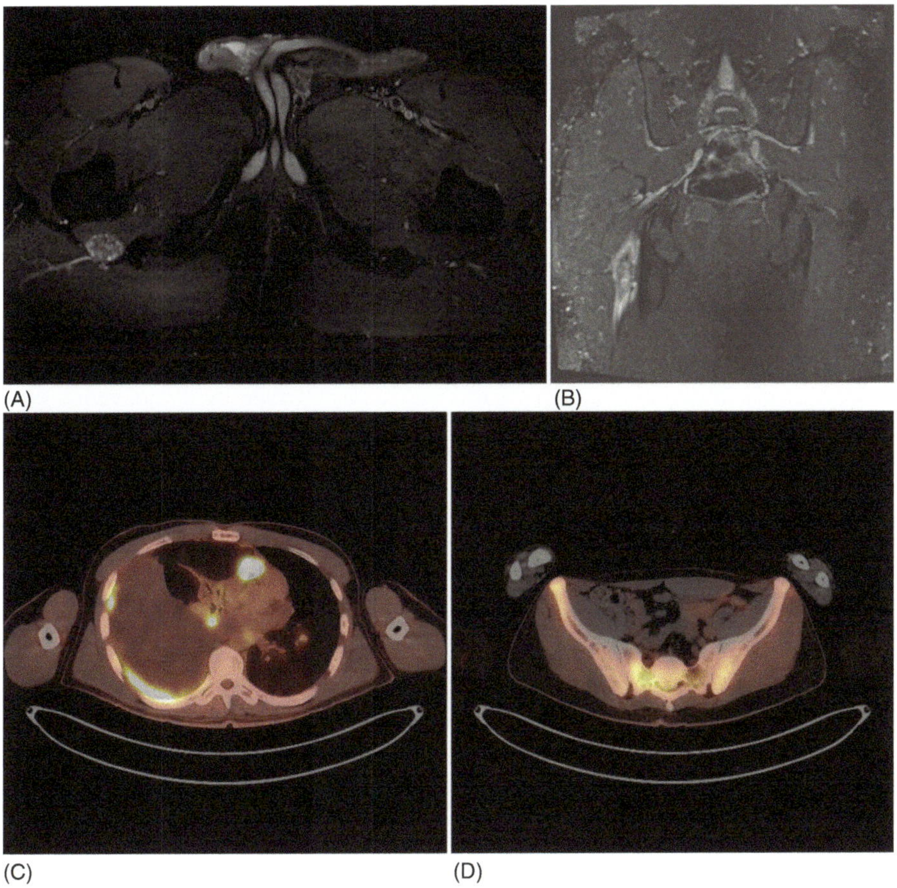

FIGURE 17.1 **Radiographic characteristics of patient with epithelioid sarcoma.** (A) T2 hyperintense and enhancing lobulated tumor within the right sciatic nerve, at the level of the hamstring tendon origins. (B) STIR sequence showing significant peritumoral edema. (C) Extensive metastatic disease with multiple pleural-based lung nodules and associated large pleural effusion. (D) Diffuse osseous metastasis with iliac and sacral involvement.

STIR, short-tau inversion recovery.

Histopathologic Features

ES is characterized by nodular aggregates of epithelioid cells immunoreactive to cytokertins (CKs), EMA, vimentin, and often CD34 positivity. There are different histologic features in the classic and proximal subtypes. In the classical form of ES, histologic features include nodular aggregates, nets, or cords of uniform epithelial cells with abundant eosinophilic cytoplasm. Nuclei have vesicular chromatin with minimal atypia and small nucleoli. Central necrosis in this subtype is prominent, giving the appearance of a granulomatous process. Epithelioid cells are located toward the center and a gradual transition to spindle morphology is seen toward the periphery. In 20% of cases, dystrophic calcification and metaplastic bone formation are seen. In the periphery, aggregates of inflammatory cells are also typical.[1,4,15]

On the other hand, the proximal subtype has multinodular sheets of larger, polygonal cells with higher degree of atypia with variable rhabdoid morphology. Pleomorphic epithelioid cells with large vesicular nuclei and prominent nucleoli are seen. Also, intralesional focus of necrosis is common, but the geographic pattern of the classic type with "granulomatous appearance" is absent. Rarely, a pattern with features of both classical and proximal subtypes exists. Other morphologic patterns are angiomatoid, large cell/rhabdoid, and fibroma-like. In these cases, immunohistochemistry (IHC) is key to identify the classic ES profiles.[1,4]

Immunophenotype by IHC is similar in classic and proximal subtypes. Both express high- and low-molecular-weight CKs with diffuse and focal patterns, most commonly, CK8, CK19, but negative or only focally positive for CK5/6. A great proportion is also positive for EMA. CD34 is positive in more than 50% of cases, which is useful to differentiate ES from carcinoma. Still, some cases show very focal or even absent CKs and CD34, and morphology may mimic other epithelial neoplasms as squamous cell carcinomas, benign fibrous histiocytomas, nodular fasciitis, and nonneoplastic lesions. In these cases, a high index of suspicion is important in order to assess the nuclear expression of *SMARCB1/INI1* by IHC and fluorescence in situ hybridization (FISH), which is a loss in over 90% of ES.[16,17]

MOLECULAR AND BIOLOGIC DRIVERS

There is significant genetic heterogeneity between ES tumors, with no identified pathognomonic cytogenetic abnormality. In karyotype analysis, the majority of cases have a complex karyotype with multiple numeric and structural abnormalities. ES has recurrent translocations involving the chromosome 22. The most common are t(8:22) (q22q11) and, in a minority of cases of proximal variant, t(10:22).[1,18,19] These observations of recurrent involvement of chromosome 22q11 lead to the identification of the loss of two tumor suppressor genes: *SMARCB1/INI1* and *NF2*. This loss has been documented in 20% of human cancers. However, only in rhabdoid tumors is this loss always driven by homozygous genetic inactivation of *SMARCB1* gene. A report from the INT National Cancer Institute of Milan, which analyzed 40 ES cases, was the first to report the gene status in ES with loss of *SMARCB1/INI1* expression. Here, homozygous gene inactivation was found for 60% of cases.[7] In other *SMARCB1/INI1* negative tumors, there is no consistent genetic alterations. Among STSs, complete loss of expression of *SMARCB1/INI1* is found in ES, myoepithelial carcinoma, and epithelioid malignant peripheral nerve sheath tumor.[1,4,20]

The *SMARCB1* gene encodes the adenosine triphosphate (ATP)-dependent subunit of SWI/SNF chromatin remodeling complex, which regulates genomic stability, cell cycle, and other signaling pathways. *SMARCB1* is associated with activation of the Hedgehog pathway, which in embryonic life is responsible for stem cell differentiation.[1,21] Furthermore, loss of *SMARCB1* also results in aberrant transcription of p16INK4a and/or p21, which is a negative regulator of cyclin D1 and CDK 4/6, hence blocking phosphorylation of Rb and consequently arresting the cell cycle.[22,23] Also important is the interaction of SWI/SNF chromatin remodeling complex with EZH2, a histone methyltransferase. EZH2 is highly active in stem cells, repressing genes associated with cell cycle arrest and promoting self-renewal. In adult tissues, EZH2 activity is opposed by SWI/SNF complex, which promotes differentiation and regulates self-renewal.[24] The latest is important, as drugs targeting EZH2 are undergoing trials for different cancer types.

It is postulated that loss of *SMARCB1/INI1* is probably an earlier event causing genomic instability and explaining the complexity of karyotypes seen in ES. Other associated pathways include PI3K/AKT/mTOR and EGFR. Yet, no positive results have been yielded from targeting this pathways.[1]

TREATMENT CONSIDERATIONS

In the localized and the metastatic setting, the rarity of ES challenges the clinical approach owing to limited evidence, which comes mainly from nonuniform retrospective series. In a series of localized ES, limitations are often due to small sample size, short follow-up periods, and inconsistency in terms of procedures and use of adjuvant treatments. From these studies, long-term survival reports range from 42% to 79%. Nonetheless, rates of local failure are considerably high: 30% to over 70% of local recurrence and over 40% progression to distant metastasis. For patients with metastatic disease, data also comes from small retrospective cohorts and small ES subset analysis from prospective clinical trials for STS. At the moment, prognosis for patients with metastatic disease is poor with 46% survival at 1 year and no patients surviving at 5 years.[5]

Management of the Primary Tumor

Controlling localized disease consists of surgical resection with some evidence supporting the use of adjuvant RT. Only small retrospective series of patients with localized ES treated with surgery with or without RT have been published. Overall, these small retrospective series have limitations due to inconsistency regarding the surgical procedures done and the use of RT. To our knowledge, there is only one series from M.D. Anderson Cancer Center (MDACC) with consistent limb sparing surgery and use of adjuvant RT. The 10-year OS rate in this series ranged from 50% to 74%.[10,25]

Chase and Enzinger in 1985 published the largest series to date involving 202 patients. They reported 77% of local recurrence despite over 50% of the patients undergoing initial amputation.[8] Other two small series at Massachusetts General Hospital and Memorial Sloan-Kettering Cancer Center reported that local failure rates were more than 50% and about 50% of patients subsequently required amputation as part of treatment. However, only a small proportion of patients in both of these series received adjuvant RT. Still, Massachusetts General Hospital series, which suggested marginal surgery with or without adjuvant RT, was associated with worse prognosis, and higher local and distant recurrence rates.[10,26] Furthermore, investigators from the Mayo Clinic reported a local recurrence rate of 38% and metastatic rate of 47% after a median follow-up of 102 months. Although they found no difference in the rates of distant metastasis, they suggested that recurrence rate decreased with increasing aggressiveness of the surgery. Yet, the metastatic rate was no different between procedures.[27] Older series of patients treated with only resection reported local recurrence rates of 75% to >90%.[28,29] Subsequently, in 1983, Shimm et al. reported the outcomes of five patients treated with adjuvant RT. In this series, four out of the five patients had no evidence of disease at follow-up (duration of follow-up 18–84 months).[30] In MDACC series of 21 patients who underwent limb sparing surgery and adjuvant RT, local recurrence was 37%, which is similar to the above-mentioned series, but all patients had limb preservation. In accordance, limb sparing surgery followed by adjuvant RT is generally recommended.

Additionally, these series identified certain prognostic factors. Patients with tumors <5 cm have a 5-year overall survival (OS) rate of 79% compared with only 25% for patients with lesions >5 cm. Furthermore, OS is significantly higher, 77% for patients for primary extremity lesions compared to 39% in nonextremity locations and at 5 years, disease-free survival (DFS) rate was around 56% in patients with extremity ES versus 0% in nonextremity locations. Furthermore, necrosis more than 30%, vascular invasion, presence of local symptoms, regional lymphadenopathy, and positive margins correlate with poor prognosis.[25,31,32]

Probable explanations for the high rate of local recurrence despite the high proportion of aggressive surgeries is the fact that macroscopic descriptions of the procedures probably do not correlate with the microscopic surgical margins. Margin status was not reported in the mentioned series. In patients treated with local surgery and adjuvant radiation, 35% of recurrences occurred within the surgical margins and within the radiation fields. For this reason, it is recommended to attempt wide surgical margins and generous RT fields. In the MDACC series, the mean marginal field was 6.7 cm (which is the difference between the largest tumor dimension and the largest RT portal dimension). For ES a marginal field of at least 10 cm may be indicated to minimize recurrence.[25]

Ultimately, even though there is no well-established role for the use of sentinel node biopsy, this may be considered for prognostic implications. In cohorts of limb STS, sentinel node biopsy was positive in 17% of cases, but false negative rates of up to 29% were reported.[33,34]

Management of Metastatic Disease

The use of systemic chemotherapy for locally advanced and metastatic ES derives from limited retrospective studies. To date, the largest cohort included 115 patients in a multi-institutional case series from 17 centers in Europe, the United States, and Japan. Cases were diagnosed between 1990 and 2016 and had available tissue for pathologic confirmation. All cases had evidence of loss of *SMARCB1/INI1*. Responses were evaluated by response evaluation criteria in solid tumors (RECIST). Systemic chemotherapy consisted of anthracycline-based regimens (85 patients), gemcitabine-based regimens (41 patients), or pazopanib (18 patients). In the anthracycline-based group, one patient (1%) had a complete response (CR), 18 patients (21%) partial response (PR), 45 patients (53%) stable disease (SD), and 21 patients (25%) had progression of disease (PD). Overall response rate (ORR) (CR + PR) was 22%, median progression-free survival (PFS) and OS were 6 and 16 months, respectively. In the gemcitabine-based group, two patients (5%) achieved CR, nine patients (22%) PR, 16 patients (39%) SD, and 14 patients (34%) PD. The response rate was 27%, and median PFS and OS were 4 and 19 months, respectively. Finally, in the pazopanib group, there were no CR or PR, but nine patients (50%) had SD with two prolonged SD of over 21 months; the other 50% of patients had PD. The median PFS and OS were 3 and 14 months, respectively.[35]

Other smaller series have also shown activity of anthracycline-based and gemcitabine-based chemotherapy as palliative treatment for ES. In a series of 21 patients, first-line palliative chemotherapy granted partial response in three patients (14%), 12 patients had SD (57%), and five patients 23% progressed. Median PFS and OS was 7 and 35 months. Both the above-mentioned series describe better responses in the classical subtype.[36] Another series of 28 patients from three German participating institutions evaluating the role of palliative chemotherapy reported best response of SD in 46% of patients treated with anthracycline-based regimen. Here, PFS for anthracycline single agent was 3 months versus 8 months for combination anthracycline/ifosfamide. In the same series, the use of gemcitabine/docetaxel showed stability of disease in 83% of patients and PFS of 8 months.[37] Lastly, the European Organization for Research and Treatment of Cancer (EORTC) analyzed the subgroup of metastatic ES derived from prospective EORTC trials for STS. They included ECORTC 62012 (doxorubicin vs.

doxorubicin/ifosfamide), 62043 (pazopanib), 62072 (pazopanib vs. placebo), and 62091 (doxorubicin vs. trabectedin). A total of 27 patients were identified, 18 patients received palliative chemotherapy as first-line treatment and nine patients as second-line treatment. In the first-line setting, four patients (22%) had PR (one treated with anthracycline/ifosfamide, two treated with pazopanib, and one treated with trabectedin), 10 patients (56%) had SD (three received doxorubicin alone, six doxorubicin/ifosfamide combination, and one trabectedin), and four patients had PD. As second-line treatment, patients were treated only with pazopanib: one patient (11%) had PR, four patients (44%) SD, and four patients (44%) PD. Median PFS and OS was 4 and 11 months, respectively, for patients who received first-line treatment versus 2.7 and 9.7 months for patients who received second-line treatment.[38]

Most recently, tazemetostat, an oral selective inhibitor of EHZ2, was approved by the FDA for the treatment of advanced and metastatic ES. Tazemetostat efficacy was evaluated in a multicenter prospective phase II study of tumors with loss of expression of SMARCB1/INI1. As previously stated, SMARCB1/INI1 is a subunit of the SWI/SWF complex, which is a negative regulator of EZH2. EZH2 is a histone methyl transferase part of polycomb repressive complex 2 (PRC2), which functions as a key epigenetic regulator for stem cell differentiation.[39] The cohort of 62 patients with ES showed an ORR of 15% (95% CI 7-26%) and disease control rate (DCR) of 26%. From the responders, over 60% had prolonged responses lasting 6 months or longer. Median OS for the cohort was 82.4 weeks (95% CI 47.4%, not estimable). Tazemetostat appears to be overall well tolerated. Most common adverse effects (AEs) are mild to moderate and include fatigue (39%), nausea (35%), and cancer-related pain (32%). Grade ≥3 AEs were reported in 10 patients (16%); most common were anemia and weight loss.[40] This is the first prospective trial for patients with ES and these results are encouraging for further investigation in the adjuvant and metastatic settings. A Phase III study for its use as first line in combination with doxorubicin is currently under way (NCT04204941).

SUMMARY

ES is a particularly rare subtype of STS that affects mainly young adults. ES initial presentation is of slow and indolent growth with significant invasion of musculoskeletal and neurovascular tissues. Mainstay treatment approach for localized disease is surgical resection with some evidence supporting the use of adjuvant RT. Nevertheless, local recurrence considerably exceeds what is seen for other sarcoma subtypes, and distant metastasis is also common. In the scenario of locally advanced or metastatic disease, ES shows response to anthracycline, gemcitabine-based chemotherapy, and targeted therapy with pazopanib; still, responses are short lived, and the disease is ultimately fatal in all patients. In over 90% of cases, loss of expression of SMARCB1/INI1 is identified. This protein is a subunit of SWI/SWF complex, a known oncogenic driver implicated in genomic stability, regulation of cell cycle, and regulation of critical differentiation pathways. Recently, tazemetostat has shown promising activity in ES. This agent targets the inhibition of EZH2, a histone methyltransferase that is overactive in the absence of functional SWI/SWF complex. Better understanding of this molecular driver is crucial for further development of better treatment approaches for these patients.

CASE STUDY

In November 2014, a 27-year-old man presented with progressive worsening pain of the right calf, hamstring, and gluteal area. Pain was later associated with paresthesia of the right foot and calf. He initially underwent MRI showing a T2 hyperintense 3.7-cm lesion at the level of the hamstring tendon origins within the right sciatic nerve. The lesion had heterogeneous postcontrast enhancement with some scattered areas that did not enhance. Sciatic neuritis seen as nerve edema in the surroundings of the tumor was present. Additionally, an ill-defined area, measuring about 2.6 cm, of intramedullary hyperintensity within the right iliac bone was noted. Subsequently, he underwent biopsy, which confirmed the diagnosis of ES. The tumor was composed of epithelioid cells positive for keratin, epithelial membrane antigen (EMA), and CD34. Expression of INI1 was lost. Owing to the epithelioid pathologic findings, he underwent lymphoscintigraphy with single photon emission computed tomography (SPECT)/CT revealing scintigraphic evidence of sentinel lymph nodes along the right internal iliac region and the right common iliac region. However, staging PET/CT showed no activity other than the primary lesion at the level of the sciatic nerve. As PET/CT scan was negative in the area of the sentinel node, and sampling in this area would be associated with morbidity, the decision was to forgo sentinel node biopsy. He then underwent preoperative intensity modulated radiation therapy (IMRT) with a total dose of 50 Gy in 25 fractions given over 5 weeks.

Subsequently, he underwent surgical resection of the mass. Pathologic findings consisted of a 2.5-cm mass, grade 2, American Joint Committee on Cancer (AJCC) stage ypT1bNx; margins were negative with the closest at 0.25 cm, and the tumor had 20% necrosis. He was then followed by surveillance with MRI of the right thigh every 6 months. Follow-up until 3 years after initial presentation showed no evidence of disease. Nonetheless, he developed a rapidly growing mass in the right scalp and right submandibular area. He initially was seen by a dermatologist, who attempted treatment with local steroids with no improvement. Subsequent biopsies showed metastatic epithelioid sarcoma, grade 2/3, similar in morphology to the initial lesion. After biopsy, the scalp lesion developed unremitting bleeding. PET/CT showed the development of multiple metastatic foci, including the right frontal scalp, right submental area, right vocal cord, multiple bilateral pulmonary nodules up to 2 cm, and diffuse osseous lesions including the right iliac area. He received palliative radiation therapy (RT) to the scalp to control the bleeding. Immediately after, he was started on palliative doxorubicin/ifosfamide. The best response achieved was a partial response (PR) at 2 months of starting chemotherapy and then stable disease (SD) at 4 months. At 7 months after initiation of palliative chemotherapy, he showed progression of disease with significant metastatic disease in the right hemothorax and development of right pleural effusion. He was switched to second-line gemcitabine/docetaxel. However, he deteriorated rapidly with worsening pulmonary function after cycle 1 of gemcitabine/docetaxel and he decided to proceed with hospice. He died 56 months after the original diagnosis and 12 months after the diagnosis of metastatic disease. This case presentation highlights the unique aggressive clinical behavior of ES, including high rates of local recurrence and metastasis. Lastly, the case exemplifies the complex, multidisciplinary approaches required for the management of this condition and the need for further preclinical and clinical research in order to improve the prognosis of patients with this disease.

REFERENCES

1. Thway K, Jones RL, Noujaim J, Fisher C. Epithelioid sarcoma: diagnostic features and genetics. *Adv Anat Pathol*. 2016;23(1):41–49. doi:10.1097/PAP.0000000000000102
2. Enzinger FM. Epithelioid sarcoma. A sarcoma simulating a granuloma or a carcinoma. *Cancer*. 1970;26(5):1029–1041. doi:10.1002/1097-0142(197011)26:5<1029::AID-CNCR2820260510>3.0.CO;2-R
3. Oda Y, Dal Cin P, Laskin WB. Epithelioid sarcoma. *Nishi Nihon Hifuka*. 1979;41(1):14–20. doi:10.2336/nishinihonhifu.41.14
4. Fletcher CDM, Bridge JA, Hogendoorn PCW, et al. *WHO classification of tumours of soft tissue and bone*. Lyon, France: International Agency for Research on Cancer; 2013. http://ebookcentral.proquest.com/lib/miami/detail.action?docID=4661026
5. Jawad MU, Extein J, Min ES, Scully SP. Prognostic factors for survival in patients with epithelioid sarcoma: 441 cases from the SEER database. *Clin Orthop Relat Res*. 2009;467(11):2939–2948. doi:10.1007/s11999-009-0749-2
6. Casanova M, Ferrari A, Collini P, et al. Epithelioid sarcoma in children and adolescents: a report from the Italian Soft Tissue Sarcoma Committee. *Cancer*. 2006;106(3):708–717. doi:10.1002/cncr.21630
7. Gasparini P, Facchinetti F, Boeri M, et al. Prognostic determinants in epithelioid sarcoma. *Eur J Cancer*. 2011;47(2):287–295. doi:10.1016/j.ejca.2010.09.003
8. Chase D, Enzinger F. Epithelioid sarcoma: diagnosis, prognostic indicators and treatments. *Am J Surg Pathol*. 1985:241–263. https://journals.lww.com/ajsp/abstract/1985/04000/epithelioid_sarcoma__diagnosis,_prognostic.1.aspx
9. Bos GD, Pritchard DJ, Reiman HM, et al. Epithelioid sarcoma. An analysis of fifty-one cases. *J Bone Joint Surg Am*. 1988;70(6):862–870. doi:10.2106/00004623-198870060-00011
10. Ross HM, Lewis JJ, Woodruff JM, Brennan MF. Epithelioid sarcoma: clinical behavior and prognostic factors of survival. *Ann Surg Oncol*. 1997;4:491–495. doi:10.1007/bf02303673
11. Hanna SL, Kaste S, Jenkins JJ, et al. Epithelioid sarcoma: clinical, MR imaging and pathologic findings. *Skeletal Radiol*. 2002;31(7):400–412. doi:10.1007/s00256-002-0509-9

12. McCarville MB, Kao SC, Dao TV, et al. Magnetic resonance and computed tomography imaging features of epithelioid sarcoma in children and young adults with pathological and clinical correlation: a report from Children's Oncology Group study ARST0332. *Pediatr Radiol*. 2019;49(7):922–932. doi:10.1007/s00247-019-04389-2
13. Yamato M, Nishimura G, Yamaguchi T, et al. Epithelioid sarcoma with unusual radiological findings. *Skeletal Radiol*. 1997;26(10):606–610. doi:10.1007/s002560050294
14. Tateishi U, Hasegawa T, Kusumoto M, et al. Radiologic manifestations of proximal-type epithelioid sarcoma of the soft tissues. *AJR Am J Roentgenol*. 2002;179(4):973–978. doi:10.2214/ajr.179.4.1790973
15. Miettinen M, Fanburg-Smith JC, Virolainen M, et al. Epithelioid sarcoma: an immunohistochemical analysis of 112 classical and variant cases and a discussion of the differential diagnosis. *Hum Pathol*. 1999;30(8):934–942. doi:10.1016/S0046-8177(99)90247-2
16. Orrock JM, Abbott JJ, Gibson LE, Folpe AL. INI1 and GLUT-1 expression in epithelioid sarcoma and its cutaneous neoplastic and nonneoplastic mimics. *Am J Dermatopathol*. 2009;31(2):152–156. doi:10.1097/DAD.0b013e31818a5c4f
17. Hornick JL, Dal Cin P, Fletcher CDM. Loss of INI1 expression is characteristic of both conventional and proximal-type epithelioid sarcoma. *Am J Surg Pathol*. 2009;33(4):542–550. doi:10.1097/PAS.0b013e3181882c54
18. Cordoba JC, Parham DM, Meyer WH, Douglass EC. A new cytogenetic finding in an epithelioid sarcoma, t(8;22)(q22;q11). *Cancer Genet Cytogenet*. 1994;72(2):151–154. doi:10.1016/0165-4608(94)90132-5
19. Lualdi E, Modena P, Debiec-Rychter M, et al. Molecular cytogenetic characterization of proximal-type epithelioid sarcoma. *Genes Chromosomes Cancer*. 2004;41(3):283–290. doi:10.1002/gcc.20086
20. Sapi Z, Papp G, Szendroi M, et al. Epigenetic regulation of SMARCB1 by miR-206, -381 and -671-5p is evident in a variety of SMARCB1 immunonegative soft tissue sarcomas, while miR-765 appears specific for epithelioid sarcoma. A miRNA study of 223 soft tissue sarcomas. *Genes Chromosomes Cancer*. 2016;55:786–802. doi:10.1002/gcc.22379
21. Li L, Fan XS, Xia QY, et al. Concurrent loss of INI1, PBRM1, and BRM expression in epithelioid sarcoma: implications for the cocontributions of multiple SWI/SNF complex members to pathogenesis. *Hum Pathol*. 2014;45(11):2247–2254. doi:10.1016/j.humpath.2014.06.027
22. Serrano M. The tumor suppressor protein p16INK4a. *Exp Cell Res*. 1997;237(1):7–13. doi:10.1006/excr.1997.3824
23. Romagosa C, Simonetti S, López-Vicente L, et al. P16Ink4a overexpression in cancer: a tumor suppressor gene associated with senescence and high-grade tumors. *Oncogene*. 2011;30(18):2087–2097. doi:10.1038/onc.2010.614
24. Makita S, Tobinai K. Targeting EZH2 with tazemetostat. *Lancet Oncol*. 2018;19(5):586–587. doi:10.1016/S1470-2045(18)30149-9
25. Callister MD, Ballo MT, Pisters PWT, et al. Epithelioid sarcoma: results of conservative surgery and radiotherapy. *Int J Radiat Oncol Biol Phys*. 2001;51(2):384–391. doi:10.1016/S0360-3016(01)01646-7
26. Steinberg B, Gelberman R, Mankin H, Rosenberg AE. Epithelioid sarcoma in the upper extremity. *J Bone Joint Surg Am*. 1992;74(1)28–35.
27. Halling AC, Wollan PC, Pritchard DJ, et al. Epithelioid sarcoma: a clinicopathologic review of 55 cases. *Mayo Clin Proc*. 1996;71(7):636–642. doi:10.1016/S0025-6196(11)63000-0
28. Bryan R, Soule E, Dobyns J, et al. Primary epithelioid sarcoma of the hand and forearm. *J Bone Joint Surg Am*. 1974;56(3):458–465.
29. Santiago H, Feinerman LK, Lattes R. Epithelioid sarcoma: a clinical and pathologic study of nine cases. *Hum Pathol*. 1972;3(1):133–147. doi:10.1016/S0046-8177(72)80064-9
30. Shimm DS, Suit HD. Radiation therapy of epithelioid sarcoma. *Cancer*. 1983;52(6):1022–1025. doi:10.1002/1097-0142(19830915)52:6<1022::AID-CNCR2820520616>3.0.CO;2-I
31. Collin C, Godbold J, Hajdu S, Brennan M. Localized extremity soft tissue sarcoma: an analysis of factors affecting survival. *J Clin Oncol*. 1987;5(4):601–612. doi:10.1200/JCO.1987.5.4.601
32. Spillane AJ, Thomas JM, Fisher C. Epithelioid sarcoma: the clinicopathological complexities of this rare soft tissue sarcoma. *Ann Surg Oncol*. 2000;7(3):218–225. doi:10.1007/BF02523657
33. Andreou D, Boldt H, Werner M, et al. Sentinel node biopsy in soft tissue sarcoma subtypes with a high propensity for regional lymphatic spread—results of a large prospective trial. *Ann Oncol*. 2013;24(5):1400–1405. doi:10.1093/annonc/mds650
34. Wright S, Armeson K, Hill EG, et al. The role of sentinel lymph node biopsy in select sarcoma patients: a meta-analysis. *Am J Surg*. 2012;204(4):428–433. doi:10.1016/j.amjsurg.2011.12.019
35. Frezza AM, Jones RL, Vullo SL, et al. Anthracycline, gemcitabine, and pazopanib in epithelioid sarcoma a multi-institutional case series. *JAMA Oncol*. 2018;4(9):1–5. doi:10.1001/jamaoncol.2018.0219
36. Jones RL, Constantinidou A, Olmos D, et al. Role of palliative chemotherapy in advanced epithelioid sarcoma. *Am J Clin Oncol*. 2012;35(4):351–357. doi:10.1097/COC.0b013e3182118cf7
37. Pink D, Richter S, Gerdes S, et al. Gemcitabine and docetaxel for epithelioid sarcoma: results from a retrospective, multi-institutional analysis. *Oncology*. 2014;87(2):95–103. doi:10.1159/000362602
38. Touati N, Schoffski P, Litiere S, et al. EORTC Soft Tissue and Bone Sarcoma Group (STBSG) experience with advanced/metastatic epithelioid sarcoma patients treated in prospective trials: clinical profile and response to systemic therapy. *Clin Oncol (R Coll Radiol)*. 2018;30(7):448–454. doi:10.1016/j.clon.2018.02.065
39. Margueron R, Reinberg D. The polycomb complex PRC2 and its mark in life. *Nature*. 2011;469(7330):343–349. doi:10.1038/nature09784
40. Stacchiotti S, Schoffski P, Jones R, et al. Safety and efficacy of tazemetostat, a first-in-class EZH2 inhibitor, in patients with epithelioid sarcoma. *J Clin Oncol*. 2019;37(15_suppl):11003. doi:10.1200/JCO.2019.37.15_suppl.11003

18

Angiosarcoma

Brian Schulte, Steven I. Robinson, Borislav A. Alexiev, and Mark Agulnik

INTRODUCTION

Angiosarcoma (AS), also known as hemangiosarcoma or lymphangiosarcoma, is a malignant tumor thought to be derived from the endothelium. The exact vascular origin is unknown, and AS likely originates from both blood vessels and lymphatics.[1] AS is an incredibly rare subtype of soft tissue sarcoma (STS), accounting for <1% of all sarcomas.[2] These tumors are characterized by an aggressive clinical behavior with frequent metastases and relapse.[3] Given their relative scarcity, the optimal treatment of AS remains somewhat of a mystery. Furthermore, AS may present in a striking variety of different anatomic locations.[4] Significant heterogeneity within the diagnosis of AS makes design and development of trials as well as therapies more difficult. As a result, there are no completed Phase III trials exclusively confined to AS, although studies are currently ongoing.[5] Much of the data utilized is either Phase II, anecdotal, or part of larger studies involving STS. This ambiguity, as well as the factors already mentioned, make AS one of the more difficult cancers to treat.

EPIDEMIOLOGY

Collectively, ASs account for 2% of STSs.[3] Given that AS is a rare subpopulation of an uncommon neoplasm, it accounts for only two to three cases per 1 million population.[2] Referencing data from the Surveillance, Epidemiology, and End Results (SEER) registries, results have shown that approximately 60% of ASs are cutaneous, located within the skin or superficial soft tissues. Among primary cutaneous AS, approximately 90% occur within the Caucasian population, with a sex ratio of 1:1. Furthermore, there is a direct correlation of incidence with increased age, with most tumors occurring around age 60.[6] When ASs do appear in childhood, they appear in an epidemiologic pattern different from that of adults—often with visceral as opposed to cutaneous manifestations.[7] In adults, lesions are typically located on the head and neck, followed by trunk, lower extremities, and upper extremities.

Despite their scarcity, AS may occur in nearly any location within the human body.[4] Most AS cases occur spontaneously, but several risk factors have been identified. Risk factors for AS include radiation, chronic lymphedema, arsenic, vinyl chloride, and familial syndromes.[3] Association of AS formation with lymphedema was first noted by Stewart and Treves in six women with a history of breast cancer.[8] The combination of lymphedema and AS later assumed the eponymous name Stewart–Treves syndrome. Although the association of AS with prior breast cancer surgery became well recognized, AS is also associated with other forms of lymphedema.[6] Numerous groups have proposed mechanisms behind the association of lymphedema and AS, including associated growth of obstructed lymphatics. Others believe that carcinogenesis occurs secondary to chronic inflammation within an immunologically privileged site that is unable to adequately remove neoplastic cells.[9]

Within the breast cancer population, radiation has also been shown to be associated with development of AS.[10] This has increasingly been seen in women, due to radiation as part of breast-conserving treatment for breast cancer.[11] The frequency of their association has bred definitions for their diagnosis. Tumors must be biopsy-proven, arising within a prior field of radiation, occurring within a latency period of several years, and arising in an area without a predominance of lymphedema.[12–14] While the breast cancer survivor population is best studied, AS is also present in a large series of childhood cancer survivors.[3] Interestingly, despite the association of radiation with AS, sun exposure has not been demonstrated to contribute to increased incidence.[15]

Other noteworthy causes of AS include toxins, such as vinyl chloride, thorium dioxide, and arsenic, which are associated with the formation of hepatic AS.[16] Anabolic steroids have also been associated.[4,6,17]

There have been case reports of AS arising in association with prosthetic joints[18–20] as well as vascular grafts.[21–23] There is insufficient data to draw meaningful conclusions about the causality of the association of AS in these cases, however. In addition to environmental exposures, several genetic abnormalities have also been linked to AS. Associations include *BRCA1* and *BRCA2*, *NF1* (neurofibromatosis type 1), *IDH1* (Maffucci syndrome), and *PIK3CA* (Klippel–Trenaunay syndrome).[3] Of note, AS is not normally associated with Li–Fraumeni syndrome, although the syndrome is associated with an increased risk of sarcoma.[24]

CLINICAL FEATURES AND PRESENTATION

Often, cutaneous AS may resemble an ecchymotic lesion or a raised purple papule that is multifocal and may easily be mistaken for a simple benign growth. Others may present with intermittent bleeding, edema, and pain.[6] These lesions typically develop on the head, neck, and face—particularly on the scalp and forehead.[6,25] As these lesions grow, edema, fungation, ulceration, and hemorrhage can develop. Even early on, AS may be multifocal—which complicates therapy and results in suboptimal initial management in many cases.[26] As described in larger case series of AS, often patients would present with an asymptomatic mass or lesion. Fewer had discomfort associated with the mass or lesion.[4] The median size of primary tumors was 3.8 cm in one of the larger case series. Primary tumors of deep soft tissue or organs were located on extremities (10/22), trunk (3/22), heart (3/22), head/neck (2/22), liver (1/22), spleen (1/22), and adrenal gland (1/22).[4]

At presentation, the primary lesion is multifocal in 10% to 15% of cases. Lymph node (LN) involvement is present at initial diagnosis in 10% to 15% of soft tissue AS, in about 5% of scalp AS, and rarely in primary breast AS. About 15% of patients present with metastatic disease at the time of diagnosis.[6,27] In a review of 82 patients with AS, 44% presented with locally advanced or unresectable disease.[4]

The 5-year overall survival (OS) rate of nonmetastatic AS is about 31% to 43%.[28] OS is highly correlated with the site of the primary AS. For instance, 10-year survival rate is about 28% for extremities, 21% for scalp, and 0% for other primary sites.[6] In a paper by Sinnamon et al. published in 2016, analyzing the OS of 821 patients with soft tissue and cutaneous AS undergoing resection, a more comprehensive analysis of risk factors was performed.[29] Factors independently associated with worse OS included increased age, black race, head and neck location, increasing size, and positive margins. Of note, qualification of this model was performed in conjunction with the American Joint Committee on Cancer (AJCC) *Cancer Staging Manual*, 7th edition, which bears some differences from the 8th edition.[30]

DIAGNOSTIC APPROACH

STSs, including AS, are staged using the AJCC system.[31] Given that AS itself only represents a small proportion of STS, this becomes a relatively imperfect model.[29] Clinical staging, as with any neoplasm, involves definition of the AS by physical examination, imaging, and diagnostic biopsies of related sites. It is based on characteristics of the tumor (T), nodes (N), metastases (M), and grade (G). Grading, in particular, is not recommended within AJCC *Cancer Staging Manual*, 8th edition. Tumors that may appear low grade may behave clinically aggressive, and many sarcoma experts approach them as they would a high-grade sarcoma. Histopathologic identification of AS is sometimes challenging because it can be mistaken for other vascular tumors. Histologic features can vary within and between cases. In a low-grade form, AS may resemble hemangioma, whereas the high-grade form may be more similar in appearance to epithelial carcinomas.[3]

Diagnosis of AS is typically made by resection or biopsy. Recent studies have shown that diagnosis of AS may be made by fine-needle aspiration (FNA), but cytologic features may be inadequate for proper diagnosis, so most sarcoma pathologists prefer a core-needle, incisional, or excisional biopsy.[32] AS histologically has a wide variety of appearances, ranging from clearly vasoformative to poorly differentiated solid tumors. Of those that are nonvasoformative, they may appear epithelioid, as spindle cells, or mixed.[33] Reticulin staining, in addition to immunohistochemistry may be useful in determining the origin of less characteristic AS. A high proportion stain for CD31, von Willebrand factor, or, albeit less specific, CD34.[1]

IMAGING

The size of the primary lesion, and presence or absence of distant metastases need to be determined prior to treatment initiation. Diagnostic assessment, in addition to tissue assessment (Figures 18.1 and 18.2), should include MRI.[3] MRI features show T1 intermediate intensity and high T2 signal

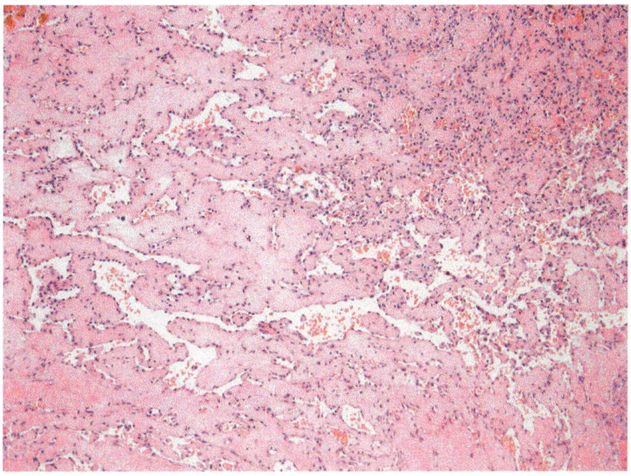

FIGURE 18.1 Infiltrative and dissecting growth of irregularly shaped and anastomosing vascular channels are present within collagenous connective tissue—this is a characteristic feature of angiosarcoma and is viewable with hematoxylin and eosin staining (H&E, x100).

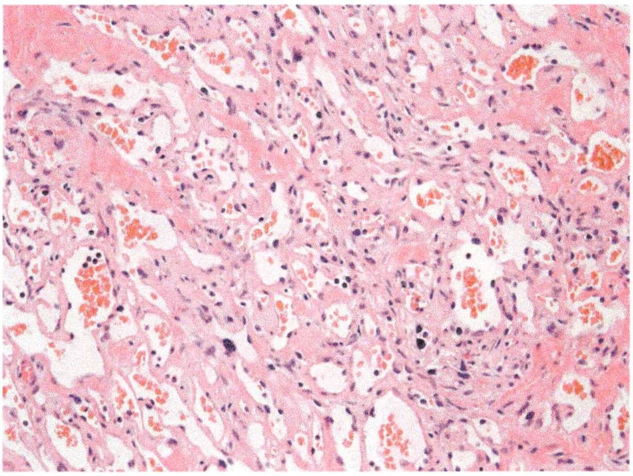

FIGURE 18.2 Higher magnification of hematoxylin and eosin staining (H&E, 200x) of angiosarcoma specimen from Figure 18.1 shows clear nuclear atypia.

intensity—which may be consistent with hemorrhage. The most diagnostic finding is the presence of high-flow serpentine vessels.[34] AS demonstrates enhancement after intravenous contrast administration. Otherwise, imaging findings are largely nonspecific, and differential diagnosis may include glioma, cavernoma, and hemorrhagic metastases.

Chest imaging, particularly CT of the thorax with contrast agent, should be performed prior to initiation of therapy to exclude metastatic disease, as the lung is the most common site of hematologic spread.[4] PET/CT can be considered for patients considered at risk for LN metastases. Patients with cardiac AS are at increased risk for intracranial dissemination and MRI of the brain should be considered.[35]

MOLECULAR ABERRATIONS

Over the last decade, our understanding of cancer genomics, not merely that of AS, has evolved significantly. We now understand that AS is a complex group of tumors with numerous associated genetic alterations. There is no one change that leads to development of all AS. In 2014, investigators found that protein tyrosine phosphatase receptor type B and phospholipase C gamma 1 are recurrently mutated in AS.[36] Previous studies had shown that knockdown resistance (KDR) mutations are present in 10%

of patients with AS.[37] *MYC* and *FLT4* mutations are seen in patients with AS secondary to radiation and lymphedema.[38] A 2015 sequencing study demonstrated that over half of AS showed genetic alterations in the mitogen-activated protein kinase (MAPK) pathway, involving *KRAS, HRAS, NRAS, BRAF, MAPK1*, and *NF1*. The most frequent genetic mutation was *TP53* with 35% of tumors.[39] In a 2015 study of 203 adolescent and young adult sarcomas, three *NTRK1* fusions were found in three tumor types, including AS.[40] This is believed to be an underestimate of total prevalence and may have important implications for targeted therapy.

GENERAL THERAPEUTIC APPROACH

There are, as of yet, no randomized controlled trials involving the treatment of localized AS. Most treatment strategies have been developed through retrospective case series. Localized AS is initially treated with surgical resection, with the goal being R0 margins, or margins shown to be clear microscopically. Involved margins (R1 or R2) are common secondary to the multifocal nature of AS. If R1 or R2 margins are obtained, guidelines recommend repeat resection for R0 margins. Excision is often difficult, with closure requiring reconstruction rather than primary closure. In one series, the average surgical defect left after excision was 14.3 cm by 11.8 cm, with the largest spanning 28 cm by 27 cm.[41] Retrospective analyses of different surgical techniques have not clearly shown superiority of any surgical approach. At a single center, there was no significant difference in OS shown between Mohs surgery and wide local excision.[33]

Given high risk of local recurrence, adjuvant radiotherapy is recommended, and may even be associated with a reduced risk of death (Table 18.1).[4,6,41] At one center, only five of 36 patients managed initially with surgery alone were rendered disease free, versus nine of 20 who received surgery as well as radiation therapy (RT).[6] In a series of 82 patients, in which 46 underwent resection of primary disease, 2/3 received adjuvant radiation. No difference in recurrence was noted between groups.[4] In a retrospective analysis of 48 patients with scalp and face AS, OS rate was 45.8% for 2 years in patients who received radiation as well as surgery.[42] For those patients who had surgery, or radiation alone, OS rate was 11.1% at 2 years. This population was abnormal, however, in that 45 of 48 patients had recurrence. Although there are no prospective clinical trials of adjuvant chemotherapy in AS patients, some sarcoma centers generalize from randomized clinical trials and meta-analyses that support the use of adjuvant/neoadjuvant chemotherapy for patients with high-grade sarcoma.[17] This approach would add three to six cycles of doxorubicin 75 to 90 mg/m^2 by 72-hour infusion plus ifosfamide 8 to 10 g/m^2 divided over 4 to 5 days to resection and/or radiation. Although a large, multicenter series suggested a benefit for the addition of a taxane to radiotherapy for cutaneous AS, other limited retrospective data seem to suggest no benefit.[4,43,44]

Surveillance Follow-Up for Localized Disease

Given the propensity of AS to recur, adequate surveillance is an important aspect of management. Although the imaging properties of AS have been studied, no definitive guidelines particular to this tumor type have been recommended.[34] Follow-up imaging may be pursued in accordance with National Comprehensive Cancer Network (NCCN) guidelines for STS. For stage I disease, at least annual chest imaging should be performed, with chest CT being preferred. For stage II/III disease, reimaging after surgery, in addition to chest imaging every 3 to 6 months for at least 2 to 3 years is recommended.

In one case series of 46 patients with localized disease, 26% had local recurrence after a median interval of 11 months (range of 1–63), and 43% had a distant recurrence at median of 8 months.[4] In another series, in which 56 patients underwent local excision, 24 developed local recurrence alone, 18 developed local recurrence and distant metastases, and 10 developed distant metastases alone.[6]

TABLE 18.1 Recurrence Rates for Local Angiosarcoma by Treatment Modality

		Local Recurrence (%)	
Local Disease Location	***N***	**Surgery Alone**	**S+RT**
All locations[6]	67	86	55
All locations[33]	55	41	31
		Two-year OS (%)	
Face[42]	48	0	25

N, number of patients; OS, overall survival; S+RT, surgery plus radiation therapy.

Factors associated with increased risk of recurrence included breast location, size >5 cm, and incomplete resection.[45]

METASTATIC DISEASE

In two larger retrospective studies, between 13% and 43% patients presented with metastatic disease.[4,6,33] As mentioned above, distant recurrence is not uncommon with AS and has been noted in numerous retrospective studies. Sites of distant metastases include the lung, bone, bowel/mesentery, liver, regional LNs, skin, brain, adrenal glands, kidney, and heart.[33,45] In one study of 99 patients with metastatic AS, diseas-specific survival rates were 40%, 29%, and 10% for 1, 2, and 5 years, respectively.[45] Overall, the outcomes for patients with metastatic AS are significantly worse than those for patients with local tumors or locally recurrent tumors.

SYSTEMIC THERAPY FOR METASTATIC DISEASE

Anthracyclines

In general, metastatic AS is considered to be a fatal and incurable disease. While there is no true standard of care, studies have been able to demonstrate the effectiveness of numerous cytotoxic and targeted therapeutic agents. Current regimens largely involve anthracyclines or taxanes.[46] In 2014, a pooled analysis of AS patients from the European Organization for Research and Treatment of Cancer (EORTC) clinical trials of first-line anthracycline-containing regimens showed similar outcomes when comparing AS to other STS histologis types.[47] A total of 108 patients with AS were included in the analysis, with 25% response rate achieved compared to 21% of the remaining STS patients. Progression-free survival (PFS) and OS were similar for AS and other STS histologic types. Median PFS for AS patients was 4.9 months, with a median OS (mOS) of 9.9 months. This is comparable to a median PFS (mPFS) of 4.3 months and OS of 12 months for other STSs. Only 41% of AS patients survive to 1 year, compared to 50% of other STS patients.

In 2016, olaratumab, in combination with doxorubicin, was approved for treatment of STS.[48] Olaratumab is a monoclonal antibody against platelet-derived growth factor receptor A (PDGFRα). A Phase II study, incorporating unresectable and metastatic STSs, randomized 1:1 to doxorubicin/olaratumab and doxorubicin alone, showed significantly increased median overall survival (mOS) with addition of olaratumab. Of note, the study population contained a total of seven AS patients and was consistent across subtype stratification (leiomyosarcoma vs. nonleiomyosarcoma). OS was only significantly improved in the first-line setting—meaning that the combination of olaratumab and doxorubicin should be utilized in the first-line setting. Unfortunately, the Phase III study did not confirm the efficacy of olaratumab, and this agent is no longer available.

In a retrospective study at one center, approximately 21 patients received pegylated liposomal doxorubicin (PLD) in the first-line setting.[49] Within this study, the response rate was similar between PLD, doxorubicin, and taxane agents within the first-line setting. Given this data, PLD may be a reasonable treatment strategy for a patient with AS, in order to mitigate the toxicity of doxorubicin.

Taxanes

Historically, sensitivity of AS to taxanes has distinguished them from other STS subtypes.[50] Numerous studies have demonstrated the effectiveness of taxanes in the first-line setting.[51,52] In particular, the Phase II ANGIOTAX trial showed an overall response rate (ORR) of 19%, with mPFS of 4 months, and an OS of 8 months with weekly paclitaxel.[53] Results from the ANGIOTAX trial were in line with prior retrospective analyses, showing similar PFS, but variable ORR.

Gemcitabine

Gemcitabine has been shown to be effective when combined with docetaxel as a second-line regimen for most STSs.[54] A retrospective study of 25 patients with advanced AS demonstrated an ORR of 68% and a mOS of 17 months.[55]

While mostly studied in combination with anthracyclines or taxanes, gemcitabine may also be considered as single-agent treatment (see Table 18.2).[55,56] In a retrospective analysis of 25 patients who received weekly gemcitabine alone, patients had an ORR (partial response + complete response) of 68%. mOS in this case series was 17 months with mPFS of 7 months. In one patient, a locally advanced

TABLE 18.2 **Efficacy of Chemotherapeutic Agents for Patients With Angiosarcoma**

Treatment	Study Type	*N*	mPFS	mOS
Anthracyclines	No specific agent; prospective, pooled analysis[47]	108	4.9 mo	9.9 mo
Taxanes	Paclitaxel: Angiotax, prospective, Phase II trial[53]	30	4 mo	8 mo
	Angiotax Plus, prospective Phase II trial, paclitaxel arm[56]	26/50	6.6 mo	19.5 mo
Paclitaxel + bevacizumab	Angiotax Plus, prospective Phase II trial, combination arm[56]	24/50	6.6 mo	15.9 mo
Gemcitabine	Retrospective analysis, gemcitabine single agent[55]	25	7 mo	17 mo

mOS, median overall survival; mPFS, median progression-free survival.

tumor was made resectable again.[55] These results were highly encouraging, particularly in light of the tolerability of the study agent.

Antiangiogenic Treatment

In vitro studies demonstrated a possible role of vascular endothelial growth factor (VEGF) and receptors in development and persistence of AS.[57,58] Bevacizumab is a recombinant humanized antibody against VEGF, which has shown to be linked to tumor growth and metastases. In a study of 32 patients with AS or epithelioid hemangioendothelioma, approximately 48% of AS patients showed stable disease.[59]

Given the success of taxane and bevacizumab therapy independently, the ANGIOTAX PLUS trial randomized 50 AS patients to receive weekly paclitaxel or combination of paclitaxel plus bevacizumab.[56] Within this trial, single-agent paclitaxel arm showed improved ORR of 45.8% compared to 28% for the combination arm. PFS was similar in both arms, but OS was longer in the paclitaxel arm at 19.5 months.

Endoglin, or CD105, is highly expressed on angiogenic and proliferative endothelial cells. Endoglin is a co-receptor for transforming growth factor receptor-β, and is upregulated in the setting of VEGF blockade, representing a potential escape mechanism that may be overcome with combination therapy.[60]

Recently, a Phase III trial of carotuximab (TRC105), a chimeric IgG1 antibody against endoglin, in addition to pazopanib, was conducted (TAPPAS).[5] Primary outcome measure was PFS, with OS and ORR as secondary endpoints.[61] Unfortunately, this study found no improvement in PFS or OS when TRC105 was added to pazopanib compared to pazopanib alone.[62]

Tyrosine Kinase Inhibitors

While less studied, tyrosine kinase inhibitors (TKIs) have been shown to have occasional effect as treatment in AS. Generally, two TKIs are considered in the treatment of AS, sorafenib, and pazopanib. Initial data for sorafenib came from a 2009 Phase II study incorporating STSs. Analysis of the data from that study demonstrated a significant response among those patients with AS in the treatment arm.[63] A Phase II trial of sorafenib was conducted specifically in AS in 2012.[64] This study stratified individuals into visceral and cutaneous AS. Ultimately, it only demonstrated a PFS of 1.8 and 3.8 months, respectively, as well as an OS of 12 and 9 months, respectively for visceral and cutaneous tumors.

Additional work has been done to study pazopanib, in particular, which has shown suppressive activity against VEGFR, PDGFR, and KDR, with overall benefit in AS patients. A retrospective analysis of 40 patients with AS performed by European Organisation for Research and Treatment of Cancer (EORTC) showed PFS of 3 months and OS of 9.9 months. These results were similar to those in the PALETTE study for all STSs.[65,66] Within the review by the EORTC, pazopanib was used as a second or later line of therapy, indicating that it might be useful for patients less able to tolerate more intensive treatment regimens, including taxanes and anthracyclines.

The effectiveness of regorafenib, an orally available inhibitor of VEGFR1, VEGFR2, VEGFR3, KIT, and PDGFR, was studied in STS population that included AS patients (REGOSARC).[67] Within this study, the mOS was 12.1 months in the treatment arm versus 9.5 months with placebo. More recently, data from an open-label Phase II study of oral regorafenib in 18 patients were announced. PFS rate at 4 months was 46%, with mPFS of 2.7 months and OS of 15 months.[68]

Nonselective Beta Blockers

The role of β-adrenergic receptors is important in numerous normal physiologic functions. These G-protein–coupled receptors are present on numerous cancers, and have been historically used in the

TABLE 18.3 Efficacy of Targeted Agents for Patients With Angiosarcoma

Treatment	Study Type	*N*	mPFS	mOS
Bevacizumab	Prospective, Phase II, single arm[59]	30	6.5 mo	31 mo
Pazopanib	Retrospective analysis[65]	40	3 mo	9.9 mo
Sorafenib	Phase II study[64]	41	1.8, 3.8 mo	12, 9.0 mo
Propranolol	Case report[78]	1	Unknown	Unknown
Checkpoint inhibition	Laboratory, case report[75,76]	1	Unknown	Unknown

mOS, median overall survival; mPFS, median progression-free survival.

treatment of infantile hemangiomas (IHs).[69] β-Receptors are present on AS, and treatment with high doses of propranolol causes apoptosis of cell lines.[70] Data are limited regarding the utilization of nonspecific β-blockade in the treatment of AS and are mostly available in case reports. In one patient, serial biopsies demonstrated a decreased proliferative index from 30% to 20%.[71] A combination of propranolol with metronomic cyclophosphamide demonstrated effectiveness in a single case as well.[72] Given the hints of benefit in case reports and the tolerability of therapy, further studies with β-blockade are likely upcoming in AS.

Checkpoint Inhibitors

Large advances have been made in the field of immunotherapy, particularly in cancers, such as melanoma.[73] More recently, immunotherapy has been considered as a potential treatment for sarcomas. In a Phase II trial of STS that unfortunately did not include AS, there was an 18% response rate.[74] A 2017 paper demonstrated that, within a sample of 24 AS, approximately 66% expressed programmed death-ligand 1 (PD-L1).[75] This information is encouraging in that PD-L1 expression has previously been shown to correlate with effectiveness of checkpoint inhibition. Case reports have demonstrated possible effectiveness of pembrolizumab in treatment of AS.[76] At present, the role of immunotherapy in treatment of AS remains undefined. In a Phase II trial of nivolumab with or without ipilimumab for treatment of metastatic sarcoma, three AS patients were included in the combined study.[77] Notably, one AS patient was among those patients with confirmed responses ($N = 6$). Given the exciting nature of these developments, it is anticipated that much additional research will be conducted regarding the role of checkpoint inhibition in treatment of AS (Table 18.3).[78]

Sequence of Therapies

The optimal sequence of anthracycline, taxane, and other therapies remains somewhat unclear at this time. There have been no randomized controlled trials directly comparing effectiveness of taxane to anthracycline treatment. Most retrospective studies demonstrate similar effectiveness, and survival rates between taxanes and anthracyclines. In 2011, a comparison of doxorubicin-containing regimens, weekly paclitaxel, and metastatectomy were analyzed by Penel et al.[79] Given that this study incorporated the outcomes associated with the treatment of 149 patients, it is one of the largest to date. mOS was 11 months in the doxorubicin-containing regimens and 13.1 months with weekly paclitaxel. Time to progression was 3.9 months with doxorubicin and 5.6 months with weekly paclitaxel. Furthermore, a comparison of 117 patients who were treated with weekly paclitaxel or doxorubicin as first-line therapy was performed in 2012.[80] In this study, there was no difference in response rate or significant difference in mOS. There was, however, a significant difference in ORR (53% vs. 29% in paclitaxel and doxorubicin, respectively, $p = .02$). Notably, there was also a larger proportion of patients with cutaneous AS in the paclitaxel group. Given the overall comparability of anthracycline and taxane regimens in the treatment of AS, there are insufficient data to recommend one form of treatment over the other as an optimal first line. It is clearly established, though, that it is reasonable to use each sequentially in the treatment of patients.

Evidence to guide subsequent lines of therapy is less clear, however, and treatment decisions often depend on patient performance status and behavior of disease. As mentioned above, pazopanib has been studied as a second or later line of treatment with modest results.[65] Furthermore, as additional data are collected regarding the roles of regorafenib, propranolol, and immunotherapy, the role for each in the hierarchy of AS treatment will become clearer. The NCCN-approved AS systemic therapies include, in addition to those already described, vinorelbine, sorafenib, sunitinib, and all other systemic therapy options per NCCN Soft Tissue Sarcoma Guidelines for nonspecific histologic types.[46]

SUMMARY

AS is a rare tumor of endothelial origin. Despite its scarcity, AS can present with local disease in nearly any organ system. Furthermore, rate of local recurrence as well as metastasis is high, making AS a difficult cancer to treat. In locoregional disease, AS is best treated with resection as well as RT. In the setting of metastatic disease, front-line therapy with anthracyclines or taxanes has been shown to be effective. Second-line therapy with taxanes or anthracyclines (whichever was not utilized in the first line) has likewise demonstrated some success. Evidence for later lines of therapy is less clear, with recent studies, however, with TKIs, nonspecific β-blockers, and immunotherapy showing some promise.

Regardless of the stage at presentation, as well as treatment, long-term prognosis is poor. Significantly more research must be performed in order to better understand the biology as well as the best means of treatment for AS.

CASE STUDY

The patient is a 40-year-old man without significant past medical history who presented to clinic for evaluation of intermediate- to high-grade metastatic AS. Imaging demonstrated a 5-cm lung mass, in addition to metastatic osseous disease. Core-needle biopsy revealed irregularly shaped blood vessels, and CD31 and FLI-1 on immunohistochemistry, suggestive of AS. The initial stage was T1bN0M1G3 and treatment was started with doxorubicin (Adriamycin) and olaratumab, for which he underwent 11 cycles (eight cycles of combined therapy, followed by olaratumab alone for a total of 33 weeks) until eventual progression of disease. During treatment, he maintained good performance status and was able to work. Following palliative radiation to the right pelvis for worsening pain, he was transitioned to gemcitabine in addition to docetaxel. His chemotherapy regimen was altered with eventual discontinuation of docetaxel after significant treatment-associated symptom burden. Single-agent gemcitabine was attempted, but again, tolerance for therapy was poor. Although his disease responded well to therapy, and was stable for 4 months, his quality of life was poor. He was eventually transitioned to paclitaxel single agent and achieved CR after eight cycles. Given worsening peripheral neuropathy, paclitaxel was discontinued, and the patient was given a drug holiday with surveillance. In total, 18 months have passed since the time of diagnosis, and he remains without evidence of disease.

This case illustrates a somewhat atypical scenario in that the patient responded so robustly to numerous lines of therapy. His OS and PFS were far longer than the mOS and mPFS for AS. Here, we see a common sequence of therapy in utilization of doxorubicin, as well as taxane in first and second lines. Later lines of treatment might incorporate TKIs or other NCCN-suggested agents.

REFERENCES

1. Fletcher CDM. *Diagnostic Histopathology of Tumors*. 4th ed. Philadelphia, PA: Saunders; 2013.
2. Rouhani P, Fletcher CDM, Devesa SS, Toro JR. Cutaneous soft tissue sarcoma incidence patterns in the U.S.: an analysis of 12,114 cases. *Cancer*. 2008;113(3):616–627. doi:10.1002/cncr.23571
3. Young RJ, Brown NJ, Reed MW, et al. Angiosarcoma. *Lancet Oncol*. 2010;11(10):983–991. doi:10.1016/S1470-2045(10)70023-1
4. Abraham JA, Hornicek FJ, Kaufman AM, et al. Treatment and outcome of 82 patients with angiosarcoma. *Ann Surg Oncol*. 2007;14(6):1953–1967. doi:10.1245/s10434-006-9335-y
5. Mehta CR, Liu L, Theuer C. An adaptive population enrichment phase 3 trial of TRC105 and pazopanib versus pazopanib alone in patients with advanced angiosarcoma (TAPPAS Trial). *Ann Oncol*. 2019;30(1):103–108. doi:10.1093/annonc/mdy464
6. Mark RJ, Poen JC, Tran LM, et al. Angiosarcoma: a report of 67 patients and a review of the literature. *Cancer*. 1996;77(11):2400–2406. doi:10.1002/(SICI)1097-0142(19960601)77:11<2400::AID-CNCR32>3.0.CO;2-Z
7. Deyrup AT, Miettinen M, North PE, et al. Angiosarcomas arising in the viscera and soft tissue of children and young adults: a clinicopathologic study of 15 cases. *Am J Surg Pathol*. 2009;33(2):264–269. doi:10.1097/PAS.0b013e3181875a5f

8. Stewart FW, Treves N. Lymphangiosarcoma in postmastectomy lymphedema; a report of six cases in elephantiasis chirurgica. *Cancer*. 1948;1(1):64–81. doi:10.1002/1097-0142(195311)6:6<1192::AID-CNCR2820060613>3.0.CO;2-#
9. Lahat G, Dhuka AR, Hallevi H, et al. Angiosarcoma: clinical and molecular insights. *Ann Surg*. 2010;251(6):1098–1106. doi:10.1097/SLA.0b013e3181dbb75a
10. Lucas DR. Angiosarcoma, radiation-associated angiosarcoma, and atypical vascular lesion. *Arch Pathol Lab Med*. 2009;133(11):1804–1809. doi:10.1043/1543-2165-133.11.1804
11. Shah S, Rosa M. Radiation-associated angiosarcoma of the breast: clinical and pathologic features. *Arch Pathol Lab Med*. 2016;140(5):477–481. doi:10.5858/arpa.2014-0581-RS
12. Virtanen A, Pukkala E, Auvinen A. Angiosarcoma after radiotherapy: a cohort study of 332 163 Finnish cancer patients. *Br J Cancer*. 2007;97(1):115–117. doi:10.1038/sj.bjc.6603805
13. Ronen S, Ivan D, Torres-Cabala CA, et al. Post-radiation vascular lesions of the breast. *J Cutan Pathol*. 2019;46(1):52–58. doi:10.1111/cup.13363
14. Cahan GW, Woodard HQ, Norman LH. Sarcoma arising in irradiated bone. *Cancer*. 1948;1(1):3–29. doi:10.1002/1097-0142(194805)1:1<3::aid-cncr2820010103>3.0.co;2-7
15. Morgan MB, Swann M, Somach S, et al. Cutaneous angiosarcoma: a case series with prognostic correlation. *J Am Acad Dermatol*. 2004;50(6):867–874. doi:10.1016/j.jaad.2003.10.671
16. Budd GT. Management of angiosarcoma. *Curr Oncol Rep*. 2002;4(6):515–519. doi:10.1007/s11912-002-0066-3
17. Florou V, Wilky BA. Current and future directions for angiosarcoma therapy. *Curr Treat Options Oncol*. 2018;19(3):14. doi:10.1007/s11864-018-0531-3
18. Mallick A, Jain S, Proctor A, Pandey R. Angiosarcoma around a revision total hip arthroplasty and review of literature. *J Arthroplasty*. 2009;24(2):323.e17–323.e20. doi:10.1016/j.arth.2008.04.007
19. Zhu W, Feng B, Ma Q, et al. Angiosarcoma around hip joint prosthesis. *Chin Med J (Engl)*. 2016;129(21):2642. doi:10.4103/0366-6999.192783
20. Visuri T, Pulkkinen P, Paavolainen P. Malignant tumors at the site of total hip prosthesis. Analytic review of 46 cases. *J Arthroplasty*. 2006;21(3):311–323. doi:10.1016/j.arth.2005.03.046
21. Milite D, Pilon F, Ferrari A, et al. Aortic epithelioid angiosarcoma after endovascular aneurysm repair. *Ann Vasc Surg*. 2016;35:207.e17–207.e21. doi:10.1016/j.avsg.2016.02.014
22. Fenton J, Veenstra M, Bove P. Angiosarcoma involving native abdominal aortic aneurysm sac after endograft repair. *Ann Vasc Surg*. 2014;28(2):490.e1–490.e4. doi:10.1016/j.avsg.2013.03.016
23. Agaimy A, Ben-Izhak O, Lorey T, et al. Angiosarcoma arising in association with vascular Dacron grafts and orthopedic joint prostheses: clinicopathologic, immunohistochemical, and molecular study. *Ann Diagn Pathol*. 2016;21:21–28. doi:10.1016/j.anndiagpath.2016.01.002
24. McBride KA, Ballinger ML, Killick E, et al. Li-Fraumeni syndrome: cancer risk assessment and clinical management. *Nat Rev Clin Oncol*. 2014;11(5):260–271. doi:10.1038/nrclinonc.2014.41
25. Prabhash K, Tandon N. Sarcomas of head and neck region. *Indian J Cancer*. 2011;48(3):282. doi:10.4103/0019-509X.84910
26. Albores-Saavedra J, Schwartz AM, Henson DE, et al. Cutaneous angiosarcoma. Analysis of 434 cases from the surveillance, epidemiology, and end results program, 1973-2007. *Ann Diagn Pathol*. 2011;15(2):93–97. doi:10.1016/j.anndiagpath.2010.07.012
27. Fayette J, Martin E, Piperno-Neumann S, et al. Angiosarcomas, a heterogeneous group of sarcomas with specific behavior depending on primary site: a retrospective study of 161 cases. *Ann Oncol*. 2007;18(12):2030–2036. doi:10.1093/annonc/mdm381
28. Fury MG, Antonescu CR, Van Zee K, et al. A 14-year retrospective review of angiosarcoma: clinical characteristics, prognostic factors, and treatment outcomes with surgery and chemotherapy. *Cancer J*. 2005;11(3):241–247. doi:10.1097/00130404-200505000-00011
29. Sinnamon AJ, Neuwirth MG, McMillan MT, et al. A prognostic model for resectable soft tissue and cutaneous angiosarcoma. *J Surg Oncol*. 2016;114(5):557–563. doi:10.1002/jso.24352
30. Fisher SB, Chiang YJ, Feig BW, et al. Comparative performance of the 7th and 8th editions of the American Joint Committee on Cancer Staging Systems for Soft Tissue Sarcoma of the Trunk and Extremities. *Ann Surg Oncol*. 2018;25(5):1126–1132. doi:10.1245/s10434-018-6378-9
31. Amin MB, Edge S, Greene F, et al. *AJCC Cancer Staging Manual*. 8th ed. New York, NY: Springer International Publishing; 2017.
32. Geller RL, Hookim K, Sullivan HC, et al. Cytologic features of angiosarcoma: a review of 26 cases diagnosed on FNA. *Cancer Cytopathol*. 2016;124(9):659–668. doi:10.1002/cncy.21726
33. Buehler D, Rice SR, Moody JS, et al. Angiosarcoma outcomes and prognostic factors: a 25-year single institution experience. *Am J Clin Oncol*. 2013;37(5):473–479. doi:10.1097/COC.0b013e31827e4e7b
34. Gaballah AH, Jensen CT, Palmquist S, et al. Angiosarcoma: clinical and imaging features from head to toe. *Br J Radiol*. 2017;90(1075):20170039. doi:10.1259/bjr.20170039
35. Shweikeh F, Bukavina L, Saeed K, et al. Brain metastasis in bone and soft tissue cancers: a review of incidence, interventions, and outcomes. *Sarcoma*. 2014;2014:475175. doi:10.1155/2014/475175
36. Behjati S, Tarpey PS, Sheldon H, et al. Recurrent PTPRB and PLCG1 mutations in angiosarcoma. *Nat Genet*. 2014;46(4):376–379. doi:10.1038/ng.2921
37. Antonescu CR, Yoshida A, Guo T, et al. KDR activating mutations in human angiosarcomas are sensitive to specific kinase inhibitors. *Cancer Res*. 2009;69(18):7175–7179. doi:10.1158/0008-5472.CAN-09-2068

38. Manner J, Radlwimmer B, Hohenberger P, et al. MYC high level gene amplification is a distinctive feature of angiosarcomas after irradiation or chronic lymphedema. *Am J Pathol*. 2010;176(1):34–39. doi:10.2353/ajpath.2010.090637
39. Murali R, Chandramohan R, Moller I, et al. Targeted massively parallel sequencing of angiosarcomas reveals frequent activation of the mitogen activated protein kinase pathway. *Oncotarget*. 2015;6(34):36041–36052. doi:10.18632/oncotarget.5936
40. Morosini D, Chmielecki J, Goldberg M, et al. Comprehensive genomic profiling of sarcomas from 267 adolescents and young adults to reveal a spectrum of targetable genomic alterations. *J Clin Oncol*. 2015;33(15_suppl):11020. doi:10.1200/jco.2015.33.15_suppl.11020
41. Pawlik TM, Paulino AF, McGinn CJ, et al. Cutaneous angiosarcoma of the scalp: a multidisciplinary approach. *Cancer*. 2003;98(8):1716–1726. doi:10.1002/cncr.11667
42. Ogawa K, Takahashi K, Asato Y, et al. Treatment and prognosis of angiosarcoma of the scalp and face: a retrospective analysis of 48 patients. *Br J Radiol*. 2012;85(1019):1127–1133. doi:10.1259/bjr/31655219
43. Köhler HF, Neves RI, Brechtbühl ER, et al. Cutaneous angiosarcoma of the head and neck: report of 23 cases from a single institution. *Otolaryngol Head Neck Surg*. 2008;139(4):519–524. doi:10.1016/j.otohns.2008.07.022
44. Buschmann A, Lehnhardt M, Toman N, et al. Surgical treatment of angiosarcoma of the scalp: less is more. *Ann Plast Surg*. 2008;61(4):399–403. doi:10.1097/SAP.0b013e31816b31f8
45. Lahat G, Dhuka AR, Lahat S, et al. Outcome of locally recurrent and metastatic angiosarcoma. *Ann Surg Oncol*. 2009;16(9):2502–2509. doi:10.1245/s10434-009-0569-3
46. von Mehren M, Randall RL, Benjamin RS, et al. Soft Tissue Sarcoma, Version 2.2018, NCCN Clinical Practice Guidelines in Oncology. *J Natl Compr Canc Netw*. 2018;16(5):536-563. doi:10.6004/jnccn.2018.0025
47. Young RJ, Natukunda A, Litière S, et al. First-line anthracycline-based chemotherapy for angiosarcoma and other soft tissue sarcoma subtypes: pooled analysis of eleven European Organisation for Research and Treatment of Cancer Soft Tissue and Bone Sarcoma Group trials. *Eur J Cancer*. 2014;50(18):3178–3186. doi:10.1016/j.ejca.2014.10.004
48. Tap WD, Jones RL, Van Tine BA, et al. Olaratumab and doxorubicin versus doxorubicin alone for treatment of soft-tissue sarcoma: an open-label phase 1b and randomised phase 2 trial. *Lancet*. 2016;388(10043):488–497. doi:10.1016/S0140-6736(16)30587-6
49. D'Angelo SP, Munhoz RR, Kuk D, et al. Outcomes of systemic therapy for patients with metastatic angiosarcoma. *Oncology*. 2015;89(4):205–214. doi:10.1159/000381917
50. Skubitz KM, Haddad PA. Paclitaxel and pegylated-liposomal doxorubicin are both active in angiosarcoma. *Cancer*. 2005;104(2):361–366. doi:10.1002/cncr.21140
51. Schlemmer M, Reichardt P, Verweij J, et al. Paclitaxel in patients with advanced angiosarcomas of soft tissue: a retrospective study of the EORTC soft tissue and bone sarcoma group. *Eur J Cancer*. 2008;44(16):2433–2436. doi:10.1016/j.ejca.2008.07.037
52. Fata F, O'Reilly E, Ilson D, et al. Paclitaxel in the treatment of patients with anglosarcoma of the scalp or face. *Cancer*. 1999;86(10):2034–2037. doi:10.1002/(SICI)1097-0142(19991115)86:10<2034::AID-CNCR21>3.0.CO;2-P.
53. Penel N, Bui BN, Bay JO, et al. Phase II trial of weekly paclitaxel for unresectable angiosarcoma: the ANGIOTAX study. *J Clin Oncol*. 2008;26(32):5269–5274. doi:10.1200/JCO.2008.17.3146
54. Maki RG, Wathen JK, Patel SR, et al. Randomized phase II study of gemcitabine and docetaxel compared with gemcitabine alone in patients with metastatic soft tissue sarcomas. *J Clin Oncol*. 2007;25(19):2755–2763. doi:10.1200/JCO.2006.10.4117
55. Stacchiotti S, Palassini E, Sanfilippo R, et al. Gemcitabine in advanced angiosarcoma: a retrospective case series analysis from the Italian rare cancer network. *Ann Oncol*. 2012;23(2):501–508. doi:10.1093/annonc/mdr066
56. Ray-Coquard IL, Domont J, Tresch-Bruneel E, et al. Paclitaxel given once per week with or without bevacizumab in patients with advanced angiosarcoma: a randomized phase II trial. *J Clin Oncol*. 2015;33(25):2797–2802. doi:10.1200/JCO.2015.60.8505
57. Ferrara N, Davis-Smyth T. The biology of vascular endothelial growth factor. *Endocr Rev*. 1997;18(1):4–25. doi:10.1210/edrv.18.1.0287
58. Itakura E, Yamamoto H, Oda Y, Tsuneyoshi M. Detection and characterization of vascular endothelial growth factors and their receptors in a series of angiosarcomas. *J Surg Oncol*. 2008;97(1):74–81. doi:10.1002/jso.20766
59. Agulnik M, Yarber JL, Okuno SH, et al. An open-label, multicenter, phase II study of bevacizumab for the treatment of angiosarcoma and epithelioid hemangioendotheliomas. *Ann Oncol*. 2013;24(1):257–263. doi:10.1093/annonc/mds237
60. Kaplon H, Reichert JM. Antibodies to watch in 2018. *MAbs*. 2013;10(2):183–203. doi:10.1080/19420862.2018.1415671
61. Sankhala KK, Attia S, Barve MA, et al. TRC105 (endoglin antibody) in combination with pazopanib in patients with advanced angiosarcoma. Presented at: *Connective Tissue Oncology Society Meeting*; November 9–12, 2016:Lisbon, Partugal.
62. Fritchie K, Attia S, Okuno SH, et al. CD105: a therapeutic target for sarcomas. *Mol Cancer Ther*. 2013;12(11 suppl):B237. doi:10.1158/1535-7163
63. Maki RG, D'Adamo DR, Keohan ML, et al. Phase II study of sorafenib in patients with metastatic or recurrent sarcomas. *J Clin Oncol*. 2009;27(19):3133–3140. doi:10.1200/JCO.2008.20.4495
64. Ray-Coquard I, Italiano A, Bompas E, et al. Sorafenib for patients with advanced angiosarcoma: a phase II trial from the French Sarcoma Group (GSF/GETO). *Oncologist*. 2012;17(2):260–266. doi:10.1634/theoncologist.2011-0237

65. Kollár A, Jones RL, Stacchiotti S, et al. Pazopanib in advanced vascular sarcomas: an EORTC Soft Tissue and Bone Sarcoma Group (STBSG) retrospective analysis. *Acta Oncol*. 2017;56(1):88–92. doi:10.1080/0284186X.2016.1234068
66. Van Der Graaf WTA, Blay JY, Chawla SP, et al. Pazopanib for metastatic soft-tissue sarcoma (PALETTE): a randomised, double-blind, placebo-controlled phase 3 trial. *Lancet*. 2012;379(9829):1879–1886. doi:10.1016/S0140-6736(12)60651-5
67. Mir O, Brodowicz T, Italiano A, et al. Safety and efficacy of regorafenib in patients with advanced soft tissue sarcoma (REGOSARC): a randomised, double-blind, placebo-controlled, phase 2 trial. *Lancet Oncol*. 2016;17(12):1732–1742. doi:10.1016/S1470-2045(16)30507-1
68. Agulnik M, Van Tine BA, Attia A, et al. Multicenter, open-label phase II study of daily oral regorafenib for chemotherapy-refractory, metastatic and locally advanced angiosarcoma. *Ann Oncol*. 2018;29(suppl 8):viii576–viii595. https://oncologypro.esmo.org/Meeting-Resources/ESMO-2018-Congress/Multicenter-Open-Label-Phase-II-Study-of-Daily-Oral-Regorafenib-for-Chemotherapy-Refractory-Metastatic-and-Locally-Advanced-Angiosarcoma
69. Wagner MJ, Ravi V, Menter DG, Sood AK. Endothelial cell malignancies: new insights from the laboratory and clinic. NPJ *Precis Oncol*. 2017;1(1):11. doi:10.1038/s41698-017-0013-2
70. Stiles JM, Amaya C, Rains S, et al. Targeting of beta adrenergic receptors results in therapeutic efficacy against models of hemangioendothelioma and angiosarcoma. *PLoS One*. 2013;8(3):e60021. doi:10.1371/journal.pone.0060021
71. Chow W, Amaya CN, Rains S, et al. Growth attenuation of cutaneous angiosarcoma with propranolol-mediated β-blockade. *JAMA Dermatol*. 2015;151(11):1226–1229. doi:10.1001/jamadermatol.2015.2554
72. Daguzé J, Saint-Jean M, Peuvrel L, et al. Visceral metastatic angiosarcoma treated effectively with oral cyclophosphamide combined with propranolol. *J Am Acad Dermatol Case Rep*. 2016;2(6):497–499. doi:10.1016/j.jdcr.2016.10.005
73. Robert C, Long GV, Brady B, et al. Nivolumab in previously untreated melanoma without *BRAF* mutation. *N Engl J Med*. 2015;372(4):320–330. doi:10.1056/NEJMoa1412082
74. Tawbi HA, Burgess M, Bolejack V, et al. Pembrolizumab in advanced soft-tissue sarcoma and bone sarcoma (SARC028): a multicentre, two-cohort, single-arm, open-label, phase 2 trial. *Lancet Oncol*. 2017;18(11):1493–1501. doi:10.1016/S1470-2045(17)30624-1
75. Botti G, Scognamiglio G, Marra L, et al. Programmed death ligand 1 (PD-L1) expression in primary angiosarcoma. *J Cancer*. 2017;8(16):3166–3172. doi:10.7150/jca.19060
76. Sindhu S, Gimber LH, Cranmer L, et al. Angiosarcoma treated successfully with anti-PD-1 therapy—a case report. *J Immunother Cancer*. 2017;5(1):1–5. doi:10.1186/s40425-017-0263-0
77. D'Angelo SP, Mahoney MR, Van Tine BA, et al. Nivolumab with or without ipilimumab treatment for metastatic sarcoma (Alliance A091401): two open-label, non-comparative, randomised, phase 2 trials. *Lancet Oncol*. 2018;19(3):416–426. doi:10.1016/S1470-2045(18)30006-8
78. Amaya CN, Perkins M, Belmont A, et al. Non-selective beta blockers inhibit angiosarcoma cell viability and increase progression free- and overall-survival in patients diagnosed with metastatic angiosarcoma. *Oncoscience*. 2018;5(3–4):124–134. doi:10.18632/oncoscience.413
79. Penel N, Italiano A, Ray-coquard I, et al. Metastatic angiosarcomas: doxorubicin-based regimens, weekly paclitaxel and metastasectomy significantly improve the outcome. *Ann Oncol*. 2012;23(2):517–523. doi:10.1093/annonc/mdr138
80. Italiano A, Cioffi A, Penel N, et al. Comparison of doxorubicin and weekly paclitaxel efficacy in metastatic angiosarcomas. *Cancer*. 2012;118(13):3330–3336. doi:10.1002/cncr.26599

19

Desmoid Tumor

Chelsea R. Horwood and Valerie P. Grignol

INTRODUCTION

Desmoid tumors, or aggressive fibromatosis, are locally aggressive soft tissue tumors that do not have the ability to metastasize. The majority are spontaneous in nature; however, they are also seen in association with familial adenomatous polyposis (FAP). Desmoid tumors can further be divided by location—intra-abdominal, extra-abdominal, and abdominal wall—and typically present as nonmobile, fixed soft tissue masses. They are more common in women and in a younger age group. Mutations leading to tumorigenesis are seen in the β-catenin or adenomatous polyposis coli (APC) genes from the Wnt/β-catenin pathway. CT, ultrasound imaging, and MRI can be utilized for diagnostic imaging and surveillance. An image-guided core-needle biopsy is necessary for diagnosis. The standard of care has been complete surgical resection. However, radiation and other systemic therapies can be used as primary, adjuvant, or neoadjuvant treatment. Watchful waiting has been used in more indolent subtypes, and a period of observation is becoming the recommendation for all types. Desmoid tumors have a high propensity for recurrence; therefore, close surveillance is essential, particularly in the first 2 years. Treatment regimens should be individualized and require a multidisciplinary approach.

EPIDEMIOLOGY

Desmoid tumors are a very rare form of soft tissue tumor that are locally aggressive in nature. They account for 3% of all soft tissue sarcomas, with an incidence of 2.4 to 4.3 per million per year.[1] Women are two times more likely to be affected than men with the average age of 25 to 35 years (range 15–60 years).[1–3] The higher propensity for women to be affected is thought to be hormonal in nature, as many stain positive for the estrogen receptor immunohistochemically.[4] There is no specific racial or ethnic group preferentially affected.

There are two primary subtypes of desmoid tumors, sporadic and familial. Sporadic tumors account for the vast majority of desmoid tumors, with ~90% of those encountered, equating to roughly 3.43 per million per year.[5] The far less common subtype, familial, is associated with FAP. FAP is estimated to occur in one to five per 10,000 individuals and accounts for <10% of all desmoid tumors.[6] Patients with desmoid tumors associated with the familial subtype have an 852 times greater risk of having a desmoid tumor than the remainder of the population.[7] This is especially prevalent in the Gardner syndrome variant of FAP, which is associated with fibromas, osteomas, sebaceous cysts, and intestinal polyps. Additionally, patients with FAP who have desmoid tumors are more likely to be male, younger, and have intra-abdominal tumors.[8,9]

MOLECULAR PATHOGENESIS

The majority of desmoid tumors arise from a mutation in the Wnt/β-catenin pathway.[1] A smaller proportion arises from derangements in the APC complex that affects the same pathway.[9,10] The Wnt/β-catenin pathway normally plays a role in developmental gene expression as well as regulating the amount of β-catenin available intracellularly.[1] The APC complex is a kinase pathway that is inhibited by the Wnt pathway. However, when activated, APC complex phosphorylates β-catenin on threonine 41 and serine 33, 37, and 45 of the β-catenin gene on exon 3. This leads to its degradation via a proteasome within the cell, ultimately leading to decreased amounts of β-catenin.[11] When inactivated by the Wnt pathway, the APC complex can no longer phosphorylate β-catenin, leading to its accumulation within the cell. This increase of β-catenin within the cell cytoplasm leads to translocation into the nucleus, where it plays a pivotal role in gene transcription of cyclin-D1 and c-myc. Cyclin-D1 and c-myc stimulate cell proliferation.[1,12]

Sporadic Subtype

Roughly 95% of "wild type" desmoid tumors have mutations in the Wnt/β-catenin pathway described previously and results in majority of extra-abdominal desmoid tumors.[13] *CTNNB1* gene mutation is the most common that is encountered in the sporadic subtype of desmoid tumors, accounting for 85% of mutations seen.[9,10,14] The *CTNNB1* gene codes for β-catenin. Three different point mutations, T41A, S45F, and S45P, are seen in β-catenin.[11,15] Many studies have shown higher recurrence rates and reduced 5-year disease-free survival for patients with mutations in β-catenin of *CTNNB1*.[9,11] Specifically, the S45F mutation, has a higher rate of recurrence after surgical excision of the primary tumor; this may also be linked to anatomic location as there is a high rate of extra-abdominal desmoids with the S45F mutation.[11,16,17] Multiple studies have evaluated the high rate of recurrence and specific gene markers. Current research is focusing on tailoring clinical care based on genetic markers.

Other aberrations have been noted in sporadic type desmoid tumors. Trisomy 8 and trisomy 20 have been seen in up to one-third of all desmoid tumors.[18,19] Roughly 64% of pediatric desmoid tumors also have mutations in *CTNNB1*; however, they also have mutations in *AKT1* E17K in 31% of tumors, *BRAF* V600E in 19% of tumors, and *TP53* R273H in 9% of tumors.[20]

Familial Subtype

The vast majority of desmoid tumors are sporadic; however, patients with FAP typically have a mutation in the APC gene complex.[9] Germ-line mutations in APC lead to the development of desmoid tumors in 10% to 25% of patients with FAP.[12,21,22] FAP is an autosomal dominant hereditary condition caused by a mutation in the APC gene complex on chromosome 5q21-q22 that leads to hundreds of polyps within the colon.[23] Owing to improvements in screening and treatment among patients with FAP, desmoid tumors have become the number one cause of death among patients who have undergone colectomy.[22] The majority of patients with APC mutations are also more likely to have intra-abdominal desmoid tumors, with high preponderance for small bowel mesentery involvement.[24] A young male with a primary intra-abdominal desmoid tumor should be referred for colonoscopy given the association with FAP.[2]

PRESENTATION

Desmoid tumors typically present as painless, nonmobile masses on the trunk or arms. They can also present with bowel obstruction, or rarely, as acute bowel ischemia or functional issues with ileoanal anastomoses in patients with FAP who have previously undergone total abdominal colectomy.[25,26] There are three primary anatomic locations: extra-abdominal, intra-abdominal, and abdominal wall. Molecular subtype and response to therapy vary by anatomic location. Location is an important consideration in treatment algorithm in patients presenting with desmoid tumors.

Extra-Abdominal

Extra-abdominal desmoid tumors occur anywhere from the head and neck, the trunk, to the extremities. Extremity desmoids occur anywhere on the arms, legs, girdles, and deep pelvis. Among extra-abdominal desmoid tumors, those in the extremity have a worse overall disease-free survival, with a 20% decreased disease-free survival rate compared to other locations.[27] These lesions typically arise from musculo-aponeurotic structures. Local growth can result in limb deformation and pain.

Intra-Abdominal

Intra-abdominal tumors are typically associated with FAP and are primarily mesenteric in location.[27] Local progression can lead to bowel obstruction, ureteral obstruction, bowel ischemia, and organ dysfunction. This anatomic site is a small subset of desmoids, accounting for only 2% to 15% of all desmoid tumors, and has up to an 88% recurrence rate.[2,21,28,29] There is a 3.5% to 32% incidence among patients with FAP; however, they can occur sporadically.[28] Therefore, an intra-abdominal desmoid should not be assumed to be associated with hereditary subtype until full pathologic evaluation. Any person who presents with an intra-abdominal desmoid tumor under 40 years of age should have a colonoscopy to evaluate for colon polyps and possible FAP.[28,30] Intra-abdominal desmoids typically arise from within the small bowel mesentery. This leads to challenging surgical resection due to the risk of bowel ischemia secondary to wide local excision of the supplying mesentery.[31] This can result in short gut syndrome and lifelong total parental nutrition (TPN) in some patients. Given these risks, medical management should be employed when a significant portion of the mesentery is compromised prior to undergoing surgical treatment.

Abdominal Wall

Patients with abdominal wall desmoid tumors typically present with a nontender, palpable abdominal wall mass. This location has the best prognosis for disease-free survival and response to therapy compared to the other locations.[32,33] Wide local excision of abdominal wall tumors can lead to difficulties in abdominal wall reconstruction. This requires a multidisciplinary approach to surgical management among the surgical oncologist and reconstructive surgeon during preoperative planning.[34,35]

Abdominal wall desmoids are also much more common among women, and pregnant women in particular. It is thought that estrogen causes an increase in disease proliferation secondary to expression of the estrogen receptor β ligand on tumor cells; however, the exact mechanism is not understood.[36,37] Despite an increase in incidence during pregnancy, it can still be managed with standard therapies including surgery or "watchful waiting." One study showed that 14% of pregnant women who underwent watchful waiting had spontaneous regression, only 27% of patients had tumor progression, and only one patient had to undergo cesarean section secondary to her disease. However, there was a higher rate of progression of the tumor among women who were pregnant.[37] There is no difference in recurrence-free survival among women with abdominal wall desmoids who are pregnant and those who are not pregnant. Pregnancy is not contraindicated in patients with history of desmoid tumors.[37,38]

IMAGING: DIAGNOSIS AND CHARACTERISTICS

Ultrasound exam, CT, and MRI are all utilized in the diagnosis, staging, and surveillance of desmoid tumors. Ultrasound can be utilized for peripheral or abdominal wall tumors. They have variable appearance on ultrasound images and either present as well-defined hypoechoic structures or ill-defined, infiltrative masses.[39] They are often identified by the "tail sign," the tumor infiltrating along fascial planes, or the "staghorn sign," which shows linear tumor extension.[40] Ultrasound is particularly useful for pregnant women with abdominal wall tumors given the lack of radiation. It can also be used to serially follow extremity/abdominal wall desmoids.

Typically, cross-sectional imaging is the initial step in diagnosis of desmoid tumors. It allows for further delineation of tumor size, surrounding anatomic involvement, and invasion into any adjacent structures. CT scan with contrast is the preferred imaging modality for intra-abdominal desmoid tumors. They usually appear as poorly defined masses with variable contrast attenuation. The amounts of collagen and myxoid components dictate the appearance on CT.[39,41] The more myxoid component, the more hypodense the lesion will appear. The more skeletal muscle, collagen, and fibrotic components, the more hyperdense the lesion will appear.[40] However, it is very rare to have necrosis or calcifications seen on CT imaging. Intra-abdominal desmoid tumors seen with FAP typically have extensions with radiating spicules into the mesentery and which can help delineate any other organ impingement or bowel obstruction.[42]

MRI, specifically T2-weighted imaging, is the modality of choice for evaluating abdominal wall and extra-abdominal desmoid tumors. It most commonly appears as low intensity of T2-weighted images and hyperintense on T1-weighted images.[40] Another typical finding on MRI is the "band sign," which is low signal, nonenhancing bands within the tumor.[40,43] Similar to CT imaging, tumors can have a heterogeneous appearance based on myxoid and collagenous components. It is also rare to see necrosis.[43] MRI is also useful in the assessment of desmoid tumors among pregnant women.

DIAGNOSTIC APPROACH

In order to diagnose desmoid tumors, an image-guided core-needle biopsy is recommended. This can be done via ultrasound for peripheral tumors or via CT-guided biopsy for intra-abdominal or deep pelvic tumors. Pathologic examination shows poorly circumscribed, infiltrating lesions that have an abundance of spindle cells within collagen. They also have low cellularity and proliferation of fibroblasts. Immunohistochemical staining is positive for muscle-specific actin (MSA) and smooth muscle actin (SMA) and negative for desmin, h-caldesmon, and S-100.[1] Additionally, 40% to 91% stain positive for β-catenin; however, some advocate that a better diagnostic marker is a mutational analysis of *CTNNB1* for diagnosis.[44,45] Differential diagnoses include scar tissue, low-grade fibromyxoid sarcoma, nodular fasciitis, myofibroma, Gardner fibroma, and collagenous fibroma.

THERAPEUTIC APPROACH

The primary treatment for desmoid tumors is surgical resection. Nonsurgical therapies include hormonal therapy, chemotherapy, tyrosine kinase inhibitors (TKI), radiation, and "watchful waiting." The watchful waiting approach is reasonable because approximately 20% of tumors undergo spontaneous regression. Treatment regimens are described in detail in the following sections. Local control still remains difficult, despite which modality used, with recurrence rates between 24% and 77%.[46,47] Table 19.1 summarizes response and recurrence rates of the various treatment modalities.

Surgery

Standard treatment for desmoid tumors is wide local excision to negative margins. Intraoperatively, the goal is wide local excision with 1-cm margins when possible.[48] However, based on location and size of the tumor, this can lead to significant morbidity and even death. Multiple studies have evaluated

TABLE 19.1 Summary of Therapies: Recurrence and Responses in Desmoid Tumors

Treatment Type	Recurrence Rate (%)	No. Patients	Tumor Types	Reference
Surgery				
R0 resection*	5-year: 75%–84%	203	Extra- and intra-abdominal	Gronchi, et al. 2003[27]
R1 resection*	5-year: 52%–81%	189	Trunk and extra-abdominal	Merchant, et al. 1999[49]
Treatment Type	**Response Rate (%)**	**No. Patients**	**Tumor types**	**Reference**
Hormonal therapy†	40%–51%	79	Intra-abdominal	Desurmont, et al. 2015[21]
NSAIDs				
Single therapy†	~27%	Meta-analysis	Extra- and intra-abdominal	Bocale, et al. 2011[65]
Conjunction with hormonal therapy†	~85%	7	Trunk and intra-abdominal	Klein, et al. 1987[66]
COX-2 inhibitors†	95%	22	Extra- and intra-abdominal	Nishida, et al. 2010[72]
Radiation				
Partial response†	~80%	44	Trunk and extra-abdominal	Keus, et al. 2013[74]
Complete response*	~13%	52	Extra- and intra-abdominal	Micke, et al. 2005[75]
Chemotherapy†	30%–80%	68	Extra- and intra-abdominal	de Camargo, et al. 2010[69] and Desurmont, et al. 2015[21]
Tyrosine kinase inhibitors				
Partial response†	65%–70%	19	Extra- and intra-abdominal	Heinrich, et al. 2006[88]
Complete response*	6%–16%	51	Extra- and intra-abdominal	Chugh, et al. 2010[89]
Novel therapies				
Limb perfusion†	~75%	25	Extra-abdominal	van Broekhoven, et al. 2015[17]
γ-Secretase inhibitor†	~30%	17	Extra- and intra-abdominal	Kummar, et al. 2017[101]

*Complete response rates = complete regression of disease.
†Partial response rates = stable or regression of disease.
COX, cyclooxygenase; NSAIDs, nonsteroidal anti-inflammatory drugs.

the recurrence rate for margin negative (R0) disease and recurrence potential. Patients with R0 resection have 5-year recurrence rates ranging from 16% to 25%.[27,49,50] Five-year recurrence rates increase with microscopically positive margins (R1) on final pathology, ranging from 19% to 48% for R1 resection.[27,49,51,52] Given the high rate of recurrence after surgical resection, several studies have evaluated prognosis with regard to R0 versus R1 resection. Some studies have shown improved prognosis with microscopically negative margins,[50,53,54] while others have shown minimal to no prognostic benefit to R0 resection.[51,55] Given these findings, the goal of surgery should be R0 resection. However, this should be limited based on organ compromise or severe limb/disfigurement from resection because the debate of margin status on prognosis is still in question. Indeed, some surgical series show that R0 margins are achieved in only a minority of patients.

Frozen section has been used intraoperatively to help determine margin status.[46,48] However, desmoid tumor is hard to distinguish from scar tissue on frozen section. Furthermore, it does not improve the rate of recurrence.[46] Therefore, frozen section analysis intraoperatively is not recommended.

As stated previously, excision of desmoid tumors can be difficult based on size and location. When addressing abdominal wall tumors, these large masses can leave significant abdominal wall defects, requiring a multimodality approach to repair. At our institution, we commonly involve plastic surgery for assistance in coverage of large defects requiring an array of soft tissue transfers and flaps. Mesh is also commonly employed. Mesh is safe to use in reconstruction of abdominal wall defects after resection of desmoid tumors, with low primary tumor recurrence and long-lasting abdominal wall repairs.[33]

For the intra-abdominal tumor location, it is important to close the peritoneum, even with staged procedures, in order to prevent fistula tract formation. Mesh is also a viable option for closure of the abdominal wall after intra-abdominal tumor resection. This location can present a particularly difficult problem when a significant portion of the mesentery is compromised or the tumor is in proximity to the origin of the superior mesenteric artery. Again, a multidisciplinary approach can be utilized with vascular surgery for involvement in bypass procedures of the superior mesenteric artery in order to obtain R0 resection.[56]

Surgical management for extremity desmoid tumors should focus on limb salvage. If the tumor is not resectable without limb loss, it is reasonable to treat the primary tumor with other modalities or the addition of adjuvant therapy with positive margins. Multiple studies have shown that limb salvage with adjuvant treatment modalities is a safe option for patients with extremity desmoid tumors.[57–59] Therefore, standard of care for extremity desmoid tumors is limb salvage, with R1 resection if necessary followed by adjuvant systemic therapy or radiation as indicated.

Isolated limb perfusion has also been utilized for extremity tumors that are unable to achieve R0 resection. Limb perfusion using tumor necrosis factor-α (TNF-α) and melphalan-based isolated limb perfusion (TM-ILP) has shown response rates as high as 75%. However, these are associated with the known side effects of epidermolysis and intractable pain.[60,61] Amputation does remain an option for patients who do not tolerate local therapy, have continued growth of the primary tumor, desire primary amputation, or have a poor functional status at baseline.

Hormonal and Nonsteroidal Anti-Inflammatory Drugs (NSAIDs)

Both NSAIDs and hormonal therapy are commonly employed as adjuvant therapy for desmoid tumors. Given the propensity for desmoid tumors to occur in females and that they have been found to stain positive for the estrogen receptor, antiestrogen agents are used; however, the exact mechanism is unknown.[2,62–64] Hormonal therapy is typically employed as adjuvant therapy and for recurrence of desmoid tumors. They have a low overall side effect profile and are typically tolerated well by patients. Most commonly, tamoxifen and raloxifene are used as first-line antiestrogen agents with partial response rates as high as 40% to 51%.[21,65] Other hormonal agents that have to be used include megestrol, progesterone, goserelin+tamoxifen, and testolactone. With regard to NSAIDs, sulindac is the most commonly employed NSAID for systemic treatment, but indomethacin is also used.[66] However, response rates to NSAIDs alone are low, ~27%.[21]

Given the low response to individual therapy with antiestrogen or NSAIDs alone, combination therapy has been used. When used in combination, response rates were as high as 85% in one study, for both patients with sporadic type and FAP-associated tumors, defined as stable disease or regression.[67] Furthermore, these agents were able to be discontinued with only one long-term recurrence. Given these sustained findings, high-dose NSAID and antiestrogen therapy can be applied in patients who were not resectable or had R1 disease. Use for many months may be required before there is any relief of symptoms or reduction in disease.[67–69]

Celecoxib (Celebrex) and other cyclooxygenase-2 (COX-2) inhibitors have been used for management of desmoid tumors, either as single therapy or in combination with other agents.[70–72] COX-2 inhibitors are thought to independently target the Wnt/β-catenin pathway that is also affected by desmoid tumor pathogenesis.[73] However, the literature to support its use is sparse, with case studies or small pilot trials. Further work needs to be done to address this possible therapeutic agent for the treatment of desmoid tumors.

Radiation Therapy

When tumor resection would lead to functional deficits or is in a location that is otherwise unresectable, radiation has been shown to be effective treatment for desmoid tumors. Rates of local control are ~80% for disease that is not amenable to surgical resection.[74,75] The European Organisation for Research and Treatment of Cancer (EORTC) performed a Phase II clinical trial, evaluating patients with unresectable disease who underwent a standardized radiation regimen with local control in ~80% of patients. Complete response was low, with only 13% of patients with complete response to radiation therapy; partial response was noted in 36.4%, and stable disease was noted in 40.9% of patients.[74] It is important to recognize that the response to radiation therapy can occur slowly over the years after completion of treatment. There is interest in combining systemic and radiation therapy for unresectable desmoid tumors. A small study evaluated imatinib with radiation therapy with promising results for local control.[76]

Radiation therapy can be used both in the neoadjuvant and adjuvant settings as well as definitive therapy for desmoid tumors that are unresectable. Two large meta-analysis studies have evaluated surgery without adjuvant radiation and adjuvant radiation therapy after surgery. One study saw superior local control of tumor for those who underwent radiation with surgery compared to surgery alone (75% vs. 68%, respectively).[77] Another study evaluated patients with R1 resection who were treated with and without adjuvant radiation therapy. The overall recurrence of desmoid tumors was higher with R1 resection, but there was an overall improvement in recurrence rate with adjuvant radiation for both primary tumors and recurrence.[78] However, there have been no prospective, randomized control trials evaluating radiation as adjuvant therapy for desmoid tumors. The rarity of desmoid tumors makes it a challenging disease in which to conduct randomized clinical trials. Furthermore, the radiation doses used in the past were variable and based on institutional practices, making evaluation of these studies difficult. Current National Comprehensive Cancer Network (NCCN) guidelines suggest 50 Gy in conventional fractionation for adjuvant radiation and 50 to 56 Gy for treatment of unresected disease. Smaller, retrospective studies have shown no benefit for surgery alone compared to surgery with radiation.[79] Radiation can also have significant side effects including skin irritation, edema, and fibrosis, although these are generally mild-moderate in modern series,[74] and also carries the risk of a radiation-associated malignancy. Given these issues, it is important to employ a multidisciplinary approach when evaluating patients for radiation therapy.

Neoadjuvant radiation therapy has also been evaluated; however, like adjuvant therapy, there have been no randomized prospective studies. Furthermore, the literature is sparse and the available studies are small and not standardized. There is a proposed benefit to improve local control and to bridge patients to resectable disease. Similar to the other adjuvant treatments described, chemotherapy has been used in conjunction with radiation with response rates as high as 90%.[80,81]

Chemotherapy

Systemic chemotherapy agents are typically used for unresectable or recurrent disease with response rates ranging from 30% to 80%, depending on agent and regimen used.[21,69,82,83] Agents include methotrexate, vinblastine, cisplatin, and (most commonly) anthracyclines. Chemotherapy is usually second-line systemic therapy given the side effect profile. However, if the disease is rapidly progressing, unresectable, or encroaching on critical adjacent structures, it can be used as first-line therapy.[83–85] Similar to NSAID and hormonal therapies, it can take multiple months prior to seeing any effect from treatment.[83]

First-line chemotherapy agents are anthracycline-based regimens due to high response rates and longer periods of progression-free survival (PFS). One study evaluated anthracycline-based chemotherapy regimens compared to other forms of systemic therapy (i.e., NSAIDs, antiestrogens, and imatinib). They found a 54% response rate with anthracycline-based chemotherapy compared to only 12% with the other treatment modalities (p = .0011), with a higher PFS for patients who did not have extremity location desmoid tumors.[83] Others have shown increased PFS of 74 months while on anthracycline-based therapy.[82] However, a trade-off is the potential cardiotoxic side effects of anthracycline-based treatment that can make this a less favorable option for some patients. Studies have also evaluated methotrexate with vinblastine for low-dose chemotherapy regimens with promising results.[86,87] However, these studies are limited given the small sample size.

Tyrosine Kinase Inhibitors

TKIs including imatinib, sunitinib, sorafenib, and pazopanib have been used for treatment of desmoid tumors with response rates of approximately 20% and minimal toxicity. Multiple Phase II clinical trials have been performed evaluating imatinib for treatment of desmoid tumors. They have shown PFS in ~65% of all patients. However, the overall response rate was low, ranging from 6% to 16% with the higher response rate seen in patients receiving higher doses of imatinib. Side effects for these trials was overall low.[88–90]

Sunitinib has also been used for treatment of desmoid tumors. It appears to be more potent than imatinib with small studies showing that sunitinib may be beneficial when imatinib was not.[91] A Phase II clinical trial showed that roughly one-fourth of all patients responded to therapy, of which, three-fourths had a 2-year PFS. However, there was significant adverse reactions to therapy with bleeding, bowel perforation, and fistula to tumor for intra-abdominal mesenteric desmoid tumors.[92] Patients being treated with sunitinib need to be counseled on the possible adverse reactions.

Sorafenib has been used for treatment of desmoid tumors; until recently it has only been studied in Phase II studies. These studies revealed partial response rates of 25% with sorafenib, with stable disease in 70% of patients.[93] A recent Phase III clinical trial of sorafenib has reported results on the first 75 patients; the response rate was 33% and PFS doubled over the placebo arm.[94] Sorafenib has also been used in conjunction with celecoxib in case studies with major responses in patients who had recurrent disease.[70]

To date, the use of pazopanib has been limited. Only one small case report has shown improved symptoms and response to pazopanib.[95–97] Similar to sorafenib, results of a recently completed clinical trial were reported but have not been finalized; improved responses and PFS were seen compared to methotrexate vincristine.[98] Final results of these studies are awaited to evaluate the overall benefit of these TKIs in the treatment of desmoid tumors.

Novel Therapy

There are several new therapies investigating recently discovered pathways and targets in desmoid tumors. A Phase I trial that is investigating PF-03084014, an oral reversible γ-secretase inhibitor, is currently ongoing. This γ-secretase inhibitor interacts with the Notch pathway. Initially developed for Alzheimer's treatment to inhibit β-amyloid accumulation, it is also being investigated in desmoid tumors. The Notch pathway involves four surface receptors that function in most cases as an oncogene. These receptors are particularly high on stromal cells, the exact mechanism with regard to desmoid tumors is unknown, but is likely due to cell cycle arrest.[99,100] The γ-secretase inhibitor has shown tumor response in desmoid tumor in ~30% of patients and additional stable disease in ~30% of patients.[101] The side effect profile is also low and well tolerated, with nausea, vomiting, hypophosphatemia, and hypertension as the most common side effects.[99] This shows promise for new novel treatment of desmoid tumors, with ongoing studies looking at the efficacy of γ-secretase inhibitor efficacy on a larger cohort of patients.[99]

Rhamm is a protein seen in wound healing and neoplastic processes that is expressed in high levels on desmoid tumors. Small animal models have shown *Rhamm* associated with cell–cell contact and proliferation.[102] It may be a new target in the treatment of desmoid tumors.

Another new therapy for desmoid tumors is targeting hyaluronan (HA), a glycosaminoglycan on mesenchymal cells. Immunochemistry has shown that HA plays a role in cell signaling and tumor proliferation. This interaction may lead to targeted therapy that inhibits this interaction.[103]

Watchful Waiting

There has been a growing body of evidence that advocates for surveillance alone of desmoid tumors, or "watchful waiting." It stems from the high rate of recurrence after surgery, the observation of spontaneous regression in some patients, and high morbidity seen with some tumor resections. This approach includes active, careful surveillance of patients on a regular schedule with appropriate imaging based on location for 2 months consecutively, then 3 months for 1 year, followed by 6 months for 5 years, and then yearly for an indefinite time period.[68] The best candidates for the watchful waiting approach are those with no symptoms and are not related to any critical anatomic structures. More aggressive management may be more appropriate for those tumors in close relation to such structures.

Watchful waiting was initially advocated in Europe and has since been more widely employed in the United States. A study in the *European Journal of Surgical Oncology* in 2008 showed that patients who were managed with surgery (R0 resection) versus those patients under surveillance with medical therapy had the same event-free survival rate of 65%. The only difference between the two groups in regard to improved event-free survival was quality of resection and location of tumor.[32] This led to a wider study to look at patients being treated with systemic therapy compared to no therapy. They found that there was no difference in PFS among the groups (49.9% vs. 58.6%, respectively).[37] The majority of recurrences were seen in the first 2 years,[53] advocating for the highest surveillance and monitoring in those early years. Some institutions are now using "watchful waiting" as first line after diagnosis of desmoid tumor and only move to other treatment modalities if the tumor is an aggressive phenotype.[28,68]

FOLLOW-UP AND SURVEILLANCE

As stated previously, the highest rate of desmoid tumor recurrence is seen within the first 2 years.[53] Patients should undergo history and physical exams along with appropriate imaging, based on location every 3 to 6 months for the first 2 to 3 years and then annually after that time.[104]

PROPENSITY TO METASTASIZE

Unlike other soft tissue tumors, desmoid tumors lack the ability to metastasize to other locations in the body, although multifocal tumors can occur, particularly in the extremities.[105,106] However, as discussed previously, they act aggressively, invading surrounding structures and recur locally even with microscopic and gross margin negative resections.

THERAPEUTIC APPROACH FOR RECURRENT DISEASE

Desmoid tumors have a very high recurrence rate, ranging from 19% to 77%.[77] For recurrent disease, surgical resection (as described previously) is standard of care if surgically resectable. However, radiation and other systemic treatment modalities can be utilized for recurrent disease. Patients with recurrent desmoid tumors should be evaluated by a multidisciplinary team and should be treated with the modality that is the most appropriate based on location, tumor biology, and associated structures involved. No single therapy has been shown to be the most effective for recurrent disease.

SUMMARY

Desmoid tumors are characterized by their infiltrative nature and propensity for recurrence. For asymptomatic patients, a period of watchful waiting to characterize the individual disease process is useful. This must be balanced against potential critical organ resection if there is progression. Particularly mesenteric desmoids should be considered for nonsurgical therapies as the majority involve a significant portion of mesenteric vasculature that can lead to intestinal compromise, fistula, and abdominal wall disasters with resection. For extremity lesions, imaging is invaluable in determining total extent of disease as often these lesions have long tails and the palpable mass on exam is only a small portion of the entire lesion. Sparing patients large morbid resections should be the strategy with initial resection, which should aim for gross total resection because recurrence rates are similar for microscopically positive or negative margins.

CASE STUDY

A 27-year-old woman presented to the sarcoma surgical oncology clinic with recurrent desmoid of the lower extremity. She initially underwent resection 7 years before. She had developed recurrence 6 years after resection and then another at 1 year prior to this most recent recurrence. Surgical resection had required skin grafting previously. She self-palpated several nodules a few months postoperatively. These nodules were associated with pain with exercise. MRI revealed several enhancing nodules along the gastrocnemius and soleus muscles totaling 12.5 cm in craniocaudal dimension (Figure 19.1). Biopsy of the lesion showed desmoid fibromatosis. Meloxicam had been started by the referring institution. Repeat imaging revealed growth during this time. The case was presented at multidisciplinary tumor board, and owing to the extent of disease, possible Achilles tendon involvement and short-term recurrence after her most recent surgery, the consensus was to begin chemotherapy with a combination of sorafenib and celecoxib. The patient reported decrease in pain after a few weeks with improvement in ability to walk long distances. After 5 months on therapy exam, an MRI revealed a decrease in size in all lesions (Figure 19.2). She will continue with this therapy until no further response clinically and radiographically is seen, at which time she will be considered for surgical resection versus observation.

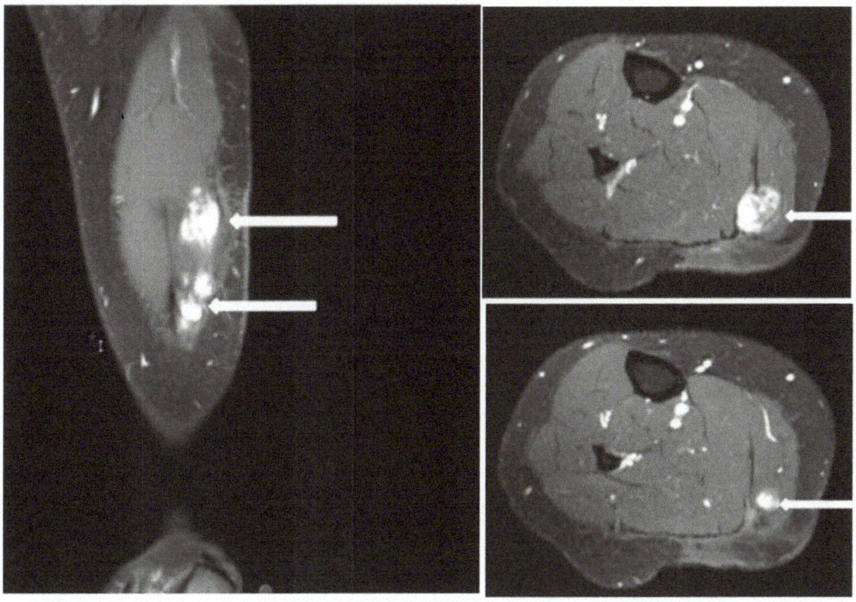

FIGURE 19.1 MRI T1 sagittal and axial views of patient with lower extremity desmoid tumor. Imaging shows multiple enhancing nodules along gastrocnemius muscle consistent with desmoid tumor.

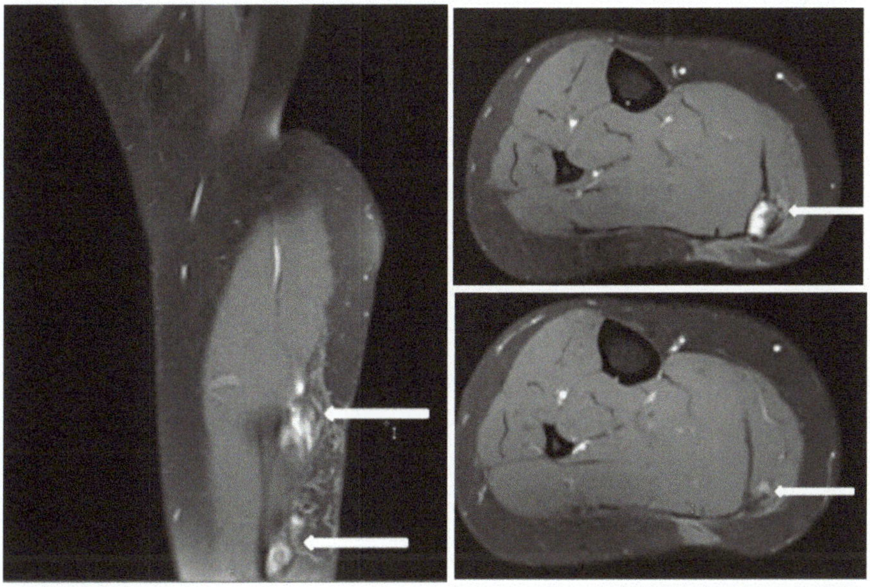

FIGURE 19.2 MRI T1 sagittal and axial views of same patient after 5 months on therapy. Imaging reveals decrease in size of all tumor nodules.

REFERENCES

1. Martínez TJ, Pajares BI, Torres RI, et al. Desmoid-type fibromatosis: who, when, and how to treat. *Curr Treat Options Oncol*. 2017;18(5):29. doi:10.1007/s11864-017-0474-0
2. Eastley NC, Hennig IM, Esler CP, Ashford RU. Nationwide trends in the current management of desmoid (aggressive) fibromatosis. *Clin Oncol (R Coll Radiol)*. 2015;27(6):362–368. doi:10.1016/j.clon.2015.02.006
3. Walczak BE, Rose PS. Desmoid: the role of local therapy in an era of systemic options. *Curr Treat Options Oncol*. 2013;14(3):465–473. doi:10.1007/s11864-013-0235-7
4. Janinis J, Patriki M, Vini L, et al. The pharmacological treatment of aggressive fibromatosis: a systematic review. *Ann Oncol*. 2003;14(2):181–190. doi:10.1093/annonc/mdg064
5. Fallen T, Wilson M, Morlan B, Lindor NM. Desmoid tumors—a characterization of patients seen at Mayo Clinic 1976-1999. *Fam Cancer*. 2006;5(2):191–194. doi:10.1007/s10689-005-5959-5
6. Nieuwenhuis MH, Vasen HFA. Correlations between mutation site in APC and phenotype of familial adenomatous polyposis (FAP): a review of the literature. *Crit Rev Oncol Hematol*. 2007;61(2):153–161. doi:10.1016/j.critrevonc.2006.07.004
7. Seow-Choen F. The management of desmoids in patients with familial adenomatous polyposis (FAP). *Acta Chir Iugosl*. 2008;55(3):83–87. doi:10.2298/aci0803083s
8. Nieuwenhuis MH, Casparie M, Mathus-Vliegen LMH, et al. A nation-wide study comparing sporadic and familial adenomatous polyposis-related desmoid-type fibromatoses. *Int J Cancer*. 2011;129(1):256–261. doi:10.1002/ijc.25664
9. Colombo C, Miceli R, Lazar AJ, et al. CTNNB1 45F mutation is a molecular prognosticator of increased postoperative primary desmoid tumor recurrence: an independent, multicenter validation study. *Cancer*. 2013;119(20):3696–3702. doi:10.1002/cncr.28271
10. Colombo C, Urbini M, Astolfi A, et al. Novel intra-genic large deletions of CTNNB1 gene identified in WT desmoid-type fibromatosis. *Genes Chromosomes Cancer*. 2018;57(10):495–503. doi:10.1002/gcc.22644
11. Dômont J, Salas S, Lacroix L, et al. High frequency of beta-catenin heterozygous mutations in extra-abdominal fibromatosis: a potential molecular tool for disease management. *Br J Cancer*. 2010;102(6):1032–1036. doi:10.1038/sj.bjc.6605557
12. Lips DJ, Barker N, Clevers H, Hennipman A. The role of APC and beta-catenin in the aetiology of aggressive fibromatosis (desmoid tumors). *Eur J Surg Oncol*. 2009;35(1):3–10. doi:10.1016/j.ejso.2008.07.003
13. Crago AM, Chmielecki J, Rosenberg M, et al. Near universal detection of alterations in CTNNB1 and Wnt pathway regulators in desmoid-type fibromatosis by whole-exome sequencing and genomic analysis. *Genes Chromosomes Cancer*. 2015;54(10):606–615. doi:10.1002/gcc.22272
14. Kim G, Kurnit KC, Djordjevic B, et al. Nuclear β-catenin localization and mutation of the CTNNB1 gene: a context-dependent association. *Mod Pathol*. 2018;31(10):1553–1559. doi:10.1038/s41379-018-0080-0
15. Kundu JK, Choi KY, Surh YJ. Beta-catenin-mediated signaling: a novel molecular target for chemoprevention with anti-inflammatory substances. *Biochim Biophys Acta*. 2006;1765(1):14–24. doi:10.1016/j.bbcan.2005.08.006
16. Lazar AJF, Tuvin D, Hajibashi S, et al. Specific mutations in the beta-catenin gene (CTNNB1) correlate with local recurrence in sporadic desmoid tumors. *Am J Pathol*. 2008;173(5):1518–1527. doi:10.2353/ajpath.2008.080475
17. van Broekhoven DLM, Verhoef C, Grünhagen DJ, et al. Prognostic value of CTNNB1 gene mutation in primary sporadic aggressive fibromatosis. *Ann Surg Oncol*. 2015;22(5):1464–1470. doi:10.1245/s10434-014-4156-x
18. Kouho H, Aoki T, Hisaoka M, Hashimoto H. Clinicopathological and interphase cytogenetic analysis of desmoid tumours. *Histopathology*. 1997;31(4):336–341. doi:10.1046/j.1365-2559.1997.2800874.x
19. Fletcher JA, Naeem R, Xiao S, Corson JM. Chromosome aberrations in desmoid tumors. Trisomy 8 may be a predictor of recurrence. *Cancer Genet Cytogenet*. 1995;79(2):139–143. doi:10.1016/0165-4608(94)00134-w
20. Meazza C, Belfiore A, Busico A, et al. AKT1 and BRAF mutations in pediatric aggressive fibromatosis. *Cancer Med*. 2016;5(6):1204–1213. doi:10.1002/cam4.669
21. Desurmont T, Lefèvre JH, Shields C, et al. Desmoid tumour in familial adenomatous polyposis patients: responses to treatments. *Fam Cancer*. 2015;14:31–39. doi:10.1007/s10689-014-9760-1
22. Sturt NJ, Clark SK. Current ideas in desmoid tumours. *Fam Cancer*. 2006;5:275–285; discussion 287–278. doi:10.1007/s10689-005-5675-1
23. Vasen HF, Velthuizen ME, Kleibeuker JH, et al. Hereditary cancer registries improve the care of patients with a genetic predisposition to cancer: contributions from the Dutch Lynch syndrome registry. *Fam Cancer*. 2016;15:429–435. doi:10.1007/s10689-016-9897-1
24. Clark SK, Neale KF, Landgrebe JC, Phillips RK. Desmoid tumours complicating familial adenomatous polyposis. *Br J Surg*. 1999;86:1185–1189. doi:10.1046/j.1365-2168.1999.01222.x
25. Church JM. Mucosal ischemia caused by desmoid tumors in patients with familial adenomatous polyposis: report of four cases. *Dis Colon Rectum*. 1998;41:661–663. doi:10.1007/BF02235279
26. Sagar PM, Möslein G, Dozois RR. Management of desmoid tumors in patients after ileal pouch-anal anastomosis for familial adenomatous polyposis. *Dis Colon Rectum*. 1998;41:1350–1355. doi:10.1007/BF02237046
27. Gronchi A, Casali PG, Mariani L, et al. Quality of surgery and outcome in extra-abdominal aggressive fibromatosis: a series of patients surgically treated at a single institution. *J Clin Oncol*. 2003;21:1390–1397. doi:10.1200/JCO.2003.05.150

28. Kasper B, Baumgarten C, Garcia J, et al. An update on the management of sporadic desmoid-type fibromatosis: a European Consensus Initiative between Sarcoma PAtients EuroNet (SPAEN) and European Organization for Research and Treatment of Cancer (EORTC)/Soft Tissue and Bone Sarcoma Group (STBSG). *Ann Oncol*. 2017;28:2399–2408. doi:10.1093/annonc/mdx323
29. Lotfi AM, Dozois RR, Gordon H, et al. Mesenteric fibromatosis complicating familial adenomatous polyposis: predisposing factors and results of treatment. *Int J Colorectal Dis*. 1989;4:30–36. doi:10.1007/BF01648547
30. Kasper B. Systemic treatment approaches for sporadic desmoid-type fibromatosis: scarce evidence and recommendations. *Oncol Res Treat*. 2015;38:244–248. doi:10.1159/000381909
31. Latchford AR, Sturt NJ, Neale K, et al. A 10-year review of surgery for desmoid disease associated with familial adenomatous polyposis. *Br J Surg*. 2006;93:1258–1264. doi:10.1002/bjs.5425
32. Bonvalot S, Eldweny H, Haddad V, et al. Extra-abdominal primary fibromatosis: aggressive management could be avoided in a subgroup of patients. *Eur J Surg Oncol*. 2008;34:462–468. doi:10.1016/j.ejso.2007.06.006
33. Wilkinson MJ, Chan KE, Hayes AJ, Strauss DC. Surgical outcomes following resection for sporadic abdominal wall fibromatosis. *Ann Surg Oncol*. 2014;21:2144–2149. doi:10.1245/s10434-014-3618-5
34. Couto Netto SD, Teixeira F, Menegozzo CAM, et al. Abdominal wall reconstruction after desmoid type fibromatosis radical resection: case series from a single institution and review of the literature. *Int J Surg Case Rep*. 2017;33:167–172. doi:10.1016/j.ijscr.2017.02.050
35. Stojadinovic A, Hoos A, Karpoff HM, et al. Soft tissue tumors of the abdominal wall: analysis of disease patterns and treatment. *Arch Surg*. 2001;136:70–79. doi:10.1001/archsurg.136.1.70
36. Deyrup AT, Tretiakova M, Montag AG. Estrogen receptor-beta expression in extraabdominal fibromatoses: an analysis of 40 cases. *Cancer*. 2006;106:208–213. doi:10.1002/cncr.21553
37. Fiore M, Coppola S, Cannell AJ, et al. Desmoid-type fibromatosis and pregnancy: a multi-institutional analysis of recurrence and obstetric risk. *Ann Surg*. 2014;259:973–978. doi:10.1097/SLA.0000000000000224
38. Cates JM. Pregnancy does not increase the local recurrence rate after surgical resection of desmoid-type fibromatosis. *Int J Clin Oncol*. 2015;20:617–622. doi:10.1007/s10147-014-0743-x
39. Ganeshan D, Amini B, Nikolaidis P, et al. Current update on desmoid fibromatosis. *J Comput Assist Tomogr*. 2018;43(1):29–38. doi:10.1097/RCT.0000000000000790
40. Braschi-Amirfarzan M, Keraliya AR, Krajewski KM, et al. Role of imaging in management of desmoid-type fibromatosis: a primer for radiologists. *Radiographics*. 2016;36:767–782. doi:10.1148/rg.2016150153
41. Murphey MD, Ruble CM, Tyszko SM, et al. From the archives of the AFIP: musculoskeletal fibromatoses: radiologic-pathologic correlation. *Radiographics*. 2009;29(7):2143–2173. doi:10.1148/rg.297095138
42. Sinha A, Hansmann A, Bhandari S, et al. Imaging assessment of desmoid tumours in familial adenomatous polyposis: is state-of-the-art 1.5 T MRI better than 64-MDCT? *Br J Radiol*. 2012;85(1015):e254–e261. doi:10.1259/bjr/42420290
43. Vandevenne JE, De Schepper AM, De Beuckeleer L, et al. New concepts in understanding evolution of desmoid tumors: MR imaging of 30 lesions. *Eur Radiol*. 1997;7(7):1013–1019. doi:10.1007/s003300050243
44. Carlson JW, Fletcher CDM. Immunohistochemistry for beta-catenin in the differential diagnosis of spindle cell lesions: analysis of a series and review of the literature. *Histopathology*. 2007;51(4):509–514. doi:10.1111/j.1365-2559.2007.02794.x
45. Koike H, Nishida Y, Kohno K, et al. Is immunohistochemical staining for β-catenin the definitive pathological diagnostic tool for desmoid-type fibromatosis? A multi-institutional study. *Hum Pathol*. 2019;84:155–163. doi:10.1016/j.humpath.2018.09.018
46. Bertani E, Testori A, Chiappa A, et al. Recurrence and prognostic factors in patients with aggressive fibromatosis. The role of radical surgery and its limitations. *World J Surg Oncol*. 2012;10:184. doi:10.1186/1477-7819-10-184
47. Escobar C, Munker R, Thomas JO, et al. Update on desmoid tumors. *Ann Oncol*. 2012;23(3):562–569. doi:10.1093/annonc/mdr386
48. Bertani E, Chiappa A, Testori A, et al. Desmoid tumors of the anterior abdominal wall: results from a monocentric surgical experience and review of the literature. *Ann Surg Oncol*. 2009;16(6):1642–1649. doi:10.1245/s10434-009-0439-z
49. Merchant NB, Lewis JJ, Woodruff JM, et al. Extremity and trunk desmoid tumors: a multifactorial analysis of outcome. *Cancer*. 1999;86(10):2045–2052. doi:10.1002/(SICI)1097-0142(19991115)86:10<2045::AID-CNCR23>3.0.CO;2-F
50. Abbas AE, Deschamps C, Cassivi SD, et al. Chest-wall desmoid tumors: results of surgical intervention. *Ann Thorac Surg*. 2004;78(4):1219–1223; discussion 1219–1223. doi:10.1016/j.athoracsur.2004.03.015
51. Gronchi A, Casali PG, Mariani L, et al. Status of surgical margins and prognosis in adult soft tissue sarcomas of the extremities: a series of patients treated at a single institution. *J Clin Oncol*. 2005;23:96–104. doi:10.1200/JCO.2005.04.160
52. Spear MA, Jennings LC, Mankin HJ, et al. Individualizing management of aggressive fibromatoses. *Int J Radiat Oncol Biol Phys*. 1998;40:637–645. doi:10.1016/S0360-3016(97)00845-6
53. Lev D, Kotilingam D, Wei C, et al. Optimizing treatment of desmoid tumors. *J Clin Oncol*. 2007;25:1785–1791. doi:10.1200/JCO.2006.10.5015
54. Harati K, Jaenisch A, Behr B, et al. Effect of surgical margins on prognosis in aggressive fibromatosis: a single-institutional analysis of 90 patients. *Oncol Lett*. 2017;14:5129–5134. doi:10.3892/ol.2017.6864

55. Salas S, Dufresne A, Bui B, et al. Prognostic factors influencing progression-free survival determined from a series of sporadic desmoid tumors: a wait-and-see policy according to tumor presentation. *J Clin Oncol.* 2011;29:3553–3558. doi:10.1200/JCO.2010.33.5489
56. Berri RN, Baumann DP, Madewell JE, et al. Desmoid tumor: current multidisciplinary approaches. *Ann Plast Surg.* 2011;67:551–564. doi:10.1097/SAP.0b013e3182084cf6
57. Stoeckle E, Coindre JM, Longy M, et al. A critical analysis of treatment strategies in desmoid tumours: a review of a series of 106 cases. *Eur J Surg Oncol.* 2009;35:129–134. doi:10.1016/j.ejso.2008.06.1495
58. Lewis JJ, Boland PJ, Leung DH, et al. The enigma of desmoid tumors. *Ann Surg.* 1999;229:866–872; discussion 872–863. doi:10.1097/00000658-199906000-00014
59. Mankin HJ, Hornicek FJ, Springfield DS. Extra-abdominal desmoid tumors: a report of 234 cases. *J Surg Oncol.* 2010;102:380–384. doi:10.1002/jso.21433
60. Broekhoven DL, Deroose JP, Bonvalot S, et al. Isolated limb perfusion using tumour necrosis factor α and melphalan in patients with advanced aggressive fibromatosis. *Br J Surg.* 2014;101:1674–1680. doi:10.1002/bjs.9659
61. Grünhagen DJ, Wilt JH, Verhoef C, et al. TNF-based isolated limb perfusion in unresectable extremity desmoid tumours. *Eur J Surg Oncol.* 2005;31:912–916. doi:10.1016/j.ejso.2005.07.002
62. Huang K, Wang CM, Chen JG, et al. Prognostic factors influencing event-free survival and treatments in desmoid-type fibromatosis: analysis from a large institution. *Am J Surg.* 2014;207:847–854. doi:10.1016/j.amjsurg.2013.08.007
63. Hansmann A, Adolph C, Vogel T, et al. High-dose tamoxifen and sulindac as first-line treatment for desmoid tumors. *Cancer.* 2004;100:612–620. doi:10.1002/cncr.11937
64. Gronchi A, Lo Vullo S, Colombo C, et al. Extremity soft tissue sarcoma in a series of patients treated at a single institution: local control directly impacts survival. *Ann Surg.* 2010;251:506–511. doi:10.1097/SLA.0b013e3181cf87fa
65. Bocale D, Rotelli MT, Cavallini A, Altomare DF. Anti-oestrogen therapy in the treatment of desmoid tumours: a systematic review. *Colorectal Dis.* 2011;13:e388–e395. doi:10.1111/j.1463-1318.2011.02758.x
66. Klein WA, Miller HH, Anderson M, DeCosse JJ. The use of indomethacin, sulindac, and tamoxifen for the treatment of desmoid tumors associated with familial polyposis. *Cancer.* 1987;60:2863–2868. doi:10.1002/1097-0142(19871215)60:12<2863::AID-CNCR2820601202>3.0.CO;2-I
67. Quast DR, Schneider R, Burdzik E, et al. Long-term outcome of sporadic and FAP-associated desmoid tumors treated with high-dose selective estrogen receptor modulators and sulindac: a single-center long-term observational study in 134 patients. *Fam Cancer.* 2016;15:31–40. doi:10.1007/s10689-015-9830-z
68. Gronchi A, Colombo C, Le Péchoux C, et al. Sporadic desmoid-type fibromatosis: a stepwise approach to a non-metastasising neoplasm—a position paper from the Italian and the French Sarcoma Group. *Ann Oncol.* 2014;25:578–583. doi:10.1093/annonc/mdt485
69. de Camargo VP, Keohan ML, D'Adamo DR, et al. Clinical outcomes of systemic therapy for patients with deep fibromatosis (desmoid tumor). *Cancer.* 2010;116:2258–2265. doi:10.1002/cncr.25089
70. Benech N, Walter T, Saurin JC. Desmoid tumors and celecoxib with sorafenib. *N Engl J Med.* 2017;376:2595–2597. doi:10.1056/NEJMc1702562
71. Yang S, Wang X, Jiang H, et al. Effective treatment of aggressive fibromatosis with celecoxib guided by genetic testing. *Cancer Biol Ther.* 2017;18(10):757–760. doi:10.1080/15384047.2017.1373215
72. Nishida Y, Tsukushi S, Shido Y, et al. Successful treatment with meloxicam, a cyclooxygenase-2 inhibitor, of patients with extra-abdominal desmoid tumors: a pilot study. *J Clin Oncol.* 2010;28(6):e107–e109. doi:10.1200/JCO.2009.25.5950
73. Xia JJ, Pei LB, Zhuang JP, et al. Celecoxib inhibits β-catenin-dependent survival of the human osteosarcoma MG-63 cell line. *J Int Med Res.* 2010;38(4):1294–1304. doi:10.1177/147323001003800411
74. Keus RB, Nout RA, Blay JY, et al. Results of a phase II pilot study of moderate dose radiotherapy for inoperable desmoid-type fibromatosis—an EORTC STBSG and ROG study (EORTC 62991-22998). *Ann Oncol.* 2013;24(10):2672–2676. doi:10.1093/annonc/mdt254
75. Micke O, Seegenschmiedt MH; German Cooperative Group on Radiotherapy for Benign Diseases. Radiation therapy for aggressive fibromatosis (desmoid tumors): results of a national Patterns of Care Study. *Int J Radiat Oncol Biol Phys.* 2005;61(3):882–891. doi:10.1016/j.ijrobp.2004.07.705
76. Moding EJ, Million L, Avedian R, et al. Concurrent imatinib and radiation therapy for unresectable and symptomatic desmoid tumors. *Sarcoma.* 2017;2017:2316839. doi:10.1155/2017/2316839
77. Nuyttens JJ, Rust PF, Thomas CR Jr, Turrisi AT 3rd. Surgery versus radiation therapy for patients with aggressive fibromatosis or desmoid tumors: a comparative review of 22 articles. *Cancer.* 2000;88(7):1517–1523. doi:10.1002/(SICI)1097-0142(20000401)88:7<1517::AID-CNCR3>3.0.CO;2-9
78. Janssen ML, van Broekhoven DLM, Cates JMM, et al. Meta-analysis of the influence of surgical margin and adjuvant radiotherapy on local recurrence after resection of sporadic desmoid-type fibromatosis. *Br J Surg.* 2017;104(4):347–357. doi:10.1002/bjs.10477
79. Guadagnolo B Ashleigh, Zagars GK, Ballo MT. Long-term outcomes for desmoid tumors treated with radiation therapy. *Int J Radiat Oncol Biol Phys.* 2008;71(2):441–447. doi:10.1016/j.ijrobp.2007.10.013
80. Francis WP, Zippel D, Mack LA, et al. Desmoids: a revelation in biology and treatment. *Ann Surg Oncol.* 2009;16(6):1650–1654. doi:10.1245/s10434-008-0285-4
81. Baliski CR, Temple WJ, Arthur K, Schachar NS. Desmoid tumors: a novel approach for local control. *J Surg Oncol.* 2002;80(2):96–99. doi:10.1002/jso.10104

82. Gega M, Yanagi H, Yoshikawa R, et al. Successful chemotherapeutic modality of doxorubicin plus dacarbazine for the treatment of desmoid tumors in association with familial adenomatous polyposis. *J Clin Oncol*. 2006;24(1):102–105. doi:10.1200/JCO.2005.02.1923
83. Garbay D, Le Cesne A, Penel N, et al. Chemotherapy in patients with desmoid tumors: a study from the French Sarcoma Group (FSG). *Ann Oncol*. 2012;23(1):182–186. doi:10.1093/annonc/mdr051
84. Okuno SH, Edmonson JH. Combination chemotherapy for desmoid tumors. *Cancer*. 2003;97(4):1134–1135. doi:10.1002/cncr.11189
85. Patel SR, Evans HL, Benjamin RS. Combination chemotherapy in adult desmoid tumors. *Cancer*. 1993;72(11):3244–3247. doi:10.1002/1097-0142(19931201)72:11<3244::aid-cncr2820721118>3.0.co;2-d
86. Toiyama Y, Konishi N, Inoue Y, et al. Successful treatment of ileal pouch desmoids using multimodal chemotherapy with low-dose vinblastine and methotrexate in a patient with familial adenomatous polyposis. *Clin J Gastroenterol*. 2009;2(3):170–174. doi:10.1007/s12328-008-0055-7
87. Weiss AJ, Lackman RD. Low-dose chemotherapy of desmoid tumors. *Cancer*. 1989;64(6):1192–1194. doi:10.1002/1097-0142(19890915)64:6<1192::aid-cncr2820640605>3.0.co;2-j
88. Heinrich MC, McArthur GA, Demetri GD, et al. Clinical and molecular studies of the effect of imatinib on advanced aggressive fibromatosis (desmoid tumor). *J Clin Oncol*. 2006;24(7):1195–1203. doi:10.1200/JCO.2005.04.0717
89. Chugh R, Wathen JK, Patel SR, et al. Efficacy of imatinib in aggressive fibromatosis: results of a phase II multicenter Sarcoma Alliance for Research through Collaboration (SARC) trial. *Clin Cancer Res*. 2010;16(19):4884–4891. doi:10.1158/1078-0432.CCR-10-1177
90. Penel N, Le Cesne A, Bui BN, et al. Imatinib for progressive and recurrent aggressive fibromatosis (desmoid tumors): an FNCLCC/French Sarcoma Group phase II trial with a long-term follow-up. *Ann Oncol*. 2011;22(2):452–457. doi:10.1093/annonc/mdq341
91. Skubitz KM, Manivel JC, Clohisy DR, Frolich JW. Response of imatinib-resistant extra-abdominal aggressive fibromatosis to sunitinib: case report and review of the literature on response to tyrosine kinase inhibitors. *Cancer Chemother Pharmacol*. 2009;64(3):635–640. doi:10.1007/s00280-009-1010-0
92. Jo JC, Hong YS, Kim KP, et al. A prospective multicenter phase II study of sunitinib in patients with advanced aggressive fibromatosis. *Invest New Drugs*. 2014;32(2):369–376. doi:10.1007/s10637-013-0059-0
93. Gounder MM, Lefkowitz RA, Keohan ML, et al. Activity of sorafenib against desmoid tumor/deep fibromatosis. *Clin Cancer Res*. 2011;17(12):4082–4090. doi:10.1158/1078-0432.CCR-10-3322
94. Gounder MM, Mahoney MR, Van Tine BA, et al. Phase III, randomized, double blind, placebo-controlled trial of sorafenib in desmoid tumors (Alliance A091105). *J Clin Oncol*. 2018;36(15_suppl):11500–11500. doi:10.1200/JCO.2018.36.15_suppl.11500
95. Szucs Z, Messiou C, Wong HH, et al. Pazopanib, a promising option for the treatment of aggressive fibromatosis. *Anticancer Drugs*. 2017;28(4):421–426. doi:10.1097/CAD.0000000000000474
96. Martin-Liberal J, Benson C, McCarty H, et al. Pazopanib is an active treatment in desmoid tumour/aggressive fibromatosis. *Clin Sarcoma Res*. 2013;3(1):13. doi:10.1186/2045-3329-3-13
97. Bulut G, Ozluk A, Erdogan AP, et al. Pazopanib: a novel treatment option for aggressive fibromatosis. *Clin Sarcoma Res*. 2016;6:22. doi:10.1186/s13569-016-0061-3
98. Toulmonde M, Ray-Coquard IL, Pulido M, et al. DESMOPAZ pazopanib (PZ) versus IV methotrexate/vinblastine (MV) in adult patients with progressive desmoid tumors (DT) a randomized phase II study from the French Sarcoma Group. *J Clin Oncol*. 2018;36(15 suppl):11501. doi:10.1200/JCO.2018.36.15_suppl.11501
99. Hughes DPM, Kummar S, Lazar AJ. New, tolerable γ-secretase inhibitor takes desmoid down a notch. *Clin Cancer Res*. 2015;21(1):7–9. doi:10.1158/1078-0432.CCR-14-1660
100. Shang H, Braggio D, Lee YJ, et al. Targeting the Notch pathway: a potential therapeutic approach for desmoid tumors. *Cancer*. 2015;121(22):4088–4096. doi:10.1002/cncr.29564
101. Kummar S, O'Sullivan CG, Do KT, et al. Clinical activity of the γ-secretase inhibitor PF-03084014 in adults with desmoid tumors (aggressive fibromatosis). *J Clin Oncol*. 2017;35(14):1561–1569. doi:10.1200/JCO.2016.71.1994
102. Tolg C, Poon R, Fodde R, et al. Genetic deletion of receptor for hyaluronan-mediated motility (Rhamm) attenuates the formation of aggressive fibromatosis (desmoid tumor). *Oncogene*. 2003;22(44):6873–6882. doi:10.1038/sj.onc.1206811
103. Briggs A, Rosenberg L, Buie JD, et al. Antitumor effects of hyaluronan inhibition in desmoid tumors. *Carcinogenesis*. 2015;36(2):272–279. doi:10.1093/carcin/bgu324
104. Ghert M, Yao X, Corbett T, et al. Treatment and follow-up strategies in desmoid tumours: a practice guideline. *Curr Oncol*. 2014;21(4):e642–9. doi:10.3747/co.21.2112
105. Alman BA, Pajerski ME, Diaz-Cano S, et al. Aggressive fibromatosis (desmoid tumor) is a monoclonal disorder. *Diagn Mol Pathol*. 1997;6(2):98–101. doi:10.1097/00019606-199704000-00005
106. Li M, Cordon-Cardo C, Gerald WL, Rosai J. Desmoid fibromatosis is a clonal process. *Hum Pathol*. 1996;27(9):939–943. doi:10.1016/s0046-8177(96)90221-x

20

Undifferentiated Pleomorphic Sarcoma/Myxofibrosarcoma/ Other Fibrosarcomas

Gabriel Tinoco and David Liebner

INTRODUCTION

Malignant fibrous histiocytoma (MFH) is a term coined in 1964 to describe a group of soft tissue sarcomas (STSs) of mixed histiocytic and fibroblastic lineage.[1] MFH was recognized for many years as the most common STS in adults and was associated with a metastatic rate of around 30% and a 5-year overall survival rate of approximately 70%.[2] However, subsequent histopathologic and molecular studies demonstrated that MFH was quite diverse, and although tumors classified as MFH shared morphologic similarities, it was soon recognized that this diagnosis encompassed a diverse group of sarcomas with distinct clinical behavior. Underscoring this was evidence of patterns of incomplete mesenchymal differentiation in tumors classified as MFH, with some demonstrating features of smooth muscle, adipose tissue, and peripheral nerve sheath.[3–6] In light of these findings, the term MFH is now considered obsolete, and the majority of cases previously classified as MFH have been reclassified as undifferentiated pleomorphic sarcoma (UPS).[7] The term UPS encompasses malignant neoplasms of mesenchymal origin, which demonstrate cellular pleomorphism and which lack evidence of cellular differentiation. Most cases do not have an apparent predisposing factor, but prior radiation is a risk factor, accounting for about 2% to 3% of UPS cases, as are hereditary cancer predisposition syndromes, such as Li–Fraumeni syndrome.[8,9] Overall, UPS constitutes 10% of adult STSs, with an incidence of around one new case per 100,000 per year and represents one of the most common STS subtypes diagnosed in older adults.[10]

Over the past decade, new light has been shed on the underpinnings of UPS, and this information will translate into new therapeutic horizons for patients suffering from this disease.

CLINICAL PRESENTATION

UPS typically presents as deep-seated lesions in the extremities or trunk, with lesions in the lower extremities being the most common. In contrast, superficial or subcutaneous lesions are rare in this sarcoma type. Clinical features of UPS are not specific, and the patients may present with a variable myriad of symptoms based on the location of the primary tumor. For example, UPS of the extremity tend to enlarge rapidly and painlessly.[11,12] In contrast, patients with retroperitoneal tumors may develop constitutional symptoms including anorexia, weight loss, malaise, fatigue, and early satiety.[11]

The most common age of diagnosis for UPS is between the ages of 50 and 70 years,[10] with cases of pediatric UPSs being infrequent.[13] The majority of evidence suggests that males and females are approximately equally affected, although a slightly increased male prevalence has also been reported.[7]

DIAGNOSTIC APPROACH

Tumor biopsy remains the gold standard for morphologic diagnosis. Numerous ancillary techniques are useful in support of morphologic diagnosis, including immunohistochemistry (IHC), classical cytogenetics, fluorescence in situ hybridization (FISH), and genetic sequencing.[31] Sarcoma diagnosis should be carried out by an experienced sarcoma pathologist.

The diagnosis of UPS is based on exclusion, as the key feature of UPS is the absence of a specific line of differentiation. Several sarcoma types show a comparable degree of cellular pleomorphism, such as sarcomatoid carcinoma (SC) and pleomorphic forms of liposarcoma, leiomyosarcoma, and rhabdomyosarcoma, among others.[11] These sarcoma types should be considered in the differential diagnosis and should be excluded to reach the diagnosis of UPS.

RADIOGRAPHIC EVALUATION

The radiologic evaluation of STS has changed over the past 30 years. Initially, the evaluation of these tumors was limited to radiographs. With the introduction of CT and MRI, the ability to accurately characterize STSs changed dramatically.[14] There are no pathognomonic radiologic findings in UPS. The radiologic evaluation of UPS follows the general approach to STS and should include CT or MRI of the primary site and imaging of the lungs to evaluate for distant metastatic spread at presentation. Whole-body PET-CT is a useful adjunct to CT/MRI of the primary tumor[31] and can be helpful for staging, prognostication, and subsequent evaluation of treatment response for patients receiving systemic therapy or radiotherapy.[15] As the risk of central nervous system (CNS) metastasis is low—1% to 8%[16]—imaging of the brain is not required at presentation unless patients demonstrate clinical symptoms suggesting CNS metastasis.

TUMOR CHARACTERISTICS

Although there have been several studies to elucidate the molecular aberrations driving UPS, the critical pathways involved in oncogenesis of UPS remain incompletely understood.[10,17–20] Early studies of UPS/MFH revealed that these tumors are characterized by complex genomic profiles with frequent gains and losses of whole chromosomes or chromosome regions as well as focal amplifications and deletions.[21–23]

Loss of tumor suppressor genes in UPS has also been reported, with 71% exhibiting at least one mutation and deletion in *p53* in a cohort of 109 patients[24] or inactivation of the *RB1* gene.[25]

Gene expression profiling has not identified significant recurrent alterations in UPS.[12] However, Wang et al. described the increased activation of Hedgehog and Notch signaling pathways in cells with stem-like tumor-initiating potential from UPS.[26] The overexpression of DKK1, an inhibitor of the Wnt canonical pathway, has also been reported.[27] Helias-Rodzewicz et al. and later the Cancer Genome Atlas Research Network (CGARN) reported *CCNE1*, *VGLL3*, and *YAP1* genes were found to be overexpressed in a subset of UPS, indicating a proportion of them may be driven by the Hippo pathway.[23,28] More recently, Delespaul et al. reported a small subset of UPS harbor fusions that involve the *TRIO* gene.[29]

Further studies are needed to understand the impact of various genomic and epigenetic events on the prognosis and optimal management of UPS.[12]

GENERAL THERAPEUTIC APPROACH

Patients should be discussed in multidisciplinary sarcoma tumor boards, as it has been shown they will have adequate radiologic tumor assessments, tumor biopsies, and better adherence with clinical recommendations compared with patients who were not discussed at the sarcoma tumor board.[30]

Wide excision plus radiotherapy remains the cornerstone of treatment of nonmetastatic tumors, and it is considered the standard of care.[31] Randomized trials have confirmed the role of these treatment modalities.[32–34]

Neoadjuvant or adjuvant anthracycline-based systemic chemotherapy is a consideration for patients with large (>5 cm), high-grade UPS per current consensus guidelines.[31] A 2008 meta-analysis of 18 randomized trials evaluating adjuvant chemotherapy in patients with STS suggested benefits in both local control and risk of distant metastasis in patients receiving systemic chemotherapy. Combination regimens using doxorubicin plus ifosfamide were associated with a 46% relative risk reduction in death (odds ratio [OR] for death 0.56, 95% confidence interval [CI] 0.36–0.85), which translated into an absolute risk reduction of 11%. Inclusion of ifosfamide appears to be important in reducing risk of death, as adjuvant chemotherapy with single-agent doxorubicin did not meet criteria for statistical significance.[35]

Tumor size and grade were subsequently demonstrated to be important factors to consider when evaluating patients for adjuvant doxorubicin plus ifosfamide chemotherapy. The European Organisation for Research and Treatment of Cancer (EORTC) 62931 study was a 351-patient randomized study of observation versus adjuvant doxorubicin plus ifosfamide chemotherapy in patients with grade 2 or 3 STS, >5 cm in size. This study only included 40 patients with UPS out of 281 cases reviewed.[36] There was no difference in progression-free survival (PFS) or overall survival for all patients included in this study. However, subset analyses suggested a possible survival benefit from adjuvant chemotherapy, for patients with large (>10 cm), high-grade (grade 3) tumors.[36] A subsequent patient-level reanalysis of the EORTC 62931 study, using the SARCULATOR nomogram to separate patients into low-, intermediate-, and high-risk cohorts, suggested that adjuvant chemotherapy may be beneficial to patients with the highest risk of recurrence following surgical resection alone.[37]

Given that doxorubicin plus ifosfamide is an intensive regimen that is not well tolerated, alternative chemotherapy regimens have been evaluated in the adjuvant setting for UPS. Recently, adjuvant chemotherapy with doxorubicin and ifosfamide was shown to be superior to gemcitabine plus docetaxel in patients with high-risk UPS.[38] Several new adjuvant approaches are currently under investigation including the addition of oral tyrosine kinase inhibitors (e.g., pazopanib),[39] other small molecule radiosensitizers (e.g., AMG-232),[40] and immunomodulatory drugs (e.g., pembrolizumab)[41] to radiation and wide excision.

For patients with resectable, localized UPS who are not being treated on a clinical trial, wide surgical excision with adjuvant or neoadjuvant radiotherapy remains the standard of care; anthracycline-based chemotherapy with doxorubicin and ifosfamide should be considered for high-risk patients with good performance status and preserved organ function.[31]

SURVEILLANCE

Essential goals of follow-up surveillance include early identification of recurrences, identification of treatment-related complications, and patient reassurance. After the definitive treatment for localized disease is completed, the patients will require periodic visits and scans (CT or MRI), because patient recurrence risk never returns to zero.[42] The follow-up interval may vary depending on the institution. There is limited data regarding the best strategy for surveillance.[43–46] The National Comprehensive Cancer Network (NCCN) guidelines outline the importance of a prudent follow-up schedule, tailored to the recurrence risk. Higher grade and larger tumors may require a more intensive follow-up.

For patients with low-risk tumors (stage I), who completed treatment with curative intent, follow-up with annual scanning of the primary site for at least 5 years is recommended.[31] Often these patients are seen every 3 to 4 months in the immediate postoperative period for the first 2 years, then every 4 to 6 months for the next 2 years, and yearly thereafter.[47]

Patients with high risk tumors (stage II–III) may have follow-up visits with imaging every 3 months for the first 1 to 2 years, then visits every 4 months for the next 1 to 2 years, followed by visits every 6 months for 1 to 2 years, and yearly visits thereafter.[47]

PROGNOSIS

Sarcoma staging is essential not only because it provides an individual patient prognosis but also because it determines treatment. The staging system most often used for STS is the American Joint Committee on Cancer (AJCC) staging system. The AJCC recently published the eighth edition of its staging system, based on a retrospective analysis of 21,396 cohorts of adult patients with STS of the extremity or trunk.[48]

Prognostic factors include tumor size, grade, and distant metastases at initial presentation.[49] The majority of UPSs are high-grade tumors, having a historical local recurrence rate ranging from 19% to 31%, a metastatic rate of 31% to 35%, and a 5-year survival rate of 65% to 70%. Only a minority of patients develop metastases after 5 years, with the common metastatic sites being lung (90%), bone (8%), and liver (1%). Regional lymph node metastases are uncommon.[2,50–52]

Several prediction tools have been developed in sarcomas. In 2002, Kattan et al. developed a nomogram, based on a prospectively followed cohort of 2,136 adult patients with primary STS who were treated at Memorial Sloan-Kettering Cancer Center (MSKCC; New York, NY). This nomogram can predict the likelihood of recurrence and overall survival for up to 12 years.[53,54]

The prognostic nomogram Sarculator (http://www.sarculator.com)[55,56] calculates the probability of overall survival and distant metastasis at 5 and 10 years after surgery. It considers patient age, tumor size, tumor grade, and tumor.[55] The Sarculator was previously retrospectively tested and validated in 1,452 and 2,300 patients, respectively[55] and further validated in a prospective randomized trial investigating perioperative anthracycline-based chemotherapy for high-risk STS of extremities and trunk wall.[57–59] Its potential use in the clinics has been recently demonstrated.[37]

METASTATIC DISEASE

For patients with oligometastatic disease, metastasectomy or other definitive local therapy for metastases should be considered as part of a multimodality approach. There is conflicting data on the potential survival benefit of metastasectomy. In a retrospective study of 48 patients, there was no improvement in the overall survival for patients treated with metastasectomy, compared with those with unresectable disease.[60] A recent retrospective study involving 112 patients with metastatic STS identified several statistically significant variables for improved overall survival including resection of metastatic disease, <4 pulmonary metastases, and the presence of lymph node metastases versus pulmonary metastases. The 5-year survival rate was 59% and 8%, respectively.[61]

A retrospective study of 66 patients with sarcoma reported that pulmonary metastasectomy led to a median survival of 25.5 months. However, recurrent metastasis was associated with poor prognosis.[62] Despite the fact, recurrence is frequent after initial metastasectomy; a study based on a large prospective review of 539 patients suggested a potential survival benefit of repeat pulmonary metastasectomy in appropriately selected patients.[63]

Currently, no data support the optimal management of patients presenting with metastatic disease; the choice of local control modality may depend on factors such as performance status, patient preference, lesion location/accessibility, ability to preserve normal tissue function, and anticipated morbidity of treatment modality.[31]

In the metastatic setting, doxorubicin as a single agent or in combination with ifosfamide is likely to be the first choice of chemotherapy.[31] The sensitivity of STS to single-agent doxorubicin was demonstrated since the early 1970s,[64] and it has remained one of the most important systemic agents to the present time. Its dose-dependent effect has been well studied.[65]

Single-agent ifosfamide has a similar response rate compared to doxorubicin, ranging between 7% and 41% in patients who previously failed a doxorubicin-based regimen.[66–70] A dose–response relationship has been shown for ifosfamide in metastatic STS with a threshold between 6 g/m^2 and 10 g/m^2.[2,68,71,72] One of the most active chemotherapy regimens, in terms of response rate, is AIM (doxorubicin/Ifosfamide/mesna),[73] but because of its potential toxicities, the use of this combination for palliation should be restricted to selected patients, for whom the specific goal is tumor shrinkage.

Other drugs such as trabectedin, gemcitabine, docetaxel, and pazopanib also have shown activity in the advanced setting.[31] These therapies represent the most commonly used regimens for patients with metastatic/locally advanced UPS. Patients with advanced UPS have the worst outcome compared with other histologic STS subtypes.[74]

Emerging data on the use of checkpoint inhibitors opens new potential treatment options for patients with advanced disease.[75] Recently, Tawbi et al. published the results of the SARC028 Phase II study of single-agent pembrolizumab (anti-programmed death-1 antibody) in multiple sarcoma types, in which four out of 10 patients with UPS had an objective response rate (ORR) of 40%.[20] A different trial evaluating the use of nivolumab, as a single agent and in combination with ipilimumab, also reported responses in patients with UPS.[76] These promising results with checkpoint inhibitors suggest that other immunotherapeutic treatments may provide benefits to UPS patients; for example, MAGE-A3 has been described as a potential therapeutic target in patients with UPS.[77] The dynamic evolution of the immunotherapy field forecasts the development of new clinical trials for UPS patients.

ATYPICAL FIBROXANTHOMA (UNDIFFERENTIATED PLEOMORPHIC SARCOMA OF THE SKIN)

This uncommon cutaneous neoplasm of mesenchymal origin was initially described in 1961.[78] The relationship between atypical fibroxanthoma (AFX), pleomorphic dermal sarcoma (PDS), and UPS is not fully understood, and some authors consider AFX a less aggressive variant within the spectrum of UPS, and others consider it a distinct malignancy.[23]

It occurs most frequently as a solitary nodule on sun-damaged skin of the elderly. Typically, it affects the superficial skin of the head and neck (particularly nose, cheek, and ear) and has been found to have low metastatic potential and excellent clinical outcomes.[79–81]

AFX most commonly arises in older adults (usually in the seventh or eighth decade of life) and has a predilection for men.[81,82]

Predisposing factors include solar exposure and radiotherapy.[79,83,84] Ultraviolet-related mutations and photoproducts have been found in these lesions.[85–87] Other risk factors reported include immunosuppressive agents[88] and HIV.[89] Children with xeroderma pigmentosum have developed ATX as well.[90] Genetically, these tumors often harbors UV signature mutations, as well as *COL11A1, ERBB4, CSMD3,* and FAT1 alterations.[91]

Patients diagnosed with ATX should have a full skin examination, including palpation of lymph nodes. Radiologic imaging may be necessary for patients with signs or symptoms suggestive of distant disease.

The mainstay of the treatment is surgical resection of the lesion with negative margins.[84,92] Radiation therapy is reserved for unresectable lesions. In individual cases, combination chemotherapy with doxorubicin (Adriamycin) and ifosfamide has been successful.[93]

FIBROSARCOMAS

Fibrosarcomas (FSs) have been traditionally defined as tumors with cells that resemble the aspect of normal fibroblasts. As the diagnostic criteria evolved over time, the reported incidence went from 12% of all adult STSs in 1974[94] to 1% in 2010.[95] This STS group is composed by several different subtypes.

Adult-Type Fibrosarcoma

Adult-type FS is the most common in the third through fifth decades of life. Bahrami et al. found that patients with this sarcoma type ranged in age from 6 to 74 years, with a median age of 50 years.[95]

Like other sarcomas, adult-type FS causes no pathognomonic symptoms. Most patients present with a solitary, slow growing, painless mass in an extremity.[11] These tumors may occur in any soft tissue site but are most common in the deep soft tissues of the lower extremities, particularly the thigh and knee, followed by the trunk and upper extremities, although some may arise in the head and neck.[11]

The diagnosis of FS is performed through an exclusion process after a tissue biopsy is obtained. FS does not exhibit any lineage-specific markers, such as cytokeratin or S-100 protein.[11] The molecular genetic alterations of adult-type FS are yet to be fully characterized, but multiple rearrangements have been reported.[96,97] In contrast to infantile FS,[98] this tumor lacks a characteristic cytogenetical abnormality. As the diagnostic criteria of FS changed over time, the analysis of the results of old series became problematic as it included other sarcoma types. For that reason, more emphasis has been placed on the results of recent studies.

A study published in 2010 showed that 12 of 24 (50%) patients with follow-up died of locally aggressive and/or metastatic disease; only six patients were alive without disease and six died of other causes.[95] Hansen et al. reported the rate of local recurrences in seven of 21 (33%) patients with follow-up, and three of 21 (14.3%) patients developed metastases and died of a tumor.[99] The lung is the principal metastatic site, followed by the axial skeleton. As in other sarcoma types, most often metastases are diagnosed within the first 2 years after diagnosis.[11]

There are several additional factors associated with FS. Tumors arising from previously irradiated fields have been reported.[95] It is not clear whether trauma is a contributing factor in the development of FS; however, multiple cases have been reported following trauma.[100–103]

As in other sarcomas, surgical resection is the most effective treatment when feasible.

Myxofibrosarcoma

The term myxofibrosarcoma (MFS) was proposed by Angervall et al. in 1997[104] and its usage has developed through time. Currently, WHO definition includes tumors with different grades, a broad range of cellularity, nuclear atypia, and varying amounts of myxoid stroma unified by the multinodular growth pattern and characteristic curvilinear vasculature.[7]

More frequently, MFS presents as a slowly enlarging, painless mass in the lower extremities of patients in the fifth to seventh decades of life. It seems to be slightly more prevalent in men rather than in women.[11,105] Like UPS, MFS does not have a specific line of differentiation; therefore, the diagnosis of MFS relies in a quantitative threshold of myxoid changes.[105] MFS does not harbor pathognomonic genetic findings.[106]

MFS displays a longitudinal mode of spreading and can infiltrate microscopically far beyond what is grossly apparent, requiring careful surgical resection. MFSs are characterized by high local recurrence rates of 50% to 60%.[107] Genetically, these tumors often have copy number alterations and mutations in *TP53, RB1, CDKN2A, CDKN2B*, and *NF1*, among others.[106]

As seen in other sarcomas, the metastatic potential is related to the histologic grade: intermediate-grade and high-grade neoplasms may develop metastases in approximately 20% to 35% of cases, whereas low-grade MFS rarely metastasizes.[4,105] The overall 5-year survival rate is 70%.[108]

The presence of more than 5% of the myxoid component has been correlated with better outcome.[109]

Sclerosing Epithelioid Fibrosarcoma

Sclerosing epithelioid fibrosarcoma (FES) is a very rare variant of FS, composed of epithelioid cells arranged in nests and cords and deposited in a densely hyalinized collagenous matrix. It was first described by Meis-Kindblom et al. in 1995.[110] Genetically, these tumors harbor multiple fusion genes, including *FUS-CREB3L2, EWSR1-CREB3L, FUS-CREM*, and *PAX5-CREB3L1*.[111]

The age of presentation is wide, with a median age of 45 years, with no clear gender predilection.[110,112] The greatest extent of patients develop a deep-seated mass affecting the lower extremity. The lesion may be painful in up to one-third of cases.[11] SEF can also develop in the trunk, upper extremities, head and neck, and rarely bone.[110,113–116]

For localized disease, wide surgical excision remains the cornerstone of therapy. Radiation therapy has been used in the adjuvant setting for non-R0 resections. In the metastatic setting, doxorubicin-based therapies remain the first-line treatment.

SUMMARY

UPSs encompass malignant neoplasms of mesenchymal origin, which demonstrate cellular pleomorphism and which lack evidence of cellular differentiation. The term UPS has been coined in replacement of the obsolete term MFH as research evidence revealed the latter constituted a diverse group of neoplasms with various differentiation (Table 20.1). FSs constitute a rare group of STSs that usually affect deep tissues.

For localized disease, the treatment of high-grade tumors includes a multimodality approach (perioperative chemotherapy, radiation therapy, and surgery), followed by close surveillance with scans and follow-up visits. For metastatic disease, these patients will require systemic therapies as well as radiation therapy and surgery in selected patients. The dynamic evolution of the immunotherapy and targeted therapy fields forecasts the development of new clinical trials for these patients.

TABLE 20.1 Genetic Findings of Undifferentiated Pleomorphic Sarcoma, Adult Fibrosarcoma, Atypical Fibroxanthoma, Myxofibrosarcoma, and Sclerosing Epithelioid Fibrosarcoma

Sarcoma Subtype	Main Genetic Alterations
UPS	Copy number alterations, TP53 deletion, RB1 inactivation DKK1, CCNE1, VGLL3, YAP1 overexpression TRIO gene fusion
Fibrosarcoma	*ETV6* and *NTRK3* gene rearrangement (infantile fibrosarcoma)
AFX	UV signature mutations, COL11A1, ERBB4, CSMD3, and FAT1 mutations
MFS	Copy number alterations,TP53, RB1, CDKN2A, CDKN2B, NF1 mutations
SEF	FUS-CREB3L2, EWSR1-CREB3L, FUS-CREM, PAX5-CREB3L1 mutations

AFX, atypical fibroxanthoma; MFS, myxofibrosarcoma; SEF, sclerosing epithelioid fibrosarcoma; UPS, undifferentiated pleomorphic sarcoma.

CASE STUDY

The patient is a 52-year-old Caucasian man who initially presented to his primary care physician with a complaint of a knot-sized mass to his right buttock, associated with pain after prolonged sitting and tingling to the posterior right thigh. Unfortunately, he was lost to follow-up for several months owing to loss of insurance. A CT scan of the pelvis performed 3 months after initial presentation demonstrated an 11-cm mass centered in the right gluteal muscles. He ultimately underwent a biopsy 7 months after initial presentation because of symptomatic progression of the mass. Final pathologic features were consistent with high-grade pleomorphic spindle cell sarcoma with focal myoid differentiation. He was referred to our tertiary sarcoma center for comprehensive multidisciplinary evaluation and management. MRI demonstrated progressive enlargement of the buttock mass, now measuring 15.8 cm in maximum diameter (Figure 20.1A). PET-CT demonstrated intense fluorodeoxyglucose (FDG) uptake in the mass (SUVmax 23.6) (Figure 20.1B); there was no evidence of distant metastatic disease. Based on presentation, his 5- and 10-year risks of developing distant metastasis were estimated at 46% and 51%, respectively, per the SARCULATOR nomogram.

Molecular profiling of the tumor identified a *TP53* mutation, but no actionable driver mutations. PD-L1 expression (Dako 22C3) on the tumor was positive, with a score of 41% to 50%.

After multidisciplinary evaluation, he elected to proceed with neoadjuvant chemotherapy with doxorubicin plus ifosfamide. Shortly after initiating systemic chemotherapy he reported reduction in pain and noted that the tumor was softer and he was able to sit with significantly less discomfort. He completed six cycles of neoadjuvant doxorubicin plus ifosfamide followed by 50 Gy of neoadjuvant radiation in 25 fractions. Subsequent MRI demonstrated that the mass was grossly stable in size, but that there was significantly less internal enhancement, consistent with treatment effect.

Five weeks after completing radiation, he underwent radical resection of his right buttock sarcoma with plastics closure with a local muscle advancement flap. Final pathologic finding was consistent with a high-grade UPS with myoid differentiation, grade 3, measuring 15.8 cm in maximum diameter; tumor necrosis/fibrosis was estimated at 75% to 80%, consistent with neoadjuvant treatment effect. Margins were negative for involvement with tumor.

Postoperatively, he was transitioned to active surveillance with CT scans of the chest and MRI of the primary site every 3 to 6 months per NCCN guidance. He remains without evidence of disease.

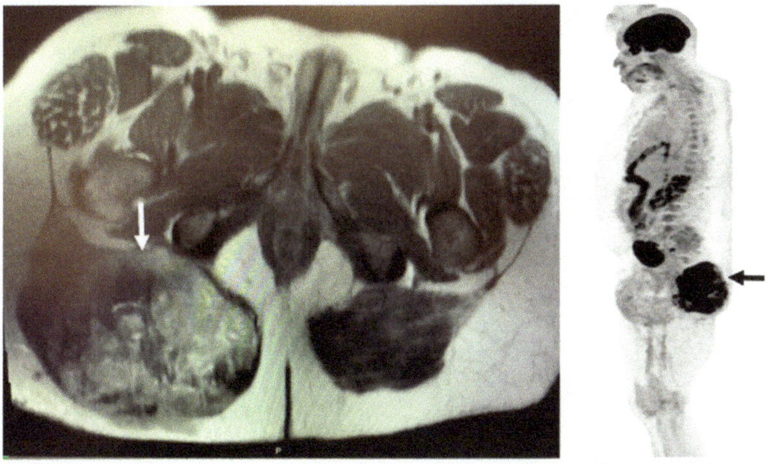

(A) (B)

FIGURE 20.1 (A) T2-Axial MRI section showing heterogeneous enhancing mass in the right gluteal musculature consistent with primary tumor site (arrow). (B) PET/CT scan imaging portraying a large soft tissue lesion in the right gluteal musculature consistent with primary tumor site (arrow) and no evidence of metastasis.

REFERENCES

1. O'Brien JE, Stout AP. Malignant fibrous xanthomas. *Cancer*. 1964;17:1445–1455. doi:10.1002/1097-0142(196411)17:11<1445::aid-cncr2820171112>3.0.co;2-g
2. Le Doussal V, Coindre J-M, Leroux A, et al. Prognostic factors for patients with localized primary malignant fibrous histiocytoma: a multicenter study of 216 patients with multivariate analysis. *Cancer*. 1996;77(9):1823–1830. doi:10.1002/(SICI)1097-0142(19960501)77:9<1823::AID-CNCR10>3.0.CO;2-1
3. Fletcher CD. Pleomorphic malignant fibrous histiocytoma: fact or fiction? A critical reappraisal based on 159 tumors diagnosed as pleomorphic sarcoma. *Am J Surg Pathol*. 1992;16(3):213–228. https://journals.lww.com/ajsp/Abstract/1992/03000/Pleomorphic_Malignant_Fibrous_Histiocytoma__Fact.1.aspx
4. Fletcher CD, Gustafson P, Rydholm A, et al. Clinicopathologic re-evaluation of 100 malignant fibrous histiocytomas: prognostic relevance of subclassification. *J Clin Oncol*. 2001;19(12):3045–3050. doi:10.1200/JCO.2001.19.12.3045
5. Oda Y, Tamiya S, Oshiro Y, et al. Reassessment and clinicopathological prognostic factors of malignant fibrous histiocytoma of soft parts. *Pathol Int*. 2002;52(9):595–606. doi:10.1046/j.1440-1827.2002.01399.x
6. Coindre JM, Mariani O, Chibon F, et al. Most malignant fibrous histiocytomas developed in the retroperitoneum are dedifferentiated liposarcomas: a review of 25 cases initially diagnosed as malignant fibrous histiocytoma. *Mod Pathol*. 2003;16(3):256–262. doi:10.1097/01.MP.0000056983.78547.77
7. Fletcher C. *WHO Classification of Tumours of Soft Tissue and Bone*. 4th ed. Lyon, France: IARC Press; 2013:468.
8. Ognjanovic S, Olivier M, Bergemann TL, Hainaut P. Sarcomas in TP53 germline mutation carriers: a review of the IARC TP53 database. *Cancer*. 2012;118(5):1387–1396. doi:10.1002/cncr.26390
9. Ballinger ML, Goode DL, Ray-Coquard I, et al. Monogenic and polygenic determinants of sarcoma risk: an international genetic study. *Lancet Oncol*. 2016;17(9):1261–1271. doi:10.1016/S1470-2045(16)30147-4
10. Henderson MT, Hollmig ST. Malignant fibrous histiocytoma: changing perceptions and management challenges. *J Am Acad Dermatol*. 2012;67(6):1335–1341. doi:10.1016/j.jaad.2012.04.013
11. Goldblum JR, Folpe AL, Weiss S. *Enzinger and Weiss's Soft Tissue Tumors*. New York, NY: Elsevier; 2014.
12. Widemann BC, Italiano A. Biology and management of undifferentiated pleomorphic sarcoma, myxofibrosarcoma, and malignant peripheral nerve sheath tumors: state of the art and perspectives. *J Clin Oncol*. 2018;36(2):160–167. doi:10.1200/JCO.2017.75.3467
13. Howlader N, Noone AM, Krapcho M, et al. eds. *SEER Cancer Statistics Review 1975–2016*. Bethesda, MD: National Cancer Institute; 2019. https://seer.cancer.gov/csr/1975_2016
14. Kransdorf MJ, Murphey MD. Radiologic evaluation of soft-tissue masses: a current perspective. *AJR Am J Roentgenol*. 2000;175(3):575–587. doi:10.2214/ajr.175.3.1750575
15. Katal S, Gholamrezanezhad A, Kessler M, et al. PET in the diagnostic management of soft tissue sarcomas of musculoskeletal origin. *PET Clin*. 2018;13(4):609–621. doi:10.1016/j.cpet.2018.05.011
16. Chaigneau L, Patrikidou A, Ray-Coquard I, et al. Brain metastases from adult sarcoma: prognostic factors and impact of treatment. A retrospective analysis from the French Sarcoma Group (GSF/GETO). *Oncologist*. 2018;23(8):948–955. doi:10.1634/theoncologist.2017-0136
17. Lee YF, John M, Edwards S, et al. Molecular classification of synovial sarcomas, leiomyosarcomas and malignant fibrous histiocytomas by gene expression profiling. *Br J Cancer*. 2003;88(4):510–515. doi:10.1038/sj.bjc.6600766
18. Baird K, Davis S, Antonescu CR, et al. Gene expression profiling of human sarcomas: insights into sarcoma biology. *Cancer Res*. 2005;65(20):9226–9235. doi:10.1158/0008-5472.CAN-05-1699
19. Carneiro A, Francis P, Bendahl PO, et al. Indistinguishable genomic profiles and shared prognostic markers in undifferentiated pleomorphic sarcoma and leiomyosarcoma: different sides of a single coin? *Lab Invest*. 2009;89(6):668–675. doi:10.1038/labinvest.2009.18
20. Tawbi HA, Burgess M, Bolejack V, et al. Pembrolizumab in advanced soft-tissue sarcoma and bone sarcoma (SARC028): a multicentre, two-cohort, single-arm, open-label, phase 2 trial. *Lancet Oncol*. 2017;18(11):1493–1501. doi:10.1016/S1470-2045(17)30624-1
21. Guillou L, Aurias A. Soft tissue sarcomas with complex genomic profiles. *Virchows Arch*. 2010;456(2):201–217. doi:10.1007/s00428-009-0853-4
22. Kresse SH, Ohnstad HO, Bjerkehagen B, et al. DNA copy number changes in human malignant fibrous histiocytomas by array comparative genomic hybridisation. *PLoS One*. 2010;5(11):e15378. doi:10.1371/journal.pone.0015378
23. Soleymani T, Hollmig ST. Conception and management of a poorly understood spectrum of dermatologic neoplasms: atypical fibroxanthoma, pleomorphic dermal sarcoma, and undifferentiated pleomorphic sarcoma. *Curr Treat Options Oncol*. 2017;18(8):50. doi:10.1007/s11864-017-0489-6
24. Perot G, Chibon F, Montero A, et al. Constant p53 pathway inactivation in a large series of soft tissue sarcomas with complex genetics. *Am J Pathol*. 2010;177(4):2080–2090. doi:10.2353/ajpath.2010.100104
25. Mairal A, Terrier P, Chibon F, et al. Loss of chromosome 13 is the most frequent genomic imbalance in malignant fibrous histiocytomas. A comparative genomic hybridization analysis of a series of 30 cases. *Cancer Genet Cytogenet*. 1999;111(2):134–138. doi:10.1016/S0165-4608(98)00227-1
26. Wang CY, Wei Q, Han I, et al. Hedgehog and Notch signaling regulate self-renewal of undifferentiated pleomorphic sarcomas. *Cancer Res*. 2012;72(4):1013–1022. doi:10.1158/0008-5472.CAN-11-2531
27. Matushansky I, Hernando E, Socci N D, et al. Derivation of sarcomas from mesenchymal stem cells via inactivation of the Wnt pathway. *J Clin Invest*. 2007;117(11):3248–3257. doi:10.1172/JCI31377

28. Helias-Rodzewicz Z, Perot G, Chibon F, et al. YAP1 and VGLL3, encoding two cofactors of TEAD transcription factors, are amplified and overexpressed in a subset of soft tissue sarcomas. *Genes Chromosomes Cancer*. 2010;49(12):1161–1171. doi:10.1002/gcc.20825
29. Delespaul L, Lesluyes T, Perot G, et al. Recurrent TRIO fusion in nontranslocation-related sarcomas. *Clin Cancer Res*. 2017;23(3):857–867. doi:10.1158/1078-0432.CCR-16-0290
30. Blay JY, Le Cesne A, Penel N, et al. The nationwide cohort of 26,883 patients with sarcomas treated in NETSARC reference network between 2010 and 2015 in France: major impact of multidisciplinary board presentation prior to 1st treatment. *Ann Oncol*. 2016;27(suppl_6):vi483. doi:10.1093/annonc/mdw388.03
31. National Comprehensive Cancer Network. *Soft Tissue Sarcoma Version 2.2019*. https://www.nccn.org/professionals/physician_gls/
32. Rosenberg SA, Tepper J, Glatstein E, et al. The treatment of soft-tissue sarcomas of the extremities: prospective randomized evaluations of (1) limb-sparing surgery plus radiation therapy compared with amputation and (2) the role of adjuvant chemotherapy. *Ann Surg*. 1982;196(3):305–315. doi:10.1097/00000658-198209000-00009
33. Pisters PW, Harrison LB, Leung DH, et al. Long-term results of a prospective randomized trial of adjuvant brachytherapy in soft tissue sarcoma. *J Clin Oncol*. 1996;14(3):859–868. doi:10.1200/JCO.1996.14.3.859
34. Yang JC, Chang AE, Baker AR, et al. Randomized prospective study of the benefit of adjuvant radiation therapy in the treatment of soft tissue sarcomas of the extremity. *J Clin Oncol*. 1998;16(1):197–203. doi:10.1200/JCO.1998.16.1.197
35. Pervaiz N, Colterjohn N, Farrokhyar F, et al. A systematic meta-analysis of randomized controlled trials of adjuvant chemotherapy for localized resectable soft-tissue sarcoma. *Cancer*. 2008;113(3):573–581. doi:10.1002/cncr.23592
36. Woll PJ, Reichardt P, Le Cesne A, et al. Adjuvant chemotherapy with doxorubicin, ifosfamide, and lenograstim for resected soft-tissue sarcoma (EORTC 62931): a multicentre randomised controlled trial. *Lancet Oncol*. 2012;13(10):1045–1054. doi:10.1016/S1470-2045(12)70346-7
37. Pasquali S, Pizzamiglio S, Touati N, et al. The impact of chemotherapy on survival of patients with extremity and trunk wall soft tissue sarcoma: revisiting the results of the EORTC-STBSG 62931 randomised trial. *Eur J Cancer*. 2019;109:51–60. doi:10.1016/j.ejca.2018.12.009
38. Gronchi A, Ferrari S, Quagliuolo V, et al. Histotype-tailored neoadjuvant chemotherapy versus standard chemotherapy in patients with high-risk soft-tissue sarcomas (ISG-STS 1001): an international, open-label, randomised, controlled, phase 3, multicentre trial. *Lancet Oncol*. 2017;18(6):812–822. doi:10.1016/S1470-2045(17)30334-0
39. Weiss AR, Chi YY, Chen YL, et al. Preoperative chemoradiation +/− pazopanib in non-rhabdomyosarcoma soft tissue sarcoma (NRSTS): a report from Children's Oncology Group (COG) and NRG Oncology. *J Clin Oncol*. 2019;37(15_suppl):11002–11002. doi:10.1200/JCO.2019.37.15_suppl.11002
40. Welliver MX, Tine BAV, Houghton P, et al. MDM2 inhibitor AMG-232 and radiation therapy in treating patients with soft tissue sarcoma with wild-type TP53: a phase IB study (NRG-DT001). *J Clin Oncol*. 2019;37(15_suppl):TPS11076–TPS11076. doi:10.1200/JCO.2019.37.15_suppl.TPS11076
41. Mowery YM, Ballman KV, Riedel RF, et al. SU2C-SARC032: a phase II randomized controlled trial of neoadjuvant pembrolizumab with radiotherapy and adjuvant pembrolizumab for high-risk soft tissue sarcoma. *J Clin Oncol*. 2018;36(15_suppl):TPS11588–TPS11588. doi:10.1200/jco.2018.36.15_suppl.tps11588
42. Lewis JJ, Leung D, Casper ES, et al. Multifactorial analysis of long-term follow-up (more than 5 years) of primary extremity sarcoma. *Arch Surg*. 1999;134(2):190–194. doi:10.1001/archsurg.134.2.190
43. Whooley BP, Mooney MM, Gibbs JF, Kraybill WG. Effective follow-up strategies in soft tissue sarcoma. *Semin Surg Oncol*. 1999;17(1):83–87. doi:10.1002/(sici)1098-2388(199907/08)17:1<83::aid-ssu11>3.0.co;2-w
44. Whooley BP, Gibbs JF, Mooney MM, et al. Primary extremity sarcoma: what is the appropriate follow-up? *Ann Surg Oncol*. 2000;7(1):9–14. doi:10.1007/s10434-000-0009-x
45. Kane JM 3rd. Surveillance strategies for patients following surgical resection of soft tissue sarcomas. *Curr Opin Oncol*. 2004;16(4):328–332. doi:10.1097/01.cco.0000127879.62254.d3
46. Patel SA, Royce TJ, Barysauskas CM, et al. Surveillance imaging patterns and outcomes following radiation therapy and radical resection for localized extremity and trunk soft tissue sarcoma. *Ann Surg Oncol*. 2017;24(6):1588–1595. doi:10.1245/s10434-016-5755-5
47. Patel SR, Zagars GK, Pisters PWT. The follow-up of adult soft-tissue sarcomas. *Semin Oncol*. 2003;30(3):413–416. doi:10.1016/s0093-7754(03)00101-5
48. Cates JMM. The AJCC 8th edition staging system for soft tissue sarcoma of the extremities or trunk: a cohort study of the SEER database. *J Natl Compr Canc Netw*. 2018;16(2):144–152. doi:10.6004/jnccn.2017.7042
49. Maretty-Nielsen K. Prognostic factors in soft tissue sarcoma. *Dan Med J*. 2014;61(11):B4957. https://ugeskriftet.dk/files/scientific_article_files/2018-11/b4957.pdf
50. Zagars GK, Mullen JR, Pollack A. Malignant fibrous histiocytoma: outcome and prognostic factors following conservation surgery and radiotherapy. *Int J Radiat Oncol Biol Phys*. 1996;34(5):983–994. doi:10.1016/0360-3016(95)02262-7
51. Salo JC, Lewis JJ, Woodruff JM, et al. Malignant fibrous histiocytoma of the extremity. *Cancer*. 1999;85(8):1765–1772. doi:10.1002/(SICI)1097-0142(19990415)85:8<1765::AID-CNCR17>3.0.CO;2-K
52. Engellau J, Anderson H, Rydholm A, et al. Time dependence of prognostic factors for patients with soft tissue sarcoma: a Scandinavian Sarcoma Group Study of 338 malignant fibrous histiocytomas. *Cancer*. 2004;100(10):2233–2239. doi:10.1002/cncr.20254

53. Kattan MW, Leung DHY, Brennan MF. Postoperative nomogram for 12-year sarcoma-specific death. *J Clin Oncol*. 2002;20(3):791–796. doi:10.1200/JCO.2002.20.3.791
54. Eilber FC, Brennan MF, Eilber FR, et al. Validation of the postoperative nomogram for 12-year sarcoma-specific mortality. *Cancer*. 2004;101(10):2270–2275. doi:10.1002/cncr.20570
55. Callegaro D, Miceli R, Bonvalot S, et al. Development and external validation of two nomograms to predict overall survival and occurrence of distant metastases in adults after surgical resection of localised soft-tissue sarcomas of the extremities: a retrospective analysis. *Lancet Oncol*. 2016;17(5):671–680. doi:10.1016/S1470-2045(16)00010-3
56. Callegaro D, Miceli R, Mariani L, et al. Soft tissue sarcoma nomograms and their incorporation into practice. *Cancer*. 2017;123(15):2802–2820. doi:10.1002/cncr.30721
57. Gronchi A, Frustaci S, Mercuri M, et al. Short, full-dose adjuvant chemotherapy in high-risk adult soft tissue sarcomas: a randomized clinical trial from the Italian Sarcoma Group and the Spanish Sarcoma Group. *J Clin Oncol*. 2012;30(8):850–856. doi:10.1200/JCO.2011.37.7218
58. Gronchi A, Stacchiotti S, Verderio P, et al. Short, full-dose adjuvant chemotherapy (CT) in high-risk adult soft tissue sarcomas (STS): long-term follow-up of a randomized clinical trial from the Italian Sarcoma Group and the Spanish Sarcoma Group. *Ann Oncol*. 2016;27(12):2283–2288. doi:10.1093/annonc/mdw430
59. Pasquali S, Colombo C, Pizzamiglio S, et al. High-risk soft tissue sarcomas treated with perioperative chemotherapy: improving prognostic classification in a randomised clinical trial. *Eur J Cancer*. 2018;93:28–36. doi:10.1016/j.ejca.2018.01.071
60. Kane JM, Finley JW, Driscoll D, et al. The treatment and outcome of patients with soft tissue sarcomas and synchronous metastases. *Sarcoma*. 2002;6(2):69–73. doi:10.1080/1357714021000022168
61. Ferguson PC, Deheshi BM, Chung P, et al. Soft tissue sarcoma presenting with metastatic disease: outcome with primary surgical resection. *Cancer*. 2011;117(2):372–379. doi:10.1002/cncr.25418
62. Okiror L, Peleki A, Moffat D, et al. Survival following pulmonary metastasectomy for sarcoma. *Thorac Cardiovasc Surg*. 2016;64(2):146–149. doi:10.1055/s-0035-1546430
63. Chudgar NP, Brennan MF, Tan KS, et al. Is repeat pulmonary metastasectomy indicated for soft tissue sarcoma? *Ann Thorac Surg*. 2017;104(6):1837–1845. doi:10.1016/j.athoracsur.2017.07.024
64. Benjamin RS, Wiernik PH, Bachur NR. Adriamycin: a new effective agent in the therapy of disseminated sarcomas. *Med Pediatr Oncol*. 1975;1(1):63–76. doi:10.1002/mpo.2950010109
65. Borden EC, Amato DA, Rosenbaum C, et al. Randomized comparison of three adriamycin regimens for metastatic soft tissue sarcomas. *J Clin Oncol*. 1987;5(6):840–850. doi:10.1200/JCO.1987.5.6.840
66. Antman KH, Ryan L, Elias A, et al. Response to ifosfamide and mesna: 124 previously treated patients with metastatic or unresectable sarcoma. *J Clin Oncol*. 1989;7(1):126–131. doi:10.1200/JCO.1989.7.1.126
67. Bramwell VH, Mouridsen HT, Santoro A, et al. Cyclophosphamide versus ifosfamide: a randomized phase II trial in adult soft-tissue sarcomas. The European Organization for Research and Treatment of Cancer [EORTC], Soft Tissue and Bone Sarcoma Group. *Cancer Chemother Pharmacol*. 1993;31(suppl 2):S180–S184.
68. Patel SR, Vadhan-Raj S, Papadopolous N, et al. High-dose ifosfamide in bone and soft tissue sarcomas: results of phase II and pilot studies—dose-response and schedule dependence. *J Clin Oncol*. 1997;15(6):2378–2384. doi:10.1200/JCO.1997.15.6.2378
69. Buesa JM, López-Pousa A, Martín J, et al. Phase II trial of first-line high-dose ifosfamide in advanced soft tissue sarcomas of the adult: a study of the Spanish Group for Research on Sarcomas (GEIS). *Ann Oncol*. 1998;9(8):871–876. doi:10.1023/a:1008474802882
70. Nielsen OS, Judson I, van Hoesel Q, et al. Effect of high-dose ifosfamide in advanced soft tissue sarcomas. A multicentre phase II study of the EORTC Soft Tissue and Bone Sarcoma Group. *Eur J Cancer*. 2000;36(1):61–67. doi:10.1016/s0959-8049(99)00240-3
71. Le Cesne A, Antoine E, Spielmann M, et al. High-dose ifosfamide: circumvention of resistance to standard-dose ifosfamide in advanced soft tissue sarcomas. *J Clin Oncol*. 1995;13(7):1600–1608. doi:10.1200/JCO.1995.13.7.1600
72. Cerny T, Leyvraz S, von Briel T, et al. Saturable metabolism of continuous high-dose ifosfamide with mesna and GM-CSF: a pharmacokinetic study in advanced sarcoma patients. Swiss Group for Clinical Cancer Research (SAKK). *Ann Oncol*. 1999;10(9):1087–1094. doi:10.1023/a:1008386000547
73. Judson I, Verweij J, Gelderblom H, et al. Doxorubicin alone versus intensified doxorubicin plus ifosfamide for first-line treatment of advanced or metastatic soft-tissue sarcoma: a randomised controlled phase 3 trial. *Lancet Oncol*. 2014;15(4):415–423. doi:10.1016/S1470-2045(14)70063-4
74. Savina M, Le CA, Blay JY, et al. Patterns of care and outcomes of patients with METAstatic soft tissue SARComa in a real-life setting: the METASARC observational study. *BMC Med*. 2017;15(1):78. doi:10.1186/s12916-017-0831-7
75. Groisberg R, Hong DS, Behrang A, et al. Characteristics and outcomes of patients with advanced sarcoma enrolled in early phase immunotherapy trials. *J Immunother Cancer*. 2017;5(1):100. doi:10.1186/s40425-017-0301-y
76. D'Angelo SP, Mahoney MR, Van Tine BA, et al. Nivolumab with or without ipilimumab treatment for metastatic sarcoma (Alliance A091401): two open-label, non-comparative, randomised, phase 2 trials. *Lancet Oncol*. 2018;19(3):416–426. doi:10.1016/S1470-2045(18)30006-8
77. Conley AP, Wang WL, Livingston JA, et al. MAGE-A3 is a clinically relevant target in undifferentiated pleomorphic sarcoma/myxofibrosarcoma. *Cancers*. 2019;11(5):677. doi:10.3390/cancers11050677
78. Helwig EB. Atypical fibroxanthoma. *Tex State J Med*. 1963;(59):664.
79. Fretzin DF, Helwig EB. Atypical fibroxanthoma of the skin. A clinicopathologic study of 140 cases. *Cancer*. 1973;31(6):1541–1552. doi:10.1002/1097-0142(197306)31:6<1541::aid-cncr2820310635>3.0.co;2-6

80. Dahl I. Atypical fibroxanthoma of the skin. A clinico-pathological study of 57 cases. *Acta Pathol Microbiol Scand A*. 1976;84(2):183–197. https://www.ncbi.nlm.nih.gov/pubmed/1258644
81. Ziemer M. Atypical fibroxanthoma. *J Dtsch Dermatol Ges*. 2012;10(8):537–550. doi:10.1111/j.1610-0387.2012.07980.x.
82. Wollina U, Schönlebe J, Ziemer M, et al. Atypical fibroxanthoma: a series of 56 tumors and an unexplained uneven distribution of cases in southeast Germany. *Head Neck*. 2015;37(6):829–834. doi:10.1002/hed.23673
83. Mirza B, Weedon D. Atypical fibroxanthoma: a clinicopathological study of 89 cases. *Australas J Dermatol*. 2005;46(4):235–238. doi:10.1111/j.1440-0960.2005.00190.x
84. Ang GC, Roenigk RK, Otley CC, et al. More than 2 decades of treating atypical fibroxanthoma at Mayo Clinic: what have we learned from 91 patients? *Dermatol Surg*. 2009;35(5):765–772. doi:10.1111/j.1524-4725.2009.01126.x
85. Dei Tos AP, Maestro R, Doglioni C, et al. Ultraviolet-induced p53 mutations in atypical fibroxanthoma. *Am J Pathol*. 1994;145(1):11–17. https://www.ncbi.nlm.nih.gov/pubmed/8030743
86. Sakamoto A, Oda Y, Itakura E, et al. Immunoexpression of ultraviolet photoproducts and p53 mutation analysis in atypical fibroxanthoma and superficial malignant fibrous histiocytoma. *Mod Pathol*. 2001;14(6):581–588. doi:10.1038/modpathol.3880354
87. Sakamoto A. Atypical fibroxanthoma. *Clin Med Oncol*. 2008;2:117–127. doi:10.4137/cmo.s506
88. Ferri E, Iaderosa GA, Armato E. Atypical fibroxanthoma of the external ear in a cardiac transplant recipient: case report and the causal role of the immunosuppressive therapy. *Auris Nasus Larynx*. 2008;35(2):260–263. doi:10.1016/j.anl.2007.04.013
89. Perrett CM, Macedo C, Francis N, et al. Atypical fibroxanthoma in an HIV-infected individual. *J Cutan Pathol*. 2011;38(4):357–359. doi:10.1111/j.1600-0560.2010.01642.x
90. Shao L, Newell B, Quintanilla N. Atypical fibroxanthoma and squamous cell carcinoma of the conjunctiva in xeroderma pigmentosum. *Pediatr Dev Pathol*. 2007;10(2):149–152. doi:10.2350/06-06-0103.1
91. Lai K, Harwood CA, Purdie KJ, et al. Genomic analysis of atypical fibroxanthoma. *PLoS One*. 2017;12(11): e0188272. doi:10.1371/journal.pone.0188272
92. Tolkachjov SN, Kelley BF, Alahdab F, et al. Atypical fibroxanthoma: systematic review and meta-analysis of treatment with Mohs micrographic surgery or excision. *J Am Acad Dermatol*. 2018;79(5):929–934.e6. doi:10.1016/j.jaad.2018.06.048
93. Miller K, Goodlad JR, Brenn T. Pleomorphic dermal sarcoma: adverse histologic features predict aggressive behavior and allow distinction from atypical fibroxanthoma. *Am J Surg Pathol*. 2012;36(9):1317–1326. doi:10.1097/PAS.0b013e31825359e1
94. Pritchard DJ, Soule EH, Taylor WF, Ivins JC. Fibrosarcoma—a clinicopathologic and statistical study of 199 tumors of the soft tissues of the extremities and trunk. *Cancer*. 1974;33(3):888–897. doi:10.1002/1097-0142(197403)33:3<888::aid-cncr2820330339>3.0.co;2-c
95. Bahrami A, Folpe AL. Adult-type fibrosarcoma: a reevaluation of 163 putative cases diagnosed at a single institution over a 48-year period. *Am J Surg Pathol*. 2010;34(10):1504–1513. doi:10.1097/PAS.0b013e3181ef70b6
96. Dal CP, Pauwels P, Sciot R, Van den BH. Multiple chromosome rearrangements in a fibrosarcoma. *Cancer Genet Cytogenet*. 1996;87(2):176–178. doi:10.1016/0165-4608(95)00280-4
97. Limon J, Szadowska A, Iliszko M, et al. Recurrent chromosome changes in two adult fibrosarcomas. *Genes Chromosomes Cancer*. 1998;21(2):119–123. doi:10.1002/(sici)1098-2264(199802)21:2<119::aid-gcc7>3.0.co;2-3
98. Chetty R. Neurotrophic tropomyosin or tyrosine receptor kinase (NTRK) genes. *J Clin Pathol*. 2019;72(3):187–190. doi:10.1136/jclinpath-2018-205672
99. Hansen T, Katenkamp K, Brodhun M, Katenkamp D. Low-grade fibrosarcoma—report on 39 not otherwise specified cases and comparison with defined low-grade fibrosarcoma types. *Histopathology*. 2006;49(2):152–160. doi:10.1111/j.1365-2559.2006.02480.x
100. Stout AP. Fibrosarcoma the malignant tumor of fibroblasts. *Cancer*. 1948;1(1):30–63. doi:10.1002/1097-0142(194805)1:1<30::aid-cncr2820010104>3.0.co;2-d
101. Ivins JC, Dockerty MB, Ghormley RK. Fibrosarcoma of the soft tissues of the extremities; a review of 78 cases. *Surgery*. 1950;28(3):495–508. https://www.ncbi.nlm.nih.gov/pubmed/14776656
102. Tanz SS. Fibrosarcoma following single trauma; report of a case. *J Int Coll Surg*. 1957;27(5 part 1):620–626. https://www.ncbi.nlm.nih.gov/pubmed/13429137
103. Morris JM, Lucas DB. Fibrosarcoma within a sinus tract of chronic draining osteomyelitis. Case report and review of literature. *J Bone Joint Surg Am*. 1964;46:853–857. doi:10.2106/00004623-196446040-00019
104. Angervall L, Kindblom LG, Merck C. Myxofibrosarcoma. A study of 30 cases. *Acta Pathol Microbiol Scand A*. 1977;85a(2):127–140. doi:10.1111/j.1699-0463.1977.tb00410.x
105. Mentzel T, Calonje E, Wadden C, et al. Myxofibrosarcoma. Clinicopathologic analysis of 75 cases with emphasis on the low-grade variant. *Am J Surg Pathol*. 1996;20(4):391–405. doi:10.1097/00000478-199604000-00001
106. Ogura K, Hosoda F, Arai Y, et al. Integrated genetic and epigenetic analysis of myxofibrosarcoma. *Nat Commun*. 2018;9(1):2765. doi:10.1038/s41467-018-03891-9
107. Carvalho SD, Pissaloux D, Crombé A, et al. Pleomorphic sarcomas: the state of the art. *Surg Pathol Clin*. 2019;12(1):63–105. doi:10.1016/j.path.2018.10.004
108. Penel N, Coindre JM, Giraud A, et al. Presentation and outcome of frequent and rare sarcoma histologic subtypes: a study of 10,262 patients with localized visceral/soft tissue sarcoma managed in reference centers. *Cancer*. 2018;124(6):1179–1187. doi:10.1002/cncr.31176

109. Lee AY, Agaram NP, Qin LX, et al. Optimal percent myxoid component to predict outcome in high-grade myxofibrosarcoma and undifferentiated pleomorphic sarcoma. *Ann Surg Oncol.* 2016;23(3):818–825. doi:10.1245/s10434-015-5063-5
110. Meis-Kindblom JM, Kindblom LG, Enzinger FM. Sclerosing epithelioid fibrosarcoma. A variant of fibrosarcoma simulating carcinoma. *Am J Surg Pathol.* 1995;19(9):979–993. doi:10.1097/00000478-199509000-00001
111. Arbajian E, Puls F, Antonescu CR, et al. In-depth genetic analysis of sclerosing epithelioid fibrosarcoma reveals recurrent genomic alterations and potential treatment targets. *Clin Cancer Res.* 2017;23(23):7426–7434. doi:10.1158/1078-0432.CCR-17-1856
112. Antonescu CR, Baren A. Spectrum of low-grade fibrosarcomas: a comparative ultrastructural analysis of low-grade myxofibrosarcoma and fibromyxoid sarcoma. *Ultrastruct Pathol.* 2004;28(5–6):321–332. doi:10.1080/019131290882259
113. Folk GS, Williams SB, Foss RB, Fanburg-Smith JC. Oral and maxillofacial sclerosing epithelioid fibrosarcoma: report of five cases. *Head Neck Pathol.* 2007;1(1):13–20. doi:10.1007/s12105-007-0002-9
114. Doyle LA, Wang WL, Dal CP, et al. MUC4 is a sensitive and extremely useful marker for sclerosing epithelioid fibrosarcoma: association with FUS gene rearrangement. *Am J Surg Pathol.* 2012;36(10):1444–1451. doi:10.1097/PAS.0b013e3182562bf8
115. Arbajian E, Puls F, Magnusson L, et al. Recurrent EWSR1-CREB3L1 gene fusions in sclerosing epithelioid fibrosarcoma. *Am J Surg Pathol.* 2014;38(6):801–808. doi:10.1097/PAS.0000000000000158
116. Wojcik JB, Bellizzi AM, Dal CP, et al. Primary sclerosing epithelioid fibrosarcoma of bone: analysis of a series. *Am J Surg Pathol.* 2014;38(11):1538–1544. doi:10.1097/PAS.0000000000000265
117. ESMO/European Sarcoma Network Working Group. Soft tissue and visceral sarcomas: ESMO Clinical Practice Guidelines for diagnosis, treatment and follow-up. *Ann Oncol.* 2014;25(suppl 3):iii102–iii112. doi:10.1093/annonc/mdu254

21

Malignant Peripheral Nerve Sheath Tumor

Jack F. Shern and Brigitte C. Widemann

INTRODUCTION

Malignant peripheral nerve sheath tumors (MPNSTs) are soft tissue sarcomas (STSs) that arise from peripheral nerve sheaths. MPNSTs are aggressive tumors and associated with high frequency of local recurrence and metastatic disease. About half of all MPNSTs arise in patients with neurofibromatosis type 1 (NF1), but tumors also develop in individuals without inherited NF1 and arise with greater incidence in areas following irradiation. To date, complete surgical resection with wide negative margins remains the cornerstone of successful therapy and is required for cure. The objective response rate of MPNSTs to chemotherapy is low and the impact of chemotherapy in the adjuvant or neoadjuvant setting on survival has not been defined. Preoperative or postoperative radiation therapy (RT) has a role in local control, especially for large tumors. However, high doses of radiation are required for the treatment of MPNSTs, which can be challenging, depending on the location of the primary tumor. Several histology-specific Phase II trials with agents targeting pathways implied in the pathogenesis and progression of MPNSTs have been conducted, but have not resulted in clinical activity to date. New insights into the molecular pathogenesis of MPNSTs as well as the availability of disease-specific preclinical models give hope for the development of more effective combination therapies for unresectable or metastatic MPNSTs. In addition, recent insights into the clinical development of NF1-associated MPNSTs may allow for earlier diagnosis of MPNST/MPNST precursor lesions and for the development of MPNST prevention strategies. Most MPNSTs in NF1 develop in preexisting plexiform neurofibromas, which are histologically benign peripheral nerve sheath tumors. In addition to biallelic loss of *NF1* in neurofibromas and plexiform neurofibromas, atypical neurofibromas are characterized by heterozygous loss of *CDKN2A/B*, which appears to be the first step toward malignant transformation. The recent clinical and imaging characterization of atypical neurofibromas may allow for earlier diagnosis of lesions at risk of transforming to MPNST, and for treatment and prevention strategies. As most atypical neurofibromas appear well defined and encapsulated on clinical evaluation and MRI, these lesions are more amenable to surgical removal compared to fully established high-grade MPNSTs. These and other anticipated advances, including the identification of biomarkers of MPNST transformation, will hopefully result in effective prevention and treatment strategies for this devastating tumor.

ESTIMATED INCIDENCE

MPNSTs account for 4% of all STSs.[1] Approximately 50% of all MPNSTs arise in patients with NF1, and the lifetime risk of MPNST for patients with NF1 ranges from 8% to 15.8%,[2,3] making MPNST the leading cause of death in patients with NF1.[3] Approximately 40% of MPNSTs are sporadic and 10% occur in patients with a history of radiation exposure. The age of diagnosis in NF1-associated MPNST is younger (typically 20–50 years old) with 10% to 20% of cases reported in children (aged 1–19 years), compared to sporadic MPNST, which typically occur in late adulthood.[4] Analyses from the Surveillance, Epidemiology, and End Results (SEER) Program indicate a slightly higher incidence of MPNST in males (55.11%) than in females (44.89%), and among all age groups there is an elevated incidence in African Americans compared to Caucasians and other ethnicities.[5]

CLINICAL PRESENTATION

MPNST typically presents as an enlarging mass, which is frequently associated with pain. Neurologic deficits or paresthesia can be associated with the involved nerves. Particular consideration should be paid to patients with NF1 and plexiform neurofibroma. These histologically benign tumors are frequently associated with pain. However, a change in pain quality and intensity should be considered as a sign of malignant transformation and trigger further evaluation. In addition, the development of pain or any mass that arises within a prior radiation field should result in consideration for MPNSTs. As complete surgical resection is the only curative therapy for MPNSTs and these tumors can develop rapidly in preexisting plexiform neurofibromas, clinical and imaging evaluation have to be performed in a timely fashion to maximize outcome.

A number of prognostic factors have been identified including large tumor size (>5 cm), truncal location, and incomplete surgical resection (reviewed by Farid et al.).[6] In several studies, NF1 status has also been associated with worse outcome compared to sporadic MPNST, but not consistently, and a more recent meta-analysis described that this effect is not present in studies after 2000, possibly owing to better surveillance and earlier diagnosis of MPNST in NF1 patients.[7]

Diagnostic Approach

A pretreatment biopsy followed by experienced pathological evaluation is necessary for accurate diagnosis, grading, and management of MPNSTs. This can be done by core-needle or open incisional technique, and ideally the biopsy site should be coordinated with the surgeon who may undertake definitive surgery. Because of the potential for sampling error, especially in MPNSTs developing in a preexisting plexiform neurofibroma, several core-needle biopsies may have to be obtained to avoid false negative results. MRI and fluorodeoxyglucose (FDG)-PET have utility in identifying the site for the biopsy. A recent consensus meeting determined that for lesions that, based on clinical and imaging evaluations, are concerning for atypical neurofibromas but clearly not high-grade MPNST, a biopsy may not be necessary to establish the diagnosis prior to surgical resection of the lesion.[8] This includes lesions with distinct nodular appearance, which do not show a recent change in clinical symptoms, rapid growth, or high FDG-PET avidity.[8,9] Given that the surgical approaches for high-grade MPNST compared to low-grade MPNST and atypical neurofibromas are different, a biopsy is recommended prior to surgery in all cases in which there is uncertainty of the diagnosis.

Pathology of Malignant Peripheral Nerve Sheath Tumors

A sarcoma can be diagnosed as MPNST when it has nerve elements or when it develops in a patient with a clinical diagnosis of NF1. Most NF1-associated MPNSTs are high-grade, which is characterized by high cellularity, high mitotic rate—at least 10 mitotic features/10 high power fields (HPFs)—nuclear atypia, and necrosis. In contrast to neurofibromas, most high-grade MPNST have lost *S100* and *CD34* expression by immunohistochemistry. In addition, loss of trimethylated histone H3 at lysine residue 27 (H3K27me3) has been described as a marker of MPNST with a frequency between 30% to 90%.[10] This marker may not be specific for MPNST because it has also been described in other tumors, in particular synovial sarcoma.[11] With the clinical and genomic characterization of atypical neurofibromas as precursor lesions to MPNST, a recent pathology consensus review focused on characterizing and providing diagnostic criteria for neurofibromas, neurofibromas with atypia, and low-grade and high-grade MPNST.[11] The consensus review proposed the term atypical neurofibromatous neoplasm of uncertain biologic potential (ANNUBP) for lesions concerning for a potentially higher risk for malignant transformation. The term ANNUBP is reserved for lesions meeting at least two of the following four criteria: cytologic atypia, loss of neurofibroma architecture, hypercellularity, and a mitotic index of ≥1/50 HPFs and <3/10 HPFs. The ANNUBP is different from low-grade MPNST, which are characterized by the absence of necrosis but have a mitotic index between 3 to 9/10 HPFs. The review also commented that the distinction between ANNUBP and low-grade MPNST can be difficult and gradual and that the clinical behavior of low-grade MPNST is similar to that of an ANNUBP in that these lesions are at low risk for local recurrence and essentially no risk for metastasis.

Radiographic Features and Recommended Imaging

In patients with sporadic MPNST, the recommended imaging and diagnostic approach is similar to that for other STSs. Imaging should include detailed imaging of the primary tumor with CT and MRI and metastatic workup including chest CT and FDG-PET scan as appropriate.

In patients with NF1, several subgroups have been identified as having a greater risk for MPNST and may benefit from more frequent imaging with the goals of identifying MPNST or MPNST precursors early. Patients with NF1 microdeletion,[12,13] high plexiform neurofibroma burden and/or known atypical neurofibroma(s) are at greater risk for developing MPNST.[8,9] The role of whole-body MRI in these patients is being studied in the research setting, including the National Cancer Institute's NF1 natural history study (NCT00924196). The advantage of whole-body MRI lies in the ability to comprehensively assess growth patterns without exposure to radiation and contrast agents.[14] Whole-body MRI also allows monitoring the entire disease burden and several areas of potential concern for malignant transformation. However, while whole-body MRI is feasible, and short tau (T1) inversion recovery (STIR) sequence has been recommended as a core sequence, whole-body MRI is not widely available. In addition, the reproducibility of whole-body MRI and the benefit from prospective longitudinal whole-body MRI is not established yet.[15] Imaging evaluation for NF1 MPNST should include MRI with and without contrast and diffusion-weighted imaging to delineate the disease. Imaging should include the surrounding plexiform neurofibroma in its entirety. CT chest/abdomen/pelvis should be performed to evaluate for metastatic disease sites including lungs, liver, and adrenals.

FDG-PET imaging has been evaluated extensively for its utility in identifying MPNSTs. Multiple studies have evaluated the qualitative and quantitative (maximal standard uptake value [SUVmax]) assessment of FDG-PET to distinguish neurofibroma from MPNST and have overwhelmingly shown that high-grade MPNST has higher FDG-avidity compared to neurofibromas and thus diagnostic utility.[16] Plexiform neurofibromas are rarely FDG-avid, while most high-grade MPNST show increased FDG-uptake with SUV cutoffs of more than 3.5[17] and 4.0[18] being proposed to distinguish between plexiform neurofibroma and MPNST. Fewer studies have reported on the FDG uptake in atypical neurofibromas and low-grade MPNST.[4,9,17,18] The SUVmax for these lesions can overlap with those seen in high-grade MPNST and plexiform neurofibromas, and more studies will be required to identify if SUVmax for high-grade MPNST and atypical neurofibromas/low-grade MPNST are sufficiently different to be of diagnostic utility. Detailed MRI evaluations have identified size, heterogeneous contrast enhancement, perilesional edema, and perilesional enhancement as predictors for MPNST versus benign nerve sheath tumors. In addition, evaluation of the apparent diffusion coefficient (ADC) has value in predicting for MPNST[19] in that lesions with ADC values $\leq 1.0 \times 10^{-3}$/s were at 150 times greater risk being an MPNST compared to lesions with ADC values $>1.0 \times 10^{-3}$/s.[20] Prospective studies comparing FDG-PET and MRI with diffusion weighted imaging and ADC values may allow further definition for the role of these imaging modalities.

MOLECULAR ABERRATIONS DRIVING MPNST

Given the high incidence of MPNST within the NF1 population, there have been significant efforts to describe the genetic and molecular mechanisms underlying the malignant transformation of plexiform neurofibroma to MPNST. These efforts have intensified over the past two decades for two reasons. First, clinical observations on the malignant transformation of plexiform neurofibromas defined atypical neurofibromas as a precursor lesion to MPNST. Second, next-generation sequencing methods allowed the complete characterization of the somatic genome underlying these lesions. Genetically, the clinical observations have been matched with mutational profiling studies that have demonstrated sequential and gradual loss of tumor suppressor genes. This work has led to a genetic model, whereby the primary driver of tumorigenesis in plexiform neurofibromas is biallelic loss of *NF1* function[21] followed by chromosome rearrangement and the loss of *CDKN2A* (the gene that encodes INK4A/p16) in atypical neurofibromas.[21,22] Finally, mutations in *EED* or *SUZ12*, components of polycomb repressive complex 2 (PRC2), lead to loss of H3K27me3 and subsequent dysregulation of transcriptional repression.[23,24] Somatic alteration of other genes such as *RAS*[25], *TP53*[23,24], and *BRAF*[26] have been reported at varying frequencies.[27]

While there are no recurrent chromosomal translocations observed in MPNST, cytogenetic and hybridization array studies have demonstrated significant aneuploidy characterizes MPNST tumors. These studies identify recurrent losses of chromosomes 1p, 9p, 11, 12p, 14q, 18, 22q and gains of chromosome 7, 8q, and 15q.[28] These findings highlight the potential that MPNSTs may contain inherently unstable genomes, a hypothesis that may have important implications in the age of immunotherapy. An interesting analysis summarizing a relatively large cohort of TCGA data reported a median of 2.5 mutations per megabase in 134 analyzed cases, with less than 10% of MPNST harboring more than 20 mutations per megabase.[29] This relatively low mutational burden may reflect the finding of low or absent expression of *PDL1* and *PD1* within these tumors[30] and a disappointing response to checkpoint inhibitors in the handful of reported MPNST treated with these agents.[31] Despite these findings, there may be some subsets of patients that will respond to these novel agents, and a Phase II trial of a PD1 inhibitor is currently underway in patients with metastatic or locally unresectable MPNST (NCT02691026).

The discovery of alteration of PRC2 members in MPNST has enlightened the understanding of the transcriptomic and epigenetic landscapes of these tumors. The PRC2 complex plays a critical cellular role in maintaining condensed chromatin, mainly by catalyzing the histone modification of H3K27me3 in specific genomic locations that are transcriptionally silent. PRC2 is involved in various biologic processes, including differentiation, maintaining cell identity and proliferation, and stem-cell plasticity.[32] There are three major protein subunits in the complex—SUZ12, EED, and the catalytic EZH2—however, only mutation of *SUZ12* and *EED* have been observed in MPNSTs. Interestingly, those patients with a germline microdeletion of the *NF1* locus have a particularly increased risk of MPNST due to concomitant loss of *SUZ12*, which sits adjacent to the *NF1* gene on chromosome 17.[24] The observation of IHC correlation between *PRC2* mutation and loss of H3K27me3 staining is currently being incorporated into the standardization of histopathologic evaluation of MPNST.[10,33] While the transcriptomic consequences of the loss of *PRC2* are currently being defined, downstream affected genes include cell specific transcription factors, imprinted genes such as *IGF2*, and genes associated with development and morphogenesis. All of these disrupted genes may be future therapeutic targets in these tumors.[23]

The overall disappointing response of MPNST to conventional chemotherapy regimens led to a concentrated effort by the field to identify molecular targets that might represent therapeutic vulnerabilities in MPNST. Given the predominance of MPNST in the NF1 population as well as the presence of somatic mutations of *NF1* in the sporadic tumors, targeting of the Ras/Raf/MAPK pathway has been extensively explored both in the preclinical models as well as in the clinic. Tantalizingly, single-agent use of the MEK inhibitor selumetinib was found to be active in plexiform neurofibromas,[34] providing further rationale for MEK inhibition to play a central role in the development of combination strategies.[35] The PI3K/MTOR/AKT signaling pathway is also hyperactive in *NF1* deficient cells[36] and multiple in vivo studies have demonstrated the potential utility of targeting this pathway in MPNST.[37,38] These preclinical efforts led to the development of a clinical trial studying the combination of selumetinib with the mTOR inhibitor sirolimus for patients with unresectable or metastatic MPNST (SARC031), which recently began enrollment (ClinicalTrials.gov Identifier: NCT03433183). Another potential therapeutic target, further downstream of activated MAPK is Aurora Kinase A (AURKA), which was found to be upregulated in MPNSTs and demonstrated activity both in vitro and in vivo.[39] Here, again, the need to develop combination strategies will be important as single-agent targeting of AURKA stabilized tumor volume and provided some improvement in PFS but still resulted in disease progression in the preclinical models. Canonical WNT and beta-catenin signaling are known to be a critical factors in both Schwann cell development and MPNST tumorigenesis[40,41] and are another attractive molecular target for therapeutic development. The tumor microenvironment is an additional target for peripheral nerve sheath tumors. Both plexiform neurofibromas and MPNST contain macrophages, which may contribute to tumor progression. Preclinical studies in MPNST models with an agent targeting *CSF1* and *KIT* (PLX3397) in combination with mTOR inhibition resulted in development of a clinical trial (ClinicalTrials.gov identifier: NCT02584647).[42] Finally, given the transcriptional dysregulation in MPNST tumors due to activated MAPK signaling and the loss of PRC2, targeting of active enhancers with bromodomain inhibitors, acting on BRD4,[43] have emerged as a unique vulnerability of MPNST. Anticipating the need for combination strategies has led to strategies co-targeting MEK or MTOR with BRD4[44] as well as the use of proteolysis-targeting chimeras (PROTACs) that simultaneously target bromodomain activity, and bromodomain and extraterminal domain (BET) protein abundance.[45]

Common Anatomic Location and General Therapeutic Approach for MPNST

MPNST can arise along any peripheral nerve. The most common locations of primary MPNST are trunk, extremities, and less frequently head and neck. NF1-associated MPNST are more frequently deep seated/truncal in comparison to sporadic MPNST, which is critical, as complete surgical resection in these locations is more difficult to accomplish.[4,46] In addition, at diagnosis NF1-associated MPNST are more frequently locally advanced compared to sporadic MPNST.[4,46] While at diagnosis, less than 10% of MPNST are metastatic,[46] MPNST has a high propensity to metastasize with the most frequent locations of metastasis in decreasing order being pulmonary, bone, liver, abdominal cavity, adrenal gland, diaphragm, mediastinal, brain, ovary, kidney, and retroperitoneum.[4,47,48]

Complete surgical resection is the only curative therapy in patients with high-grade MPNST.[49,50] The surgical goal is wide local resection, which can be difficult and associated with significant morbidity. Amputation, may be required in cases in which negative margins cannot be achieved otherwise, in particular in MPNST arising from major nerves.[51]

The role of RT has not been studied in prospective trials for MPNST to date. However, a prospective randomized trial of radiation for STSs demonstrated a delay in progression-free but not overall survival in patients receiving radiation.[52] Several retrospective studies have described improvement in local control of MPNST with radiation,[53] and there is consensus to administer radiation, if feasible, to high-grade MPNST, especially if the tumor is larger than 5 cm in diameter.[8] Similar to the role of radiation for other STSs, preoperative radiation should be considered, as it has the advantage of a smaller radiation field compared to postoperative radiation.[54] The role of proton beam therapy is being studied in STSs, but no studies in MPNST have been reported to our knowledge.[55]

The role of chemotherapy in MPNST has been prospectively evaluated in very few trials and the impact of chemotherapy on survival in patients with MPNST is not known.[1,56] Several retrospective studies have described responses to standard chemotherapy agents, such as doxorubicin and ifosfamide used to treat other STSs.[1,4,57] Notably, a retrospective analysis of 12 European Organization for Research and Treatment of Cancer Soft Tissue and Bone Sarcoma Trials analyzed the outcomes of 175 patients with MPNST out of 2,675 eligible STSs. The outcomes were similar for MPNST and other STSs with a response rate, median progression-free survival, and overall survival of 21% versus 22%, 17 versus 16 weeks, and 48 versus 51 weeks, respectively. Compared to single-agent doxorubicin, the combination of doxorubicin and ifosfamide achieved the best response.[58] This study did not compare response for NF1 associated versus sporadic MPNST. However, worse chemotherapy response in NF1 associated MPNST compared to sporadic MPNST has been described in several prior studies and was also associated with worse survival in NF1 patients.[49,59] A recent prospective study (SARC006, ClinicalTrials.gov Identifier: NCT00304083) evaluated the role of standard STS chemotherapy in high-grade unresectable MPNST. Patients were stratified by sporadic versus NF1-associated MPNST, with the primary endpoint of determining objective response (complete and partial response) using WHO criteria after two cycles of doxorubicin and ifosfamide followed by two cycles of ifosfamide and etoposide. Etoposide was included in this trial because it is active in pediatric STSs and because topoisomerase IIα, the drug's target, has been reported as the most overexpressed gene in MPNST compared to benign neurofibromas.[60] No complete responses were observed, and the partial response rate was lower in NF1-associated MPNST (17.2%) compared to sporadic MPNST (33%).[1] However, this trial did not complete enrollment and was not powered to detect a difference in response rates between the two strata. Importantly, in contrast to trials with targeted agents (see later discussion) chemotherapy resulted in disease stabilization in most patients, with very few patients experiencing disease progression after four cycles of chemotherapy.

Given the poor outcome of unresectable and metastatic MPNST, histology specific trials with targeted agents have been developed. Objective responses were not observed in single agent trials with erlotinib (EGFR inhibitor), sorafenib, imatinib, dasatinib (inhibitors of several receptor tyrosine kinases), alisertib (aurora kinase inhibitor), or in combination trials of bevacizumab and everolimus (VEGF and mTOR inhibition), and ganetespib and sirolimus (HSP90 and mTOR inhibition).[56,61,62] In addition to lack of objective responses, in most trials, the progression-free survival was short, with most patients experiencing disease progression after two treatment cycles. Several current treatment trials therefore define success as the clinical benefit rate, defined as objective imaging response or disease stability after 4 months (approximately four treatment cycles).

Preclinical models and genetically engineered mouse models (GEMMs) of NF1-related benign and MPNST, which recapitulate the human disease, have become available and are being used to conduct preclinical trials of targeted agents (reviewed by Kim et al.).[56] The hope is that these models will facilitate the selection of active agents and combination of agents for clinical trials. Concerted preclinical efforts have been joined by clinical trials coordinated through sarcoma-specific cooperative groups such as the Sarcoma Alliance for Research through Collaboration (SARC) and the Department of Defense sponsored NF Clinical Trials Consortium. These resources and infrastructure will accelerate the timely conduct and completion of clinical trials with strong scientific rationale and hopefully lead to identification of active therapies for patients with MPNST.

Atypical Neurofibromas as Precursor Lesions to MPNST

Atypical neurofibromas, which are defined by pathologic characteristics, such as nuclear atypia, increased cellularity, and loss of neurofibroma architecture,[11] have been identified as precursor lesions for MPNST. The genetic model proposed to describe the malignant transformation from plexiform neurofibroma to MPNST through atypical neurofibroma also supports this definition based on the loss of *CDKN2A* observed in most cases of atypical neurofibromas.[22] The recent clinical and imaging characterization of atypical neurofibromas allows for recognition of this malignant precursor lesion and through early resection possibly for the prevention to the development of high-grade MPNST.[8,9] Atypical neurofibromas have a distinct nodular appearance on STIR MRI and can develop within and outside plexiform neurofibromas. The growth rate of atypical neurofibromas frequently exceeds the growth rate of plexiform neurofibromas, and in contrast to plexiform neurofibromas, most atypical neurofibromas are

TABLE 21.1 Therapeutic Approach to Malignant Peripheral Nerve Sheath Tumors (MPNSTs)

Tumor	Treatment Modality			
	Surgery	**Radiation**	**Chemotherapy**	**Investigational Agents**
Atypical neurofibroma and low-grade MPNST	If feasible without major morbidity. Wide negative margins not needed (marginal margins sufficient)	No	No	Currently no trials specifically for atypical neurofibromas available; consider for unresectable or multiple tumors
MPNST high-grade, nonmetastatic, resectable	Yes, with wide negative margins by an experienced sarcoma/neurosurgeon	Preoperative (preferred) or postoperative for tumors >5 cm or for microscopic positive margins	No evidence; institution specific pre- and/or post surgery (include doxorubicin and ifosfamide)	Currently no investigational trials for completely resected MPNST available
MPNST high-grade, nonmetastatic unresectable	If feasible after neoadjuvant chemotherapy	If tumor shrinkage allows for surgery or in palliative setting	Neoadjuvant chemotherapy with goal to shrink tumor for potential resection	Consider after neoadjuvant chemotherapy
MPNST high-grade, metastatic	With palliative intent	With palliative intent	No evidence; institution specific	Yes

MPNST, malignant peripheral nerve sheath tumors.

PET-FDG avid. Clinically, many atypical neurofibromas are associated with pain and palpable atypical neurofibromas are firm.[9] In contrast to high-grade MPNST, atypical neurofibromas do not require resection with wide negative margins, which is surgically less challenging and results in less morbidity to patients.[9,63,64] Limited data available to date suggest that atypical neurofibromas and low-grade MPNST are at low risk for recurrence after marginal resection. Given the great challenges in the treatment of high-grade MPNST, a future focus of clinical care and research should be in the identification of MPNST precursor lesions and surgical resection, if feasible, with the goal of preventing malignant transformation. A recent State of the Science meeting for MPNST recommended conducting prospective clinical and imaging studies to further define diagnostic and therapeutic strategies for atypical neurofibromas.[8]

Recommended Follow-Up After Definitive Therapy for Primary Sarcoma

There are no published guidelines for follow-up of MPNST patients after definitive therapy; however, as noted, local or metastatic relapses of MPNST are common and there are reports of early detection and subsequent gross total resection of relapse.[65] Therefore, our practice is for close interval follow-up with detailed physical exam, and imaging performed every 3 months initially, similar to the evaluation of other STSs. Imaging should include MRI of primary site as well as imaging of the lungs by CT scan. As noted previously, FDG-PET scan is potentially useful, in particular for patients with high plexiform neurofibroma burden, as it may allow for easier identification of lesions concerning for recurrence or new disease sites. At the NCI, as part of the NF1 natural history study, noncontrast whole-body MRI using STIR sequence is also being evaluated and appears helpful in patients who have high neurofibroma burden and possibly more than one distinct nodular lesion. The development of a circulating tumor DNA assay such as that developed for other STSs,[66] which could be used for noninvasive diagnostics, monitoring response to systemic therapy, and surveying for disease recurrence, would be a useful addition to clinical practice.

SUMMARY

Caveats, Pearls, Pitfalls, Solutions: The NCI Pediatric Oncology Branch Experience

MPNST diagnosis: New or increasing pain in a patient with NF1 should prompt expedited workup for MPNST. Experienced clinical evaluation, pathology review and genomic workup are valuable to aid in both diagnosis and selection of therapeutic options. Longitudinal (whole-body) MRI may aid in the diagnosis of lesions concerning for MPNST in patients with substantial plexiform neurofibroma burden.

Atypical neurofibroma management: Atypical neurofibromas are precursor lesions for MPNST and surgical resection is a strategy to prevent high-grade MPNST. Atypical neurofibromas and low-grade

MPNST do not require surgery with wide negative margins and should be considered if feasible without significant morbidity. While atypical neurofibromas have a distinct clinical and imaging appearance there is some overlap with low-grade and high-grade MPNST. Therefore, biopsy should be considered to determine the optimal surgical approach.

High-grade MPNST management: For high-grade MPNST, complete surgical resection with wide negative margins is the only curative therapeutic modality. Radiation has value in local control of high-grade MPNST. Preoperative radiation can be administered with a smaller radiation field compared to postoperative radiation. There is no consensus on the use of neoadjuvant and adjuvant chemotherapy for high-grade MPNST, and its role on progression-free and overall survival should be studied prospectively in the national consortium clinical trial setting. Trials in preclinical models of MPNST will aid in the selection and prioritization of agents for clinical trials. The development of histology-specific clinical trials with agents targeting genomic alterations, the tumor microenvironment, and possibly immunologic targets has the potential to alter the course for patients with unresectable, metastatic, or relapsed MPNST.

CASE STUDIES

Case 1

A 17-year-old young woman with NF1 presents to the National Health Institute (NIH) for enrollment in the NF1 natural history study. She complained of a painful, firm right neck nodular lesion. Her diagnostic imaging with axial STIR MRI is described in Figure 21.1A–D. In comparison to a normal neck MRI at age 13 years and 4 months (Figure 21.1A), MRI at age 17 years and 7 months old showed a distinct nodular lesion (Figure 21.1B). Follow-up imaging at age 18 years and 8 months showed progressive growth of the lesion (Figure 21.1C), which was avid on FDG-PET with SUVmax 8.0 (Figure 21.1D). The clinical diagnosis of a likely atypical neurofibroma was made. No biopsy was performed and the lesion was surgically resected by removing the encapsulated lesion without clinical morbidity. Pathology confirmed an ANNUBP (Figure 21.1E). Characteristics for the ANNUBP: Intraneural/plexiform neurofibroma, with hypercellularity and nuclear atypia in Schwann cells, one mitotic feature found per 50 HPFs. Not shown: Retention of S100-positive Schwann cells and CD34-positive fibroblasts with slight reduction of the latter focally. Loss of CDKN2A in the Schwann cell population and retention in fibroblasts. p53 is not typically increased. MIB1-labeling is about 5% to 7% at the most. The lesion has not recurred on follow-up imaging for more than 2 years after resection. We hypothesize that surgical resection of this lesion may have prevented the transformation to high-grade MPNST.

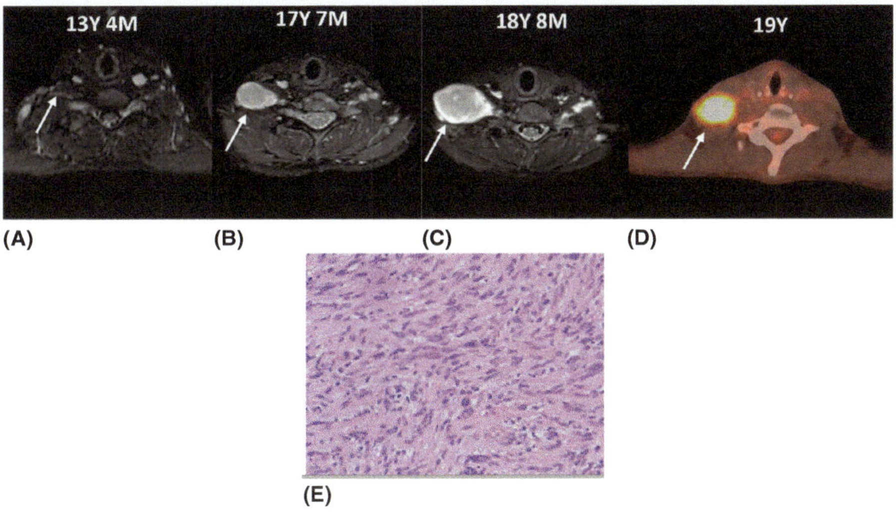

FIGURE 21.1 Development and progressive growth of atypical neurofibromatous neoplasm of uncertain biologic potential (ANNUBP) in teenager with neurofibromatosis type 1.

Case 2

A 7-year-old girl with NF1 and germline NF1 whole-gene deletion is enrolled in a clinical trial with a MEK inhibitor for a left paraspinal plexiform neurofibroma. (Figure 21.2A, orange arrow: plexiform neurofibroma, white arrow: small nodular lesion). She experienced a partial response in the plexiform neurofibroma based on volumetric MRI analysis. MRI at age 9 years and 7 months shows minimal change (Figure 21.2B). At age 10 years and 3 months, while still on the MEK inhibitor, she presented with new left flank pain. STIR MRI at that time demonstrates an enlarging nodular lesion (Figure 21.2C, white arrow) compared to prior imaging. The plexiform neurofibroma component is unchanged (Figure 21.2C, orange arrow). The rapid lesion growth combined with new pain, FDG-avidity with SUVmax of 5.4 (Figure 21.2D, white arrow), young age, and history of NF1 whole-gene deletion raised concern for potential MPNST versus atypical neurofibroma. A biopsy confirmed high-grade MPNST (Figure 21.2E). Characteristics: High-grade MPNST arising in a diffuse plexiform neurofibroma: 27 mitoses/10 HPF, tumor necrosis 10%. Not shown: Notable loss of CD34, S100 protein, SOX10, and trimethylation of histone 3 at codon 27 (H3K27me3) in the high-grade tumor component, while present in the neurofibroma components.

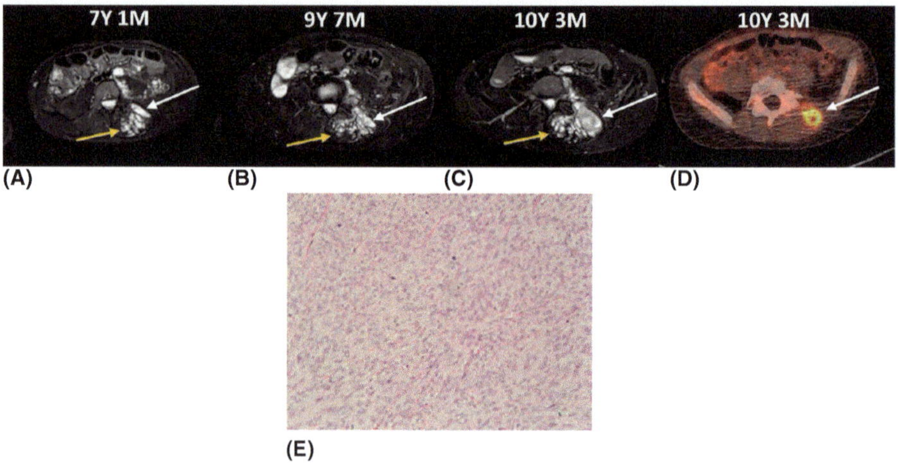

FIGURE 21.2 Development of high-grade MPNST in a child with NF1 and preexisting plexiform neurofibroma.

The MPNST was subsequently resected. This case demonstrates the difficulty in using imaging characteristics alone to determine the pathologic diagnosis. A combination of clinical and imaging findings raised concern for MPNST, which was confirmed. If in doubt, we recommend image-guided biopsy prior to surgery and close consultation with an experienced sarcoma surgeon.

REFERENCES

1. Higham CS, Steinberg SM, Dombi E, et al. SARC006: Phase II trial of chemotherapy in sporadic and neurofibromatosis type 1 associated chemotherapy-naive malignant peripheral nerve sheath tumors. *Sarcoma*. 2017;2017:8685638. doi:10.1155/2017/8685638
2. Evans DGR, Baser ME, McGaughran J, et al. Malignant peripheral nerve sheath tumours in neurofibromatosis 1. *J Med Genet*. 2002;39(5):311–314. doi:10.1136/jmg.39.5.311
3. Uusitalo E, Rantanen M, Kallionpää RA, et al. Distinctive cancer associations in patients with neurofibromatosis type 1. *J Clin Oncol*. 2016;34(17):1978–1986. doi:10.1200/JCO.2015.65.3576
4. Meany H, Widemann B, Ratner N. Malignant peripheral nerve sheath tumors: prognostic and diagnositc markers and therapeutic targets. In: Upadhyaya M, Cooper DN, eds. *Neurofibromatosis Type 1: Molecular and Cellular Biology*. Heidelberg, Germany: Springer-Verlag; 2012:445–468.
5. Peckham-Gregory EC, Montenegro RE, Stevenson DA, et al. Racial/ethnic disparities and incidence of malignant peripheral nerve sheath tumors: results from the Surveillance, Epidemiology, and End Results Program, 2000-2014. *J Neurooncol*. 2018;139(1):69–75. doi:10.1007/s11060-018-2842-4

6. Farid M, Demicco EG, Garcia R, et al. Malignant peripheral nerve sheath tumors. *Oncologist*. 2014;19(2):193–201. doi:10.1634/theoncologist.2013-0328
7. Kolberg M, Høland M, Agesen TH, et al. Survival meta-analyses for >1800 malignant peripheral nerve sheath tumor patients with and without neurofibromatosis type 1. *Neuro Oncol*. 2013;15(2):135–147. doi:10.1093/neuonc/nos287
8. Reilly KM, Kim A, Blakely J, et al. Neurofibromatosis type 1-associated MPNST state of the science: outlining a research agenda for the future. *J Natl Cancer Inst*. 2017;109(8):djx124. doi:10.1093/jnci/djx124
9. Higham CS, Dombi E, Rogiers A, et al. The characteristics of 76 atypical neurofibromas as precursors to neurofibromatosis 1 associated malignant peripheral nerve sheath tumors. *Neuro Oncol*. 2018;20(6):818–825. doi:10.1093/neuonc/noy013
10. Cleven AH, Al Sannaa GA, Briaire-de Bruijn I, et al. Loss of H3K27 tri-methylation is a diagnostic marker for malignant peripheral nerve sheath tumors and an indicator for an inferior survival. *Mod Pathol*. 2016;29:1113. doi:10.1038/modpathol.2016.103
11. Miettinen MM, Antonescu CR, Fletcher CDM, et al. Histopathologic evaluation of atypical neurofibromatous tumors and their transformation into malignant peripheral nerve sheath tumor in patients with neurofibromatosis 1-a consensus overview. *Hum Pathol*. 2017;67:1–10. doi:10.1016/j.humpath.2017.05.010
12. De Raedt T, Brems H, Wolkenstein P, et al. Elevated risk for MPNST in NF1 microdeletion patients. *Am J Hum Genet*. 2003;72(5):1288–1292. doi:10.1086/374821
13. Kehrer-Sawatzki H, Mautner VF, Cooper DN. Emerging genotype-phenotype relationships in patients with large NF1 deletions. *Hum Genet*. 2017;136(4):349–376. doi:10.1007/s00439-017-1766-y
14. Salamon J, Mautner VF, Adam G, Derlin T. Multimodal imaging in neurofibromatosis type 1-associated nerve sheath tumors. *Rofo*. 2015;187(12):1084–1092. doi:10.1055/s-0035-1553505
15. Ahlawat S, Fayad LM, Khan MS, et al. Current whole-body MRI applications in the neurofibromatoses: NF1, NF2, and schwannomatosis. *Neurology*. 2016;87(7 Suppl 1):S31–S39. doi:10.1212/WNL.0000000000002929
16. Chirindel A, Chaudhry M, Blakeley JO, Wahl R. 18F-FDG PET/CT qualitative and quantitative evaluation in neurofibromatosis type 1 patients for detection of malignant transformation: comparison of early to delayed imaging with and without liver activity normalization. *J Nucl Med*. 2015;56(3):379–385. doi:10.2967/jnumed.114.142372
17. Ferner RE, Golding JF, Smith M, et al. [18F]2-fluoro-2-deoxy-D-glucose positron emission tomography (FDG PET) as a diagnostic tool for neurofibromatosis 1 (NF1) associated malignant peripheral nerve sheath tumours (MPNSTs): a long-term clinical study. *Ann Oncol*. 2008;19(2):390–394. doi:10.1093/annonc/mdm450
18. Tsai LL, Drubach L, Fahey F, et al. [18F]-Fluorodeoxyglucose positron emission tomography in children with neurofibromatosis type 1 and plexiform neurofibromas: correlation with malignant transformation. *J Neuro Oncol*. 2012;108(3):469–475. doi:10.1007/s11060-012-0840-5
19. Well L, Salamon J, Kaul MG, et al. Differentiation of peripheral nerve sheath tumors in patients with neurofibromatosis type 1 using diffusion-weighted magnetic resonance imaging. *Neuro Oncol*. 2019;21(4):508–516. doi:10.1093/neuonc/noy199
20. Ahlawat S, Fayad LM. Imaging cellularity in benign and malignant peripheral nerve sheath tumors: utility of the "target sign" by diffusion weighted imaging. *Eur J Radiol*. 2018;102:195–201. doi:10.1016/j.ejrad.2018.03.018
21. Pemov A, Hansen NF, Sindiri S, et al. Low mutation burden and frequent loss of CDKN2A/B and SMARCA2, but not PRC2, define pre-malignant neurofibromatosis type 1-associated atypical neurofibromas. *Neuro Oncol*. 2019;21:981–992. doi:10.1093/neuonc/noz028
22. Beert E, Brems H, Daniëls B, et al. Atypical neurofibromas in neurofibromatosis type 1 are premalignant tumors. *Genes Chromosomes Cancer*. 2011;50(12):1021–1032. doi:10.1002/gcc.20921
23. Lee W, Teckie S, Wiesner T, et al. PRC2 is recurrently inactivated through EED or SUZ12 loss in malignant peripheral nerve sheath tumors. *Nat Genet*. 2014;46(11):1227–1232. doi:10.1038/ng.3095
24. Zhang M, Wang Y, Jones S, et al. Somatic mutations of SUZ12 in malignant peripheral nerve sheath tumors. *Nat Genet*. 2014;46(11):1170–1172. doi:10.1038/ng.3116
25. Perrone F, Da Riva L, Orsenigo M, et al. PDGFRA, PDGFRB, EGFR, and downstream signaling activation in malignant peripheral nerve sheath tumor. *Neuro Oncol*. 2009;11(6):725–736. doi:10.1215/15228517-2009-003
26. Bottillo I, Ahlquist T, Brekke H, et al. Germline and somatic NF1 mutations in sporadic and NF1-associated malignant peripheral nerve sheath tumours. *J Pathol*. 2009;217(5):693–701. doi:10.1002/path.2494
27. Brohl AS, Kahen E, Yoder SJ, et al. The genomic landscape of malignant peripheral nerve sheath tumors: diverse drivers of Ras pathway activation. *Sci Rep*. 2017;7(1):14992. doi:10.1038/s41598-017-15183-1
28. Carroll SL. The challenge of cancer genomics in rare nervous system neoplasms: malignant peripheral nerve sheath tumors as a paradigm for cross-species comparative oncogenomics. *Am J Pathol*. 2016;186(3):464–477. doi:10.1016/j.ajpath.2015.10.023
29. Chalmers ZR, Connelly CF, Fabrizio D, et al. Analysis of 100,000 human cancer genomes reveals the landscape of tumor mutational burden. *Genome Med*. 2017;9(1):34. doi:10.1186/s13073-017-0424-2
30. Shurell E, Singh AS, Crompton JG, et al. Characterizing the immune microenvironment of malignant peripheral nerve sheath tumor by PD-L1 expression and presence of CD8+ tumor infiltrating lymphocytes. *Oncotarget*. 2016;7(39):64300–64308. doi:10.18632/oncotarget.11734
31. Paoluzzi L, Cacavio A, Ghesani M, et al. Response to anti-PD1 therapy with nivolumab in metastatic sarcomas. *Clin Sarcoma Res*. 2016;6:24. doi:10.1186/s13569-016-0064-0

32. Margueron R, Reinberg D. The Polycomb complex PRC2 and its mark in life. *Nature*. 2011;469:343–349. doi:10.1038/nature09784
33. Prieto-Granada CN, Wiesner T, Messina JL, et al. Loss of H3K27me3 expression is a highly sensitive marker for sporadic and radiation-induced MPNST. *Am J Surg Pathol*. 2016;40(4):479–489. doi:10.1097/PAS.0000000000000564
34. Dombi E, Baldwin A, Marcus LJ, et al. Activity of selumetinib in neurofibromatosis type 1-related plexiform neurofibromas. *N Engl J Med*. 2016;375(26):2550–2560. doi:10.1056/NEJMoa1605943
35. Gross AM, Wolters PL, Dombi E, et al. Selumetinib in children with inoperable plexiform neurofibromas. *N Engl J Med*. 2020;382(15):1430–1442. doi:10.1056/NEJMoa1912735
36. Johannessen CM, Reczek EE, James MF, et al. The NF1 tumor suppressor critically regulates TSC2 and mTOR. *Proc Natl Acad Sci U S A*. 2005;102(24):8573–8578. doi:10.1073/pnas.0503224102
37. Johansson G, Mahller YY, Collins MH, et al. Effective in vivo targeting of the mammalian target of rapamycin pathway in malignant peripheral nerve sheath tumors. *Mol Cancer Ther*. 2008;7(5):1237–1245. doi:10.1158/1535-7163.MCT-07-2335
38. Zou CY, Smith KD, Zhu QS, et al. Dual targeting of AKT and mammalian target of rapamycin: a potential therapeutic approach for malignant peripheral nerve sheath tumor. *Mol Cancer Ther*. 2009;8(5):1157–1168. doi:10.1158/1535-7163.MCT-08-1008
39. Patel AV, Eaves D, Jessen WJ, et al. Ras-driven transcriptome analysis identifies aurora kinase A as a potential malignant peripheral nerve sheath tumor therapeutic target. *Clin Cancer Res*. 2012;18(18):5020–5030. doi:10.1158/1078-0432.CCR-12-1072
40. Watson AL, Rahrmann EP, Moriarity BS, et al. Canonical Wnt/β-catenin signaling drives human schwann cell transformation, progression, and tumor maintenance. *Cancer Discov*. 2013;3(6):674–689. doi:10.1158/2159-8290.CD-13-0081
41. Rahrmann EP, Watson AL, Keng VW, et al. Forward genetic screen for malignant peripheral nerve sheath tumor formation identifies new genes and pathways driving tumorigenesis. *Nat Genet*. 2013;45(7):756–766. doi:10.1038/ng.2641
42. Patwardhan PP, Surriga O, Beckman MJ, et al. Sustained inhibition of receptor tyrosine kinases and macrophage depletion by PLX3397 and rapamycin as a potential new approach for the treatment of MPNSTs. *Clin Cancer Res*. 2014;20(12):3146–3158. doi:10.1158/1078-0432.CCR-13-2576
43. De Raedt T, Beert E, Pasmant E, et al. PRC2 loss amplifies Ras-driven transcription and confers sensitivity to BRD4-based therapies. *Nature*. 2014;514:247–251. doi:10.1038/nature13561
44. Varin J, Poulain L, Hivelin M, et al. Dual mTORC1/2 inhibition induces anti-proliferative effect in NF1-associated plexiform neurofibroma and malignant peripheral nerve sheath tumor cells. *Oncotarget*. 2016;7(24):35753–35767. doi:10.18632/oncotarget.7099
45. Le LQ, Cooper JM, Patel AJ, et al. Overcoming BET inhibitor resistance in malignant peripheral nerve sheath tumors. *Clin Cancer Res*. 2019;25(11):3404-3416. doi:10.1158/1078-0432.CCR-18-2437
46. Valentin T, Le Cesne A, Ray-Coquard I, et al. Management and prognosis of malignant peripheral nerve sheath tumors: the experience of the French Sarcoma Group (GSF-GETO). *Eur J Cancer*. 2016;56:77–84. doi:10.1016/j.ejca.2015.12.015
47. Ducatman BS, Scheithauer BW, Piepgras DG, et al. Malignant peripheral nerve sheath tumors. A clinicopathologic study of 120 cases. *Cancer*. 1986;57(10):2006–2021. doi:10.1002/1097-0142(19860515)57:10<2006::aid-cncr2820571022>3.0.co;2-6
48. Meis JM, Enzinger FM, Martz KL, Neal JA. Malignant peripheral nerve sheath tumors (malignant schwannomas) in children. *Am J Surg Pathol*. 1992;16(7):694–707. doi:10.1097/00000478-199207000-00008
49. Carli M, Ferrari A, Mattke A, et al. Pediatric malignant peripheral nerve sheath tumor: the Italian and German soft tissue sarcoma cooperative group. *J Clin Oncol*. 2005;23(33):8422–8430. doi:10.1200/JCO.2005.01.4886
50. Ferner RE, Gutmann DH. International consensus statement on malignant peripheral nerve sheath tumors in neurofibromatosis. *Cancer Res*. 2002;62(5):1573–1577. https://cancerres.aacrjournals.org/content/62/5/1573
51. Vauthey JN, Woodruff JM, Brennan MF. Extremity malignant peripheral nerve sheath tumors (neurogenic sarcomas): a 10-year experience. *Ann Surg Oncol*. 1995;2(2):126–131. doi:10.1007/bf02303627
52. Yang JC, Chang AE, Baker AR, et al. Randomized prospective study of the benefit of adjuvant radiation therapy in the treatment of soft tissue sarcomas of the extremity. *J Clin Oncol*. 1998;16(1):197–203. doi:10.1200/JCO.1998.16.1.197
53. Bradford D, Kim A. Current treatment options for malignant peripheral nerve sheath tumors. *Curr Treat Options Oncol*. 2015;16(3):328. doi:10.1007/s11864-015-0328-6
54. Kaushal A, Citrin D. The role of radiation therapy in the management of sarcomas. *Surg Clin North Am*. 2008;88(3):629–646, viii. doi:10.1016/j.suc.2008.03.005
55. Frisch S, Timmermann B. The evolving role of proton beam therapy for sarcomas. *Clin Oncol (R Coll Radiol)*. 2017;29(8):500–506. doi:10.1016/j.clon.2017.04.034
56. Kim A, Stewart DR, Reilly KM, et al. Malignant peripheral nerve sheath tumors state of the science: leveraging clinical and biological insights into effective therapies. *Sarcoma*. 2017;2017:7429697. doi:10.1155/2017/7429697
57. Hirbe AC, Cosper PF, Dahiya S, Van Tine BA. Neoadjuvant ifosfamide and epirubicin in the treatment of malignant peripheral nerve sheath tumors. *Sarcoma*. 2017;2017:3761292. doi:10.1155/2017/3761292

58. Kroep JR, Ouali M, Gelderblom H, et al. First-line chemotherapy for malignant peripheral nerve sheath tumor (MPNST) versus other histological soft tissue sarcoma subtypes and as a prognostic factor for MPNST: an EORTC soft tissue and bone sarcoma group study. *Ann Oncol*. 2011;22(1):207–214. doi:10.1093/annonc/mdq338
59. Ferrari A, Miceli R, Rey A, et al. Non-metastatic unresected paediatric non-rhabdomyosarcoma soft tissue sarcomas: results of a pooled analysis from United States and European groups. *Eur J Cancer*. 2011;47(5):724–731. doi:10.1016/j.ejca.2010.11.013
60. Skotheim RI, Kallioniemi A, Bjerkhagen B, et al. Topoisomerase-II alpha is upregulated in malignant peripheral nerve sheath tumors and associated with clinical outcome. *J Clin Oncol*. 2003;21(24):4586–4591. doi:10.1200/JCO.2003.07.067
61. Widemann BC, Lu Y, Reinke D, et al. Targeting sporadic and neurofibromatosis type 1 (NF1) related refractory malignant peripheral nerve sheath tumors (MPNST) in a phase II study of everolimus in combination with bevacizumab (SARC016). *Sarcoma*. 2019;2019:7656747. doi:10.1155/2019/7656747
62. Kim A, Lu Y, Okuno S, et al. Targeting refractory sarcomas and malignant peripheral nerve sheath tumors in a phase I/II study of sirolimus in combination with ganetespib (SARC023). *Sarcoma*. 2020;2020:5784876. doi:10.1155/2020/5784876
63. Bernthal NM, Putnam A, Jones KB, et al. The effect of surgical margins on outcomes for low grade MPNSTs and atypical neurofibroma. *J Surg Oncol*. 2014;110(7):813–816. doi:10.1002/jso.23736
64. Salloway S, Sperling R, Fox NC, et al. Two phase 3 trials of bapineuzumab in mild-to-moderate Alzheimer's disease. *N Engl J Med*. 2014;370(4):322–333. doi:10.1056/NEJMoa1304839
65. Lee CS, Huh JS, Chang JW, Park JK. The early detection of recurrence of malignant peripheral nerve sheath tumor by frequent magnetic resonance imaging. *J Korean Neurosurg Soc*. 2010;47(1):51–54. doi:10.3340/jkns.2010.47.1.51
66. Hemming ML, Klega KS, Rhoades J, et al. Detection of circulating tumor DNA in patients with leiomyosarcoma with progressive disease. *JCO Precis Oncol*. 2019;2019:1–11. doi:10.1200/PO.18.00235

22

Extraskeletal Myxoid Chondrosarcoma

Silvia Stacchiotti, Giacomo Giulio Baldi, Carlo Morosi, Angelo Paolo Dei Tos, and Alessandro Gronchi

INTRODUCTION AND EPIDEMIOLOGY

Extraskeletal myxoid chondrosarcoma (EMC) is an exceedingly rare soft tissue sarcoma (STS) accounting for <3% of all STSs. It usually arises in adults with a peak incidence in the fifth decade and has a a male predominance (M/F ratio 2:1), with few cases described in childhood and adolescence.[1]

EMC is a morphologically distinctive neoplasm, described for the first time in 1953 by Stout and Verner[2] under the name of chondrosarcoma of the extraskeletal soft tissue and formally defined as a distinctive entity under the name of EMC by Enzinger and Shiraki in 1972.[3] EMC is classified by World Health Organization (WHO) as a tumor of uncertain differentiation.[1,4] In fact, despite the name, there is no convincing evidence of cartilaginous differentiation, with no clinicopathologic or genetic features in common with any chondrosarcoma subtype. Some molecular studies had shown neuroendocrine properties, raising the possibilities of multiphenotypic differentiation.[5,6]

EMC arises in deep soft tissues of the proximal extremities and limb girdle in approximately 80% of cases, thigh being the most common site and accounting for 30% to 40% of all cases. Less commonly involved anatomic locations include the head and neck region, the paraspinal soft tissue, the trunk (mostly chest wall and abdominal wall), and the pelvis.[4] Pediatric cases of EMC seem to have the propensity to occur in uncommon locations such as scalp, parotid gland, urethra, and sacrococcygeal region. Exceptionally, EMC can arise primarily in bone.[7–9]

Clinically, EMC usually presents as an enlarging, deep-seated soft tissue mass, often accompanied by pain and tenderness; in some cases, EMC can mimic a hematoma, and when arising around joints, it can produce functional impairment.

DIAGNOSTIC APPROACH

The recommended imaging of the primary tumor is MRI. Because lymph node involvement is more frequent than observed in the other STSs, regional lymph node status assessment through CT/MRI is advisable.

Radiographically, because of the presence of a rich myxoid matrix, EMC usually appears as a low attenuation lesion on CT scan and displays hyperintense signal with hypointense internal septa on T2-weighted MRI, which is reflective of a high water content. They also have pronounced lobular architecture often invading extracompartmental, bony, and vascular structures. As the tumor may undergo hemorrhagic and necrotic degeneration, signal characteristics on T1-weighted MRI can vary, ranging from low-, intermediate- and high-intensity features compared to muscle.[10–12] Peripheral/septal enhancement was observed in nearly one-third of the cases after the administration of contrast medium. In addition, serpentine high-flow vessels may be seen: they correspond to the hemangiopericytoma-like areas, which can be identified histologically (see Figure 22.1).

Similar to other STSs, a chest and abdomen CT scan is mandatory for staging purposes; metastases are usually pulmonary, but extrapulmonary metastases can less commonly occur. Fluorodeoxyglucose (FDG)-PET/CT imaging may be useful in selected cases to investigate tumor aggressiveness.[11] As for all sarcomas, pathologic diagnosis is mandatory. Usually a core-needle biopsy taken within a sarcoma reference center is considered the best approach.

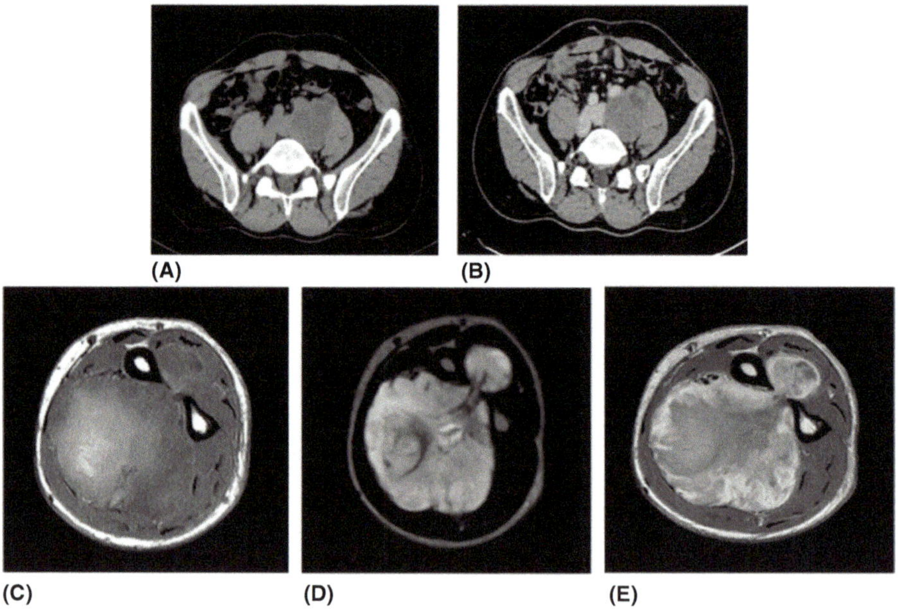

FIGURE 22.1 (A–B) Primary retroperitoneal extraskeletal myxoid chondrosarcoma (EMC) on axial pre- and postcontrast administration on CT scan. (C) Primary left forearm EMC on T1-weighted MRI shows a focus of high signal intensity within the tumor resulting from hemorrhage. (D) Primary left forearm extraskeletal myxoid chondrosarcoma on T2-weighted MRI shows hyperintense signaling with hypointense internal septa. (E) Primary left forearm extraskeletal myxoid chondrosarcoma on T1-weighted MRI after contrast administration with typical peripheral/septal enhancement.

PATHOLOGY AND MOLECULAR BIOLOGY

Microscopically, EMC typically features multinodular architecture defined by fibrous septa that divide the tumor into hypocellular lobules with abundant pale blue myxoid or chondromyxoid matrix.[1] The stroma is strikingly hypovascular. The cells characteristically grow in cords, strands, and even more complex trabecular or cribriform arrays (Figure 22.2). Cytoplasm is eosinophilic to vacuolated and harbors uniform round to oval nuclei. Mitotic activity is usually low. Some tumors have prominent rhabdoid cytoplasmic inclusions. Rare cases are hypercellular with decreased myxoid matrix and have higher grade, often epithelioid cytomorphology.[13,14] Well-formed hyaline cartilage is virtually never seen.

From the molecular standpoint, EMC is characterized by the rearrangement of the *NR4A3* gene, also known as *NOR1*. *NR4A3* gene rearrangement represents an important tool to enable differential

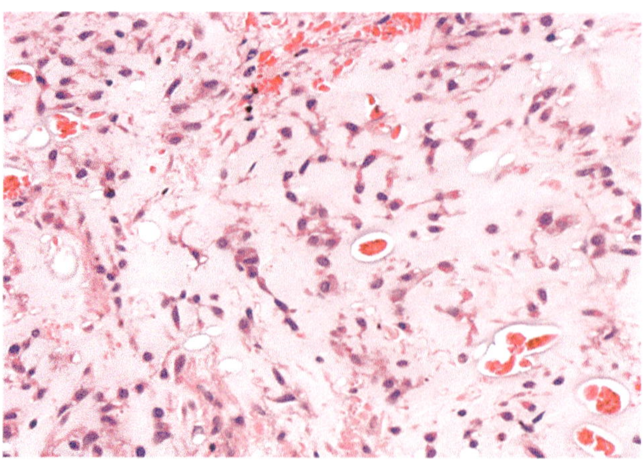

FIGURE 22.2 Extraskeletal myxoid chondrosarcoma neoplastic cells typically grow in cords set in abundant chondromyxoid matrix (hematoxylin & eosin stain).

diagnosis with other mimics, in particular myoepithelial neoplasms. *NR4A3* has been implicated in regulating key cellular functions, including proliferation, cell survival, and inflammation.[15–17] In most cases, the *NR4A3* gene is rearranged with the *EWSR1* gene (approximately 70% of cases) as a result of a t(9;22)(q22;q12) translocation. Less frequently, *NR4A3* has been found rearranged with other genes and in particular *TAF15* (17q12), more rarely *TCF12* (15q21), *TGF* (3q12.2), or *FUS* (16p11.2). The spectrum of *NR4A3* rearrangements is, however, evolving in EMC, and recently *HSPA8* was also identified as a novel fusion partner of *NR4A3*.[18–21] While the *EWSR1-NR4A3* and *TAF15-NR4A3* fusion proteins are strong transcriptional activators, the *HSPA8-NR4A3* could act as a transcriptional repressor,[22] assuming different pathogenetic mechanisms of the disease based on the presence of different translocations.

A clear correlation between *NR4A3* gene fusion variants with morphology and clinical outcome has not been identified to date, though retrospective studies showed that *TAF15-NR4A3* subtype had more aggressive features. In particular, *TAF15-NR4A3* positive EMC showed a higher incidence of rhabdoid phenotype, high-grade morphology (solid pattern of growth, marked nuclear atypia, high mitotic activity), and a more aggressive clinical outcome compared to the *EWSR1–NR4A3* cases.[23] Recently to highlight this issue and to provide grounds for better risk stratification criteria, a set of EMC samples and cell models expressing either *EWSR1* or the *TAF15* fusion transcript were molecularly profiled by RNA-seq showing that the two EMC molecular variants display a distinct transcriptional profile with axon guidance and neurogenesis pathways as major discriminants. In particular, class 4 to 6 semaphorins with a pro-tumorigenic activity were more often expressed in *TAF15-NR4A3* tumors, while class 3 semaphorins that convey growth inhibitory signals were more abundant in *EWSR1-NR4A3* tumors. These results suggest that the type of *NR4A3* fusion could dictate an axon guidance switch and impact on tumor cell biology.[24]

Finally, deletions or mutations involving the *SMARCB1* gene have been identified in a small subset of EMC, particularly in cases with rhabdoid morphology.[25,26]

GENERAL THERAPEUTIC APPROACH

Currently the only curative option for EMC, when feasible, is wide local resection with negative margins (remove the tumor with a rim of normal tissue around it), that is the standard surgical procedure as for the all patients with an adult type, localized STS.[27,28] A surgeon specifically trained in the treatment of this rare disease must carry it out.

The use of radiation therapy (RT) for localized disease in the adjuvant or neoadjuvant setting is still debated, because the impact of RT has largely gone understudied in this histotype, and historically, it has been considered a chemotherapy- and RT-resistant tumor.

A retrospective study of 87 patients with EMC treated at two referral institutions between 1975 and 2008 showed a high rate of local recurrence in patients who underwent surgical resection without RT (35% at a median follow-up of 2.2 years).[29] Recently, a propensity score weighted, population-based analysis of the Surveillance, Epidemiology and End Results (SEER) database was performed to examine the effect of external beam RT (EBRT) on cancer-specific survival for 156 patients with localized EMC as first malignancy.[30] There were 147 patients (94%) who received surgery and 50 patients (32%) who received EBRT. Forty-five patients (29%) received both surgical resection and EBRT. At a median follow-up of 33 months, the authors observed a cancer-specific survival rate of 97% versus 85% and 94% versus 85% in favor of EBRT at 3 and 5 years, respectively. In this analysis tumor size, locoregional lymph node involvement, and type of surgery significantly correlated with cancer-specific survival.

Based on these results, we could extrapolate that therapeutic strategies that include aggressive local treatment with surgical resection and EBRT should be considered in localized disease, in particular for surgically removed large lesions and/or cases with locoregional nodal involvement. Neoadjuvant RT is preferable when tumor shrinkage is needed for a surgical downstaging when function preservation is the goal.

By contrast, there are no data to support the use of adjuvant/neoadjuvant chemotherapy in the disease unless high-grade features are seen.[27,29,31–33] In this case, chemotherapy is still not standard, but may be offered as an option for shared decision-making with the patient.[34]

In our experience, some patients with locally advanced and marginally resectable disease treated with chemotherapy and RT, also in combination in the preoperative setting, experienced significant responses, despite this tumor being commonly believed to be resistant to chemotherapy and RT; this kind of response allowed us in some cases to perform less extensive surgery than originally planned, especially for critical anatomic sites.

TABLE 22.1 Clinicopathologic Studies and Main Prognostic Factors in Extraskeletal Myxoid Chondrosarcoma

Reference	Years	Number of Pts	OS (%)		Prognostic Factor
			5 Years	10 Years	
Enzinger and Shiraki[3]	1972	34	83	83	Cellularity
Saleh et al.[13]	1992	10	80	60	NA
Meis-Kindblom et al.[5]	1999	99	90	70	Age, tumor size and location, metastasis
Oliveira et al.[35]	2000	23	91	78	None
McGrory et al.[32]	2001	16	87	63	Tumor size, histologic factors (cellularity, Ki-67, atypia)
Drilon et al.[29]	2008	87	82	65	Tumor size, metastasis
Ogura et al.[33]	2012	23	91	84	Tumor size, metastasis

NA, not available; Pts, patients; OS, overall survival.

PROGNOSTIC FACTORS AND PROPENSITY TO METASTASIZE

EMC have usually an indolent natural history, but a more aggressive course is observed in high-grade and/or dedifferentiated cases. The rate of both local recurrence (range from 35% to 50%) and distant metastasis (range from 25% to 50%) is high in EMC, although metastases often occur late after the diagnosis of primary tumor (Table 22.1)[2,3,13,14,27,29,35]

Ten-year survival ranges between 85% and 65% and 5-year survival is approximately 90%.[29,33] As already discussed, the most common sites of metastasis are the lung, lymph nodes, bone, and other soft tissue sites. Based on the few data available, older age, proximal extremity location, larger tumor size (>10 cm), and high-grade confer a worse prognosis.[4,32]

There are few published data to indicate the optimal routine follow-up policy for surgically treated STS patients with localized disease[36] and in particular for EMC patients. Given the risk of local recurrence and distant metastasis, regular follow-up after excision of primary disease, especially for the high-grade variant of EMC, is advisable.

The recommended follow-up should include a CT scan of thorax and abdomen and an MRI of the primary tumor site. Because metastatic disease can occur late in EMC, with more than 70% of local recurrences and first metastases of EMC happening beyond 5 years, longer follow-up is suggested.

THERAPEUTIC APPROACH FOR METASTATIC DISEASE

As for all STS, surgical resection can be a reasonable option with curative intent, taking into accont the expected morbidity in cases of limited, resectable, slow growing lung metastases.[37]

By contrast, patients with advanced disease not amenable to surgical resection cannot be cured and may need medical treatment, expecially with evidence of disease progression. Data available in the literature on the activity of anticancer agents in EMC are few and mostly retrospective.

While retrospective series published some years ago reported very limited activity of chemotherapeutic agents generally used for STS (for example, anthracycline-based, dacarbazine-based or ifosfamide-based regimens) (Table 22.2),[29,31–33] more recently, a retrospective study on a small series of molecularly confirmed EMC patients treated with anthracycline-based chemotherapy,[38] showed better results. In this study, four partial responses by the Response Evaluation Criteria in Solid Tumors (RECIST) of 10 evaluable patients, with a median progression-free survival (PFS) of 8 months were described. Although to be confirmed prospectively and/or on larger series, a possible explanation for the different results observed in this study compared to the previous ones is the selection of cases with a diagnosis confirmed by the presence of the *NR3A4* fusion.

Other medical options include antiangiogenic agents. The first evidence on the activity of an antiangiogenic agent in EMC was reported in 2012, and consisted of a RECIST partial response[39] observed to sunitinib in two patients with an *NR4A3-EWS* positive, progressive metastatic EMC. Afterward, sunitinib activity in the same patient population was confirmed in a retrospective series of 10 patients,[40] with six of 10 partial responses and with median PFS not reached at a median follow-up of 8.5 months. Curiously, all responsive cases were *EWSR1-NR4A3* positive while the 2/10 cases carrying the *TAF15-NR4A3* fusion progressed.

TABLE 22.2 Outcomes of Treatments of Extraskeletal Myxoid Chondrosarcoma With Chemotherapy and Target Therapy

Reference	Study type	No. of Pts	Clinical Settings	Median Follow-Up (months)	Regimen	PR+SD (*n*)	Median PFS	Median OS
Patel et al.[31]	Retrospective	11	Metastatic	5 yr	Anthra- and DTIC-based	0	NA	NA
Drilon et al.[29]	Retrospective	21	Metastatic	3.6 yr	Mainly anthra-based	0	5.2 mo	17.8 mo
Ogura et al.[33]	Retrospective	4	Metastatic	9 yr	IFX-based	0	NA	NA
McGrory et al.[32]	Retrospective	6	Metastatic	7.4 yr	NA	2	NA	45 mo
Stacchiotti et al.[38]	Retrospective	10	Metastatic	30 mo	Anthra-based	7	8 mo	50 mo
Morioka et al.[47]	Prospective	2	Metastatic	22.7 mo	Trabectedin	2	10.2 mo	18.4 mo
Stacchiotti et al.[40]	Retrospective	10	Metastatic	8.5 mo	Sunitinib	6	Not reached	NA
Stacchiotti et al.[41]	Prospective	25	Metastatic/ locally advanced	27 mo	Pazopanib	21	13.5 mo	Not reached

Anthra, anthracycline; DTIC, dacarbazine; IFX, ifosfamide; OS, overall survival; NA, nat available; PFS, progression-free survival; PR, partial response; Pts, patients; SD, stable disease.

Following these results, a prospective, investigator initiated, multicentric, European Phase II trial investigated the antitumor effect of pazopanib, which is the only antiangiogenic agent formally approved for second-line treatment of STS, in advanced progressive and translocated EMCs (Figure 22.3). This study confirmed that pazopanib is also active in this tumor type. The overall response rate (ORR) by RECIST was inferior to that observed with sunitinib, that is, 18% (4/22 evaluable patients) but 55% (12/22) of patients had evidence of tumor shrinkage. Even with pazopanib, disease control was prolonged, with a median PFS of 19 months, at a median follow-up of 27 months. In this series, all responsive patients also carried the *EWSR1-NR4A3* fusion gene.[41] Although the molecular basis for the responses is still unknown, these results surely support the use of antiangiogenics in this disease.[42]

Recent clinical data show effectiveness of trabectedin against translocation-related sarcoma (TRS),[43,44] since one of the complex mechanisms of action of this drug is the interference with the transcription of the oncogenic fusion proteins of TRS.[45,46] The only data available on trabectedin in EMC come from the subanalysis of EMC and mesenchymal chondrosarcoma (MCS) patients included in a Japanese randomized Phase II trial comparing trabectedin versus best-supportive care. In this study, one EMC patient was randomized to trabectedin with stable disease, which lasted over 1 year.[47] Additional data on a larger number of patients are needed to better understand the role of trabectedin in the disease.

Among new medical agents, the EZH2 inhibitor tazemetostat was investigated in EMC in an international multicentric Phase II study with negative results. Finally, no data are available on immunotherapy yet, although recent data on the immune profile of the disease[41] suggests that it would be rational to investigate immunotherapy.

SUMMARY

In summary, EMC is one of the rarest sarcoma subtypes, mostly arising from soft tissue and rarely also from bone. Despite its rarity, the radiographic features, morphology, immunohistochemistry, and

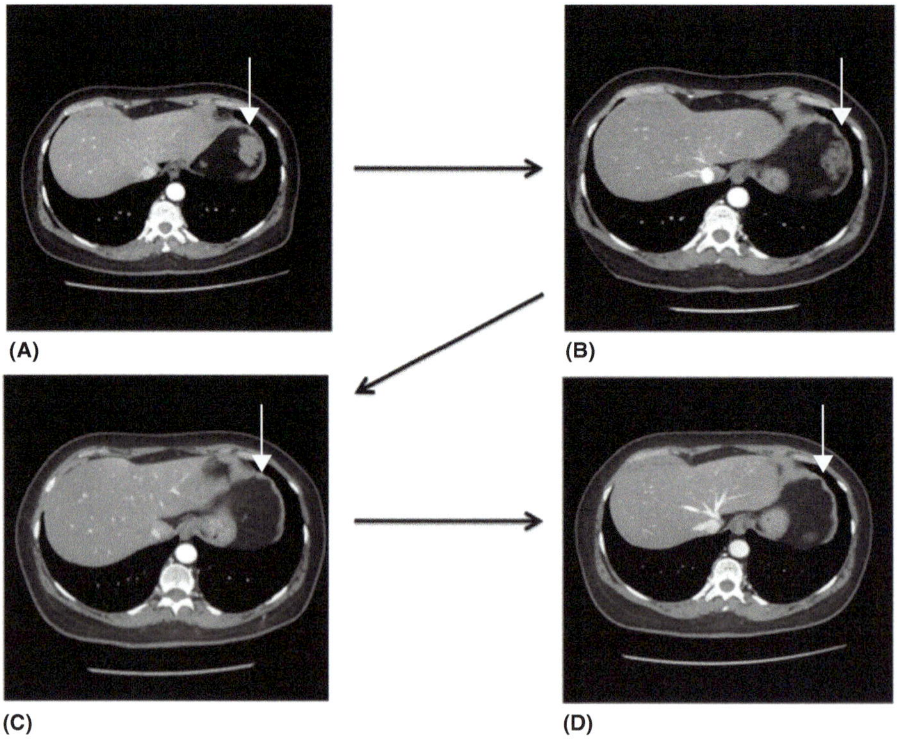

FIGURE 22.3 Complete and prolonged radiologic response with sunitinib in abdominal multiple lesions from primary retroperitoneal extraskeletal myxoid chondrosarcoma. (A) Basal CT scan showing one progressive subdiaphragmatic abdominal lesion. (B) Partial radiologic response after 6 months with sunitinib. (C) Complete radiologic response after 2 years, maintained (D) at 4 years from treatment start.

molecular biology of the disease are today quite well known and make a reliable diagnosis possible. Of course, expert pathologic validation of the diagnosis is required in all cases, as suggested in clinical practice guidelines for treatment of STS.[48] The natural history, prognostic factors, the role of adjuvant/neoadjuvant chemotherapy and radiotherapy in localized cases, the optimal sequence of medical treatments in advanced disease phase, and patterns of response are not yet well defined, so further research efforts are needed in this disease.

Because patients with advanced disease are not curable and medical options are limited, there is an urgent need to identify alternative therapeutic strategies when surgery or RT is no longer feasible.

Several promising new drugs and new therapeutic strategies are currently under study within ongoing clinical trials that address specific subtypes leading to more personalization of sarcoma treatment. International collaboration should be promoted in this regard, above all for these rare histotypes, as that networking is important to improve quality of care for rare cancers.

CASE STUDY

A 64-year-old woman presented to our sarcoma service in September 2013 for a slow growing painless and palpable mass of the left thigh of about 14 cm imaged by ultrasound. We ordered a total-body CT scan that excluded metastatic disease and an MRI of the left thigh that confirmed the presence of a neoplastic mesenchymal lesion in the thigh with hyperintense signaling and hypointense internal septa on T2-weighted imaging and with hypointense signaling on T1-weighted sequences compared to muscle with a global lobular architecture (Figure 22.4). After administration of contrast material, we observed peripheral inhomogeneous enhancement.

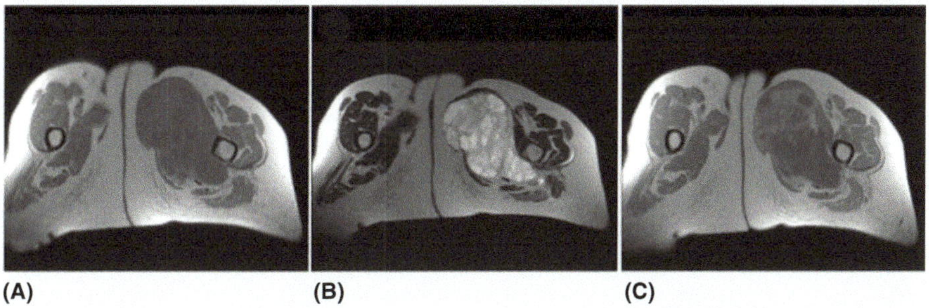

FIGURE 22.4 MRI of the primary lesion of the left thigh. (A) T1-weighted MRI; (B) T2-weighted MRI shows typical hyperintense signaling with hypointense internal septa; (C) T1-weighted MRI after contrast administration with inhomogeneous enhancement.

We performed an ultrasound-guided core-needle biopsy of the lesion and the histopathology report confirmed the diagnosis of a high-grade EMC.

We discussed the case in our multidisciplinary sarcoma board: surgery was technically feasible with a wide excision of the adductor muscles en-bloc with ileopubic and ischiopubic bone resection.

Despite the histopathologic diagnosis, given the high-grade and the local extension of the disease, resectable with a major surgery, we decided to share with the patient the possibility of a preoperative treatment with concomitant chemo-radiation therapy to try to obtain local down-staging of the disease to be followed by potentially less extensive surgery.

In December 2013, the patient started chemotherapy with epirubicin and ifosfamide. After the first cycle of chemotherapy, the patient experienced an objective reduction of the mass in the left thigh. In January 2014, the patient started RT concomitant with chemotherapy. The patient received in total three cycles of full-dose epirubicin and ifosfamide chemotherapy together with RT to the left thigh for a total fractionated dose of 50 Gy, without any treatment-related serious adverse events. The MRI performed in March 2014 showed an almost complete regression of the left thigh neoplastic lesion with a residual nodule of approximately 1 cm with hyperintense signaling on the middle and peripheral enhancement after administration of contrast material (see Figure 22.5).

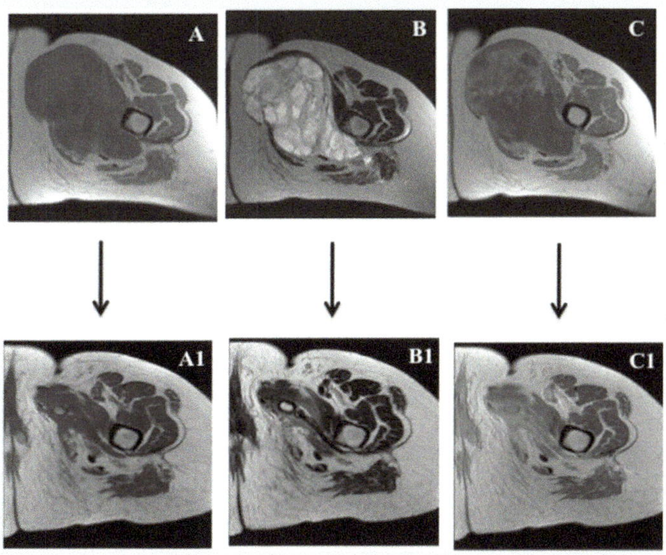

FIGURE 22.5 MRI of the primary lesion of the left thigh before and after three cycles of chemotherapy concomitant to radiotherapy showing an impressive dimensional response. (A–A1) T1-weighted MRI before and after treatment. (B–B1) T2-weighted MRI before and after treatment. (C–C1) T1-weighted MRI after before and after contrast administration.

We discussed again the case in our multidisciplinary sarcoma board and we decided to perform surgery with wide excision of the lesion en-bloc with the adductor muscles and only curettage of the cortical bone, without resection.

The final histopathological diagnosis was R0 excision of EMC with residual viable tumor in only 1% of the surgical specimen and 99% of fibrosis and necrosis without cortical bone involvement.

The patient started clinicoradiologic follow-up, and today, 6 years after diagnosis, is disease-free.

In conclusion, chemotherapy and RT, even concurrent, are feasible and can be active in EMC for marginally resectable cases arising from critical anatomic sites, and could be an option to consider in conjunction with surgery to achieve better local control and improve the treatment outcome for our patients.

REFERENCES

1. Lucas DR, Stenman G. Extraskeletal myxoid condrosarcoma. In: Fletcher CDM, Bridge JA, Hogendoorn P, Mertens F, eds. *World Health Organization (WHO) Classification of Tumours of Soft Tissue and Bone*. 4th ed. Lyon, France: IARC Press; 2013:223–224.
2. Stout AP, Verner EW. Chondrosarcoma of the extraskeletal soft tissues. *Cancer*. 1953;6(3):581–590. doi:10.1002/1097-0142(195305)6:3<581::aid-cncr2820060315>3.0.co;2-t
3. Enzinger FM, Shiraki M. Extraskeletal myxoid chondrosarcoma. An analysis of 34 cases. *Hum Pathol*. 1972;3(3):421–435. doi:10.1016/s0046-8177(72)80042-x
4. Lucas DR, Heim S. Extraskeletal myxoid condrosarcoma. In: Fletcher CDM, Unni KK, Mertens F, eds. *World Health Organization Classification of Tumours: Pathology and Genetics of Tumours of Soft Tissue and Bone*. Lyon, France: IARC Press; 2002:213–215.
5. Meis-Kindblom JM, Bergh P, Gunterberg B, Kindblom LG. Extraskeletal myxoid chondrosarcoma: a reappraisal of its morphologic spectrum and prognostic factors based on 117 cases. *Am J Surg Pathol*. 1999;23(6):636–650. doi:10.1097/00000478-199906000-00002
6. Filion C, Labelle Y. Identification of genes regulated by the EWS/NR4A3 fusion protein in extraskeletal myxoid chondrosarcoma. *Tumour Biol*. 2012;33(5):1599–1605. doi:10.1007/s13277-012-0415-2
7. Demicco EG, Wang WL, Madewell JE, et al. Osseous myxochondroid sarcoma: a detailed study of 5 cases of extraskeletal myxoid chondrosarcoma of the bone. *Am J Surg Pathol*. 2013;37(5):752–762. doi:10.1097/PAS.0b013e3182796e46
8. Finos L, Righi A, Frisoni T, et al. Primary extraskeletal myxoid chondrosarcoma of bone: report of three cases and review of the literature. *Pathol Res Pract*. 2017;2013(5):461–466. doi:10.1016/j.prp.2017.02.008
9. Antonescu CR, Argani P, Erlandson RA, et al. Skeletal and extraskeletal myxoid chondrosarcoma: a comparative clinicopathologic, ultrastructural, and molecular study. *Cancer*. 1998;83(8):1504–1521. doi:10.1002/(sici)1097-0142(19981015)83:8<1504::aid-cncr5>3.0.co;2-b
10. Murphey MD, Walker EA, Wilson AJ, et al. From the archives of the AFIP: imaging of primary chondrosarcoma: radiologic-pathologic correlation. *Radiographics*. 2003;23(5):1245–1278. doi:10.1148/rg.235035134
11. Kapoor N, Shinagare AB, Jagannathan JP, et al. Clinical and radiologic features of extraskeletal myxoid chondrosarcoma including initial presentation, local recurrence, and metastases. *Radiol Oncol*. 2014;48(3):235–242. doi:10.2478/raon-2014-0005
12. Tateishi U, Hasegawa T, Nojima T, et al. MRI features of extraskeletal myxoid chondrosarcoma. *Skeletal Radiol*. 2006;35:27–33. doi:10.1007/s00256-005-0021-0
13. Saleh G, Evans HL, Ro JY, Ayala AG. Extraskeletal myxoid chondrosarcoma. A clinicopathologic study of ten patients with long-term follow-up. *Cancer*. 1992;70(12):2827–2830. doi:10.1002/1097-0142(19921215)70:12<2827::aid-cncr2820701217>3.0.co;2-v
14. Lucas DR, Fletcher CD, Adsay NV, Zalupski MM. High-grade extraskeletal myxoid chondrosarcoma: a high-grade epithelioid malignancy. *Histopathology*. 1999;35(3):201–208. doi:10.1046/j.1365-2559.1999.00735.x
15. Brody RI, Ueda T, Hamelin A, et al. Molecular analysis of the fusion of EWS to an orphan nuclear receptor gene in extraskeletal myxoid chondrosarcoma. *Am J Pathol*. 1997;150(3):1049–1058. https://www.ncbi.nlm.nih.gov/pmc/articles/PMC1857890
16. Martínez-González J, Rius J, Castelló A, et al. Neuron-derived orphan receptor-1 (NOR-1) modulates vascular smooth muscle cell proliferation. *Circ Res*. 2003;92(1):96–103. doi:10.1161/01.es.0000050921.53008.47
17. Pei L, Castrillo A, Chen M, et al. Induction of NR4A orphan nuclear receptor expression in macrophages in response to inflammatory stimuli. *J Biol Chem*. 2005;280(32):29256–29262. doi:10.1074/jbc.M502606200
18. Flucke U, Tops BBJ, Verdijk MAJ, et al. NR4A3 rearrangement reliably distinguishes between the clinicopathologically overlapping entities myoepithelial carcinoma of soft tissue and cellular extraskeletal myxoid chondrosarcoma. *Virchows Arch*. 2012;460(6):621–628. doi:10.1007/s00428-012-1240-0

19. Labelle Y, Zucman J, Stenman G, et al. Oncogenic conversion of a novel orphan nuclear receptor by chromosome translocation. *Hum Mol Genet*. 1995;4(12):2219–2226. doi:10.1093/hmg/4.12.2219
20. Panagopoulos I, Mertens F, Isaksson M, et al. Molecular genetic characterization of the EWS/CHN and RBP56/CHN fusion genes in extraskeletal myxoid chondrosarcoma. *Genes Chromosomes Cancer*. 2002;35(4):340–352. doi:10.1002/gcc.10127
21. Broehm CJ, Wu J, Gullapalli RR, Bocklage T. Extraskeletal myxoid chondrosarcoma with a t(9;16)(q22;p11.2) resulting in a NR4A3-FUS fusion. *Cancer Genet*. 2014;207(6):276–280. doi:10.1016/j.cancergen.2014.06.024
22. Urbini M, Astolfi A, Pantaleo MA, et al. HSPA8 as a novel fusion partner of NR4A3 in extraskeletal myxoid chondrosarcoma. *Genes Chromosomes Cancer*. 2017;56(7):582–586. doi:10.1002/gcc.22462
23. Stricher F, Macri C, Ruff M, Muller S. HSPA8/HSC70 chaperone protein: structure, function, and chemical targeting. *Autophagy*. 2013;9(12):1937–1954. doi:10.4161/auto.26448
24. Brenca M, Stacchiotti S, Fassetta K, et al. NR4A3 fusion proteins trigger an axon guidance switch that marks the difference between EWSR1 and TAF15 translocated extraskeletal myxoid chondrosarcomas. *J Pathol*. 2019;249(1):90–101. doi:10.1002/path.5284
25. Agaram NP, Zhang L, Sung YS, et al. Extraskeletal myxoid chondrosarcoma with non-EWSR1-NR4A3 variant fusions correlate with rhabdoid phenotype and high-grade morphology. *Hum Pathol*. 2014;45(5):1084–1091. doi:10.1016/j.humpath.2014.01.007
26. Kohashi K, Oda Y, Yamamoto H, et al. SMARCB1/INI1 protein expression in round cell soft tissue sarcomas associated with chromosomal translocations involving EWS: a special reference to SMARCB1/INI1 negative variant extraskeletal myxoid chondrosarcoma. *Am J Surg Pathol*. 2008;32(8):1168–1174. doi:10.1097/PAS.0b013e318161781a
27. Kawaguchi S, Wada T, Nagoya S, et al. Extraskeletal myxoid chondrosarcoma: a multi-institutional study of 42 cases in Japan. *Cancer*. 2003;97(5):1285–1292. doi:10.1002/cncr.11162
28. Enneking WF, Spainer SS, Goodman MA. A system for the surgical staging of muscoloskeletal sarcoma. *Clin Orthop Relat Res*. 2003;415:4–18. doi:10.1097/01.blo.0000093891.12372.0f
29. Drilon AD, Popat S, Bhuchar G, et al. Extraskeletal myxoid chondrosarcoma: a retrospective review from 2 referral centers emphasizing long-term outcomes with surgery and chemotherapy. *Cancer*. 2008;113(12):3364–3371. doi:10.1002/cncr.23978
30. Kemmerer EJ, Gleeson E, Poli J, et al. Benefit of radiotherapy in extraskeletal myxoid chondrosarcoma: a propensity score weighted population-based analysis of the SEER database. *Am J Clin Oncol*. 2018;41(7):674–680. doi:10.1097/COC.0000000000000341
31. Patel SR, Burgess MA, Papadopoulos NE, et al. Extraskeletal myxoid chondrosarcoma. Long-term experience with chemotherapy. *Am J Clin Oncol*. 1995;18(2):161–163. doi:10.1097/00000421-199504000-00014
32. McGrory JE, Rock MG, Nascimento AG, Oliveira AM. Extraskeletal myxoid chondrosarcoma. *Clin Orthop Relat Res*. 2001;382:185–190. doi:10.1097/00003086-200101000-00025
33. Ogura K, Fujiwara T, Beppu Y, et al. Extraskeletal myxoid chondrosarcoma: a review of 23 patients treated at a single referral center with long-term follow-up. *Arch Orthop Trauma Surg*. 2012;132(10):1379–1386. doi:10.1007/s00402-012-1557-9
34. Casali PG, Abecassis N, Bauer S, et al. Soft tissue and visceral sarcomas: ESMO-EURACAN clinical practice guidelines for diagnosis, treatment and follow-up. *Ann Oncol*. 2018;29(suppl 4):iv51–iv67. doi:10.1093/annonc/mdy096
35. Oliveira AM, Sebo TJ, McGrory JE, et al. Extraskeletal myxoid chondrosarcoma: a clinicopathologic, immunohistochemical, and ploidy analysis of 23 cases. *Mod Pathol*. 2000;13(8):900–908. doi:10.1038/modpathol.3880161
36. Rothermundt C, Whelan JS, Dileo P, et al. What is the role of routine follow-up for localised limb soft tissue sarcomas? A retrospective analysis of 174 patients. *Br J Cancer*. 2014;110(10):2420–2426. doi:10.1038/bjc.2014.200
37. Blackmon SH, Shah N, Roth JA, et al. Resection of pulmonary and extrapulmonary sarcomatous metastases is associated with long-term survival. *Ann Thorac Surg*. 2009;88(3):877–884; discussion 884–885. doi:10.1016/j.athoracsur.2009.04.144
38. Stacchiotti S, Dagrada GP, Sanfilippo R, et al. Anthracycline-based chemotherapy in extraskeletal myxoid chondrosarcoma: a retrospective study. *Clin Sarcoma Res*. 2013;3(1):16. doi:10.1186/2045-3329-3-16
39. Stacchiotti S, Dagrada GP, Morosi C, et al. Extraskeletal myxoid chondrosarcoma: tumor response to sunitinib. *Clin Sarcoma Res*. 2012;2(1):22. doi:10.1186/2045-3329-2-22
40. Stacchiotti S, Pantaleo MA, Astolfi A, et al. Activity of sunitinib in extraskeletal myxoid chondrosarcoma. *Eur J Cancer*. 2014;50(9):1657–1664. doi:10.1016/j.ejca.2014.03.013
41. Stacchiotti S, Ferrari S, Redondo A, et al. Pazopanib for treatment of advanced extraskeletal myxoid condrosarcoma: a multicentre, single-arm, phase 2 trial. *Lancet Oncol*. 2019;20(9):1252–1262. doi:10.1016/S1470-2045(19)30319-5
42. van der Graaf WTA, Blay JY, Chawla SP, et al. Pazopanib for metastatic soft-tissue sarcoma (PALETTE): a randomised, double-blind, placebo-controlled phase 3 trial. *Lancet*. 2012;379(9829):1879–1886. doi:10.1016/S0140-6736(12)60651-5
43. Le Cesne A, Cresta S, Maki RG, et al. A retrospective analysis of antitumour activity with trabectedin in translocation-related sarcomas. *Eur J Cancer*. 2012;48(16):3036–3044. doi:10.1016/j.ejca.2012.05.012
44. Blay JY, Leahy MG, Nguyen BB, et al. Randomised phase III trial of trabectedin versus doxorubicin-based chemotherapy as first-line therapy in translocation-related sarcomas. *Eur J Cancer*. 2014;50(6):1137–1147. doi:10.1016/j.ejca.2014.01.012

45. Forni C, Minuzzo M, Virdis E, et al. Trabectedin (ET-743) promotes differentiation in myxoid liposarcoma tumors. *Mol Cancer Ther*. 2009;8(2):449–457. doi:10.1158/1535-7163.MCT-08-0848
46. Grohar PJ, Griffin LB, Yeung C, et al. Ecteinascidin 743 interferes with the activity of EWS-FLI1 in Ewing sarcoma cells. *Neoplasia*. 2011;13(2):145–153. doi:10.1593/neo.101202
47. Morioka H, Takahashi S, Araki N, et al. Results of a sub-analysis of a phase 2 study on trabectedin treatment for extraskeletal myxoid chondrosarcoma and mesenchymal chondrosarcoma. *BMC Cancer*. 2016;16:479. doi:10.1186/s12885-016-2511-y
48. Ray-Coquard I, Montesco MC, Coindre JM, et al. Sarcoma: concordance between initial diagnosis and centralized expert review in a population-based study within three European regions. *Ann Oncol*. 2012;23(9):2442–2449. doi:10.1093/annonc/mdr610

23

Endometrial Stromal Sarcoma

Stéphanie Gaillard and Angeles Alvarez Secord

INTRODUCTION

Endometrial stromal sarcoma (ESS) represents a very rare subset of uterine mesenchymal neoplasms and endometrial stromal tumors. Overall, ESSs represent 0.2% to 1% of all uterine malignant neoplasms and account for approximately 10% to 20% of uterine sarcomas.[1–3] Endometrial stromal tumors are grouped according to World Health Organization (WHO) 2014 classification system into four distinct categories: (a) endometrial stromal nodules, (b) low-grade endometrial stromal sarcoma (LG-ESS), (c) high-grade endometrial stromal sarcoma (HG-ESS), and (d) undifferentiated uterine sarcoma (UUS).[1] The focus of this chapter is on the ESS comprising LG-ESS and HG-ESS.

LG-ESS and HG-ESS subtypes are defined by divergent morphologic appearance, molecular aberrations with distinctive gene translocations, therapeutic management, and prognosis. LG-ESS are malignant tumors composed of nonneoplastic endometrial stromal cells with myometrial and vascular "tongue-like" infiltration patterns. The sarcomas typically have uniform cells, characteristic of endometrial stromal differentiation with minimal cellular pleomorphism and mild nuclear atypia. Common molecular alterations include the rearrangements of the *JAZF1* and *PHF1* genes. LG-ESSs tend to have a more indolent course and are treated with hormonal therapies. In comparison, HG-ESSs have high-grade nuclear atypia and mitotic activity with a more destructive infiltrative pattern of myometrial and lymphovascular invasion. HG-ESSs are more likely to demonstrate tumor cell necrosis. They are characterized by *YWHAE/FAM22* translocations and BCL6 corepressor (BCOR) alterations. HG-ESSs are associated with a more aggressive clinical behavior and worse survival outcomes.[1]

This chapter will focus on LG-ESS and HG-ESS and review distinctive clinicopathologic features, underlying molecular biology, management, and survival outcomes.

TERMINOLOGY OF ENDOMETRIAL STROMAL NEOPLASMS

Historically, the nomenclature for endometrial stromal tumors has been confusing because of the use of numerous diagnostic terms including stromal adenomyosis, stromatosis, endolymphatic stromal myosis, and stromal sarcoma. In 1966, Norris and Taylor, described a new classification system for endometrial stromal tumors based on clinicopathologic features of 53 tumors. The authors classified tumors using two groups based on the type of margin. The tumors with pushing margins were denoted as stromal nodules and were considered benign. The other main type of tumor was characterized by infiltrating margins and was referred to as either endolymphatic stromal myosis (low-grade) or stromal sarcoma (high-grade) based on mitotic activity. Endolymphatic stromal myosis had less than 10 mitotic figures in 10 high-power fields (HPFs) and had a clinically indolent course with an excellent prognosis of 100% 5-year survival. In contrast, stromal sarcomas were characterized by greater than 10 mitotic figures in 10 HPFs and had a more aggressive phenotype with worse survival.[4]

The arbitrary division of ESS into low-grade and high-grade based on mitotic count was later abandoned, as mitotic activity was deemed irrelevant with regard to prognosis.[5] In 2003, WHO proposed a two-type classification system: (a) ESS that included low-grade tumors characterized by proliferative endometrial stroma and (b) undifferentiated endometrial sarcoma, which consisted of pleomorphic tumors that did not resemble endometrial stromal cells.[5] However, the undifferentiated endometrial sarcomas included a heterogeneous subset of tumors with a different clinical phenotype, a novel gene rearrangement, and survival outcomes intermediate between the low-grade ESS and undifferentiated sarcomas.[5] The recognition of this distinct cohort of tumors led to the second WHO iteration of endometrial stromal neoplasm classification and inclusion of HG-ESS into the terminology.

The 2014 WHO classification for endometrial stromal neoplasms incorporated molecular findings into the classification system and includes four specific categories: (a) endometrial stromal nodule (which is a benign tumor), (b) LG-ESS, (c) HG-ESS, and (d) UUS.[1] The evolving terminology and classification for endometrial stromal neoplasms can lead to difficulty reviewing and interpreting the literature. For instance, older literature of uterine tumor resembling ovarian sex cord tumor may include cases now classified as LG-ESS; tumors previously categorized as undifferentiated endometrial or high-grade undifferentiated uterine sarcomas are now classified as HG-ESS; and the term undifferentiated endometrial sarcoma is no longer used.[6]

The focus of this chapter will review the two invasive endometrial stromal neoplasms, referred to as LG-ESS and HG-ESS. The pathologic, molecular characteristics, therapeutic recommendations, and surveillance are based on the 2014 WHO classification system. Aligning classification appropriately to the current terminology is challenging and reference may be made to literature using older terminology.

ESTIMATED INCIDENCE PER YEAR AND EPIDEMIOLOGY

Overall, ESSs represent 0.2% to 1% of all uterine malignant neoplasms and account for approximately 10% to 20% of uterine sarcomas.[1–3] Patients typically present with abnormal vaginal bleeding, postmenopausal bleeding, enlarged uterus or uterine mass, dysmenorrhea, pelvic pressure, or pain.[2,6] These tumors may also be asymptomatic in as many of 25%, or may be mistakenly diagnosed as leiomyoma.[3] Endometrial sarcomas are often not suspected and commonly are diagnosed following hysterectomy or myomectomy.

LG-ESS is more common than HG-ESS. LG-ESS typically develops in women between 40 and 55 years of age, >50% occur in premenopausal women, and they have been reported in young women or adolescents.[1,3] LG-ESS has been associated with prolonged estrogen exposure, tamoxifen use, and pelvic radiation.[1] LG-ESSs typically are indolent tumors characterized by excellent prognosis. Overall, the survival rates are 65% to 76% at 10 years.[6,7] However, the 5-year survival estimates for women with stage I and II disease are excellent and greater than 90%. In comparison, those with advanced disease have a higher incidence of recurrent disease and 5-year survival outcomes ranging from 40% to 50%.[1] Approximately 30% of patients will have extrauterine disease at presentation (most commonly to the ovary). Recurrence rates range from 30% to 56%, late recurrences being common, and 15% to 25% of patients succumb to recurrent disease.[3,7,8]

HG-ESSs occur at a mean age of 50 years (range 28–67 years) and often are symptomatic with abnormal vaginal bleeding, an enlarged uterus, or a pelvic mass.[3] HG-ESS has worse survival rates compared to LG-ESS and typically presents with advanced stage disease.[1] Patients with HG-ESS are more likely to develop recurrent disease within an earlier time frame.[3] The median overall survival ranges from 11 to 23 months.[9] HG-ESS has a favorable prognosis compared to undifferentiated uterine sarcomas.

DIAGNOSTIC APPROACH

When patients present with abnormal or postmenopausal bleeding and uterine mass, the evaluation should comprise a complete history, physical examination including pelvic exam, endometrial biopsy, and pelvic imaging. The differential diagnosis is extensive and includes leiomyoma, endometrial stromal nodules, endometrial stromal sarcoma subtypes, leiomyosarcoma; solitary fibrous tumors or hemangiopericytoma, undifferentiated endometrial carcinomas, uterine tumor resembling ovarian sex cord tumors, and undifferentiated uterine sarcomas.[1] Pelvic examination cannot differentiate between a benign uterine mass, such as leiomyoma, and uterine sarcoma.

Diagnostic approaches, such as endometrial sampling via biopsy or curettage can be performed. However, the accuracy of endometrial samples for ESS is uncertain owing to the rare frequency of this disease. In a report of 938 patients, only two had stromal sarcomas and both were identified on preoperative endometrial sampling.[10] Other modes of biopsy, either transcervical or transperitoneal, have been considered. Transcervical biopsy limits the risk of peritoneal spread, but may not reach all masses.[11]

Imaging features of endometrial sarcomas can be distinct from leiomyoma, but diagnosis requires heightened suspicion as discussed in the next section, "Radiographic Features and Recommended Imaging."

If the diagnosis is made preoperatively, a complete blood count and chemistry panel to assess liver and renal function as well as chemistry profile should be considered.[12] However, often the diagnosis is made postoperatively after hysterectomy or myomectomy for presumed benign disease. If diagnosed postoperatively, obtain expert pathologic review, request estrogen receptor (ER)/progesterone receptor (PR) testing, and perform imaging to assess for metastatic and unresected disease.[12]

RADIOGRAPHIC FEATURES AND RECOMMENDED IMAGING

Radiologic imaging typically includes pelvic ultrasound and pelvic MRI. On ultrasound exam, ESS has a nonspecific pattern or appearance of a heterogeneous hypoechoic endometrial mass (Figure 23.1A), with myometrial involvement. On Doppler ultrasound, low-resistance intralesional arteries and increased vasculature, which can be central or peripheral, are seen (Figure 23.1B). Key diagnostic findings of low-flow resistance within the intralesional arteries and the structural findings should increase suspicion for malignancy.[2]

On MRI, these neoplasms may appear as large polypoid masses that expand the endometrial cavity. The masses can be diffusely infiltrative and have irregular margins, and are characterized by multiple nodular lesions or masses and intramyometrial nodule extensions. A key feature characterized by a low-intensity rim on T2-weighted images may indicate hemorrhage and raise index of suspicion for ESS. Another important characteristic of ESS are the "worm-like" invasive projections that can be seen along the vasculature and ligaments on diffusion-weighted imaging.[2] MRI is useful to evaluate for locally metastatic tumor, pelvic extension of disease, and residual disease in cases of incomplete resection, intraperitoneal morcellation, or tumor fragmentation.[12] Examples of incomplete resection include supracervical hysterectomy and myomectomy.

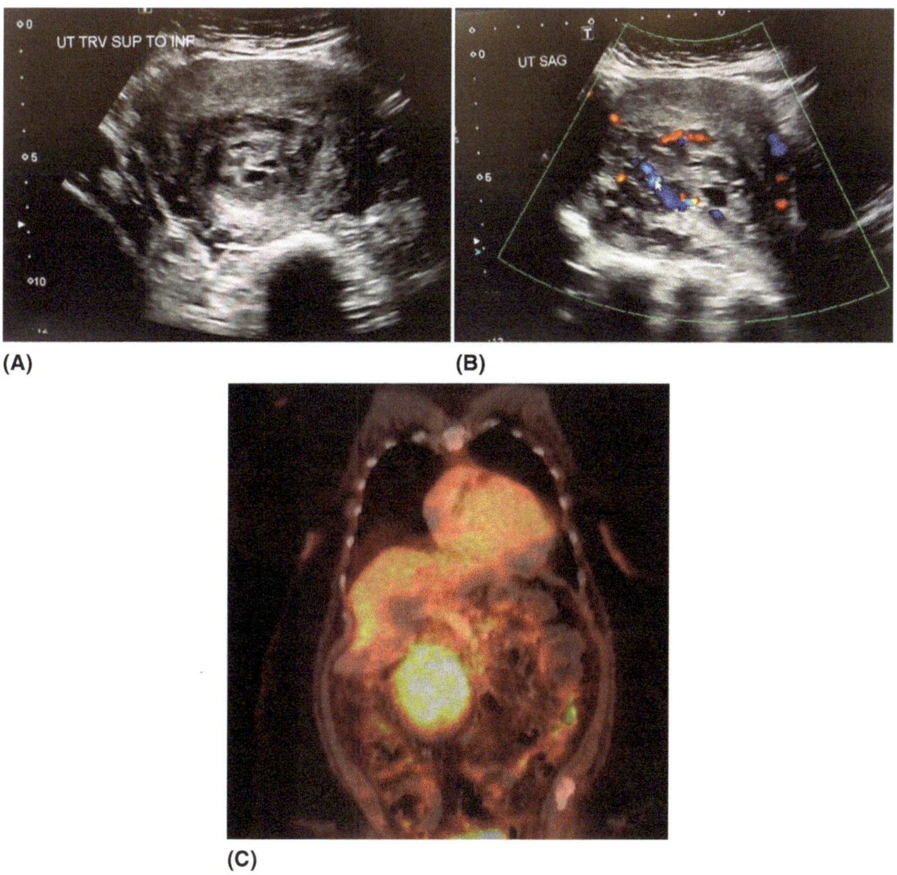

FIGURE 23.1 Radiologic imaging of endometrial stromal sarcomas. Nonspecific pattern or appearance of a heterogeneous hypoechoic endometrial mass on ultrasound (A) with low-resistance increased peripheral vasculature (B). Metastatic endometrial stromal sarcoma involving para-aortic node with high maximum standardized uptake value (SUVmax) (C).

CT scans can be useful to assess for metastatic disease. PET with or without CT can be utilized to clarify ambiguous findings.[12] There are limited data regarding PET in ESS; often the studies group the various sarcomas. PET may be useful to distinguish between uterine sarcomas and leiomyoma (Figure 23.1C). A small study including 15 uterine sarcomas and 19 leiomyomas demonstrated that the median maximum standardized uptake value (SUVmax) for these tumors was significantly different. Uterine sarcomas have higher median SUVmax of 12 compared to leiomyoma with a median SUVmax of 4.1.[13] PET imaging with a novel tracer, [^{18}F]-fluoroestradiol (FES) labeling, has been reported in patients receiving hormonal therapy demonstrating a correlation between decreased FES uptake on imaging and disease response.[14]

PATHOLOGIC FINDINGS OF ENDOMETRIAL STROMAL SARCOMAS

The anatomic location of ESS is similar for both low- and high-grade types. ESSs are intrauterine tumors and have propensity to invade the myometrium and vasculature. Distinguishing between endometrial stromal nodules, LG-ESS, HG-ESS, and other types of sarcomas can be challenging. Therefore, expert pathologic review is strongly recommended. Immunohistochemistry to assess protein and receptor expression as well as molecular characterization of the tumors for diagnostic purposes is helpful. These additional tests can be utilized to distinguish endometrial sarcomas from other mesenchymal neoplasms as well as LG-ESS from HG-ESS.

While endometrial stromal nodule is not the focus of this chapter, discussing the pathologic features of this neoplasm is important in order to distinguish from LG-ESS. Endometrial stromal nodules are benign tumors. The majority of endometrial stromal nodules are isolated yellow myometrial masses without endometrial involvement. They are typically well defined and circumscribe with a softer consistency compared to leiomyoma.[15] Histologically, endometrial stromal nodules have similar features as compared to LG-ESS and are characterized by proliferative endometrium appearance. Moreover, immunostaining and molecular abnormalities are similar in both endometrial stromal nodules and LG-ESS. In contrast to LG-ESS, endometrial stromal nodules do not display lymphovascular invasion, and the absence of invasion is the diagnostic hallmark to distinguish between LG-ESS and endometrial stromal nodules.[15]

Pathologic Characteristics of LG-ESS

LG-ESSs are low-grade sarcomas characterized by uniform cells characteristic of endometrial stromal differentiation with minimal cellular pleomorphism and mild nuclear atypia (Table 23.1). Mitotic figures may be present but do not appear to confer a worse prognosis. LG-ESSs also demonstrate myometrial and/or vascular invasion.[15] Grossly they are often recognized at the time of hysterectomy specimen evaluation by the characteristic "tongue-like" or "finger-like" pattern of myometrial invasion and involvement of the vasculature. As noted above, they have similar histologic features of endometrial stromal nodules. The differential diagnosis may include endometrial stromal nodule, intravascular leiomyomatosis, leiomyosarcoma, uterine tumors with ovarian sex cord-like features, fibromyxosarcoma, solitary fibrous tumor/hemangiopericytoma, and gastrointestinal stromal tumors. Diagnosis can be challenging owing to the presence of various histologic findings, including collagen bands, smooth muscle, skeletal muscle, cholesterol clefts, histiocytes, sex cord, glandular components, fibromyxoid, and rhabdoid features.[1,6,15] Smooth muscle differentiation is present in approximately 45% of cases and about 25% exhibit sex cord-like differentiation. LG-ESS may also mimic fibromyxosarcoma, solitary fibrous tumor/hemangiopericytoma, and gastrointestinal stromal tumor with spindled tumor cells appearing fibroblastic or myofibroblastic-like. Even more challenging, metastatic LG-ESS may appear different from the primary tumor.[1] The "tongue-like" invasive pattern helps distinguish LG-ESS from leiomyosarcomas that have a more destructive infiltrative pattern.[6,15]

LG-ESSs commonly express estrogen receptors (ERs) alpha, progesterone receptors (PRs) and androgen receptors (ARs). These tumors are often strongly positive for CD10 (75%–90%), usually exhibit positive staining for smooth-muscle actin and WT-1, less commonly for desmin (30%) and nuclear beta-catenin expression (40%). LG-ESSs are negative for h-caldesmon and HDAC8. Ki67 is less than 5%.[3,15,16]

Pathologic Characteristics of HG-ESS

HG-ESSs are malignant neoplasms notable for endometrial stroma differentiation and characterized by high-grade nuclear atypia.[1,15] The nuclei are larger, more angulated, and irregular compared

TABLE 23.1 Pathologic Characteristics, Immunohistochemical Staining, and Molecular Abnormalities of Endometrial Stromal Sarcomas

<table>
<tr><th>Endometrial Stromal Sarcoma Type</th><th colspan="2">Pathologic Characteristics</th><th>Immunohistochemical Profile</th><th>Molecular Abnormalities</th></tr>
<tr><td>Low-grade endometrial stromal sarcoma</td><td colspan="2">• Uniform cells characteristic of endometrial stromal differentiation
• Minimal cellular pleomorphism
• Mild nuclear atypia
• Myometrial and/or vascular invasion described as “tongue-like,” “finger-like,” or “wormlike”</td><td>• ER alpha, PR, AR positive
• CD10 positive
• Desmin, caldesmon +/–
• Cyclin D1 negative or 5% focal positive
• BCOR +/–
• Ki67 <5%</td><td>JAZF1/SUZ12, JAZF1/PHF1, EPC1/PHF1, EPC2/PHF1, MEAF6/PHF1, MBTD1/Cxorf67</td></tr>
<tr><td>High-grade endometrial stromal sarcoma</td><td colspan="4"></td></tr>
<tr><td>YWHAE-altered</td><td rowspan="2">• Endometrial stroma differentiation
• High-grade nuclear atypia
• Destructive myometrial and/ or vascular invasion similar
• High mitotic activity</td><td>• May be associated with LG-ESS morphology</td><td>• ER, PR, CD10 negative except in areas of LG-ESS morphology
• Desmin, caldesmon +/–
• Cyclin D1 positive
• BCOR positive
• May be KIT positive, but DOG1 negative
• CD56, CD99 positive diffuse
• Ki67 ≥5%,</td><td>YWHAE/NUTM2A/B fusion</td></tr>
<tr><td>BCOR-altered</td><td>• Myxoid background; spindled and round cell morphology
• BCOR ITD–round cell morphology</td><td>• CD10 positive (BCOR fusion)
• CD10+/– (BCOR ITD)
• ER, PR +/–
• Desmin, caldesmon +/–
• Cyclin D1 positive
• BCOR ±
• Ki67 ≥5%</td><td>ZC3H7B–BCOR fusion

BCOR ITD</td></tr>
</table>

AR, androgen receptor; ER, estrogen receptor; ITD, internal tandem duplication; LG-ESS, low-grade endometrial stromal sarcoma; PR, progesterone receptor.

Source: From Parra-Herran C, Howitt BE. Uterine mesenchymal tumors: update on classification, staging, and molecular features. *Surg Pathol Clin*. 2019;12(2):363–396. doi:10.1016/j.path.2019.01.004; Juckett LT, Lin DI, Madison R, et al. A pan-cancer landscape analysis reveals a subset of endometrial stromal and pediatric tumors defined by internal tandem duplications of BCOR. *Oncology*. 2019;96(2):101–109. doi:10.1159/000493322; McCluggage WG, Lee CH. YWHAE-NUTM2A/B translocated high-grade endometrial stromal sarcoma commonly expresses CD56 and CD99. *Int J Gynecol Pathol*. 2019;38:528–532. doi:10.1097/pgp.0000000000000554; Brunetti M, Gorunova L, Davidson B, et al. Identification of an fusion transcript in low-grade endometrial stromal sarcoma. *Oncotarget*. 2018;9(27):19203–19208. doi:10.18632/oncotarget.24969.

to those in LG-ESS.[1] These tumors may also demonstrate the “finger-like” invasive pattern into the myometrium analogous to LG-ESS, but demonstrate more extensive and destructive invasion. Mitotic activity is common and consistently >10 per 10 HPFs. HG-ESSs more commonly demonstrate tumor cell necrosis. The histologic variations seen in LG-ESS, such as glandular and sex cord-like patterns, are rarely present.[1,6] The morphology of HG-ESS varies based on the molecular subtype (Table 23.1).

HG-ESS are subclassified based on molecular alterations and the different subtypes may have distinguishing morphology: (a) YWHAE-NUTMN2 altered HG-ESS and (b) BCL6 corepressor (BCOR) altered HG-ESS.[15] The *BCOR* altered tumors represent a second form of HG-ESS and may be due to either *ZC3H7B-BCOR* gene fusions or *BCOR* internal tandem duplication (ITD).[17] The *YWHAE-NUTMN2* HG-ESSs have uniform epithelial cells arranged in nests associated by a delicate and branching vasculature. They are associated with typical LG-ESS morphologic appearance. The nuclei may exhibit increased pleomorphism and mitoses are present, but bizarre atypia should not be present. In contrast, the *BCOR* altered tumors have a different microscopic appearance, characterized by spindle cells and a prominent myxoid stroma. *ZC3H7B-BCOR* associated HG-ESS is characteristic of a new subset of myxoid HG-ESSs, which share morphologic overlap with myxoid LMS.[18] The *BCOR* ITD sarcomas often have a round cell component.[19]

HG-ESS are typically negative or have limited ER alpha, PR, and AR expression. HG-ESSs exhibit strong and diffuse cyclin D1 immunostaining.[16] HG-ESSs have been reported to staining positively for c-KIT, but negative for DOG1.[3] The two HG-ESS subtypes have different staining patterns (Table 23.1). For example, the *YWHAE-NUTMN2* HG-ESS may exhibit CD10, ER, and PR staining in the low-grade component. In contrast, CD10, ER, and PR staining is absent or only focally positive in the high-grade component of these tumors. *YWHAE-NUTMN2* HG-ESSs are strongly positive cyclin D1 in the high-grade areas, c-KIT negative, and demonstrate Ki67 ≥5%. Positive diffuse staining for CD56 and CD99 has also been reported.[20] *BCOR* altered tumors may be due to either *ZC3H7B/ BCOR* fusion or *BCOR* ITD. *BCOR* altered HG-ESS exhibit strongly positive cyclin D1 staining and higher Ki67 ≥5%. They may have limited ER/PR positivity. *BCOR* fusion HG-ESSs are strongly positive for CD10, while *BCOR* internal tandem duplication exhibit either focal/patchy CD10 positivity or are CD10 negative. Both *YWHAE-NUTMN2* and *BCOR* altered HG-ESSs demonstrate BCOR expression.[5,15]

MOLECULAR ABERRATIONS OF ENDOMETRIAL STROMAL SARCOMAS

Molecular genomic characterization in ESS can be very helpful to distinguish between low- and high-grade disease. Gene rearrangements, such as translocations, are common in both types of endometrial sarcomas.[15] However, the types of translocation, generation of fusion proteins, and oncologic potential of the aberration varies in LG-ESS compared to HG-ESS. The research continues to evolve, with several new translocations reported recently.

Molecular Aberrations of LG-ESS

LG-ESS have molecular features characterized by gene translocations. There are several of these translocations resulting in gene fusions, and most commonly the *JAZF1* gene is involved.[15] Translocations frequently involve chromosomes 6p, 7p, and 17q. One such translocation, t(7;17), *JAZF1/SUZ12* (formerly *JAZF1/JJAZ1)* is present in up to 50% of LG-ESS. The translocation is the result of the fusion of two zinc finger genes, *JAZF1* and *SUZ12* (formerly *JJAZ1*), and creation of the JAZF1/SUZ12 fusion protein.[1,15] While commonly seen in LG-ESS, this translocation has not been found in other uterine sarcomas or smooth-muscle neoplasms.

Other translocations and gene fusion proteins have been identified in LG-ESS and often involve the *PHF1* gene. These rearrangements include t(6;7), t(6;10), t(2;6), t(1;6), t(5;6) and their resulting fusion gene products: JAZF1/PHF1, EPC1/PHF1, EPC2/PHF1, MEAF6/PHF1, BRD8/PHF1, respectively.[15,21] When translocations are present, the type and frequency are as follows: *JAZF1/SUZ12* (80%); *JAZF1/PHF1* (6%), *EPC1/PHF1* (4%), *MEAF6/PHF1* (3%), *MBTD1/Cxorf67* (2%).[15]

Molecular Aberrations of HG-ESS

HG-ESS are characterized by molecular aberrations, and it was the discovery of the *YWHAE-NUTM2* fusion genes (formerly known as *YWHAE/FAM22A/B*) gene rearrangement that helped redefine the HG-ESS category in the WHO 2014 classification system.[1] HG-ESSs are subclassified by type of molecular alterations: the *YWHAE*-altered HG-ESS and *BCOR*-altered HG-ESS. *BCOR*-altered HG-ESS comprise tumors that have either *ZC3H7B-BCOR* gene fusions or *BCOR* ITD.[15,17,19] *YWHAE-NUTM2* fusion genes represent a common t(10;17) translocation.[15] Molecular testing to identify fusion transcripts may be very helpful to distinguishing between LG-ESS, HG-ESS, and other types of mesenchymal neoplasms as well as assist in the diagnosis of the ESS subtypes, *YWHAE-NUTM2* and *BCOR* altered tumors. *BCOR*-associated ESSs have been classified as low-grade as well as high-grade ESS tumors.[22] The clinical relevance of the molecular alterations is not fully understood. Given the literature reports regarding a more aggressive clinical course, the *BCOR*-associated ESS will be considered in the HG-ESS category. Other novel gene rearrangements, for example, *EPC1-SUZ12*, *EPC1-BCOR*, and *NTRK* fusions, have been reported.[17,23]

STAGING FOR ENDOMETRIAL STROMAL SARCOMAS

Historically uterine sarcomas were staged using a staging system proposed for endometrial cancers in 1988. In 2009, a new International Federation of Gynecology and Obstetrics (FIGO) staging system was developed specifically for uterine sarcomas. This new staging system had two divisions, one for ESS and leiomyosarcoma, and the other one for adenosarcoma.[3] Currently, staging for ESS utilizes the

TABLE 23.2 Staging of Uterine Sarcomas: Leiomyosarcomas and Endometrial Stromal Sarcomas

TNM	FIGO	Definition
T1	I	Tumor confined to the uterus
T1a	IA	Tumor is 5 cm or less in greatest dimension
T1b	IB	Tumor is more than 5 cm in greatest dimension
T2	II	Tumor extends beyond the uterus, within the pelvis
T2a	IIA	Tumor involves adnexa
T2b	IIB	Tumor involves other pelvic tissue
T3	III	Tumor involves abdominal tissues (not just protruding into the abdomen)
T3a	IIIA	Tumor extends to one abdominal site
T3b	IIIB	Tumor extends to more than one abdominal site
N1	IIIC	Tumor involves pelvic and/or para-aortic lymph nodes
T4	IVA	Tumor invades bladder and/or rectal mucosa
M1	IVB	Distant metastases, excluding adnexa, pelvic, and abdominal tissues

FIGO, Federation of Gynecology and Obstetrics staging system; TNM, tumor, node, metastasis staging system.
Source: National Comprehensive Cancer Network. *Uterine Neoplasms Version 3.2019*. https://www.nccn.org/professionals/physician_gls/

2017 Tumor, Node, Metastasis (TNM) staging system of the combined American Joint Committee on Cancer/Union for International Cancer Control (AJCC/UICC) and the FIGO staging system (Table 23.2). Importantly, ESS are not surgically staged and lymphadenectomy does not have therapeutic value and is not routinely recommended for staging purposes.[3,8,11]

In the eighth edition of the AJCC *Cancer Staging Manual*, the grading of ESS follows a two-tier system of low- and high-grade and uses the prior staging definitions as per the TNM and FIGO systems. Staging for ESS is based on tumor size, given that these tumors by definition invade the myometrium. The cut-off for tumor size for staging purposes is 5 cm; stage IA, <5 cm; stage IB, >5 cm. Tumor size measurements can be compromised by tumor fragmentation or distortion. Thus, correlation with imaging and intraoperative findings to allow estimation of tumor size is imperative.[15]

GENERAL THERAPEUTIC APPROACH FOR NEWLY DIAGNOSED ENDOMETRIAL STROMAL SARCOMAS

Surgery

The surgical management of LG-ESS and HG-ESS is similar. A diagnosis of ESS should elicit an expert pathologic review for confirmation. Whether the malignancy is diagnosed preoperatively or postoperatively, ER/PR testing and imaging can be helpful to determine the type of procedure and surgical approach. CT imaging of the chest, abdomen, and pelvis can assess for distant metastases and direct surgical planning.[12]

Primary Surgical Management

Primary surgical management for disease limited to the uterus includes total hysterectomy. In patients undergoing hysterectomy for a known biopsy-confirmed diagnosis of uterine sarcoma, morcellation should be avoided. Bilateral salpingo-oophorectomy is preferred, especially in those with LG-ESS and ER positive disease. The decision to perform oophorectomy is challenging in premenopausal women, as extrauterine disease has been reported in approximately 30%, commonly with ovarian metastases, at the time of initial presentation.[8] However, this data must be interpreted cautiously as these studies were conducted prior to the 2014 change in uterine stromal neoplasm classification.

If metastatic disease is identified intraoperatively, additional surgical resection may be considered.[12] However, there is limited literature regarding the role of surgery in patients with extrauterine disease conducted after the 2014 WHO classification system. Moreover, prior studies have been too small to have adequate power to determine the benefit of surgery in this patient population.[24] Therefore, the management of extrauterine disease should be individualized based on National Comprehensive Cancer Network (NCCN) guidelines.[12] When extrauterine disease is known or suspected, surgical resection is based on extent of disease, resectability, and symptoms. If the disease is amenable to resection, total hysterectomy with or without bilateral salpingo-oophorectomy and metastasectomy should be considered. In some situations surgical resection is not possible or the patient is not a candidate for primary surgery.[12]

In most cases, diagnosis of LG-ESS or HG-ESS is made following hysterectomy or myomectomy. As mentioned previously, expert pathologic review, ER/PR testing, and imaging to assess for metastatic disease are helpful for surgical planning. If supracervical hysterectomy was performed, surgical evaluation and trachelectomy can be considered. If the ovaries were preserved at the time of hysterectomy, a repeat surgical procedure to remove the ovaries is controversial.[12] There are conflicting data regarding ovarian preservation and survival outcomes (see "Fertility Preservation"). According to NCCN guidelines, oophorectomy can be considered, especially in LG-ESS or ER-positive tumor. If diagnosis was made after an uncontained morcellation procedure or fragmentation of tumor, reexploration can be considered, especially if there is concern for disease on imaging. If a second surgery is performed, some experts also recommend peritoneal and omental biopsies, but surgery for staging purposes only is not recommended.[12]

Role of Lymphadenectomy

Lymphadenectomy for staging purposes is not recommended for ESS.[8] The probability of lymph node metastases in early-stage ESS is less than 10% (range: 2.2%–33%).[1,5,11] However, the reports with higher rates of lymphatic disease were performed prior to the 2014 classification system change and probably do not reflect rates for ESS. Nodal metastases do portend a worse progress; however, lymphadenectomy does not seem to enhance survival outcomes.[6] A meta-analysis of 11 studies in women with ESS concluded that lymphadenectomy was not associated with improved survival outcomes.[18]

Radiation

Radiation therapy can be utilized in several settings in women with ESS. In general, radiation can be used to treat those with unresectable metastatic disease or patients who are not candidates for primary surgical management as well as in the adjuvant setting for women with select stages. Adjuvant radiation is not typically recommended in women with stage I disease.[12] Radiation can be considered for those with stage II-IV LG-ESS; however, there is no clear evidence that radiation therapy will improve survival.[12] Given the excellent prognosis of LG-ESS, conflicting data regarding adjuvant radiotherapy, and the long-term risks of radiation (for example, fibrosis, stricture, fistula, and second malignancies), the use of adjuvant radiation therapy should be individualized.[12] Adjuvant radiation therapy with or without systemic chemotherapy is more commonly considered for women with stage II, III, and IV HG-ESS because of the high risk of recurrence with this disease. Palliative radiation is considered for those women with unresectable, or stage IVB disease.[12] A prospective Phase III trial of adjuvant pelvic radiation was performed in women with uterine sarcoma. However, the ESS cohort was too small to confidently interpret the results.[25]

Hormonal Therapy

Hormonal therapy, also referred to as endocrine therapy is the cornerstone of management for women with LG-ESS.[12] Hormonal adjuvant therapy is recommended for women with stage II–IV disease, as well as for treatment for those with advanced or recurrent disease. In comparison, endocrine therapy in not typically recommended for HG-ESS. There are several options for hormonal therapy in LG-ESS including the following: progestin therapy with either medroxyprogesterone acetate, megestrol acetate; aromatase inhibitors; and gonadotropin-releasing hormone analogs. There is also a report of disease stabilization with fulvestrant, a pure ER-antagonist.[12,14] Selective estrogen receptor modulators (SERMs), such as tamoxifen, and estrogen replacement therapy are generally contraindicated as they may increase the risk of tumor progression and recurrence.[5]

For those with stage II-IV LG-ESS, NCCN guidelines include adjuvant hormonal therapy based on retrospective studies and increased risk of recurrence in women with locally advanced and advanced stage disease.[6,12,26] The retrospective series are limited by small numbers, but did demonstrate a reduction in recurrence with use of adjuvant hormonal therapy. A review by Zang et al. reported seven retrospective studies; six concluded that adjuvant progestin therapy yielded a lower recurrence rate compared to those who had surgery only. In one study, patients with either stage I disease (14.3% vs. 38.5%), or in all stages (33% vs. 50%) treated with adjuvant progestins had a lower recurrence rate compared to no adjuvant therapy. The recurrence-free interval ranged from 18 to 56 months.[7] A small retrospective study evaluating adjuvant progestins and aromatase inhibitors in women with stage I LG-ESS reported a significant reduction of recurrence with either progestins (7.7%) or aromatase inhibitors (14.3%) compared to no adjuvant therapy (70%). The study is too small to compare the efficacy of progestins to aromatase inhibitors. However, 69% of patients decreased or discontinued progestin therapy because of toxicity. In contrast, none of the patients taking aromatase inhibitors prematurely discontinued therapy.[26]

The duration of adjuvant hormonal therapy has not been formally evaluated. For stage I disease, adjuvant therapy may be offered for at least 2 years. The duration for those with stage II–IV disease may be extended up to 5 years or indefinitely.[6] The duration of adjuvant hormonal therapy should be based on stage of disease, status of disease, and importantly, patient tolerability. Consideration of long-term hormonal therapy and side effects should be reviewed. For instance, progestin therapy toxicity includes depression, weight gain, and thromboembolism complications, while aromatase inhibitors are notable for hot flashes, fatigue, arthralgia, and osteoporosis.[7]

Chemotherapy

Chemotherapy may be used in women with ESS as adjuvant therapy to prevent recurrence as well as in those with metastatic or recurrent disease. Chemotherapy is more commonly used for women with HG-ESS, but may be considered in women with LG-ESS who have persistent/recurrent disease and no longer are responding to hormonal therapy.[6] According to NCCN guidelines, management options for stage I disease include consideration of adjuvant chemotherapy, but observation is the preferred strategy. In addition, consideration of systemic adjuvant chemotherapy with or without radiation therapy is appropriate for patients with stage II–III HG-ESS disease due to the high risk for relapse.[12] Unfortunately, robust prospective clinical trials of adjuvant therapy in HG-ESS are lacking. However, a Phase III randomized trial that compared adjuvant chemotherapy (gemcitabine/docetaxel followed by doxorubicin) versus observation (allowed hormonal therapy) in patients with high-grade stage I and II uterine leiomyosarcoma did not demonstrate improved survival with chemotherapy compared to observation.[27] The trials was stopped prematurely because of lack of enrollment and was closed for futility. A restricted mean survival time analysis was conducted and demonstrated overall survival of 34.3 months with chemotherapy compared to 46.4 months in the observation arm.

Chemotherapy with or without radiation is typically recommended for those with stage IVB disease, incomplete resection, or metastatic disease.[12] Recommendations for chemotherapy regimens for HG-ESS are based on studies in soft tissue sarcomas and uterine leiomyosarcoma. Further detail regarding chemotherapy is provided in the section "Therapeutic Approach for Metastatic Disease."

FERTILITY PRESERVATION

Fertility preservation may be an issue in premenopausal women with ESS. Desire for future fertility should be discussed at the initial consultation visit and referral to a specialist in Reproductive Endocrinology and Fertility should be strongly considered. With regard to ovarian and uterine preservation, there are limited and controversial data. There are conflicting guidelines regarding oophorectomy for women with ESS. The NCCN clinical practice guidelines suggest consideration for oophorectomy for patients with LG-ESS.[12] European Society for Medical Oncology–European Reference Network (ESMO–EURACAN) Clinical Practice Guidelines state that the value of bilateral salpingo-oophorectomy is not yet established.[28] The Gynecologic Cancer InterGroup (GCIG) recommends consideration for ovarian preservation in young women with small tumors.[29]

Ovarian preservation may increase risk of recurrence, but has not been found to negatively affect survival.[6,29–32] One study reported on patients with LG-ESS treated from 1985 to 2014 and found a non-significant longer progression-free survival for those who underwent bilateral salpingo-oophorectomy compared with those who preserved their ovaries (38 vs. 11 months, p = .071).[31] A study using the National Cancer Institute's Surveillance, Epidemiology, and End Results (SEER) database included women younger than 50 years of age with uterine sarcomas from 1988 to 2013. For the 520 women with LG-ESS, ovarian preservation was not associated with worse overall survival (p = .41) or cancer-specific survival (p = .56).[29] In a systematic review of the literature and meta-analysis, 17 studies and 786 patients (190 with ovarian preservation and 501 with oophorectomy) were included to assess recurrence and survival outcomes. The ovarian preservation group had a significantly increased recurrence rate (46.8% vs. 24.2%; odds ratio [OR] 2.70, 95% confidence interval [CI] 1.39 to 5.28), but no difference in death rates (OR 0.80, 95% CI 0.18 to 3.47) compared with the oophorectomy group.[32]

Premenopausal patients who underwent a myomectomy may express interest in uterine preservation. There is limited literature to inform management decisions. There may be a higher risk of recurrence in women who undergo myomectomy compared to hysterectomy. Specifically, Bai et al. reported a retrospective study of 19 women who underwent myomectomy compared to 134 who underwent hysterectomy using the 2003 WHO classification system. The findings indicated a higher risk of relapse in the myomectomy group (79% vs. 25%).[30] However, there was no difference for survival outcomes. A literature review identified eight studies that included women with uterine preservation and incorporated adjuvant progestin therapy for women potentially desiring fertility. Of the 25 women, 15 pregnancies were conceived, with 14 successful deliveries. Assisted reproductive techniques were employed in three of the 15 pregnancies (20%). Eight women developed recurrent disease and one died of disease.[7] Myomectomy may be offered as an option for patients with LG-ESS who strongly desire fertility and after extensive counseling regarding risk of recurrence and long-term surveillance. Other options such as surrogacy should also be discussed. Once childbearing is complete or fertility is no longer an issue, hysterectomy should be strongly considered.

RECOMMENDED FOLLOW-UP

Patients should be counseled regarding their risk of recurrence; symptoms and signs of recurrence; and surveillance recommendations. Patients experiencing abnormal symptoms should contact their care providers expeditiously. Symptoms of recurrence include abnormal vaginal or rectal bleeding, hematuria, pain, loss of appetite, cough, shortness of breath, and abdominal swelling.[12] Surveillance for patients with ESS includes history with physical examination every 3 to 4 months for the first 2 to 3 years and then every 6 to 12 months. Imaging surveillance is recommended and should include CT scans of the chest, abdomen, and pelvis every 3 to 6 months for the first 3 years and then every 6 to 12 months for the next 2 years.[12] After 5 years, surveillance history and physical exam may be extended to every 12 months. The role of continued CT scans surveillance imaging should be based on histology, grade, and stage at the time of initial diagnosis. Moreover, the risk of recurrence versus increased radiation exposure risk from CT imaging should be considered and discussed with the patient.

PROGNOSIS, PROPENSITY TO METASTASIZE, AND COMMON METASTATIC SITES

The literature regarding the prognosis for ESS is complicated because of the changing nomenclature. Despite these limitations, the prognosis for women with LG-ESS is significantly better compared to those with HG-ESS. HG-ESSs are more aggressive tumors and are more likely to recur. HG-ESSs have a worse prognosis with higher risk for death compared to LG-ESS, but better prognosis compared to undifferentiated uterine sarcomas.[6]

LG-ESSs typically present with intrauterine disease; however, metastatic disease has been reported in 30%. Recurrence rates range from 30% to 56%, late recurrences being common, and 15% to 25% of patients succumb to recurrent disease.[3,7,8,16] The most common sites are in the abdomen/pelvis (40%–50%) and lung (25%). However, lymphatic and spinal metastases as well as hematologic recurrences have also been reported.[6] Lymph node metastases range from 2.2% to 33% of patients.[1,5,30] However, some of this data was reported prior to the change in the 2014 classification and one study also included patients with recurrent disease.[33] Therefore, the higher rate of lymph node metastases in older studies may not be representative for LG-ESS.

HG-ESS are more likely to present with advanced stage, develop recurrent disease within a year, and have a shorter median overall survival (range, 11–23 months).[3,6,9,34] In one study, 42.5% presented with stage 1 disease, while almost 60% had metastatic disease at the time of diagnosis. Over 70% of patients developed recurrent disease with abdominopelvic sites (42.5%) and distant metastasis (30%) including lung, liver, brain, and spine. Prognostic clinicopathologic features for HG-ESS also include elevated cancer antigen 125 (CA125), endometriosis, larger tumor size, and postmenopausal status, which are associated with worse survival outcomes.[34] Prognosis for HG-ESS varies based on type of molecular alterations.[15]

Tumor grade and stage are the most significant prognostic factors for ESS. A SEER analysis of ESS attempted to assess survival outcomes based on 2003 WHO classification by separating tumors by grade (1–3). Grades 1 and 2 disease was used to define LG-ESS, while grade 3 represented HG-ESS and UUS. Independent pathologic confirmation was not performed. The 5-year disease-free survival rate by grade was 91.4% for grade 1 disease; 95.4%, grade 2; and 42.1%, grade 3.[35]

Molecular alterations, such as, *YWHAE* altered and *BCOR* fusion HG-ESS have a more aggressive clinical phenotype compared with LG-ESS.[15] Patients with the *YWHAE-FAM22* translocation, which is characteristic of HG-ESS, have worse survival outcomes compared to those with *JAZF1* rearrangements, which are present in LG-ESS. Specifically, of 10 patients with *YWHAE-FAM22* alteration, two died of disease within 2 years; seven were alive with disease, and only one had no evidence of disease.[6,36] In comparison, in 17 patients with *JAZF1*-associated LG-ESS, 13 had no evidence of disease with an average follow up of 10 years, two were alive with disease, and two had died of disease. Of the two who died of disease, one expired within 1 month, while the other patient succumbed 9 years after her initial diagnosis).[6,37,38] *BCOR* ITD sarcomas may be more indolent and have a favorable clinical prognosis compared to other HG-ESS.[15]

Uncontained morcellation in women with LG-ESS who underwent uterine morcellation had an increased recurrence rate (31.4% vs. 7.4%) and decreased 5-year disease-free survival compared with those who did not have a morcellation (55% vs. 84%; OR 4.03, 95% CI 1.06–15.3). However, no significant impact on overall survival (OS) was reported.[6,39] In another study, laparoscopic hysterectomy and transvaginal scalpel morcellation of unsuspected ESS did not appear to increase intraperitoneal dissemination or recurrence risk.[40] However, these studies contain a small number of patients with limited follow-up. Manual morcellation that is not contained within a protective bag and power morcellation should be avoided in the setting of known biopsy-confirmed diagnosis of uterine sarcoma.

THERAPEUTIC APPROACH FOR METASTATIC DISEASE

The therapeutic approach for women with recurrent or metastatic disease ESS differs based on the low- or high-grade classification. Treatment options include surgery, hormonal therapy, chemotherapy, and/or radiation. Hormonal therapy is preferred for LG-ESS, while chemotherapy is the recommended option for systemic therapy in women with HG-ESS. Consideration for clinical trial participation should strongly be considered for patients with disseminated metastatic disease. Novel therapeutic options including biologic therapy and immunologic approaches are being considered. Further studies are needed to explore innovative combinations of known treatment options (radiation, endocrine therapy, and chemotherapy) with immunologic and biologic therapeutic strategies.

Therapy for Metastatic LG-ESS

Hormonal therapy is the cornerstone of treatment for women with LG-ESS. Treatment for stage II, III, and IV LG-ESS includes recommendation for estrogen-blockade in the front-line setting either alone or combined with external beam radiation therapy. Commonly used hormonal therapies are listed in the section "General Therapeutic Approach for Newly Diagnosed Endometrial Stromal Sarcomas." In brief, there are numerous hormonal therapies comprising the following options: progestin therapy (medroxyprogesterone acetate and megestrol acetate); aromatase inhibitors; gonadotropin-releasing hormone analogs; and an ER-antagonist.[6,7,12,14]

A review of hormonal therapy for treatment of recurrent or metastatic LG-ESS indicated disease control rates (response rate plus disease stabilization) of 87% to 89% with either progestin therapy or aromatase inhibitors.[7] Long-term responders are common. Appropriate sequencing and combination of hormonal therapy is unknown, and there is not sufficient prospective comparison of these therapies to inform treatment management. However, the toxicity profile may drive treatment recommendations. A small retrospective study of adjuvant hormonal therapy revealed a higher rate of dose reduction or premature discontinuation in patients taking progestin therapy compared to aromatase inhibitors (69% vs 0%, respectively).[26]

Hormonal therapy should still be considered beyond front-line treatment in those who progress. A small study of patients with LG-ESS previously treated with hormonal therapy demonstrated a 100% disease control rate as manifested by stable disease >6 months with second-line hormonal therapy.[6,41] For patients with LG-ESS who progress despite endocrine therapy, systemic chemotherapy or biologic therapy may be considered. See the section "Therapy for Metastatic HG-ESS" for discussion of chemotherapy regimens.

Therapy for Metastatic HG-ESS

Current guidelines recommend consideration of systemic adjuvant chemotherapy with or without radiation for patients with stage II–IVA HG-ESS. Chemotherapy is also recommended for patients with IVB disease and those with metastatic disease. Chemotherapy regimens are based on data extrapolated from soft tissue sarcoma and uterine leiomyosarcoma. Preferred first-line regimens are doxorubicin plus ifosfamide, single-agent doxorubicin, and gemcitabine plus docetaxel.[12] The GeDDiS trial was a randomized controlled Phase III trial comparing doxorubicin (control arm) to the combination gemcitabine plus docetaxel (experimental arm). There was no significant difference in progression-free survival rates at 24 weeks (46.3% vs. 46.4%) and median progression-free survival (23.3 weeks vs. 23.7 weeks) between those who received doxorubicin versus those who received gemcitabine and docetaxel.[42] Doxorubicin plus ifosfamide has nearly twice the response rate and a superior progression-free survival than single-agent doxorubicin in patients with soft tissue sarcoma.[12] The findings support doxorubicin plus ifosfamide or as single agent for the frail or elderly as the standard first-line treatment for patients with advanced soft tissue sarcoma.

Other chemotherapy options include dacarbazine, gemcitabine, epirubicin, ifosfamide, liposomal doxorubicin, pazopanib, temozolomide, vinorelbine, eribulin, and docetaxel. Combination regimens such as combination doxorubicin with dacarbazine; or gemcitabine with either dacarbazine or vinorelbine may be considered.[12]

Biologic and immunologic agents are also of interest. Tuyaerts and Amant provided a rationale to support immunotherapy approaches (vaccination, adoptive transfer of tumor-infiltrating lymphocytes, and T-cells engineered with a translocation breakpoint-specific T-cell receptor strategies) to treat ESS given the presence of translocation fusion breakpoints characteristic of both low- and high-grade ESS.[9] Further understanding of the underlying molecular biology, tumor microenvironment, and immunogenicity in ESS will help direct biologic, immunologic, and combination therapies in the future.

Surgery for Metastatic Endometrial Stromal Sarcoma

Surgery is a reasonable option for women with isolated metastatic recurrent disease.[12] Surgery is more likely to be considered in women with recurrent LG-ESS, given the more indolent nature of this disease.[6,43] Women with HG-ESS and isolated metastatic disease may also be candidates for surgery, especially those with long recurrence-free intervals.[6]

Radiation for Metastatic Endometrial Stromal Sarcoma

Palliative radiation is considered for those women with stage IVB disease, unresectable recurrent disease, or disseminated recurrent metastatic disease.[12] In the event of radiologically isolated metastasis, the use of radiation is dependent on location of disease, status of resectability, and prior radiation history. External beam radiation therapy either alone or in conjunction with systemic chemotherapy may be considered for those with unresectable disease or postoperatively for patients managed with surgical resection.[12] For those with isolated vaginal or pelvic recurrences, vaginal brachytherapy can be added, however, the use of brachytherapy and dosing is dependent on prior radiation history. In select cases intraoperative radiation can be an option for patients who undergo surgical exploration and resection. Reirradiation may be considered for some previously radiated patients, but that depends on site of disease, prior radiation fields, and radiation doses.[12]

SUMMARY

In conclusion, ESS is a rare subset of uterine mesenchymal neoplasms that account 0.2% to 1% of all uterine malignant neoplasms and approximately 10% to 20% of uterine sarcomas. The 2014 WHO classification system recognizes four categories of endometrial stromal neoplasms including (a) endometrial stromal nodule (ESN), (b) LG-ESS, (c) HG-ESS, and (d) UUS. LG-ESS and HG-ESS both may resemble proliferative endometrial stroma and demonstrate myometrial and vascular invasion with "tongue-like" appearance. In contrast to its low-grade counterpart, HG-ESSs tend to demonstrate high-grade nuclear atypia, pleomorphism, higher mitotic activity, and necrosis. Moreover, HG-ESSs have a more destructive and invasive growth pattern.

The majority of ESS cases are diagnosed postoperatively after hysterectomy or myomectomy. An important clinical pearl is to have a high index of suspicion in women with abnormal radiologic features. On ultrasound exam, a nonspecific pattern or appearance of a heterogeneous hypoechoic endometrial mass with myometrial involvement and increased central or peripheral vasculature should raise the index of suspicion for ESS. Key diagnostic findings on MRI include low-intensity rim on T2-weighted images indicative of hemorrhage, or "worm-like" invasive projections on diffusion-weighted imaging.

Expert pathologic review is essential to correctly diagnose LG- and HG-ESS, which can be distinguished based on morphologic features, immunostaining patterns, and molecular aberrations. LG-ESS typically are indolent tumors characterized by excellent prognosis. Overall, the survival rates are 65% to 76% at 10 years. However, the 5-year survival estimates for women with stage I and II disease is greater than 90%. In contrast, recurrence and overall survival rates for HG-ESS are worse compared to LG-ESS. Therefore, postoperative adjuvant therapy is recommended for select patients, and the type of treatment is based on histologic subtype. Adjuvant hormonal therapy is the cornerstone for treatment for women with stage II–IVA LG-ESS in order to enhance relapse-free survival. In contrast, systemic adjuvant chemotherapy is suggested for women with HG-ESS.

Close and long-term surveillance for women with ESS is important. For those with recurrent disease, there are several treatment options including surgical resection, radiation, hormonal therapy, and chemotherapy. The therapeutic management is dependent on the classification, recurrence-free interval, extent of disease, and prior therapy. Chemotherapy recommendations for women with ESS is extrapolated from available data for soft tissue sarcomas or uterine leiomyosarcomas. Consideration for clinical trial participation should strongly be considered for patients with disseminated metastatic disease.

Future directions include enhanced understanding of the molecular biology of ESS, prognostic role of gene alterations, and potential to explore novel treatment combinations including immunologic and biologic therapies.

CASE STUDY

A 50-year-old female presented for consultation and management of HG-ESS. She had been advised to initiate adjuvant chemotherapy and to consider radiation therapy by her medical oncologist. She presented with perimenopausal bleeding and a pelvic ultrasound study demonstrated an intrauterine mass felt to represent an enlarged leiomyoma with uterine size of 12 cm. She underwent vaginal hysterectomy at an outside facility with uncontained transvaginal manual morcellation. Her pathology report described an HG-ESS measuring 8 cm, with 10 mitoses/HPF, deep myometrial invasion, and lymphovascular space invasion. A complete history and physical exam was performed. The pelvic mass was negative for vaginal nodularity and adnexal masses. Consultation recommendations included CT of the chest, abdomen, and pelvis; pathologic review; and follicle-stimulating hormone. The CT scan was negative for metastatic disease and follicle-stimulating hormone was >50 IU/L. Expert pathologic review demonstrated low-grade atypia, 3 mitoses/10 HPFs, and no necrosis. Immunostaining showed positivity for CD10, ER alpha, and PR. The histologic diagnosis was LG-ESS, which was supported by molecular testing demonstrating a *JAZF1/SUZ12* fusion gene. She opted for surgical exploration and oophorectomy. Findings at the time of surgery were negative for gross evidence of disseminated disease. Bilateral salpingo-oophorectomy, omentectomy, and peritoneal biopsies were performed. Final pathologic review revealed metastatic parenchymal disease to both ovaries. There was no evidence of surface ovarian involvement. The remainder of the pathology specimens was negative. She was treated with adjuvant progestin therapy. Owing to side effects of weight gain, she opted to switch therapy to an aromatase inhibitor. She is being followed closely with surveillance exams, imaging, and dual-energy x-ray absorptiometry (DEXA) scans to assess for osteoporosis. She has been without evidence of progressive disease.

REFERENCES

1. Conklin CMJ, Longacre TA. Endometrial stromal tumors: the new WHO classification. *Adv Anat Pathol*. 2014;21(6):383–393. doi:10.1097/PAP.0000000000000046
2. Oh J, Park SB, Park HJ, Lee ES. Ultrasound features of uterine sarcomas. *Ultrasound Q*. 2019;35(4):376–384. doi:10.1097/RUQ.0000000000000454
3. Prat J, Mbatani N. Uterine sarcomas. *Int J Gynaecol Obstet*. 2015;131 (suppl 2):S105–S110. doi:10.1016/j.ijgo.2015.06.006
4. Norris HJ, Taylor HB. Mesenchymal tumors of the uterus. I. A clinical and pathological study of 53 endometrial stromal tumors. *Cancer*. 1966;19(6):755–766. doi:10.1002/1097-0142(196606)19:6<755::aid-cncr2820190604>3.0.co;2-u
5. Ali RH, Rouzbahman M. Endometrial stromal tumours revisited: an update based on the 2014 WHO classification. *J Clin Pathol*. 2015;68(5):325–332. doi:10.1136/jclinpath-2014-202829
6. Gaillard S, Secord AA. Staging, treatment, and prognosis of endometrial stromal sarcoma and related tumors and uterine adenosarcoma. In: Goff B, Garcia RL, Dizon DS, eds. *UpToDate*. 2019. https://www.uptodate.com/contents/staging-treatment-and-prognosis-of-endometrial-stromal-sarcoma-and-related-tumors-and-uterine-adenosarcoma

7. Zang Y, Dong M, Zhang K, et al. Hormonal therapy in uterine sarcomas. *Cancer Med*. 2019;8(4):1339–1349. doi:10.1002/cam4.2044
8. Mbatani N, Olawaiye AB, Prat J. Uterine sarcomas. *Int J Gynaecol Obstet*. 2018;143(suppl 2):51–58. doi:10.1002/ijgo.12613
9. Tuyaerts S, Amant F. Endometrial stromal sarcomas: a revision of their potential as targets for immunotherapy. *Vaccines (Basel)*. 2018;6(3):56. doi:10.3390/vaccines6030056
10. Bansal N, Herzog TJ, Burke W, et al. The utility of preoperative endometrial sampling for the detection of uterine sarcomas. *Gynecol Oncol*. 2008;110(1):43–48. doi:10.1016/j.ygyno.2008.02.026
11. Ghirardi V, Bizzarri N, Guida F, et al. Role of surgery in gynaecological sarcomas. *Oncotarget*. 2019;10(26):2561–2575. doi:10.18632/oncotarget.26803
12. National Comprehensive Cancer Network. *Uterine Neoplasms Version 3.2019*. https://www.nccn.org/professionals/physician_gls/
13. Kusunoki S, Terao Y, Ujihira T, et al. Efficacy of PET/CT to exclude leiomyoma in patients with lesions suspicious for uterine sarcoma on MRI. *Taiwan J Obstet Gynecol*. 2017;56(4):508–513. doi:10.1016/j.tjog.2017.05.003
14. van Kruchten M, Hospers GAP, Glaudemans AWJM, et al. Positron emission tomography imaging of oestrogen receptor-expression in endometrial stromal sarcoma supports oestrogen receptor-targeted therapy: case report and review of the literature. *Eur J Cancer*. 2013;49(18):3850–3855. doi:10.1016/j.ejca.2013.08.005
15. Parra-Herran C, Howitt BE. Uterine mesenchymal tumors: update on classification, staging, and molecular features. *Surg Pathol Clin*. 2019;12(2):363–396. doi:10.1016/j.path.2019.01.004
16. Park JY, Baek MH, Park Y, et al. Investigation of hormone receptor expression and its prognostic value in endometrial stromal sarcoma. *Virchows Arch*. 2018;473(1):61–69. doi:10.1007/s00428-018-2358-5
17. Ferreira J, Félix A, Lennerz JK, Oliva E. Recent advances in the histological and molecular classification of endometrial stromal neoplasms. *Virchows Arch*. 2018;473(6):665–678. doi:10.1007/s00428-018-2470-6
18. Gantzer J, Ray-Coquard I. Gynecological sarcomas: what's new in 2018, a brief review of published literature. *Curr Opin Oncol*. 2018;30(4):246–251. doi:10.1097/CCO.0000000000000462
19. Juckett LT, Lin DI, Madison R, et al. A pan-cancer landscape analysis reveals a subset of endometrial stromal and pediatric tumors defined by internal tandem duplications of BCOR. *Oncology*. 2019;96(2):101–109. doi:10.1159/000493322
20. McCluggage WG, Lee CH. YWHAE-NUTM2A/B translocated high-grade endometrial stromal sarcoma commonly expresses CD56 and CD99. *Int J Gynecol Pathol*. 2019;38:528–532. doi:10.1097/pgp.0000000000000554
21. Brunetti M, Gorunova L, Davidson B, et al. Identification of an fusion transcript in low-grade endometrial stromal sarcoma. *Oncotarget*. 2018;9(27):19203–19208. doi:10.18632/oncotarget.24969
22. Mansor S, Kuick CH, Lim SL, et al. ZC3H7B-BCOR-rearranged endometrial stromal sarcomas: a distinct subset merits its own classification? *Int J Gynecol Pathol*. 2019;38:420–425. doi:10.1097/pgp.0000000000000523
23. Dickson BC, Lum A, Swanson D, et al. Novel EPC1 gene fusions in endometrial stromal sarcoma. *Genes Chromosomes Cancer*. 2018;57(11):598–603. doi:10.1002/gcc.22649
24. Leath CA 3rd, Huh WK, Hyde J Jr, et al. A multi-institutional review of outcomes of endometrial stromal sarcoma. *Gynecol Oncol*. 2007;105(3):630–634. doi:10.1016/j.ygyno.2007.01.031
25. Reed NS, Mangioni C, Malmström H, et al. Phase III randomised study to evaluate the role of adjuvant pelvic radiotherapy in the treatment of uterine sarcomas stages I and II: an European Organisation for Research and Treatment of Cancer Gynaecological Cancer Group Study (protocol 55874). *Eur J Cancer*. 2008;44(6):808–818. doi:10.1016/j.ejca.2008.01.019
26. Deshmukh U, Black J, Perez-Irizarry J, et al. Adjuvant hormonal therapy for low-grade endometrial stromal sarcoma. *Reprod Sci*. 2019;26(5):600–608. doi:10.1177/1933719118778801
27. Hensley ML, Enserro D, Hatcher H, et al. Adjuvant gemcitabine plus docetaxel followed by doxorubicin versus observation for high-grade uterine leiomyosarcoma: a Phase III NRG Oncology/Gynecologic Oncology Group Study. *J Clin Oncol*. 2018;36:3324–3330. doi:10.1200/jco.18.00454
28. Casali PG, Abecassis N, Aro HT, et al. Soft tissue and visceral sarcomas: ESMO-EURACAN Clinical Practice Guidelines for diagnosis, treatment and follow-up. *Ann Oncol*. 2018;29(suppl 4):iv268–iv269. doi:10.1093/annonc/mdy321
29. Nasioudis D, Chapman-Davis E, Frey M, Holcomb K. Safety of ovarian preservation in premenopausal women with stage I uterine sarcoma. *J Gynecol Oncol*. 2017;28(4):e46. doi:10.3802/jgo.2017.28.e46
30. Bai H, Yang J, Cao D, et al. Ovary and uterus-sparing procedures for low-grade endometrial stromal sarcoma: a retrospective study of 153 cases. *Gynecol Oncol*. 2014;132(3):654–660. doi:10.1016/j.ygyno.2013.12.032
31. Stewart LE, Beck TL, Giannakopoulos NV, et al. Impact of oophorectomy and hormone suppression in low grade endometrial stromal sarcoma: a multicenter review. *Gynecol Oncol*. 2018;149(2):297–300. doi:10.1016/j.ygyno.2018.03.008
32. Nasioudis D, Ko EM, Kolovos G, et al. Ovarian preservation for low-grade endometrial stromal sarcoma: a systematic review of the literature and meta-analysis. *Int J Gynecol Cancer*. 2019;29(1):126–132. doi:10.1136/ijgc-2018-000063
33. Riopel J, Plante M, Renaud MC, et al. Lymph node metastases in low-grade endometrial stromal sarcoma. *Gynecol Oncol*. 2005;96(2):402–406. doi:10.1016/j.ygyno.2004.10.021
34. Zhang YY, Li Y, Qin M, et al. High-grade endometrial stromal sarcoma: a retrospective study of factors influencing prognosis. *Cancer Manag Res*. 2019;11:831–837. doi:10.2147/CMAR.S187849

35. Chan JK, Kawar NM, Shin JY, et al. Endometrial stromal sarcoma: a population-based analysis. *Br J Cancer*. 2008;99(8):1210–1215. doi:10.1038/sj.bjc.6604527
36. Lee CH, Mariño-Enriquez A, Ou W, et al. The clinicopathologic features of YWHAE-FAM22 endometrial stromal sarcomas: a histologically high-grade and clinically aggressive tumor. *Am J Surg Pathol*. 2012;36(5):641–653. doi:10.1097/PAS.0b013e31824a7b1a
37. Chew I, Oliva E. Endometrial stromal sarcomas: a review of potential prognostic factors. *Adv Anat Pathol*. 2010;17(2):113–121. doi:10.1097/PAP.0b013e3181cfb7c2
38. Tse KY, Crawford R, Ngan HYS. Staging of uterine sarcomas. *Best Pract Res Clin Obstet Gynaecol*. 2011;25(6):733–749. doi:10.1016/j.bpobgyn.2011.05.011
39. Park JY, Kim DY, Kim JH, et al. The impact of tumor morcellation during surgery on the outcomes of patients with apparently early low-grade endometrial stromal sarcoma of the uterus. *Ann Surg Oncol*. 2011;18(12):3453–3461. doi:10.1245/s10434-011-1751-y
40. Zhang J, Li T, Zhang J, et al. Clinical characteristics and prognosis of unexpected uterine sarcoma after hysterectomy for presumed myoma with and without transvaginal scalpel morcellation. *Int J Gynecol Cancer*. 2016;26(3):456–463. doi:10.1097/IGC.0000000000000638
41. Thanopoulou E, Aleksic A, Thway K, et al. Hormonal treatments in metastatic endometrial stromal sarcomas: the 10-year experience of the sarcoma unit of Royal Marsden Hospital. *Clin Sarcoma Res*. 2015;5:8. doi:10.1186/s13569-015-0024-0
42. Seddon B, Strauss SJ, Whelan J, et al. Gemcitabine and docetaxel versus doxorubicin as first-line treatment in previously untreated advanced unresectable or metastatic soft-tissue sarcomas (GeDDiS): a randomised controlled phase 3 trial. *Lancet Oncol*. 2017;18(10):1397–1410. doi:10.1016/S1470-2045(17)30622-8
43. Anraku M, Yokoi K, Nakagawa K, et al. Pulmonary metastases from uterine malignancies: results of surgical resection in 133 patients. *J Thorac Cardiovasc Surg*. 2004;127(4):1107–1112. doi:10.1016/j.jtcvs.2003.10.011

24

Chordoma

Jomjit Chantharasamee, Francis Hornicek, and Arun S. Singh

INTRODUCTION

Chordomas are rare bone tumors accounting for ~4% of all bony malignancies. The incidence of chordoma is approximated to be just under one case per million people and there are approximately 300 cases diagnosed per year in the United States.[1–3] Chordomas are more common in men than women and typically affect people in the fourth decade of life. The 5-year overall survival (OS) rate is reported to range from 50% to 67%, depending on the stage of the disease and the presence of relapsed or metastatic disease.[3,4]

There are various hypotheses about the pathogenesis of chordomas. One prevailing theory is that chordomas derive from the remnants of the notochord, a midline embryonal structure that plays a role in neuronal differentiation, which usually regresses during fetal development.[5–7] Currently, the molecular drivers of chordoma are still under investigation. Brachyury, vascular endothelial growth factor receptor (VEGFR), and c-KIT are putative oncogenic drivers.[8,9]

Clinically, these tumors typically grow slowly, but act in a locally invasive manner and usually occur along the axial and para-axial bones. Common locations of chordoma are the sacro-coccygeal spine, mobile spine, and skull base. Common clinical presentations, such as pain, mass effect, or cranial neuropathy vary based on the location and degree of tumor extension.[4,10–12]

The clinical management of chordomas requires a multidisciplinary approach to optimize the diagnosis and treatment plan. Expert pathologic consultation is required for this rare diagnosis. Curative surgery remains the standard treatment of chordomas. En bloc resection in conjunction with radiation is considered to be the most effective approach for localized disease.[13–17] In patients with technically inoperable disease or in patients who decline resection, high-dose radiation is an option but may have a higher rate of local progression than the combination of surgery and radiation.[17–20] Distant metastasis has been reported in 10% to 40% of patients and systemic chemotherapy has shown limited efficacy, but these have seen some promising results with the use of targeted therapy.[21–25]

PATHOGENESIS AND MOLECULAR PATHWAY

The pathogenesis of chordomas remains unclear. Various hypotheses have been proposed and the prevailing notion is that these tumors develop from notochordal remnants. The notochord is formed on day 17 of embryogenesis and migrates cranially between the ectoderm and endoderm. During fetal development, the notochord is surrounded by adjacent neuro-ectodermal tissue and is replaced by cartilage cells. Its regression remnant becomes the nucleus pulposus of the intervertebral discs. Currently, several aberrant genetic changes have been proposed to be the oncogenic drivers of chordoma.

Chromosomal Abnormalities

Theoretically, the well-known gene called "T-gene" or brachyury was considered to play a major role of both familial and sporadic chordoma development. Duplications of the brachyury gene on chromosome7, polysomy-7, or chromosome7 translocations all can cause a gain-of-function of this proto-oncogene, which induces abnormal cell growth and inhibits apoptosis within notochordal remnant cells.[26–29] Moreover, Patrick et al. have reported mutations in chromatin remodeling genes, such as *CDKN2A* and *SETD2*, in chordoma sequencing experiments.[27,30]

Mutations in Chordomas

A series of mutations have been found in chordomas, and it is unclear as yet how many are "driver" and how many are "passenger" mutations. Receptor tyrosine kinase overexpression has been detected in 77% to 99% cases.[8,9,31–34] The platelet-derived growth factor receptor (PDGFR-α and -β), c-KIT, and VEGFR can be detected in endothelial cells and various types of normal or inflammatory tissues, but rarely is expressed in normal bone or chondrocytes. These mutations have been targeted in several small studies discussed later in the chapter. Several studies reported activating mutations in the PI3K/AKT/MTOR pathway in approximately 16% of chordomas. Mutations in this pathway are a potential predictive biomarker for PI3K/MTOR inhibitor treatment.[27]

The LYST (lysosomal trafficking regulator protein) regulates intracellular protein trafficking to the endosome. It was also discovered to be a novel gene that regulates the development of chordoma in approximately 10% of cases. Abnormal regulation of this gene has been shown to result in transcription variants.

Epigenetic Change

Epigenetic changes in chordoma cell lines and tissues have been documented. However, it is unclear at this time how to take advantage of these epigenetic changes. Abnormal DNA methylation of cytosine adjacent guanine (CpG) was identified in chordoma cell lines, resulting in the silencing of several tumor suppressor genes. Hyper/hypomethylation and acetylation of histones are also found in chordoma tissues. Finally, dysregulation of microRNA has been identified; putatively, abnormal expression of specific microRNAs could initiate chordoma and facilitate tumor progression and invasion.[35–37]

CLINICAL PRESENTATION

The clinical presentation of chordomas is variable and depends on the tumor location and its extension into adjacent structures. Chordomas that arise in the mobile spine, sacrococcygeal area, and skull base all have different presentations. Typically, the clinical presentation is insidious, and most patients present with localized disease. The most common sites of metastatic disease include the lung, bone, or soft tissues, and metastasis most often occurs in patients with large primary tumors.[18] Metastatic disease can also occur late. One caveat is that the dedifferentiated variant typically has a more aggressive behavior and often presents with metastatic disease.

Spinal and Sacrococcygeal Tumor

The most common site of chordoma is S4–S5 in the sacrum. An early stage sacral chordoma can be asymptomatic or present with nonspecific pain. Patients usually experience deep pain upon tumor progression and more extensive destruction of bone. With later presentation, neurologic deficits such as weakness, paresthesias, neuropathic pain, cauda equina syndrome or bowel/bladder sphincter dysfunction can be present. Constipation can occur from rectal compression. Signs and symptoms of tumor arising in the mobile spine are similar to those for other spinal tumors. When extraosseous extension occurs, usually from the vertebral body posteriorly into the spinal canal or neural foramina, back pain, leg weakness, sensory deficit, radicular pain, abnormal deep tendon reflexes, and bowel bladder dysfunction can be present. Patients with cervical spine tumor can present with Horner syndrome due to tumor compression of the cervical sympathetic chain.[1,12,14,38]

Intracranial Tumor

Intracranial chordoma typically arises from the clivus. Headache and diplopia are the most common presenting symptoms in this situation. If the tumor extends superiorly, cavernous sinus syndrome can occur. Destructive skull base tumors can enlarge posteriorly leading to cranial neuropathies such as ophthalmopathy, trigeminal neuralgia, or facial numbness. Cerbrospinal fluid (CSF) rhinorrhea is less common. Epistaxis can occur if the tumor grows anteriorly into the nasopharynx.[10,39,40] Intracranial hemorrhage, hypopituitarism, and pituitary apoplexy have also been reported.[41]

RADIOGRAPHIC FINDINGS

CT and MRI are useful to assess the location and extension of tumor. The morphologic and contrast enhancement pattern can discriminate chordomas from the benign bone lesions, such as notochordal remnants, hematomas, bone cysts, and malignant bone tumors.

CT Scan With Contrast

CT is a highly sensitive and accurate imaging technique for bony lesions. Chordomas appear as a homogeneous mass isodense to adjacent soft tissue structures. In the contrast phase, the tumor develops heterogeneous enhancement. Calcification from bone sequestration or calcified tumor is a less common finding. These tumors are mostly central, are well circumscribed within expanded bone, and can have adjacent soft tissue extension. Bony destruction with marginal sclerosis is also common.[10,42,43]

MRI

MRI is preferred to assess soft tissue extension and neurovascular bundle involvement over CT scan but is less sensitive to detect calcification and bony osteolysis. On MRI, chordomas show low to intermediate signal intensity in T1-weighted sequences and a vivid hypersignal intensity in T2-weighted images. With gadolinium, the tumor shows heterogeneous intratumoral enhancement with a pathognomonic "honeycomb" appearance corresponding to a low signal intensity in noncontrast T1-weighted images. Some specific radiographic findings in chordomas include expansion of bone, trabeculation, and rarefaction.[10,43–45]

FDG-PET/CT

Little data is available on fluorodeoxyglucose (FDG)-PET in chordoma. Its role in tumor assessment, staging, and response evaluation is still to be defined.[46] The accuracy of FDG-PET/CT for distinguishing between low-grade malignant bone tumor and benign tumors is still under investigation. Moreover, metastases smaller than 8 mm can cause false negative readings.[47,48]

DIAGNOSTIC APPROACH

The current National Comprehensive Cancer Network (NCCN) recommendations are that chordomas and other bone malignancies should be evaluated by a multidisciplinary team at a high-volume center. Differentiating chordomas from common bone diseases is a first step in management. Tissue diagnosis is required before proceeding with curative intent. Core-needle biopsies are preferred over fine-needle aspirates as they allow the pathologist a better evaluation of the tissue architecture and help to discriminate from other bone tumors. Naturally, the biopsy technique depends on the tumor location but should be discussed in detail with the multidisciplinary team who will manage the patient to avoid inappropriate biopsy approach that may compromise planned surgery and/or radiation. Spinal tumors are readily accessible via CT-guidance or open biopsy; CT-guided core biopsy is preferred to avoid spillage of tumor. Intracranial tumors may require an endoscopic biopsy.

PATHOLOGY

Chordomas are classified into four different variants: conventional, chondroid, dedifferentiated, and poorly differentiated.

Conventional variant is the most common subtype. Pathologic findings include lobules of cells arrange in cords and cohesive nests within a mucinous matrix. By immunohistochemistry, conventional chordomas typically express epithelial membrane antigen and epithelial markers. Most tumor cells are positive for S-100. Positive immunostaining for brachyury combined with cytokeratin provides a sensitivity and specificity of 98% to 100%.[28,49]

Chondroid variant is defined as the tumor containing an area of conventional chordoma next to a low-grade hyaline-type chondrosarcoma. Immunohistochemistry staining is often similar to the conventional subtype.[50]

Dedifferentiated variant is a very rare subtype reported in approximately 5% of cases.[51] It contains a region of conventional chordoma with the areas of high-grade or poorly differentiated spindle cell sarcoma. Dedifferentiated chordomas can arise within de novo chordoma or change from the conventional type after recurrence or treatment. The tumor loses expression of brachyury and cytokeratin by immunohistochemistry. Dedifferentiated chordoma should be suspected in the cases of biopsy-proven conventional chordoma with aggressive clinical features.[50]

Poorly differentiated variant is a recently described subset of chordoma with an absence of *INI1* (*SNF5/SMARCB1*) expression. It is prevalent in the pediatric population and has an aggressive clinical course.[52]

STAGING

Complete staging is recommended before definite treatment. CT imaging should be done to exclude distant metastasis to the common sites, such as the lung, soft tissue, and bone. MRI for screening of whole spine should be done because drop metastasis along the cerebrospinal axis can occur in skull base patients and other notochordal tumors, including synchronous chordoma, or benign notochordal tumors can be seen in some patients.[53] Bone scans are considered a standard staging modality in malignant bone tumors.

DIFFERENTIAL DIAGNOSIS

The differential diagnosis for a chordoma includes benign bone lesions, malignant bone tumors, and bone metastases. MRI findings of chondrosarcomas can be similar to those for chordomas, but chondrosarcomas are more commonly located in the thoracic spine rather than the sacrococcygeal region. Ring or arc calcifications are characteristic of chondrosarcoma, but not as common in chordomas.[54] Giant cell tumors of bone can be found in the sacrum but on MRI, they possess more heterogeneous signal intensity on T2-weighted imaging without marginal sclerosis or calcification.[55] The differential diagnosis of skull base tumors includes chondrosarcoma of the skull base, but this is usually located in the paramidline region.[56] Pituitary macroadenomas mostly shows isodensity on T1-weighted and T2-weighted MRI with area of necrosis or hemorrhage.[57] Notochordal hamartomas of the skull base have similar imaging findings to chordomas, but the presence of stalk-like lesions at the prepontine region are more suggestive of hamartomas than chordomas.[58] Bony metastases often involve multiple sites, show varying enhancement, and decreased signal intensity on T1-weighted MRI.[59,60] Lymphomas are also usually multifocal, but primary bone lymphomas should be ruled out as well; lymphomas typically will exhibit high FDG uptake on PET scans. Plasmacytomas can occur as solitary bone or paramidline masses in the spine, sacrococcygeal region, or skull base with classic punched-out lesions with an associated extraosseous mass concurrent with or without clinical findings consistent with multiple myeloma.[61]

Histologically, chordomas are difficult to differentiate from benign notochordal tumors. The chondroid-type chordoma can be misdiagnosed as chondrosarcoma, which is negative for cytokeratins and brachyury by immunostaining.[50]

PROGNOSTIC FACTORS

Properly validated prognostic factors for chordomas are limited by the rarity of this disease. The literature in this area mostly consists of retrospective analyses of clinical and molecular features of chordomas. Most studies in the literature are an amalgamation of cases from different primary locations, surgical approaches, rate of clear surgical margins, and varying adjuvant radiation doses. Several of these retrospective analyses revealed that tumor size, location of primary tumor, demographic data, and surgical margin are important prognostic factors. The analysis of the California Cancer Registry Database[4] identified that in 409 chordoma patients, larger tumors were independently associated with a 2.5-fold increased risk of death. Hispanic race, high socioeconomic status, and patients undergoing surgery were reported to have a favorable outcome. The primary tumor location was not correlated with survival. Other studies have indicated that the location of primary tumor could impact survival as different locations place limits on the extent and type of surgeries that can be done. The 5-year OS in patients with intracranial primaries (67%–78%) was shorter than spinal primaries (90%–92%).[4,62–65] The negative surgical margin (R0 resection) was an independent favorable prognostic factor compared to incomplete surgery, in line with most bone and soft tissue sarcoma series.[62]

Molecular prognostic markers have been analyzed to correlate the molecular profiles with recurrence of disease and survival. The expression of brachyury and increased copy number gain of 1q or 2p of T-gene were associated with significant shorter disease-free survival (DFS) and OS.[66,67] MGMT promoter methylation was found to have a higher recurrent rate of clival chordoma compare to unmethylated tumor.[68] The overexpression of p53 or CDK4 significantly correlated with poor OS.[67] Homozygous 9p21 deletions and 1p36 deletions were found to be independent prognostic factors in clival chordoma.[69]

TREATMENT

The foundation of treatment for a chordoma is radical resection. The approach to each patient is individualized, but the goal should be to achieve negative margins with minimal surgical morbidity. However, this needs to be balanced with the fact that chordomas are usually deeply located and are locally invasive, so margin negativity need not be achieved if significant morbidity would result. Adjuvant radiation is also included in the NCCN guidelines. Radiation alone without surgery is associated with an inferior outcome compared to some surgical series, although this option may be chosen by some patients with upper sacral and cervical chordomas who are neurologically intact and might choose a lower rate of local control and avoidance of potential acute surgical morbidity Some radiation alone series, in fact, show better outcome than the frequently used paradigm of surgery and postoperative radiation, although the use of preoperative radiation as a component of high-dose proton-based radiation appears to be better than either definitive radiation or surgery with postoperative radiation.[16,17,19,20,70] There is no current data for effective adjuvant systemic treatment. Systemic treatment should be considered for patients with recurrent or disseminated disease or in the setting of a clinical trial.

SURGERY

Spinal and Sacrococcygeal Tumor

Several studies support a survival advantage with adequate surgery.[13–15] A retrospective study of 501 patients demonstrated a significantly longer DFS after wide excision than marginal resection (75% vs. 33%).[13] The surgical margin was regarded to be the most important prognostic factor and the majority of the patients with negative surgical margin remained disease-free long-term. On the contrary, all of the patients who underwent intralesional excision or inadequate dose radiation alone had recurrent disease within 2 years.[14] More recent data have reported a 92% 5-year OS after surgery with significant longer DFS among patients with R0 resection.[62] Recent data for definite radiation with high dose proton-based radiation therapy (RT) for unresected chordomas, primarily sacrococcygeal, reported 5-year local control of 85%.[20] Similar efficacy has been reported for carbon ion radiotherapy for unresected sacral chordoma.[71] An ongoing single-institution Phase II trial (ISAC/NCT01811394) being conducted in Heidelberg, Germany, randomizes patients with sacral chordoma (either unresected or following R2 resection) to scanned proton versus carbon ion RT, treating to 64 GyRBE in 16 fractions.

Skull Base/Intracranial Tumor

Intracranial chordomas are a technically challenging problem. Although radical resections provide long-term survival, surgical complications including neurologic morbidity and bleeding must be weighed against radicality of the surgical approach. Surgical complications that have been reported include cranial nerve palsy, swallowing dysfunction, intracranial hematoma, CSF leakage, hydrocephalus, and infection with an overall complication rate of approximately 10% to 25%. Only a small number of fatal complications have been reported in the literature.[15,64,65,72,73] At the moment, surgical techniques for skull-based tumors vary according to tumor location, surgical expertise, and institutional preference.

Radiation

The local recurrence rate has been reported to be as high as 40% to 50% with radical surgery for chordomas.[14,15,64,72] Effective RT may have a role to eradicate microscopic disease and diminish recurrence rate, although it is still not known how to best select patients for RT. Biologically, chordomas are relatively radioresistant tumors. Conventional doses of x-ray therapy are not felt to be effective and in general, high doses of radiation are used in the adjuvant setting. A systematic review reported the efficacy and safety of adjuvant RT in the patient with spinal and sacral chordoma.[74] The study by Zabel-du Bois et al. demonstrated the patients receiving intensity-modulated photon-beam radiation (IMRT) dose over 60 Gy had a significant lower rate of local recurrence and improved OS compared to doses below 60 Gy.[75] A prospective Phase II study by DeLaney et al. reported 5-year local control rate with combination adjuvant photon/proton radiotherapy was 94% at the median radiation dose of 76 cobalt Gy equivalent.[76] Timing of adjuvant radiation may affect the local recurrence rate. One retrospective study found 5-year local control rate was 88% in early radiation group compared with 9% in the patients who received radiation for salvage or recurrence disease.[77]

High-dose single or hypofractionated RT has also been reported to be effective for this relatively radioresistant tumor. A study by Yamada et al. revealed the 2-year local control rate of 95% of adjuvant single fraction RT with median dose 2,400 cGy.[78] However, delivery of high-dose photon beam can cause increased toxicity to surrounding tissues. Studies of proton beam therapy were conducted to allow a higher radiation dose to the target volume with minimized doses to surrounding structures. DeLaney et al. demonstrated that the local control rate among 36 patients with primary spine sarcomas, including chordoma, was 88% at 8 years with median radiation dose of 76.6 Gy. Recurrence occurred in only one of 23 patients with primary chordomas treated with adjuvant, neoadjuvant, or definitive high-dose proton/photon radiation.[76] However, surgical hardware can potentially affect the accuracy of the proton dose to the target volume. Several studies reported a higher 5-year local recurrence rate in the patients who had titanium-based stabilization hardware.[76,79] Heavy ion particle radiation may have higher biologic effectiveness because of higher linear energy transfer along the particle track, resulting in denser DNA damage, more double-stranded DNA breaks, and greater effectiveness against hypoxic cells. Studies with carbon ions report local control of 85% to 89% at 2 to 5 years.[71,80]

In patient with intracranial chordomas, the benefit of adjuvant radiation remains unclear. Retrospective studies by Choy et al. revealed that adjuvant RT improved 5-year local control from 20% to 62% in patients with subtotal resection of clival chordoma.[81] Another study showed the 4-year local control rate of 56% with adjuvant photon/proton radiation at median dose of 67 Gy.[82]

The toxicities of RT depend on the location and kind of radiation treatment (that is, particle vs. photon). Acutely, these may include fatigue, mucositis, and diarrhea. Late bowel–bladder dysfunction related to cauda equina or sacral nerve injury and other kinds of neurotoxicity, while possible, are uncommon in the modern treatment era. DeLaney et al. reported no nerve injuries among 25 patients treated in the adjuvant radiation setting with median dose of 70.2 Gy and four nerve injuries (two grade 3 sacral neuropathies and two others [grade 2 in one and grade 3 in the other]) and erectile dysfunction among 25 patients with gross disease after surgery or biopsy, treated to 77.4 Gy, many of whom had upper sacral tumors, where resection would have resulted in 100% chance of nerve injury.[76] Other potential late effects of radiation include sacral insufficiency fracture, rectal bleeding, pituitary dysfunction, and (rare) radiation associated secondary malignancy.

FOLLOW-UP AND SURVEILLANCE

The 2019 NCCN guidelines for surveillance after treatment of chordoma include history and physical examination every 6 months out to 5 years and then annually. Surveillance chest imaging is recommended every 6 months and may include an annual CT for 5 years and annually thereafter, but there may be some variations in practice among different institutions. Imaging of primary site includes x-ray studies or MRI as clinically indicated.

MANAGEMENT OF DISEASE RECURRENCE

Loco-Regional Treatment

The most common site of recurrence is in the loco-regional area. According to the best practice for management of loco-regionally recurrent chordoma by the Global Consensus Group, salvage resection should aim to achieve gross total removal with negative margins. The success rate of re-resection varies among retrospective analyses ranging from 32% to 100%. The 5-year OS depends on the quality of surgery with or without radiation, but it is uniformly acknowledged to be less successful than that achieved at the time of initial treatment.[70] Adjuvant radiation is recommended in patients without prior RT. In the patient with no prior RT, high-dose radiation with curative intent as an alternative to surgery or combined with maximal tumor resection or RT alone is indicated. No direct comparison data exist to determine the advantage of single versus combined treatment modality in this setting. A retrospective data report noted the impact of high-dose proton/photon beam RT on recurrent tumor; the 5-year DFS was 43% and 25% with surgery and nonsurgery, respectively.[16]

In patients with recurrence disease after primary adjuvant radiation, reirradiation can cause dose-limiting toxicity to adjacent organs. Reirradiation can be considered if the projected radiation dose to target volume is judged adequate for disease control with an acceptable risk toxicity. McDonald et al. reported proton reirradiation of 13 patients with an estimated 2-year rate of local control of 85%, although late toxicity included grade 3 bitemporal lobe radionecrosis in one patient that improved with hyperbaric oxygen, a grade 4 CSF leak with meningitis in one patient, and a grade 4 ischemic brainstem stroke (out of radiation field) in one patient, with subsequent neurologic recovery.[83] If definitive radiation and/or surgery is judged not feasible, palliative radiation or palliative surgery followed by radiation for symptom alleviation is reasonable.

Systemic Treatment

For patients with locally advanced disease or distant metastasis who are not candidates for loco-regional treatment, systemic therapy is indicated, although the timing for systemic therapy must be carefully considered, because curative therapy is not currently available and patients, particularly with metastatic disease, are often asymptomatic and there is often an initially indolent rate of growth. Because growth is often indolent, clinicians and patients may have the luxury to delay treatment until patients have clearly measurable disease to assess the effectiveness of any therapy as well as the opportunity to investigate and participate in available clinical trials that can generally be accessed through the clinicaltrials.gov website. As noted below, "response" assessment in chordoma may be a challenge because of the often indolent rate of tumor growth, and "activity" may be manifested only in a change in tumor growth kinetics, including cessation of growth.

The time from diagnosis to metastasis was reported in one series to range from 0.2 to 13 years.[84] The median OS from diagnosis of metastasis to death was 22.1 months regardless of treatment modality.[21] The rationale for the choice of systemic may be based on the molecular characteristics of chordomas. Conventional chordomas are generally insensitive to cytotoxic chemotherapy. However, a single Phase II study by Chugh et al. using 9-nitro-camptothecin in 15 advanced chordoma patients reported a median time to tumor progression of 9.9 weeks and objective response rate of 7%.[85] A case series by Dhall et al. showed four patients with durable disease control for 9 to 13 years after subtotal resection of conventional clival chordoma followed by ifosfamide plus etoposide.[86] Fleming et al. showed a complete response in a dedifferentiated chordoma patient with lung metastasis using a six-drug regimen of etoposide, cisplatin, vincristine, dacarbazine, cyclophosphamide without recurrence with 24 months of follow up.[87] Several cases reports using multiple drugs including carboplatin/paclitaxel, liposomal doxorubicin/thalidomide, and VAC/IE (vincristine, doxorubicin, cyclophosphamide, followed by ifosfamide and etoposide) had a durable response (complete or partial response) up to 12 months.[88–90]

Discovery of oncogenic tyrosine kinase receptor pathways led to the development of clinical trials of targeted therapy. VEGFR, PDGFR, c-KIT, or MTOR pathways have been implicated in chordoma oncogenesis, which can be targeted by various TKIs. Imatinib, a multi-kinase inhibitor, has the most promising clinical activity for metastatic chordoma. A prospective Phase II study was conducted by Stacchiotti et al. using imatinib 400 mg twice daily in 56 patients with PDGFR/PDGR positive tumors. The objective response rate was only 2%, but the disease stabilization rate was 72%. The median PFS was 9.2 months and the median OS was 34.9 months.[23] Another prospective study using dual blockade with imatinib plus everolimus was recently published and included 43 patients with progressive imatinib-pretreated advanced chordomas. The data showed a clinical benefit rate (patients responding or demonstrating absence of growth) of 88%. The median PFS was 14 months and the median OS was 47 months.[91] This clinical data indicate that imatinib should be considered as a possible first-line systemic option for advanced/unresectable disease. In addition, epidermal growth factor receptor (EGFR) and HER-2 expression was found to be a predictive biomarker for the use of EGFR targeting TKIs. The efficacy of lapatinib was reported in a Phase II prospective trial of 18 imatinib-pretreated patients who had EGFR overexpression tumor. Lapatinib at a dose of 1,500 mg/day offered a disease control rate of 72%[24] (Tables 24.1 and 24.2).

TABLE 24.1 Efficacy Data of Chemotherapy in Patients With Locally Advanced/Metastatic Chordoma

Author	Site	*n*	Subtype	Chemotherapy	Response	Duration of Disease Control
Chugh[85]	Any	15	N/A	9-Nitro-camptothecin	ORR 7% (1 PR)	mTTP 9 weeks mOS 24 months
Dhall[86]	Clivus	4	3 NOS, 1 dedifferentiated	Ifosfamide/etoposide after subtotal resection	SD	9–13 years
Fleming[87]	Sacrum	2	Dedifferentiated	Multi-drug Etoposide/cisplatin/vincristine/dacarbazine/cyclophosphamide/doxorubicin	1 CR 1 PR	6 months 12 months

CR, complete response; mTTP, median time to tumor progression; N/A, not available; NOS, not otherwise specified; ORR, objective response rate; mOS, median overall survival; PR, partial response; SD, stable disease.

TABLE 24.2 Efficacy Data of Tyrosine Kinase Inhibitor in Patients With Metastatic Chordoma

Author	Drug/Dose	n	Eligibility	ORR (RECIST) DCR	PFS	OS
Stacchotti[23]	Imatinib 800 mg/day	56	Positive PDGFRB/PDGFB expression	ORR = 2% DCR = 64%	9 months	34.9 months
Stacchotti[91]	Imatinib 400 mg/day plus everolimus 2.5 mg/day	43	Imatinib-pretreated	ORR = 2.3% DCR = 88%	14 months	47 months
Stacchotti[24]	Lapatinib 1,500 mg/day	18	Imatinib-pretreated with EGFR expression/mutation	DCR = 72% by Choi criteria	8 months	-

DCR, disease control rate; EGFR, epidermal growth factor receptor; ORR, objective response rate; OS, overall survival; PDGFRB, platelet-derived growth factor receptor-β; PFS, progression-free survival; RECIST, response evaluation criteria in solid tumors.

Immunotherapy

Currently, the use of immunotherapy is in its infancy. The rationale of using immunotherapy for metastatic chordoma is based on preclinical and clinical data. The abundant of matrix surrounding tumor cells can retard the delivery of systemic drug into chordoma cells. Mathios et al. reported upregulation of PD-1 and PD-L1 in chordoma cell lines by activating tumor-specific cytokines that provided the rationale for use of a PD-L1 inhibitor for chordoma treatment.[92] In clinical data, the prevalence of PD-L1 expression in chordoma is higher than 90%.[93] Several case reports of using nivolumab and pembrolizumab in imatinib-resistant chordoma demonstrate clinical benefit with disease control of 6 to 9 months.[94] Prospective studies of immune checkpoint inhibitors in chordoma are ongoing. Lastly, vaccines have been developed against brachyury, which is nearly uniformly expressed in chordomas. The goal of this approach is to develop a chordoma-specific immune response and trials using this approach are also ongoing at this time.[95–97]

SUMMARY

Chordomas, because of their rarity; curability with complex surgery performed by experienced surgeons; relative radiation resistance requiring high-tech, high-dose radiation in close proximity to the brain, spinal cord, spinal/sacral nerves, and/or other critical normal tissues; and subtle and variable responses to systemic therapies, should be managed by multidisciplinary teams at high volume tertiary care centers. Radical surgery is the standard treatment for localized chordoma. Adjuvant or neoadjuvant radiation is recommended because of the high recurrence rate, especially in the patients with positive surgical margins. High-dose radiation alone or with decompressive surgery that does not violate tumor capsule is indicated if curative surgery is not feasible. Re-resection remains a modestly effective approach for some patients with recurrent disease. RT for locally recurrent tumor is an option in the radiation-naïve patient or the patient with disease judged to be amenable to reirradiation with acceptable risk of toxicity to adjacent normal tissues. Targeted therapy for locally advanced or metastatic disease is effective for tumor stabilization but has a low response rate using standard response evaluation criteria in solid tumors (RECIST). Novel targeted drugs and immunotherapy remain under investigation in preclinical and clinical studies. Progress in treatment will be facilitated by enrollment of eligible patients into available clinical trials. It should be mentioned that there is a Chordoma Foundation that has provided excellent resources for chordoma patients, their families, clinicians, and researchers.

CASE STUDY

A 46-year-old woman, without significant medical history, presented with progressive occipital headaches radiating to her jaws, teeth, and posterior neck in a bilateral fashion that began in March 2017. She denied associated dysphagia, odynophagia, hemoptysis, voice changes, or visual changes. She had both an MRI and a CT angiogram of the head and neck, which showed a destructive lesion centered in the inferior clivus extending to the odontoid process and bilateral occipital condyles. The mass breached the posterior cortex of the clivus with soft tissue extension into the premedullary cistern and impinged upon the proximal basilar artery. A CT scan of the chest showed no evidence of pulmonary metastasis. Nasal endoscopy with clival mass biopsy in November 2017 revealed a proliferation of cells in a lobulated and chord-like growth pattern separated by fibrous tissues and myxoid stroma. The cells had a vacuolated (physaliferous) eosinophilic cytoplasm with hyperchromatic pleomorphic nuclei and conspicuous nucleoli with positive immunohistochemical staining for brachyury, epithelial membrane antigen (EMA), pankeratin, and S-100 in tumor nuclei compatible with chordoma. Her case was discussed at a multidisciplinary sarcoma tumor board and, given the potential morbidity of surgery and RT, she initially received imatinib 400 mg twice daily with gradual improvement of her neck pain. The following MRI demonstrated a decrease in size of chordoma, for example, the prepontine cistern component decreased from 13 × 27 mm to 8 × 14 mm. After 17 months of treatment, MRI demonstrated increased size of the clival mass, particularly the component extending into the prepontine cistern. The lesion impinged on the basilar artery and ventral surface of the pons. She was evaluated by neurosurgery and radiation oncology and was advised about potential clinical trials. She elected to participate in an immunotherapy trial for chordoma of nivolumab and relatlimab for this disease. She noted an improvement of headache symptoms after cycle 1. Unfortunately, after cycle 2, she complained of worsening headache, double vision, facial pain, and positive signs of increased intracranial pressure. A restaging MRI showed an interval increase in the size of her clival tumor, which encased the cavernous and petrous internal carotid artery (ICA) and progressive mass effect on the brainstem. Immunotherapy was discontinued because of clinical and radiologic disease progression. Craniotomy with subtotal tumor resection was performed because of the mass effect. The following endoscopic endonasal transclival transsphenoidal resection of clival chordoma with complex reconstruction of skull base was done to maximize tumor removal. The patient reported that her double vision, facial pain, and migraine-like headache resolved following surgery. Recent skull base CT scan 8 weeks after the initial surgery revealed stable residual postsurgical changes for debulking of skull base tumor.

In summary, this patient had a 17-month duration of disease control by imatinib, which was longer than the average benefit noted in the literature. Whether immunotherapy could be a potential therapy for unresectable/advanced chordoma continues to be aggressively investigated. Long-term follow-up is needed to assess the outcome of maximum tumor removal. She is currently being evaluated for adjuvant RT. Future therapeutic options for this patient include proton therapy, brachyury vaccine trials, and other systemic agents.

REFERENCES

1. Healey JH, Lane JM. Chordoma: a critical review of diagnosis and treatment. *Orthop Clin North Am*. 1989;20(3):417–426. https://www.ncbi.nlm.nih.gov/pubmed/2662114
2. Walcott BP, Nahed BV, Mohyeldin A, et al. Chordoma: current concepts, management, and future directions. *Lancet Oncol*. 2012;13(2):e69–e76. doi:10.1016/S1470-2045(11)70337-0
3. Pan Y, Lu L, Chen J, et al. Analysis of prognostic factors for survival in patients with primary spinal chordoma using the SEER Registry from 1973 to 2014. *J Orthop Surg Res*. 2018;13(1):76. doi:10.1186/s13018-018-0784-3
4. Lee J, Bhatia NN, Hoang BH, et al. Analysis of prognostic factors for patients with chordoma with use of the California Cancer Registry. *J Bone Joint Surg Am*. 2012;94(4):356–363. doi:10.2106/JBJS.J.01784
5. Horwitz T. *The Human Notochord: A Study of Its Development and Regression, Variations, and Pathologic Derivative, Chordoma*. Indianapolis, IN: Horwitz; 1977.
6. Corallo D, Trapani V, Bonaldo P. The notochord: structure and functions. *Cell Mol Life Sci*. 2015;72(16):2989–3008. doi:10.1007/s00018-015-1897-z
7. Stemple DL. Structure and function of the notochord: an essential organ for chordate development. *Development*. 2005;132(11):2503–2512. doi:10.1242/dev.01812
8. de Castro CV, Guimaraes G, Aguiar S Jr, et al. Tyrosine kinase receptor expression in chordomas: phosphorylated AKT correlates inversely with outcome. *Hum Pathol*. 2013;44(9):1747–1755. doi:10.1016/j.humpath.2012.11.024
9. Tamborini E, Miselli F, Negri T, et al. Molecular and biochemical analyses of platelet-derived growth factor receptor (PDGFR) B, PDGFRA, and KIT receptors in chordomas. *Clin Cancer Res*. 2006;12(23):6920–6928. doi:10.1158/1078-0432.CCR-06-1584
10. Erdem E, Angtuaco EC, Van Hemert R, et al. Comprehensive review of intracranial chordoma. *Radiographics*. 2003;23(4):995–1009. doi:10.1148/rg.234025176

11. Murphey MD, Andrews CL, Flemming DJ, et al. From the archives of the AFIP. Primary tumors of the spine: radiologic pathologic correlation. *Radiographics*. 1996;16(5):1131–1158. doi:10.1148/radiographics.16.5.8888395
12. Williams BJ, Raper DMS, Godbout E, et al. Diagnosis and treatment of chordoma. *J Natl Compr Canc Netw*. 2013;11(6):726–731. doi:10.6004/jnccn.2013.0089
13. Ahmed T, Abdel-Rahman O, Morsy M, et al. Management of sacrococcygeal chordoma: a systematic review and meta-analysis of observational studies. *Spine*. 2018;43(19):E1157–E1169. doi:10.1097/BRS.0000000000002638
14. Boriani S, Bandiera S, Biagini R, et al. Chordoma of the mobile spine: fifty years of experience. *Spine*. 2006;31(4):493–503. doi:10.1097/01.brs.0000200038.30869.27
15. Chibbaro S, Cornelius JF, Froelich S, et al. Endoscopic endonasal approach in the management of skull base chordomas—clinical experience on a large series, technique, outcome, and pitfalls. *Neurosurg Rev*. 2014;37(2):217–224; discussion 224–225. doi:10.1007/s10143-013-0503-9
16. Park L, DeLaney TF, Liebsch NJ, et al. Sacral chordomas: impact of high-dose proton/photon-beam radiation therapy combined with or without surgery for primary versus recurrent tumor. *Int J Radiat Oncol Biol Phys*. 2006;65(5):1514–1521. doi:10.1016/j.ijrobp.2006.02.059
17. Rotondo RL, Folkert W, Liebsch NJ, et al. High-dose proton-based radiation therapy in the management of spine chordomas: outcomes and clinicopathological prognostic factors. *J Neurosurg Spine*. 2015;23(6):788–797. doi:10.3171/2015.3.SPINE14716
18. Gupta T, Wadasadawala T, Master Z, et al. Encouraging early clinical outcomes with helical tomotherapy-based image-guided intensity-modulated radiation therapy for residual, recurrent, and/or progressive benign/low-grade intracranial tumors: a comprehensive evaluation. *Int J Radiat Oncol Biol Phys*. 2012;82(2):756–764. doi:10.1016/j.ijrobp.2010.12.044
19. Chen YL, Liebsch N, Kobayashi W, et al. Definitive high-dose photon/proton radiotherapy for unresected mobile spine and sacral chordomas. *Spine*. 2013;38(15):E930–E936. doi:10.1097/BRS.0b013e318296e7d7
20. Kabolizadeh P, Chen YL, Liebsch N, et al. Updated outcome and analysis of tumor response in mobile spine and sacral chordoma treated with definitive high-dose photon/proton radiation therapy. *Int J Radiat Oncol Biol Phys*. 2017;97(2):254–262. doi:10.1016/j.ijrobp.2016.10.006
21. Young VA, Curtis KM, Temple HT, et al. Characteristics and patterns of metastatic disease from chordoma. *Sarcoma*. 2015;2015:517657. doi:10.1155/2015/517657
22. McPherson CM, Suki D, McCutcheon IE, et al. Metastatic disease from spinal chordoma: a 10-year experience. *J Neurosurg Spine*. 2006;5(4):277–280. doi:10.3171/spi.2006.5.4.277
23. Stacchiotti S, Longhi A, Ferraresi V, et al. Phase II study of imatinib in advanced chordoma. *J Clin Oncol*. 2012;30(9):914–920. doi:10.1200/JCO.2011.35.3656
24. Stacchiotti S, Tamborini E, Lo Vullo S, et al. Phase II study on lapatinib in advanced EGFR-positive chordoma. *Ann Oncol*. 2013;24(7):1931–1936. doi:10.1093/annonc/mdt117
25. Schwab JH, Healey JH, Rose P, et al. The surgical management of sacral chordomas. *Spine*. 2009;34(24):2700–2704. doi:10.1097/BRS.0b013e3181bad11d
26. Pillay N, Plagnol V, Tarpey PS, et al. A common single-nucleotide variant in T is strongly associated with chordoma. *Nat Genet*. 2012;44(11):1185. doi:10.1038/ng.2419
27. Tarpey PS, Behjati S, Young MD, et al. The driver landscape of sporadic chordoma. *Nat Commun*. 2017;8(1):890. doi:10.1038/s41467-017-01026-0
28. Oakley GJ, Fuhrer K, Seethala RR. Brachyury, SOX-9, and podoplanin, new markers in the skull base chordoma vs chondrosarcoma differential: a tissue microarray-based comparative analysis. *Mod Pathol*. 2008;21(12):1461. doi:10.1038/modpathol.2008.144
29. Nelson AC, Pillay N, Henderson S, et al. An integrated functional genomics approach identifies the regulatory network directed by brachyury (T) in chordoma. *J Pathol*. 2012;228(3):274–285. doi:10.1002/path.4082
30. Choy E, MacConaill LE, Cote GM, et al. Genotyping cancer-associated genes in chordoma identifies mutations in oncogenes and areas of chromosomal loss involving CDKN2A, PTEN, and SMARCB1. *PLoS ONE*. 2014;9(7):e101283. doi:10.1371/journal.pone.0101283
31. Suzuki S, Dobashi Y, Hatakeyama Y, et al. Clinicopathological significance of platelet-derived growth factor (PDGF)-B and vascular endothelial growth factor-A expression, PDGF receptor-β phosphorylation, and microvessel density in gastric cancer. *BMC Cancer*. 2010;10(1):659. doi:10.1186/1471-2407-10-659
32. Duffy AM, Bouchier-Hayes DJ, Harmey JH. Vascular endothelial growth factor (VEGF) and its role in non-endothelial cells: autocrine signalling by VEGF. In: Harmey JH, ed. *VEGF and Cancer*. New York, NY: Springer Publishing Company; 2004:133–144. doi:10.1007/978-1-4419-9148-5_13
33. Enomoto H, Inoki I, Komiya K, et al. Vascular endothelial growth factor isoforms and their receptors are expressed in human osteoarthritic cartilage. *Am J Pathol*. 2003;162(1):171–181. doi:10.1016/S0002-9440(10)63808-4
34. Ikeda M, Hosoda Y, Hirose S, et al. Expression of vascular endothelial growth factor isoforms and their receptors Flt-1, KDR, and neuropilin-1 in synovial tissues of rheumatoid arthritis. *J Pathol*. 2000;191(4):426–433. doi:10.1002/1096-9896(2000)9999:9999<::AID-PATH649>3.0.CO;2-E
35. Bayrak OF, Gulluoglu S, Aydemir E, et al. MicroRNA expression profiling reveals the potential function of microRNA-31 in chordomas. *J Neurooncol*. 2013;115(2):143–151. doi:10.1007/s11060-013-1211-6
36. Long C, Jiang L, Wei F, et al. Integrated miRNA-mRNA analysis revealing the potential roles of miRNAs in chordomas. *PLoS ONE*. 2013;8(6):e66676. doi:10.1371/journal.pone.0066676

37. Chen K, Chen H, Zhang K, et al. MicroRNA profiling and bioinformatics analyses reveal the potential roles of microRNAs in chordoma. *Oncol Lett*. 2017;14(5):5533–5539. doi:10.3892/ol.2017.6839
38. York JE, Kaczaraj A, Abi-Said D, et al. Sacral chordoma: 40-year experience at a major cancer center. *Neurosurgery*. 1999;44(1):74–79. doi:10.1097/00006123-199901000-00041
39. Weber A, Liebsch N, Sanchez R, Sweriduk J S. Chordomas of the skull base. Radiologic and clinical evaluation. *Neuroimaging Clin North Am*. 1994;4(3):515–527
40. Zou MX, Lv GH, Zhang QS, et al. Prognostic factors in skull base chordoma: a systematic literature review and meta-analysis. *World Neurosurg*. 2017;100:692–694. doi:10.1016/j.wneu.2016.10.105
41. Mohindra S, Kapoor A, Kursa GK, et al. Apoplexy in an intradural clival chordoma causing intraventricular bleed. *Surg Neurol Int*. 2016;7(suppl 1):S17. doi:10.4103/2152-7806.173562
42. Meyer JE, Oot RF, Lindfors KK. CT appearance of clival chordomas. *J Comput Assist Tomogr*. 1986;10(1):34–38. doi:10.1097/00004728-198601000-00007
43. Farsad K, Kattapuram SV, Sacknoff R, et al. Sacral chordoma. *Radiographics*. 2009;29(5):1525–1530. doi:10.1148/rg.295085215
44. Doucet V, Peretti-Viton P, Figarella-Branger D, et al. MRI of intracranial chordomas. Extent of tumour and contrast enhancement: criteria for differential diagnosis. *Neuroradiology*. 1997;39(8):571–576. doi:10.1007/s002340050469
45. Rosenthal DI, Scott JA, Mankin HJ, et al. Sacrococcygeal chordoma: magnetic resonance imaging and computed tomography. *AJR Am J Roentgenol*. 1985;145(1):143–147. doi:10.2214/ajr.145.1.143
46. Stacchiotti S, Sommer J, Chordoma Global Consensus Group. Building a global consensus approach to chordoma: a position paper from the medical and patient community. *Lancet Oncol*. 2015;16(2):e71–83. doi:10.1016/S1470-2045(14)71190-8
47. Hoshi M, Oebisu N, Takada J, et al. Role of FDG-PET/CT for monitoring soft tissue tumors. *Oncol Lett*. 2014;7(4):1243–1248. doi:10.3892/ol.2014.1876
48. Tateishi U, Hosono A, Makimoto A, et al. Accuracy of 18F fluorodeoxyglucose positron emission tomography/computed tomography in staging of pediatric sarcomas. *J Pediatr Hematol Oncol*. 2007;29(9):608–612. doi:10.1097/MPH.0b013e318142b5ab
49. Vujovic S, Henderson S, Presneau N, et al. Brachyury, a crucial regulator of notochordal development, is a novel biomarker for chordomas. *J Pathol*. 2006;209(2):157–165. doi:10.1002/path.1969
50. Jo Vickie Y, Fletcher CDM. WHO classification of soft tissue tumours: an update based on the 2013 (4th) edition. *Pathology*. 2014;46(2):95–104. doi:10.1097/PAT.0000000000000050
51. Batista KMP, Reyes KYA, Lopez FP, et al. Immunophenotypic features of dedifferentiated skull base chordoma: an insight into the intratumoural heterogeneity. *Contemp Oncol (Pozn)*. 2017;21(4):267–273. doi:10.5114/wo.2017.72385
52. Shih AR, Cote GM, Chebib I, et al. Clinicopathologic characteristics of poorly differentiated chordoma. *Mod Pathol*. 2018;31(8):1237–1245. doi:10.1038/s41379-018-0002-1
53. Sebro R, DeLaney TF, Hornicek F, et al. Frequency and risk factors for additional lesions in the axial spine in subjects with chordoma: indications for screening. *Spine*. 2017;42(1):E37–E40. doi:10.1097/BRS.0000000000001723
54. Murphey MD, Walker EA, Wilson AJ, et al. From the archives of the AFIP: imaging of primary chondrosarcoma: radiologic-pathologic correlation. *Radiographics*. 2003;23(5):1245–1278. doi:10.1148/rg.235035134
55. Murphey MD, Nomikos GC, Flemming DJ, et al. From the archives of AFIP. Imaging of giant cell tumor and giant cell reparative granuloma of bone: radiologic-pathologic correlation. *Radiographics*. 2001;21(5):1283–1309. doi:10.1148/radiographics.21.5.g01se251283
56. Meyers SP, Hirsch WL Jr, Curtin HD, et al. Chondrosarcomas of the skull base: MR imaging features. *Radiology*. 1992;184(1):103–108. doi:10.1148/radiology.184.1.1609064
57. Davis PC, Hoffman JC Jr, Spencer T, et al. MR imaging of pituitary adenoma: CT, clinical, and surgical correlation. *AJR Am J Roentgenol*. 1987;148(4):797–802. doi:10.2214/ajr.148.4.797
58. Ng SH, Ko SF, Wan YL, et al. Cervical ecchordosis physaliphora: CT and MR features. *Br J Radiol*. 1998;71(843):329–331. doi:10.1259/bjr.71.843.9616246
59. Rodallec MH, Feydy A, Larousserie F, et al. Diagnostic imaging of solitary tumors of the spine: what to do and say. *Radiographics*. 2008;28(4):1019–1041. doi:10.1148/rg.284075156
60. Guillevin R, Vallee JN, Lafitte F, et al. Spine metastasis imaging: review of the literature. *J Neuroradiol*. 2007;34(5):311–321. doi:10.1016/j.neurad.2007.05.003
61. Ooi GC, Chim JCS, Au WY, Khong PL. Radiologic manifestations of primary solitary extramedullary and multiple solitary plasmacytomas. *AJR Am J Roentgenol*. 2006;186(3):821–827. doi:10.2214/AJR.04.1787
62. Radaelli S, Stacchiotti S, Ruggieri P, et al. Sacral chordoma: long-term outcome of a large series of patients surgically treated at two reference centers. *Spine*. 2016;41(12):1049–1057. doi:10.1097/BRS.0000000000001604
63. Jawad MU, Scully SP. Surgery significantly improves survival in patients with chordoma. *Spine*. 2010;35(1):117–123. doi:10.1097/BRS.0b013e3181b44387
64. Tzortzidis F, Elahi F, Wright D, et al. Patient outcome at long-term follow-up after aggressive microsurgical resection of cranial base chordomas. *Neurosurgery*. 2006;59(2):230–237; discussion 230–267. doi:10.1227/01.NEU.0000223441.51012.9D

65. Di Maio S, Temkin N, Ramanathan D, Sekhar LN. Current comprehensive management of cranial base chordomas: 10-year meta-analysis of observational studies. *J Neurosurg*. 2011;115(6):1094–1105. doi:10.3171/2011.7.JNS11355
66. Kitamura Y, Sasaki H, Kimura T, et al. Molecular and clinical risk factors for recurrence of skull base chordomas: gain on chromosome 2p, expression of brachyury, and lack of irradiation negatively correlate with patient prognosis. *J Neuropathol Exp Neurol*. 2013;72(9):814–821. doi:10.1097/NEN.0b013e3182a065d0
67. Sun X, Hornicek F, Schwab JH. Chordoma: an update on the pathophysiology and molecular mechanisms. *Curr Rev Musculoskelet Med*. 2015;8(4):344–352. doi:10.1007/s12178-015-9311-x
68. Marucci G, Morandi L, Mazzatenta D, et al. MGMT promoter methylation status in clival chordoma. *J Neurooncol*. 2014;118(2):271–276. doi:10.1007/s11060-014-1445-y
69. Zenonos GA, Fernandez-Miranda JC, Mukherjee D, et al. Prospective validation of a molecular prognostication panel for clival chordoma. *J Neurosurg*. 2019;130(5):1. doi:10.3171/2018.3.JNS172321
70. Stacchiotti S, Gronchi A, Fossati P, et al. Best practices for the management of local-regional recurrent chordoma: a position paper by the Chordoma Global Consensus Group. *Ann Oncol*. 2017;28(6):1230–1242. doi:10.1093/annonc/mdx054
71. Imai R, Kamada T, Tsuji H, et al. Effect of carbon ion radiotherapy for sacral chordoma: results of Phase I-II and Phase II clinical trials. *Int J Radiat Oncol Biol Phys*. 2010;77(5):1470–1476. doi:10.1016/j.ijrobp.2009.06.048
72. Sen C, Triana AI, Berglind N, et al. Clival chordomas: clinical management, results, and complications in 71 patients. *J Neurosurg*. 2010;113(5):1059–1071. doi:10.3171/2009.9.JNS08596
73. Pamir MN, Kiliç T, Türe U, Ozek MM. Multimodality management of 26 skull-base chordomas with 4-year mean follow-up: experience at a single institution. *Acta Neurochir (Wien)*. 2004;146(4):343–354. doi:10.1007/s00701-004-0218-3
74. Pennicooke B, Laufer I, Sahgal A, et al. Safety and local control of radiation therapy for chordoma of the spine and sacrum: a systematic review. *Spine*. 2016;41(suppl 20):S186–S192. doi:10.1097/BRS.0000000000001831
75. Zabel-du Bois A, Nikoghosyan A, Schwahofer A, et al. Intensity modulated radiotherapy in the management of sacral chordoma in primary versus recurrent disease. *Radiother Oncol*. 2010;97(3):408–412. doi:10.1016/j.radonc.2010.10.008
76. DeLaney TF, Liebsch NJ, Pedlow FX, et al. Long-term results of Phase II study of high dose photon/proton radiotherapy in the management of spine chordomas, chondrosarcomas, and other sarcomas. *J Surg Oncol*. 2014;110(2):115–122. doi:10.1002/jso.23617
77. Hug EB, Fitzek MM, Liebsch NJ, Munzenrider JE. Locally challenging osteo-and chondrogenic tumors of the axial skeleton: results of combined proton and photon radiation therapy using three-dimensional treatment planning. *Int J Radiat Oncol Biol Phys*. 1995;31(3):467–476. doi:10.1016/0360-3016(94)00390-7
78. Yamada Y, Laufer I, Cox BW, et al. Preliminary results of high-dose single-fraction radiotherapy for the management of chordomas of the spine and sacrum. *Neurosurgery*. 2013;73(4):673–680. doi:10.1227/NEU.0000000000000083
79. Staab A, Rutz HP, Ares C, et al. Spot-scanning-based proton therapy for extracranial chordoma. *Int J Radiat Oncol Biol Phys*. 2011;81(4):e489–e496. doi:10.1016/j.ijrobp.2011.02.018
80. Uhl M, Welzel T, Jensen A, et al. Carbon ion beam treatment in patients with primary and recurrent sacrococcygeal chordoma. *Strahlenther Onkol*. 2015;191(7):597–603. doi:10.1007/s00066-015-0825-3
81. Choy W, Terterov S, Ung N, et al. Adjuvant stereotactic radiosurgery and radiation therapy for the treatment of intracranial chordomas. *J Neurol Surg B Skull Base*. 2016;77(1):38–46. doi:10.1055/s-0035-1554907
82. Noël G, Feuvret L, Calugaru V, et al. Chordomas of the base of the skull and upper cervical spine. One hundred patients irradiated by a 3D conformal technique combining photon and proton beams. *Acta Oncol*. 2005;44(7):700–708. doi:10.1080/02841860500326257
83. McDonald MW, Linton OR, Shah MV. Proton therapy for reirradiation of progressive or recurrent chordoma. *Int J Radiat Oncol Biol Phys*. 2013;87(5):1107–1114. doi:10.1016/j.ijrobp.2013.09.038
84. Bergh P, Kindblom LG, Gunterberg B, et al. Prognostic factors in chordoma of the sacrum and mobile spine: a study of 39 patients. *Cancer*. 2000;88(9):2122–2134. doi:10.1002/(sici)1097-0142(20000501)88:9<2122::aid-cncr19>3.0.co;2-1
85. Chugh R, Dunn R, Zalupski MM, et al. Phase II study of 9-nitro-camptothecin in patients with advanced chordoma or soft tissue sarcoma. *J Clin Oncol*. 2005;23(15):3597–3604. doi:10.1200/JCO.2005.02.170
86. Dhall G, Traverso M, Finlay JL, et al. The role of chemotherapy in pediatric clival chordomas. *J Neurooncol*. 2011;103(3):657–662. doi:10.1007/s11060-010-0441-0
87. Fleming GF, Heimann PS, Stephens JK, et al. Dedifferentiated chordoma. Response to aggressive chemotherapy in two cases. *Cancer*. 1993;72(3):714–718. doi:10.1002/1097-0142(19930801)72:3<714::aid-cncr2820720314>3.0.co;2-1
88. Schönegger K, Gelpi E, Prayer D, et al. Recurrent and metastatic clivus chordoma: systemic palliative therapy retards disease progression. *Anticancer Drugs*. 2005;16(10):1139–1143. doi:10.1097/00001813-200511000-00015
89. Al-Rahawan MM, Siebert JD, Mitchell CS, Smith SD. Durable complete response to chemotherapy in an infant with a clival chordoma. *Pediatr Blood Cancer*. 2012;59(2):323–325. doi:10.1002/pbc.23297
90. Lee MH, Kim SR, Jeong JS, et al. Pulmonary metastatic chordoma improved by platinum-based chemotherapy. *Lung Cancer*. 2012;76(2):255–257. doi:10.1016/j.lungcan.2012.02.007
91. Stacchiotti S, Morosi C, Lo VS, et al. Imatinib and everolimus in patients with progressing advanced chordoma: a phase 2 clinical study. *Cancer*. 2018;124(20):4056–4063. doi:10.1002/cncr.31685
92. Mathios D, Ruzevick J, Jackson CM, et al. PD-1, PD-L1, PD-L2 expression in the chordoma microenvironment. *J Neurooncol*. 2015;121(2):251–259. doi:10.1007/s11060-014-1637-5

93. Feng Y, Shen J, Gao Y, et al. Expression of programmed cell death ligand 1 (PD-L1) and prevalence of tumor-infiltrating lymphocytes (TILs) in chordoma. *Oncotarget*. 2015;6(13):11139–11149. doi:10.18632/oncotarget.3576
94. Migliorini D, Mach N, Aguiar D, et al. First report of clinical responses to immunotherapy in 3 relapsing cases of chordoma after failure of standard therapies. *Oncoimmunology*. 2017;6(8):e1338235. doi:10.1080/2162402X.2017.1338235
95. Hamilton DH, David JM, Dominguez C, Palena C. Development of cancer vaccines targeting brachyury, a transcription factor associated with tumor epithelial-mesenchymal transition. *Cells Tissues Organs (Print)*. 2017;203(2):128–138. doi:10.1159/000446495
96. Heery CR, Palena C, McMahon S, et al. Phase I study of a poxviral TRICOM-based vaccine directed against the transcription factor brachyury. *Clin Cancer Res*. 2017;23(22):6833–6845. doi:10.1158/1078-0432.CCR-17-1087
97. Heery CR, Singh BH, Rauckhorst M, et al. Phase I trial of a yeast-based therapeutic cancer vaccine (GI-6301) targeting the transcription factor brachyury. *Cancer Immunol Res*. 2015;3(11):1248–1256. doi:10.1158/2326-6066.CIR-15-0119

25

Myxoid Liposarcoma

Roberta Giovanna Sanfilippo, Chiara Fabbroni, Angelo Paolo Dei Tos, and Alessandro Gronchi

INTRODUCTION

Myxoid liposarcoma (MLS) accounts for about 30% to 35% of liposarcomas and approximately 10% of all adult soft tissue sarcomas (STSs). According to the most recent WHO classification, MLS can be morphologically divided into high and low grades. The degree of aggressiveness depends on the percentage of the hypercellular component within the tumor.[1,2] These neoplasms harbor two characteristic chromosomal translocations, namely a t(12;16)(q13; p11), resulting in the fusion of *TLS–DDTI3* genes, and a rarer t(12;22)(q13;q12), resulting in the fusion of *EWS* and *DDTI3* (Figure 25.1).

So far, different molecular variants of the *TLS–DDIT3* fusion have been described, although with an undefined impact on clinical outcome.[3,4] MLS has a peculiar natural history: in contrast with other sarcoma subtypes, which primarily metastasize to the lung, they tend to spread to serosal membranes, the abdominal cavity, soft tissues, and bone.[5] Regarding the treatment of this histotype, the mainstay for localized disease is surgery, alone or in combination with radiation therapy (RT). Unfortunately, despite adequate local treatment, approximately 40% of patients relapse, and median survival following first documented metastasis is about 2 years.[6] Chemotherapy is used in patients with unresectable advanced disease.[7–9] A higher sensitivity to standard chemotherapy and RT compared to the other STS histologic types has been suggested, but long-term tumor control is far from optimal.[10,11]

When recurrence develops, surgery is an option, although the appropriate candidates must be carefully selected. Multimodality therapy is frequently used in these situations.

For patients with unresectable and/or metastatic disease, the systemic therapy option is chemotherapy. Several newer drugs including immunotherapy are under investigation.

MLS is a young adult disease, with the age at presentation on average a decade younger than that for the other histologic subtypes of liposarcoma. It has a peak of incidence in the fourth and fifth decades of life, and although very rare, it is the commonest form of liposarcoma in patients younger than 20 years of age. There is no gender predilection.[2]

MOST COMMON PRESENTING SYMPTOMS

MLS typically occurs as a large painless mass within the deep soft tissues of the limbs while, in contrast with the well-differentiated group, the retroperitoneal location seems to be exceptional.[2]

A diagnosis of primary MLS in the retroperitoneum should be regarded with suspicion, as most such cases represent either metastatic MLS or well-differentiated/dedifferentiated liposarcoma with myxoid stromal change. Metastatic sites that could cause presenting symptoms include bone (pain or fracture), lung (dyspnea), and fatty tissue (peritoneal, pericardiac, paratracheal, etc).

DIAGNOSTIC APPROACH

Accurate diagnosis of MLS including tumors arising in the extremity and trunk, usually consists of MRI. However, there are pitfalls, and expertise from a radiologist familiar with the disease is critical.

For patients with suspected or confirmed MLS, staging should be done with a contrast-enhanced chest and abdomen CT scan and MRI of the vertebral column, as bone, mediastinum, and abdominal

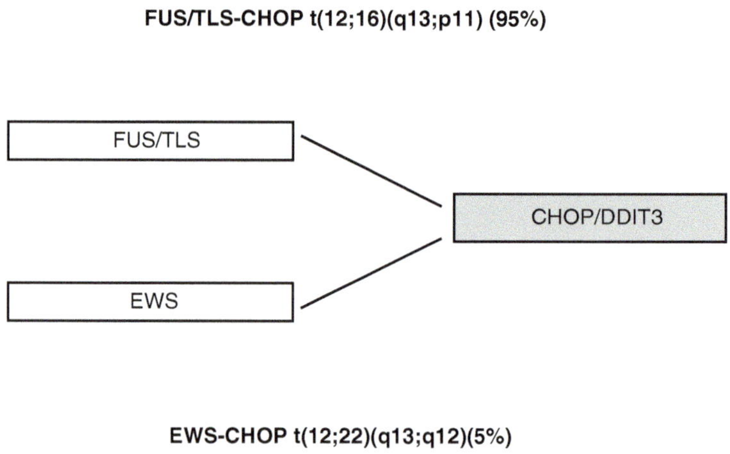

FIGURE 25.1 Specific chromosomal translocations of myxoid liposarcomas.
CHOP/DDIT3, fusion gene; FUS/TLS, gene; EWS, gene.

cavity are the most common metastatic sites.[6] The roles of PET or whole-body MRI remain to be determined. MLS indeed may or may not have a metabolic activity on PET scan and whether this correlates with disease aggressiveness is currently under investigation. Whole-body MRI may detect earlier metastatic disease, particularly to the bone. However, the impact of early metastases detection is far from being demonstrated as critical for cure.

Ultimately, to establish a diagnosis, the gold standard is histologic examination of tumor tissue. In the preoperative setting, tissue is most commonly obtained through core-needle biopsy. In the past, MLS was separated from round cell liposarcoma (RCL); however, strong morphologic as well as genetic data have led to the classification of myxoid and RCL together as part of a morphologic continuum, which includes hypercellular neoplasms composed of oval to round neoplastic cells. Cytogenetics and molecular genetics have greatly contributed to such a conceptual reappraisal by demonstrating that both myxoid and RCLs contain the same genetic abnormalities (that is, balanced translocations), most commonly t(12;16)(q13;p11), which fuses the *DDIT3* (*CHOP*) gene on 12q13 with the *FUS* (*TLS*) gene on 16p11.[2]

The classic myxoid variant shows low cellularity, conspicuous vascular network, and myxoid stroma, whereas the cellular variant shows high cellularity, made up of closely packed roundish cells, little or no intervening stroma, and a capillary pattern not easily visualized. Diagnosis of a high-grade variant requires the presence of a cellular component exceeding 5%.[1] This amount is of prognostic relevance because within the myxoid liposarcoma (MLS) spectrum, the 5-year survival rate varies between 20% and 70%, and the cellular variant falls in the shortest survival time. However, the 5% cutoff is far from being perfect to distinguish two separate entities and may lead to under- or overestimation of risk. The risk increases continuously with the rate of hypercellularity rather than by a binary classification. In summary, the higher the cellularity, the greater the risk of recurrence, metastasis, and death.

As the extent of hypercellularity predicts the risk of metastatic spread, extensive sampling of the surgical specimen is critical. Microscopically, pure MLS is remarkably hypocellular, featuring a bland spindle cell proliferation set in an abundant myxoid background. Lipoblasts are most often monovacuolated and tend to cluster around vessels or at the periphery of the lesion. The most helpful morphologic clue is the presence of a thin-walled, capillary-sized vascular network, organized in a distinctive plexiform pattern. High-grade MLS (formerly RCL) is defined by the presence of hypercellularity. Adipocytic differentiation in pure RCL is rarely appreciable, but in such circumstances the presence of S-100 immunopositivity may be diagnostically helpful.[2]

MLS is characterized by two main karyotypic aberrations: more than 95% of cases carry a specific t(12;16)(q13;p11), which fuses the *DDIT3* (*CHOP*) gene on 12q13 (a member of the CCAAT/enhancer binding protein family involved in adipocyte differentiation), with the *FUS* (*TLS*) gene on 16p11. Approximately 5% of MLSs harbor a t(12;22) (q13;q12), which fuses *DDIT3* with *EWSR1* on 22q12. *PIK3CA* mutations have also been detected in a subset of cases; this may represent a valuable additional target for future molecularly driven therapies.[12]

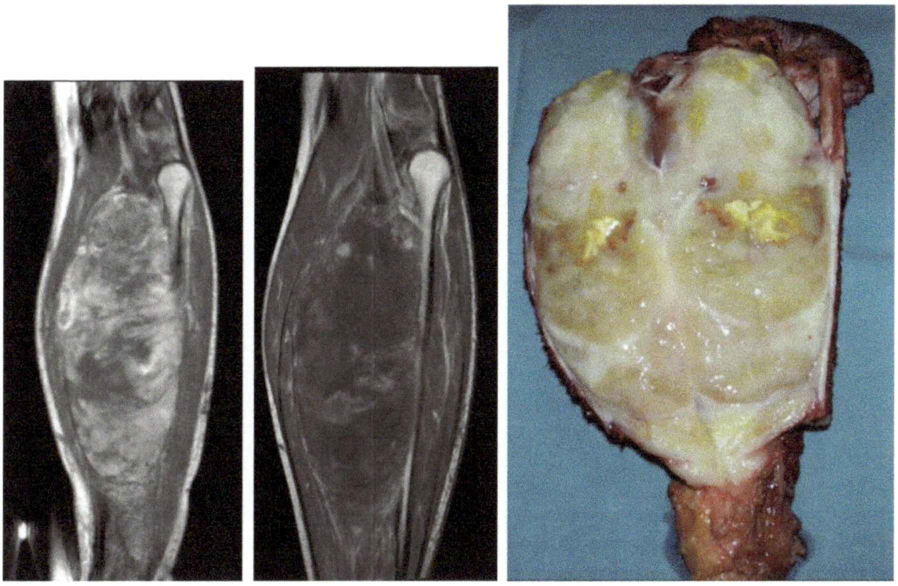

(A) (B) (C)

FIGURE 25.2 Case example of high-grade myxoid liposarcoma treated with five cycles of epirubicin and ifosfamide and concomitant radiation therapy. The pathologic specimen after the surgery showed a complete pathologic response. (A) MRI of a high-grade myxoid liposarcoma, (B) MRI with a radiological response, (C) pathologic specimen after surgery.

COMMON ANATOMIC LOCATION OF PRIMARY MLS

MLS occurs with predilection in the deep soft tissues of the extremities, and in more than two-thirds of cases arises within the musculature of the thigh. MLS rarely arises primarily in the retroperitoneum or in subcutaneous tissue. Surgery is the mainstay of treatment in patients with localized disease, alone or in combination with RT. To optimize local control, RT eventually in combination with systemic chemotherapy given before surgery may be of benefit, in order to obtain a cytoreduction and to improve the prognosis.[6] In particular, it has been repeatedly observed that the presence of hypercellularity or round cell differentiation is associated with worsening of prognosis. The 90% 5-year survival rate of MLS decreases to 20% for patients with RCLs.[6] Thus, for patients with high-grade MLS, even after complete resection, there remains a high risk for recurrence and death. Therefore, high-grade MLS may benefit from the above-mentioned multimodality treatment, either before or after surgery[7] (Figure 25.2).

Overall, the utility of systemic treatment and the sequence of therapy for each patient with MLS should be discussed within a multidisciplinary conference at a sarcoma reference center. Neoadjuvant therapy (RT and/or systemic treatment) may facilitate resectability in borderline cases, especially if tumor shrinkage can be achieved and improve the prognosis. Neoadjuvant combined chemotherapy-RT has been extensively explored in localized STS. A recent randomized trial showed a benefit of neoadjuvant anthracycline and ifosfamide doublet (AI) versus a histology-driven chemotherapy in terms of overall survival (OS) and recurrence-free survival (RFS), thus pointing to efficacy of neoadjuvant treatment as such in a subset of STS. In the MLS stratum of this trial, the interim analysis showed the noninferiority of trabectedin, with a much better toxicity profile. This study is still recruiting in the MLS stratum and is expected to complete the accrual in a year.[13] Trabectedin was recently shown also to be combinable with RT in patients affected by locally advanced MLS, with promising results.[14] If trabectedin proves to be equivalent to AI, its use alone or in combination to RT may well become the preferred approach in treatment of localized high-risk MLS.

RECOMMENDED FOLLOW-UP

Given the risk of recurrence, close surveillance is important in patients with MLS. Although consensus recommendations (National Comprehensive Cancer Network [NCCN], European Society of Medical

Oncology [ESMO]) exist for surveillance in STSs in general, there are no validated guidelines specific for MLS.[15] Most sarcoma centers recommend initial contrast-enhanced CT of the chest and abdomen at 3 to 4 months after surgery, and every 4 to 6 months for at least 2 to 3 years and up to 5 years. A similar schedule of interval imaging should be followed with contrast-enhanced MRI. Whole-body MRI has been suggested as an alternative, to offer patients to be staged with a single modality, without radiation exposure, and with high sensitivity in detecting recurrences of this disease at all sites, including bone. For superficial tumors, ultimately MRI may be replaced with ultrasound imaging. Surveillance should be modified based on personalized risk and anticipated pattern of recurrence. Late recurrences can occur, particularly in low-grade MLS.

When recurrence develops (usually detected by surveillance imaging), decision-making and overall management can be complex and multimodality therapy is frequently used. Surgery is always considered and is ultimately performed in most patients with a localized recurrence. Currently, there are no laboratory tests that are useful to detect recurrence in MLS.

PROPENSITY TO METASTASIZE

MLS is prone to recur locally, and one-third of patients develop distant metastases, but the probability of developing distant metastases depends on the histologic grade. In contrast to other types of liposarcoma or other sarcomas of the extremities, MLS tends to metastasize to unusual soft tissue (such as retroperitoneum, opposite extremity, axilla, etc.) or bone (with predilection to spine) locations, even before spread to the lung.[5] In a significant number of cases, MLS patients present clinically with synchronous or metachronous multifocal disease. This unusual clinical phenomenon most likely represents a pattern of hematogenous metastases to other sites by tumor cells seemingly incompetent to seed the lungs. The extent of hypercellularity predicts the risk of metastatic spread.

THERAPEUTIC APPROACH FOR METASTATIC DISEASE

Treatment options for patients with unresectable and metastatic disease are limited. In STS in general, front-line treatment for unresectable/metastatic disease is usually systemic therapy with doxorubicin, alone or in combination with ifosfamide, with a reported objective response rate (ORR) in the range of 20% to 40%.[7–9] The combination of doxorubicin and ifosfamide is superior to doxorubicin alone.

MLSs are known to be particularly sensitive to chemotherapy compared with other STSs,[9,10] especially to anthracycline-based combinations and trabectedin. The response rates to the front-line combination of an anthracycline and ifosfamide is approximately 65%. On the other hand, the expected response rate of MLS to trabectedin, approved for second-line therapy, is around 80%, with a mechanism of action thought to be due to binding to the fusion transcript and target genes.[16–19]

The extra activity of trabectedin in MLS was observed quite late in the development of the drug in sarcomas. In 2007, we were able to report on 51 patients with MLS who had been treated on a compassionate basis at five institutions in Europe and the United States. In this series of MLS, the response rate according to dimensional criteria was approximately 50%, and the 6-month PFS was about 80%.[20] Thus, the drug showed a major antitumor impact, in a heavily pretreated patient population, which was substantially different from what observed in other STS, including the most sensitive leiomyosarcoma and well-differentiated/dedifferentiated liposarcoma. At a longer follow-up, we updated this series regarding the subgroup of 32 patients treated in Milan. The median PFS was confirmed to be prolonged, that is, 17 months. Treatment was continued for a long time in several patients. Indeed, long progression-free intervals were observed also in patients who discontinued their treatment with trabectedin after achieving an objective response or stable disease. When they progressed, a re-challenge with trabectedin induced further responses, with relatively long progression-free intervals.[21] Some patients underwent surgery of residual disease, following the practice of surgery of extrapulmonary metastases in low-grade MLS, given the relatively indolent course of disease. However, the added value of metastasectomy is doubtful when the medical therapy has been ineffective.

An intriguing clinical observation was that tumor responses could be nondimensional initially, before giving rise to tumor shrinkage at a later time. The hallmark in these cases is a decrease in tumor contrast enhancement and radiodensity.[21] Fortunately, the sarcoma clinical community had learned the lesson deriving from gastrointestinal stromal tumors (GISTs) treated with targeted therapies, so we were ready to appreciate this type of response.[22,23] Clinicians should be aware of this pattern of tumor response in MLS, to avoid mistakes. However, this also led us to suspect that a different mechanism of action could be in place, in other words that such a pattern of tumor response, which we are used to observe with molecularly targeted therapies, could point to a kind of "targeted" mechanism of action also for a chemotherapeutic agent like trabectedin.

Preclinical studies performed in an MLS cell line indicate that trabectedin modulates transcription, presumably interfering with transcription factors that are deregulated in some sarcomas. In particular, MLSs are marked by the fusion gene *FUS-CHOP*. In the presence of trabectedin, it is transcribed normally, but is not able to activate the transcription of target genes. Thus, the mechanism of action of trabectedin is highly selective, with a depression in the expression of genes that are crucial for the late phase of adipocytic differentiation.[24]

Recently, another marine-derived drug, eribulin, was shown to be effective in metastatic adipocytic sarcomas, with a significant improvement in OS, which led to its approval by the U.S. Food and Drug Administration (FDA) and the European Medicines Agency (EMA).[25–27] However, its activity in MLS compared to pleomorphic and well-differentiated/dedifferentiated liposarcoma is still not defined. No other agents commonly used for treatment of advanced STS (e.g., gemcitabine, dacarbazine, and pazopanib) have been demonstrated to be active in MLS.

Continuous infusion, high-dose ifosfamide (icHDIFX), which is another treatment option active in advanced well-differentiated/dedifferentiated liposarcoma patients, seems not to be active in MLS.[28]

In conclusion, the more active drugs for advanced MLS are anthracyclines-based regimens (usually ifosfamide) and trabectedin.

Other treatment options are under investigation, including immunotherapy such as checkpoint inhibitors and cellular therapy. Indeed, most patients with MLS have homogeneous expression of the highly immunogenic tumor-associated antigen NY-ESO-1 or MAGE. Furthermore, while these patients have rare NY-ESO-1 or MAGE-specific T cells circulating in their blood, they lack a robust inflammatory response and generally have relatively few T cells infiltrating the tumor.[29] Agents and strategies with the ability to induce a robust endogenous tumor-specific T-cell population have the potential to dramatically activate the immune response against this neoplasm and are under investigation.

SUMMARY

In conclusion, MLS comprises a spectrum of disease with a spectrum of aggressivity that parallels the percent cellular component. Localized disease, especially for high-grade MLS, requires a multidisciplinary approach as the combination of RT and chemotherapy are recommended in the preoperative setting. The exceptional activity of trabectedin in this neoplasm encourages exploration of the efficacy of the drug in first line and in the preoperative setting. Unfortunately, up to now, even if MLS seems to be sensitive to chemotherapy, no other options are active in the advanced setting beyond the use of anthracycline-based combinations (usually ifosfamide) and trabectedin. Treatment options using adaptive immunotherapy look promising and are under investigation.

CASE STUDY

A 46-year-old man presented with a posteromedial lesion of the right thigh rapidly growing in the past 4 months (Figure 25.3). The staging chest and abdomen CT scan did not show evidence of distant metastatic disease.

A core-needle biopsy was performed. The pathology was consistent with classic MLS. Thus, the lesion was completely surgically resected. The final pathology was diagnostic for MLS (round cell 40%). Therefore, given the high risk of distant metastatic disease, the decision was made to give postoperative systemic therapy, which consisted of doxorubicin and ifosfamide for five cycles and concomitant RT (50 Gy).

The patient has since been under surveillance with chest and abdomen CT scan, and clinic visits every 3 months.

One year later, the CT scan revealed a pelvic relapse. Patient started a systemic treatment with trabectedin 1.3 mg/m^2 that he continued for 17 cycles with a partial response (Figure 25.4).

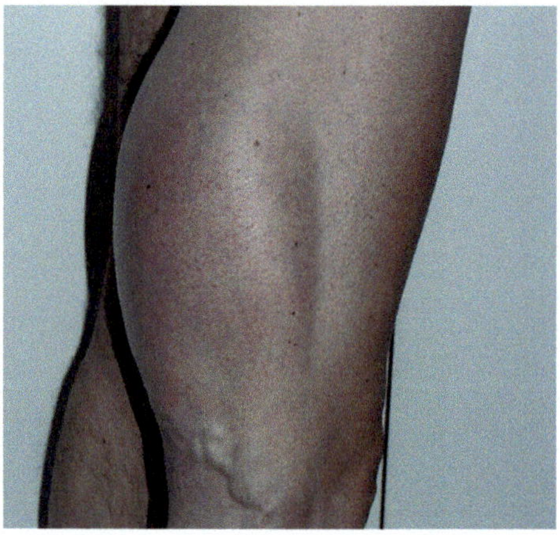

FIGURE 25.3 Clinical presentation of posteromedial lesion of the right thigh.

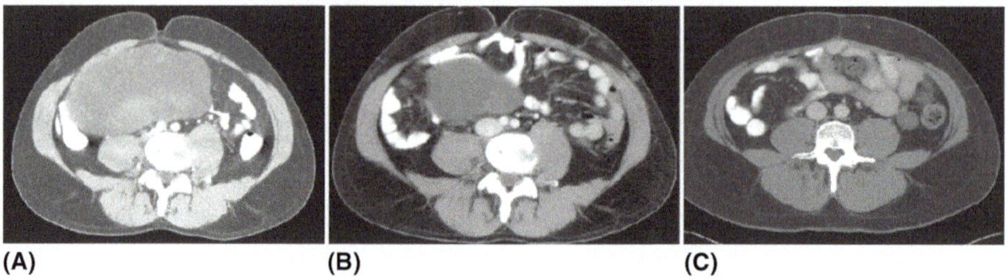

FIGURE 25.4 Radiologic response: (A) basal at relapse, (B) after 10 cycles, (C) after 17 cycles.

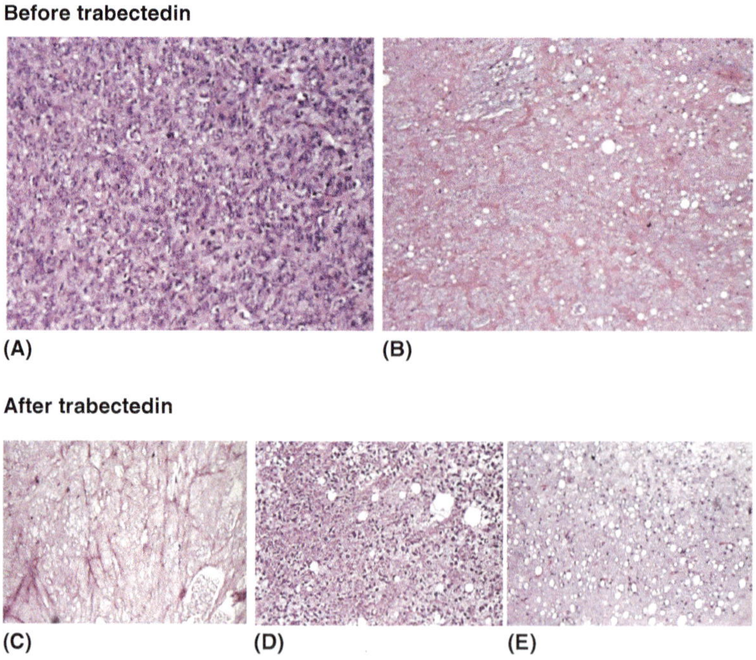

FIGURE 25.5 Changes in pathological specimens before and after trabectedin treatment with the regression of both cellular and vascular component after chemotherapy and the presence of mature component and coagulative necrosis. Before trabectedin: (A) cellular component 40%, (B) mature lipoblasts featuring cells 5%. After trabectedin: (C) cellular and vascular depletion 10%, (D) mature lipoblast featuring cell 30%, (E) necrosis 60%.

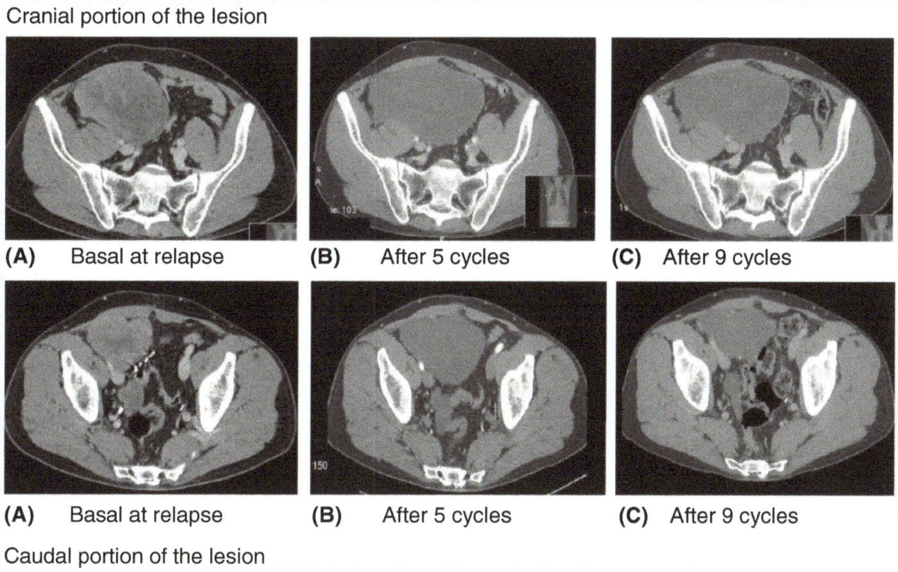

FIGURE 25.6 Radiologic response: (A) basal at relapse, (B) after five cycles, (C) after nine cycles.

Then, the case was discussed at multidisciplinary sarcoma tumor board and it was decided to surgically remove the single metastatic lesion.

The pathologic examination revealed a pathologic response to treatment with regression of both cellular and vascular component <90%, presence of mature component and coagulative necrosis (Figure 25.5).

After 3 years under surveillance, the patient presented again with abdominal/pelvic multifocal relapse, so we resumed chemotherapy with trabectedin. He did 27 additional cycles, obtaining a decrease in density shown at CT scan associated with a subsequent dimensional response (Figure 25.6).

After a total of 50 cycles of trabectedin, the patient progressed. The subsequent rapid deterioration of his general condition constrained us not to administer further lines of therapy.

REFERENCES

1. Fletcher CDM, Bridge JA, Hogendoorn P, Mertens F, eds. *World Health Organization Classification of Tumours. Pathology and Genetics of Tumours of Soft Tissue and Bone*. Paris, France: IARC Press; 2013.
2. Dei Tos AP. Liposarcomas: diagnostic pitfalls and new insights. *Histopathology*. 2014;64(1):38–52. doi:10.1111/his.12311
3. Panagopoulos I, Mertens F, Isaksson M, Mandahl N. A novel FUS/CHOP chimera in MLS. *Biochem Biophys Res Commun*. 2000;279(3):838–845. doi:10.1006/bbrc.2000.4026
4. Antonescu CR, Elahi A, Healey JH, et al. Monoclonality of multifocal myxoid liposarcoma: confirmation by analysis of *TLS-CHOP* or *EWS-CHOP* rearrangements. *Clin Cancer Res*. 2000;6(7):2788–2793. https://clincancerres.aacrjournals.org/content/6/7/2788.full-text.pdf
5. Spillane AJ, Fisher C, Thomas JM. Myxoid liposarcoma—the frequency and the natural history of nonpulmonary soft tissue metastases. *Ann Surg Oncol*. 1999;6(4):389–394. doi:10.1007/s10434-999-0389-5
6. Fiore M, Grosso F, Lo Vullo S, et al. Myxoid/round cell and pleomorphic liposarcomas: prognostic factors and survival in a series of patients treated at a single institution. *Cancer*. 2007;109(12):2522–2531. doi:10.1002/cncr.22720
7. Singer S, Demetri GD, Baldini EH, Fletcher CD. Management of soft-tissue sarcomas: an overview and update. *Lancet Oncol*. 2000;1:75–85. doi:10.1016/s1470-2045(00)00016-4
8. Keohan ML, Taub RN. Chemotherapy for advanced sarcoma: therapeutic decisions and modalities. *Semin Oncol*. 1997;24(5):572–579. https://www.ncbi.nlm.nih.gov/pubmed/9344324
9. Van Glabbeke M, van Oosterom AT, Oosterhuis JW, et al. Prognostic factors for the outcome of chemotherapy in advanced soft tissue sarcoma: an analysis of 2,185 patients treated with anthracycline-containing first-line regimens—a European Organization for Research and Treatment of Cancer Soft Tissue and Bone Sarcoma Group Study. *J Clin Oncol*. 1999;17(1):150–157. doi:10.1200/JCO.1999.17.1.150

10. Jones RL, Fisher C, Al-Muderis O, Judson IR. Differential sensitivity of liposarcoma subtypes to chemotherapy. *Eur J Cancer*. 2005;41(18):2853–2860. doi:10.1016/j.ejca.2005.07.023
11. Patel SR, Burgess MA, Plager C, et al. Myxoid liposarcoma. Experience with chemotherapy. *Cancer*. 1994;74(4):1265–1269. doi:10.1002/1097-0142(19940815)74:4<1265::aid-cncr2820740414>3.0.co;2-x
12. Sanfilippo R, Dei Tos AP, Casali PG. Myxoid liposarcoma and the mammalian target of rapamycin pathway. *Curr Opin Oncol*. 2013;25(4):379–383. doi:10.1097/CCO.0b013e32836227ac
13. Gronchi A, Ferrari S, Quagliuolo V, et al. Histotype-tailored neoadjuvant chemotherapy versus standard chemotherapy in patients with high-risk soft-tissue sarcomas (ISG-STS 1001): an international, open-label, randomised, controlled, phase 3, multicentre trial. *Lancet Oncol*. 2017;18(6):812–822. doi:10.1016/S1470-2045(17)30334-0
14. Gronchi A, Hindi N, Cruz J, et al. Trabectedin and radiotherapy in soft tissue sarcoma (TRASTS): results of a phase I study in myxoid liposarcoma from Spanish (GEIS), Italian (ISG), French (FSG) Sarcoma Groups. *EClinicalMedicine*. 2019;9:35–43. doi:10.1016/j.eclinm.2019.03.007
15. Casali PG, Abecassis N, Aro HT, et al. Soft tissue and visceral sarcomas: ESMO-EURACAN Clinical Practice Guidelines for diagnosis, treatment and follow-up. *Ann Oncol*. 2018;29(suppl 4):iv51–iv67. doi:10.1093/annonc/mdy096
16. Morgan A, Chow S. The economic impact of implementing an ergonomic plan. *Nurs Econ*. 2007;25(3):150–156. https://www.ncbi.nlm.nih.gov/pubmed/17802997
17. Garcia-Carbonero R, Supko JG, Manola J, et al. Phase II and pharmacokinetic study of ecteinascidin 743 in patients with progressive sarcomas of soft tissues refractory to chemotherapy. *J Clin Oncol*. 2004;22(8):1480–1490. doi:10.1200/JCO.2004.02.098
18. Le Cesne A, Blay JY, Judson I, et al. Phase II study of ET-743 in advanced soft tissue sarcomas: a European Organisation for the Research and Treatment of Cancer (EORTC) soft tissue and bone sarcoma group trial. *J Clin Oncol*. 2005;23(3):576–584. doi:10.1200/JCO.2005.01.180
19. Garcia-Carbonero R, Supko JG, Maki RG, et al. Ecteinascidin-743 (ET-743) for chemotherapy-naive patients with advanced soft tissue sarcomas: multicenter phase II and pharmacokinetic study. *J Clin Oncol*. 2005;23(24):5484–5492. doi:10.1200/JCO.2005.05.028
20. Grosso F, Jones RL, Demetri GD, et al. Efficacy of trabectedin (ecteinascidin-743) in advanced pretreated myxoid liposarcomas: a retrospective study. *Lancet Oncol*. 2007;8(7):595–602. doi:10.1016/S1470-2045(07)70175-4
21. Grosso F, Sanfilippo R, Virdis E, et al. Trabectedin in myxoid liposarcomas (MLS): a long-term analysis of a single-institution series. *Ann Oncol*. 2009;20(8):1439–44. doi:10.1093/annonc/mdp004
22. Casali PG, Bertulli R, Fumagalli E, et al. Some lessons learned from imatinib mesylate clinical development in gastrointestinal stromal tumors. *J Chemother*. 2004;16 (suppl 4):55–58. doi:10.1179/joc.2004.16.Supplement-1.55
23. Casali PG, Messina A, Stacchiotti S, et al. Imatinib mesylate in chordoma. *Cancer*. 2004;101(9):2086–2097. doi:10.1002/cncr.20618
24. Forni C, Minuzzo M, Virdis E, et al. Trabectedin (ET-743) promotes differentiation in myxoid liposarcoma tumors. *Mol Cancer Ther*. 2009;8(2):449–457. doi:10.1158/1535-7163.MCT-08-0848
25. Schöffski P, Ray-Coquard IL, Cioffi A, et al. Activity of eribulin mesylate in patients with soft-tissue sarcoma: a phase 2 study in four independent histological subtypes. *Lancet Oncol*. 2011;12(11):1045–1052. doi:10.1016/S1470-2045(11)70230-3
26. Schöffski P, Chawla S, Maki RG, et al. Eribulin versus dacarbazine in previously treated patients with advanced liposarcoma or leiomyosarcoma: a randomised, open-label, multicentre, phase 3 trial. *Lancet*. 2016;387(10028):1629–1637. doi:10.1016/S0140-6736(15)01283-0
27. Chawla SP, Schöffski P, Grignani G, et al. Subtype-specific activity in liposarcoma (LPS) patients (pts) from a phase 3, open-label, randomized study of eribulin (ERI) versus dacarbazine (DTIC) in patients with advanced LPS and leiomyosarcoma (LMS). *J Clin Oncol*. 2016;34(suppl_6):11037. doi:10.1200/JCO.2016.34.15_suppl.11037
28. Colia V, Fumagalli E, Provenzano S, et al. High-dose ifosfamide chemotherapy in a series of patients affected by myxoid liposarcoma. *Sarcoma*. 2017;2017:3739159. doi:10.1155/2017/3739159
29. Pollack SM, He Q, Yearley JH, et al. T-cell infiltration and clonality correlate with programmed cell death protein 1 and programmed death-ligand 1 expression in patients with soft tissue sarcomas. *Cancer*. 2017;123(17):3291–3304. doi:10.1002/cncr.30726

26

Perivascular Epithelioid Cell Sarcoma

Emily E. Jonczak

INTRODUCTION

Perivascular epithelioid cell neoplasms (PEComas) are a rare family of mesenchymal tumors, composed of histologically and immunohistochemically distinctive cells known as perivascular epithelioid cells (PECs) as defined by World Health Organization (WHO).[1] PEComas are notable for tumor cells that demonstrate a focal association with blood vessel walls and commonly express myogenic and melanocytic markers, including actin and/or desmin and HMB-45 and/or melan-A, respectively.[1] This family of tumors consists of angiomyolipoma (AML), lymphangioleiomyomatosis (LAM), clear-cell "sugar" tumor of the lung and extra pulmonary sites (CCST), clear-cell myomelanocytic tumor of the falciform ligament/ligamentum teres, and rare histologically and immunophenotypically similar tumors arising from a variety of soft tissue and visceral sites.[1–5] Pea and Bonetti et al. are credited with coining the term "perivascular epithelioid cell" in 1992 after first describing the presence of this unique cell with "prominent cytoplasmic borders and clear to granular, eosinophilic cytoplasm" in a perivascular distribution in both AML and CCST. They then suggested this cell was further distinguished in part by strong positivity of the melanocytic marker HMB-45, a common link among these rare tumors.[2,5,6] Furthermore, genetic alterations in the tuberous sclerosis complex (TSC), leading to losses of *TSC1* (9q34) or *TSC2* (16p13.3) genes have been described in both sporadic cases and in patients with the autosomal dominant disease, tuberous sclerosis, which is characterized by mental retardation, seizures, and cellular proliferations, that is, AML and LAM.[1,3,4]

Clinically, many PEComas are benign and indolent in nature, but subsets of these tumors have a malignant potential and an aggressive course, and therefore it is important that these patients are identified and treated. Historically, treatment was mainly based on surgical resection as conventional doxorubicin-based chemotherapy typically employed in other soft tissue sarcomas (STS) has largely been ineffective. Given the rarity of PEComas, the majority of our understanding of the disease comes from small case series, retrospective analysis, and clinical experience. The identification of the alterations in TSC and its relationship to the mammalian target of rapamycin (mTOR) pathway has opened doors to the exploration of mTOR inhibitors as a means to treat these patients. In this chapter, we will review the epidemiology, clinical presentation, diagnostic approach, molecular drivers, and treatment options for PEC sarcomas.

EPIDEMIOLOGY

PEComas are exceedingly rare; in fact there is no Surveillance, Epidemiology, and End Results (SEER) data to track the benign or malignant PEComas.[7] Per WHO publication as of 2013, there were approximately 200 reported cases of non-AML and non-LAM PEComas.[1] Most commonly, PEComas are present in young to middle-aged adults (mean age 45 years). PEComas are markedly more frequent in females compared to males, with a female-to-male ratio of approximately 6:1. No links to a particular race or ethnicity have been reported.[1,3,8]

CLINICAL PRESENTATION AND NATURAL HISTORY

PEComas are exceedingly rare and can present in a number of different soft tissue and visceral organs, leading to an array of presenting symptoms from asymptomatic to pain and bleeding, based on the primary location of the tumor. AML presenting classically of the kidney can occur in association with tuberous sclerosis or sporadically. AML cases associated with tuberous sclerosis are reported in both sexes with a female predominance, occurring in the third and fourth decades of life, as bilateral, small, multiple lesions, generally asymptomatic and benign. Sporadic cases tend to occur later in life, present as single lesions, unilateral, and larger. Complications can include renal failure and hemorrhage with a relatively low malignant potential.[4] LAM, another member of this family of tumors, can occur sporadically, but is frequently seen in patients with TSC. This is a rare progressive disease affecting the lungs, predominately afflicting women. The natural history of the disease is a slow progression to respiratory failure with median survival of 8 to 10 years, and the only therapy is lung transplantation. CCST is generally a benign condition in which the vast majority of cases are sporadic.[4,6]

The remainder of this chapter will focus on the tumors in this family, which have come to be referred to in literature as PEComa not otherwise specified (PEComa-NOS). PEComas have been described in case reports and series in a variety of different anatomic locations including the colon,[9–11] pancreas,[12–14] retroperitoneum,[15,16] heart,[17] adrenal gland,[18,19] breast,[20] eye,[21,22] biliary tract,[23] bone,[24,25] urinary bladder,[26–28] genitourinary tract,[29,30] skull base,[31] liver,[32–34] uterus,[35,36] cervix,[37,38] skin,[39,40] and soft tissues.[41] The clinical presentation varies based on anatomic location of the primary tumor. Patients presenting abdominopelvic PEComas describe progressive abdominal pain and weight loss. Patients presenting with genitourinary tract lesions frequently mention pain and hematuria as their chief complaint.[29] Uterine and cervical tumors often present with vaginal bleeding and those of the gastrointestinal (GI) tract with GI bleeding.

Our understanding of the natural history and prognostic features of these tumors is largely based on reviews of reported case studies and series. In 2005, Folpe et al. published the largest review to date at the time of 26 patients with PEComas of soft tissue and gynecologic origin.[42] The median age was reported as 46 years (range, 15–97); there was a marked female predominance (22 females, four males), and the sites of involvement included omentum/mesentery (six cases), uterus (four cases), pelvic soft tissue (three cases), abdominal wall (two cases), uterine cervix (two cases), and vagina, retroperitoneum, thigh, falciform ligament, scalp, broad ligament, forearm, shoulder, and neck (one case each). They evaluated the characteristics of the tumors including size, histology (epithelioid, spindled, or mixed), grade, mitotic activity, presence of necrosis, and immunohistochemistry (IHC) results to assess the predictive and clinical features of these tumors. Of note, no patients in the series had a history of tuberous sclerosis. Based on their analysis, they suggested that PEComas could be classified as "benign," "of uncertain malignant potential," or "malignant." High-risk features included size >5 cm, infiltrative growth pattern, high nuclear grade and cellularity, mitotic rate >1/50 high power fields (HPF), necrosis, and vascular invasion. Those classified as "benign" had <2 high-risk features and size <5 cm. Those classified in the "uncertain malignant potential" category had size ≥5 cm with no other high-risk features or nuclear pleomorphism/multinucleated giant cells only. Finally, those classified in the "malignant" category had two or more high-risk features. Recurrence and/or metastasis was strongly associated with tumor size >5 cm, mitotic activity greater than 1/50 HPF, and necrosis.[42] In 2012, Bleeker et al. published a review of 234 cases of PEComa-NOS in English literature, evaluating information regarding diagnostic features, treatment approaches, and outcomes.[2] Based on their multivariate analysis, primary tumor size ≥5 cm ($p = .02$) and high (1/50 HPF) mitotic rate ($p <$ 0001) were the only factors significantly associated with recurrence following surgical resection.[2]

DIAGNOSTIC APPROCH

High clinical suspicion is necessary for accurate diagnosis of these rare tumors. Like any soft tissue mass, early evaluation with imaging is critical to identify the primary location of the mass and metastatic disease. Evaluation with gadolinium-enhanced MRI and CT has been utilized in the diagnosis of these tumors. Referral to a multidisciplinary sarcoma center for initial management, including biopsy, pathology review, and surgical resection for localized disease is paramount for the best outcomes. Initial staging should include a high quality contrast-enhanced CT scan of the lungs, as well as abdomen, pelvis, and bone scan. PET/CT scan may be useful to identify occult lesions, particularly in advanced disease, but early lung metastases are often sub-centimeter in size and below the threshold of PET detection.

RADIOGRAPHIC FEATURES

On CT imaging, PEComas may appear heterogeneous with heterogeneous enhancement. On MRI imaging, they often exhibit low T1 signal and high T2 signal intensity with increased vascularity and heterogeneous enhancement.[7] One review of 22 patients with hepatic PEComas described the lesions as well-defined, heterogeneous, arterial enhanced masses with dysmorphic vessels on CT, MRI, and ultrasound images.[32]

HISTOPATHOLOGIC FEATURES

The hallmark of PEComas is the presence of the distinctive PECs. They are characterized by their perivascular location, often forming a radial arrangement of cells around the vascular lumen. PEComa-NOS tumors tend to comprise both epithelioid and spindle cell components in various degrees of proportion. The epithelioid cells are more commonly located in the immediate perivascular area, whereas the spindle cells resembling smooth muscle cells are often located away from the vessels. The PECs are described as having a clear to granular, lightly eosinophilic cytoplasm; small, centrally located, normochromatic, round to oval nuclei with small nucleoli; and slight atypia with sparse mitotic activity. However, a significant number of reported PEComas have increased mitotic activity and considerable atypical features, including nuclear atypia with hyperchromasia and irregularity.[43]

Immunohistochemically, PEC are characterized for expressing myogenic and melanocytic markers. The myogenic markers can include desmin, smooth muscle actin (SMA), muscle-specific actin/all muscle actin/HHF-35, muscle myosin and calponin. Desmin expression can be seen in approximately 30% of PEComas.[8] The melanocytic markers include HMB-45, melan-A/ART-1, tyrosinase, and micropthalmia transcription factor. The most sensitive melanocytic markers for PEComa are HMB-45 and Melan-A. S-100 protein is reported as positive in approximately 30% of PEComas, and its presence does not necessarily imply a melanocytic malignancy.[8] Cytokeratin expression is usually negative.[43] Estrogen and progesterone receptors are frequently positive in renal AML, but have been rarely shown to be positive in PEComa-NOS.[1,8,43]

MOLECULAR AND BIOLOGIC DRIVERS

Alterations in the *TSC* genes have been reported in both sporadic and in PEComas related to tuberous sclerosis. The most common abnormality observed is the loss of heterozygosity of the *TSC2* gene on 16p13. Genetic alterations on *TSC1* gene on 9q34 have also been appreciated. The *TSC* genes play an important role in regulation of the Rheb/mTOR/p70S6K pathway and therefore have been a focus for targeted therapy. Increasing studies suggest this pathway is complex with multiple protein components, but at the core of the pathway are four key proteins, including TSC1, TSC2, Rheb, and mTOR (mammalian target of rapamycin). Rheb protein is a member of the ras family of GTPases and when bound to guanosine triphosphate (GTP), it interacts with mTOR forming the activated complex termed mTORC1. This activation drives the mTOR/p70S6K pathway leading to downstream events, such as ribosome biogenesis, protein synthesis, and cell growth. Therefore, the loss of TSC1/TSC2 can have significant effects on the mTORC1 complex and result in cell growth.

There is limited data on other genetic alterations observed in PEComas. *TFE3* gene rearrangements have been increasingly observed in cases.[20,44] Interestingly, 80% of *TFE3* fusion negative PEComas have been shown to have *TSC2* mutations, whereas those harboring *TFE3* fusions lack *TSC2* mutations.[44,45]

TREATMENT CONSIDERATIONS

Complete surgical resection when feasible has historically been the mainstay of treatment. Surgery is not attempted in patients who are metastatic at the time of presentation or if the primary lesion is deemed unresectable. In 2012, Bleeker et al. reviewed 234 cases of PEComa, of which the majority, 95%, underwent surgical resection. Only 18% of patients had additional therapy beyond surgery. A minority of patients received neoadjuvant chemotherapy, radiotherapy, or combined chemoradiation with mixed response. Only one reported case had a robust response, the remaining either progressed or had minimal evidence of efficacy in the resected tumor. The role of adjuvant therapy is also unclear. The chemotherapy regimens typically utilized an anthracycline backbone typically used in other STS.[2,43]

In the metastatic setting, chemotherapy has shown little benefit. There has been enthusiasm for targeted therapies, most notably with mTOR inhibitors. Nanoparticle albumin-bound sirolimus (nab-sirolimus), an mTOR inhibitor, received Breakthrough Therapy designation from the Food and Drug Administration (FDA) based on preliminary data from the AMPECT trial presented at the American

Society of Clinical Oncology (ASCO) 2019 meeting. This is the first prospective clinical trial in advanced PEComa to date. The trial was conducted in nine U.S. cities and enrolled 34 adult patients, 31 evaluable patients with confirmed PEComa. Involved sites included uterus, pelvis, retroperitoneum, lung, kidney, liver, brain, muscle, ovary, aorta, and small bowel. The primary objective was overall response rate (ORR). Interim analysis showed 42% had an interim analysis, 69% of the partial responses (PR) were ongoing, and the median progression-free survival (mPFS) was 8.9 months. Of the 25 patients with known mutational status, five had mutations in *TSC1* and nine had mutations in *TSC2*. PR was achieved in 100% of patients with a *TSC2* mutation (9/9), 20% (1/5) of those with a *TSC1* mutation, and 9% (1/11) of patients without a mutation in *TSC1* or *TSC2*[46] (NCT02494570).

Anti-PD-1 therapy may play a role in the future. In one case report, a 46-year-old man with a PEComa located in the right popliteal fossa was initially treated with sirolimus, but was unable to tolerate the side effects. A year after his diagnosis, he presented with metastatic disease to the lungs, rib cage, and a fungating mass in the right popliteal fossa. He underwent an amputation and video-assisted thoracoscopic surgery (VATs) to confirm metastatic disease. He was subsequently treated with pazopanib and progressed. He was subsequently started on nivolumab, a PD-L1 inhibitor and imaging done at 2 and 5 months revealed significant disease response. At 12 months, he was progression-free with no identifiable metastatic lesions.[47]

SUMMARY

PEComas are an exceedingly rare subset of STS. They vary widely in clinical behavior from benign to aggressively malignant lesions. Significant progress has been made with regard to the molecular mechanism underlying the disease and understanding of histopathology and IHC for disease diagnosis. The risk assessment remains imprecise, but large tumors >5 cm and high mitotic rate of 1/50 HPF are widely accepted as risk factors for more aggressive disease. The mainstay of treatment remains surgical resection when feasible. In recurrent/metastatic disease, chemotherapy and radiation have been used with mixed to minimal benefit. The first prospective clinical trial has led to the first breakthrough therapy designation by the FDA for nab-sirolimus in the management of these patients. More needs to be learned about these unique tumors.

CASE STUDY

A 54-year-old woman with a past medical history significant for thyroid cancer following thyroidectomy and radioactive iodine in 2006, hyperlipidemia, coronary artery disease, diabetes mellitus type 2, and uterine fibroids initially presented to medical attention in May 2018 complaining of gradual weight loss and difficulty concentrating, which she attributed to her thyroid medications needing adjustment. Her primary care physician ultimately evaluated her in September 2018, when lab work was done and the only noted abnormality was thrombocytosis. She then noted progressive pelvic and back pain, and underwent CT imaging, which revealed a uterine myometrial lesion, measuring 10 cm along with external iliac lymphadenopathy measuring 2.0 x 1.7 cm and right iliac lymph node measuring 1.7 x 1.3 cm. She underwent biopsy of the endometrium, lymph node, and bone marrow. The bone marrow biopsy revealed a cellular marrow (50%) with maturing trilineage hematopoiesis. The endometrial biopsy of the anterior uterine wall was determined to be epithelioid PEComa with focal sclerosing pattern. The IHC revealed that the tumor cells were diffusely positive for cathepsin K and many cells were positive for desmin and melan-A, and negative for SOX-10 and TFE3. The proliferation rate in the cellular epithelioid area was approximately 20%. The endometrial biopsy also revealed highly atypical mucinous proliferation, most consistent with low-grade endometrial mucinous adenocarcinoma. The right iliac chain lymph node biopsy revealed metastatic malignant PEComa, high grade with IHC showing tumor cells diffusely positive for a pan melanocyte antibody cocktail, focally positive for S-100, calretinin, desmin, and SMA, and negative for SOX-10, epithelial membrane antigen (EMA), inhibin, myogen, PAX-8, and pancytokeratin. This pattern suggested a diagnosis of metastatic PEComa with a uterine mass as the primary lesion. Staging PET/CT scan was completed in January 2019 and was consistent with a 10-cm hypermetabolic uterine mass (SUV 8.2) and hypermetabolic right iliac and right common iliac lymph nodes. CT imaging done prior to initiating therapy additionally revealed bilateral lung nodules and mildly enlarged retroperitoneal and pelvic lymphadenopathy. She was evaluated by both gynecology, oncology, and the medical oncology sarcoma team and given the high-grade nature of the PEComa and low-grade mucinous adenocarcinoma. It was felt that the management of PEComa should take precedence. She was started on an mTOR inhibitor, everolimus in February 2019. She initially had difficulty with everolimus, complaining of mouth sores, rash, fatigue, and metallic taste. Her tolerance for the medication has since improved and serial imaging with CT chest, abdomen, and pelvis every 3 months has demonstrated stable disease to date.

REFERENCES

1. Fletcher CDM, Bridge JA, Hogendoorn P, Mertens, F, eds. *World Health Organization (WHO) Classification of Tumors of Soft Tissue and Bone Pathology and Genetics*. Lyon, France: IARC Press; 2013.
2. Bleeker JS, Quevedo JF, Folpe AL. "Malignant" perivascular epithelioid cell neoplasm: risk stratification and treatment strategies. *Sarcoma*. 2012;2012:541626. doi:10.1155/2012/541626
3. Fletcher CDM, Bridge JA, Hogendoorn P, Mertens F, eds. *WHO Classification of Tumours of Soft Tissue and Bone*. 4th ed. Lyon, France: IARC Press; 2013:230–231.
4. Martignoni G, Pea M, Reghellin D, et al. PEComas: the past, the present and the future. *Virchows Arch*. 2008;452(2):119–132. doi:10.1007/s00428-007-0509-1
5. Pea M, Bonetti F, Zamboni G, et al. Clear cell tumor and angiomyolipoma. *Am J Surg Pathol*. 1991;15(2):199–202. doi:10.1097/00000478-199102000-00020
6. Bonetti F, Pea M, Martignoni G, Zamboni G. PEC and sugar. *Am J Surg Pathol*. 1992;16(3):307–308. doi:10.1097/00000478-199203000-00013
7. Bocklage TJ, Quinn RH, Schmit BP, Verschraegen CF. *Bone and Soft Tissue Tumors a Multidisciplinary Review with Case Presentations*. London, UK: JP Medical Publishers; 2014.
8. Folpe AL, Kwiatkowski DJ. Perivascular epithelioid cell neoplasms: pathology and pathogenesis. *Hum Pathol*. 2010;41(1):1–15. doi:10.1016/j.humpath.2009.05.011
9. Neuhaus L, Probst A, Messmann H, et al. Invagination as manifestation of a perivascular epithelioid cell neoplasm (PEComa) of the colon. *Am J Gastroenterol*. 2018;113(8):1115. doi:10.1038/s41395-018-0147-z
10. Iwamoto R, Kataoka TR, Furuhata A, et al. Perivascular epithelioid cell tumor of the descending colon mimicking a gastrointestinal stromal tumor: a case report. *World J Surg Oncol*. 2016;14(1):285. doi:10.1186/s12957-016-1046-7
11. Baek JH, Chung MG, Jung DH, Oh JH. Perivascular epithelioid cell tumor (PEComa) in the transverse colon of an adolescent: a case report. *Tumori*. 2007;93(1):106–108. doi:10.1177/030089160709300120
12. Zhang S, Chen F, Huang X, et al. Perivascular epithelial cell tumor (PEComa) of the pancreas: a case report and review of literature. *Medicine (Baltimore)*. 2017;96(22):e7050. doi:10.1097/MD.0000000000007050
13. Zizzo M, Ugoletti L, Tumiati D, et al. Primary pancreatic perivascular epithelioid cell tumor (PEComa): a surgical enigma. A systematic review of the literature. *Pancreatology*. 2018;18(3):238–245. doi:10.1016/j.pan.2018.02.007
14. Jiang H, Ta N, Huang XY, et al. Pancreatic perivascular epithelioid cell tumor: a case report with clinicopathological features and a literature review. *World J Gastroenterol*. 2016;22(13):3693–3700. doi:10.3748/wjg.v22.i13.3693
15. Sharafeddine H, Bali B, Aoun J, Najjar MW. Retroperitoneal PEComa related to the femoral nerve. *J Neurosurg Sci*. 2017;61(1):109–112. doi:10.23736/S0390-5616.16.03219-7
16. Koenig AM, Quaas A, Ries T, et al. Perivascular epitheloid cell tumour (PEComa) of the retroperitoneum—a rare tumor with uncertain malignant behaviour: a case report. *J Med Case Rep*. 2009;3:62. doi:10.1186/1752-1947-3-62
17. Niu H, Wang FW, Zhang PJ, Bing Z. Cardiac epithelioid PEComa: report of two cases and review of the literature. *Case Rep Med*. 2012;2012:521678. doi:10.1155/2012/521678
18. Pant L, Kalita D, Chopra R, et al. Malignant perivascular epithelioid cell tumor (PEComa) of the adrenal gland: report of a rare case posing diagnostic challenge with the role of immunohistochemistry in the diagnosis. *Endocr Pathol*. 2015;26(2):129–134. doi:10.1007/s12022-015-9360-0
19. Zarineh A, Silverman JF. Adrenal perivascular epithelioid cell tumor: a case report with discussion of differential diagnoses. *Arch Pathol Lab Med*. 2011;135(4):499–502. doi:10.1043/2010-0202-CR.1
20. Kim H, Kim J, Lee SK, et al. TFE3-expressing perivascular epithelioid cell tumor of the breast. *J Pathol Transl Med*. 2019;53(1):62–65. doi:10.4132/jptm.2018.08.30
21. Alam MS, Mukherjee B, Krishnakumar S, Biswas J. Malignant perivascular epithelioid cell tumor of the orbit: Report of a case and review of literature. *Indian J Ophthalmol*. 2017;65(9):889–891. doi:10.4103/ijo.IJO_331_17
22. Varan A, Bayhan T, Kiratli H, et al. An orbital perivascular epithelioid cell tumor in a 7-year-old boy: case report and review of the literature. *J AAPOS*. 2017;21(4):325.e1–328.e1. doi:10.1016/j.jaapos.2017.05.022
23. Zhao L, Anders KH. Malignant perivascular epithelioid cell tumor of the gallbladder: a case report and review of literature. *Arch Pathol Lab Med*. 2014;138(9):1238–1241. doi:10.5858/arpa.2013-0092-CR

24. Yamashita K, Fletcher CDM. PEComa presenting in bone: clinicopathologic analysis of 6 cases and literature review. *Am J Surg Pathol*. 2010;34(11):1622–1629. doi:10.1097/PAS.0b013e3181f5974f
25. Gebhart M, Coltofeanu A. PEComa of the talus: a unique case of a soft tissue tumor within bone. *Acta Chir Belg*. 2019;119(2):118–122. doi:10.1080/00015458.2017.1394658
26. Xuesong D, Hong G, Weiguo Z. Bladder perivascular epithelioid cell tumor: dynamic CT and MRI presentation of 2 cases with 2-year follow-up and review of the literature. *Clin Genitourin Cancer*. 2019;17(5):e916–e922. doi:10.1016/j.clgc.2019.06.016
27. Tian C, Li Z, Gao D. Bladder PEComa: a case report and literature review. *Radiol Case Rep*. 2019;14(10):1293–1296. doi:10.1016/j.radcr.2019.07.012
28. Sarti A, Rubilotta E, Balzarro M, et al. Bladder perivascular epithelioid cell tumor (PEComa): a case report and literature review. *Urologia*. 2015;82(2):120–123. doi:10.5301/urologia.5000045
29. Martignoni G, Pea M, Zampini C, et al. PEComas of the kidney and of the genitourinary tract. *Semin Diagn Pathol*. 2015;32(2):140–159. doi:10.1053/j.semdp.2015.02.006
30. Eken A, Saglican Y. Primary perivascular epithelioid cell tumour (PEComa) of the prostate. *Can Urol Assoc J*. 2014;8(5–6):E455–E457. doi:10.5489/cuaj.1752
31. Lehman NL. Malignant PEComa of the skull base. *Am J Surg Pathol*. 2004;28(9):1230–1232. doi:10.1097/01.pas.0000128668.34934.81
32. Nie P, Wu J, Wang H, et al. Primary hepatic perivascular epithelioid cell tumors: imaging findings with histopathological correlation. *Cancer Imaging*. 2019;19(1):32. doi:10.1186/s40644-019-0212-x
33. Schaeffer DF, Poulin MP. Primary hepatic perivascular epithelioid tumor (PEComa). *Ann Hepatol*. 2016;15(3):436–437. doi:10.5604/16652681.1198822
34. Liu Z, Qi Y, Wang C, et al. Hepatic perivascular epithelioid cell tumor: five case reports and literature review. *Asian J Surg*. 2015;38(1):58–63. doi:10.1016/j.asjsur.2012.06.010
35. Musella A, De Felice F, Kyriacou AK, et al. Perivascular epithelioid cell neoplasm (PEComa) of the uterus: a systematic review. *Int J Surg*. 2015;19:1–5. doi:10.1016/j.ijsu.2015.05.002
36. Cossu A, Paliogiannis P, Tanda F, et al. Uterine perivascular epithelioid cell neoplasms (PEComas): report of two cases and literature review. *Eur J Gynaecol Oncol*. 2014;35(3):309–312. http://www.irog.net/archives
37. Kovac O, Babal P, Kajo K, et al. Perivascular epithelioid cell tumor (PEComa) of the uterine cervix: a case report of a 43-yr-old woman with abnormal uterine bleeding treated with hysterectomy. *Int J Gynecol Pathol*. 2018;37(5):492–496. doi:10.1097/PGP.0000000000000436
38. Kudela E, Biringer K, Kasajova P, et al. Perivascular epithelioid cell tumors of the uterine cervix. *Pathol Res Pract*. 2016;212(8):667–671. doi:10.1016/j.prp.2016.03.010
39. Stuart LN, Tipton RG, DeWall MR, et al. Primary cutaneous perivascular epithelioid cell tumor (PEComa): five new cases and review of the literature. *J Cutan Pathol*. 2017;44(8):713–721. doi:10.1111/cup.12972
40. Walsh SN, Sangüeza OP. PEComas: a review with emphasis on cutaneous lesions. *Semin Diagn Pathol*. 2009;26(3):123–130. doi:10.1053/j.semdp.2009.09.002
41. Mai KT, Belanger EC. Perivascular epithelioid cell tumour (PEComa) of the soft tissue. *Pathology*. 2006;38(5):415–420. doi:10.1080/00313020600922504
42. Folpe AL, Mentzel T, Lehr HA, et al. Perivascular epithelioid cell neoplasms of soft tissue and gynecologic origin: a clinicopathologic study of 26 cases and review of the literature. *Am J Surg Pathol*. 2005;29(12):1558–1575. doi:10.1097/01.pas.0000173232.22117.37
43. Armah HB, Parwani AV. Perivascular epithelioid cell tumor. *Arch Pathol Lab Med*. 2009;133(4):648–654. doi:10.1043/1543-2165-133.4.648
44. Thway K, Fisher C. PEComa: morphology and genetics of a complex tumor family. *Ann Diagn Pathol*. 2015;19(5):359–368. doi:10.1016/j.anndiagpath.2015.06.003
45. Agaram NP, Sung YS, Zhang L, et al. Dichotomy of genetic abnormalities in PEComas with therapeutic implications. *Am J Surg Pathol*. 2015;39(6):813–825. doi:10.1097/PAS.0000000000000389
46. Wagner AJ, Ravi V, Ganjoo KN, et al. ABI-009 (*nab*-sirolimus) in advanced malignant perivascular epithelioid cell tumors (PEComa): preliminary efficacy, safety, and mutational status from AMPECT, an open label phase II registration trial. *J Clin Oncol*. 2019;37:11005–11005. doi:10.1200/JCO.2019.37.15_suppl.11005
47. Anti-PD-1 therapy with nivolumab in the treatment of metastatic malignant PEComa. *Sarcoma J*. 2018;2:7–9. https://www.mdedge.com/sarcomajournal/article/164039/rare-sarcomas/anti-pd-1-therapy-nivolumab-treatment-metastatic

27

Synovial Sarcoma

John Charlson, Meena Bedi, David Ilan Suster, A. Craig Mackinnon, and David M. King

INTRODUCTION

Synovial sarcoma has unique features that distinguish it from other soft tissue sarcoma subtypes. It is diagnosed in both pediatric and adult patients. Under the microscope, it can manifest a variety of histologic features, ranging from epithelial cells to small, round cells. It is driven by a characteristic chromosomal translocation, which can serve as an important diagnostic feature. There are various chemotherapy options for treatment of synovial sarcoma. In addition, it frequently expresses an antigen that has placed it at the leading edge of cellular immunotherapy research in sarcoma.

EPIDEMIOLOGY

Synovial sarcoma accounts for 5% to 10% of soft tissue sarcoma cases, with an incidence of approximately 0.13 per 100,000 person-years.[1–3] Peak incidence of synovial sarcoma is in the third or fourth decade of life. It is the most common non-rhabdomyosarcoma soft tissue sarcoma among children and adolescents; one-third of synovial sarcoma cases occur in the adolescent-young adult (AYA) age group.[1,4,5] Male and female incidence is similar.[2,6]

CLINICAL PRESENTATION

Typically, synovial sarcoma arises in the deep soft tissues of the extremities. Less commonly, these tumors originate from the trunk, thorax, and head/neck.[5–7] Like other sarcoma types, synovial sarcoma can arise almost anywhere in the body, with rare presentations, including, pleuropulmonary,[8] cardiac,[9] renal, gastrointestinal tract,[10] prostate,[11] and skeletal[12,13] primary sites. Extremity synovial sarcoma typically presents as an enlarging mass. In a Surveillance, Epidemiology, and End Results (SEER) analysis of synovial sarcoma cases, 66% of patients presented with localized disease.[6] Regional lymph node involvement is reported but uncommon.[14] Despite the nomenclature, synovial sarcomas are not associated with the synovium and rarely involve the joint.

DIAGNOSTIC APPROACH

A pretreatment biopsy should be obtained to determine a tissue diagnosis and facilitate multidisciplinary treatment planning. This should be performed by an experienced surgeon or radiologist. The method of biopsy in synovial sarcoma depends on the location of primary disease. Historically, open biopsy was done to diagnose and grade sarcomas; however, in the extremity, core-needle biopsy is a reliable method for accurate diagnosis. Advantages of image-guided percutaneous biopsy include decreased cost, time, and complications compared to open biopsy.[15–17] Excisional biopsy should not be performed, as the likelihood of positive margins is high, which may compromise management of the disease process.[17] In addition, percutaneous biopsy for sarcoma minimizes the amount of tissue excised during resection of the biopsy tract at the time of surgical management.[18]

Like their extremity counterpart, retroperitoneal synovial sarcomas are diagnosed with image-guided core biopsy. However, if biopsy or imaging findings are inconclusive, resection may be performed to acquire a definitive diagnosis.

RADIOGRAPHIC FEATURES

Radiographically, synovial sarcomas may have calcifications located within the primary tumor, but typically do not have additional distinctive features from other subtypes. Imaging of the primary site with MRI or, if unable to obtain an MRI, CT scan is integral to determine disease extent and resectability of the tumor. MRI delineates not only tumor extent, but adjacent swelling as well. On MRI, synovial sarcomas are classically dark on T1-weighted sequences and bright on T2-weighted images. Although synovial sarcomas may occur in the retroperitoneum, the incidence is uncommon.[19] In this anatomic location, both CT and MRI may be helpful to demarcate the entirety of disease and infiltration or impingement on adjacent structures.[20]

Chest imaging, with a chest CT without contrast (preferred) or chest x-ray study, should also be performed to evaluate for metastasis.[21] When clinically warranted, PET/CT may be useful to characterize lung nodules and highlight other areas of disease not seen on CT.[22]

PATHOLOGIC FEATURES

Origin

Both neural and myogenic progenitor cells are candidate cells of origin for synovial sarcoma. Recent molecular studies correlating H3K4me3 levels and oncogenic gene activation in synovial sarcoma support a myogenic origin.[23]

Histology

Synovial sarcomas appear as relatively nonspecific soft tissue masses, which present as relatively circumscribed tan-yellow, sometimes pink or bluish masses, which can have nonspecific areas of edema, hemorrhage, and calcifications.[24] Synovial sarcoma has two main histologic appearances—biphasic and monophasic.

Monophasic Synovial Sarcoma

Monophasic synovial sarcoma accounts for approximately 70% of synovial sarcomas.[25] Monophasic synovial sarcoma is a spindle cell sarcoma, composed of a very monotonous population of spindle cells devoid of any glandular elements (Figures 27.1 and 27.2). The spindle cells in synovial sarcoma usually grow forming fascicles and may adopt a wide variety of histologic appearances, including herringbone, storiform, hemangiopericytic, palisading, and sclerosing patterns. The tumor cells are characterized by the absence of nuclear pleomorphism or bizarre tumor cells. The spindle cells are usually small with carrot-shaped hyperchromatic nuclei. Mitotic activity may vary considerably in these tumors and can range from 1 to >10 per 10 high power fields; the majority, however, have low mitotic activity.[24] Other features include stromal calcifications, abundant collagen, sclerotic changes, and myxoid degenerative changes. The appearance can be variable, and the diagnosis of monophasic synovial sarcoma needs to be eliminated in any tumor that resembles solitary fibrous tumor/hemangiopericytoma (SFT) because the

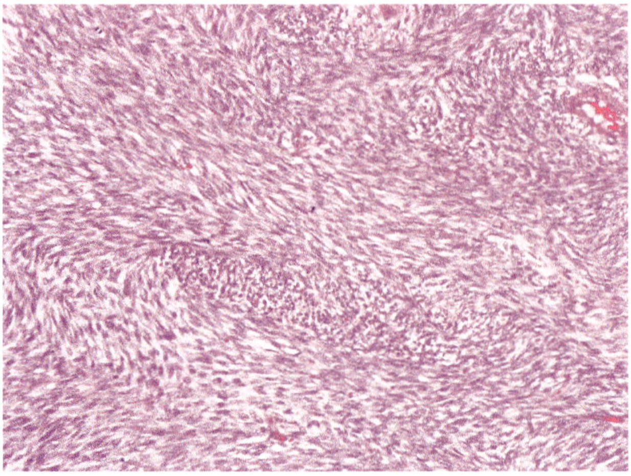

FIGURE 27.1 Monophasic synovial sarcoma shows fascicles of monotonous spindle cells with little intervening stroma.

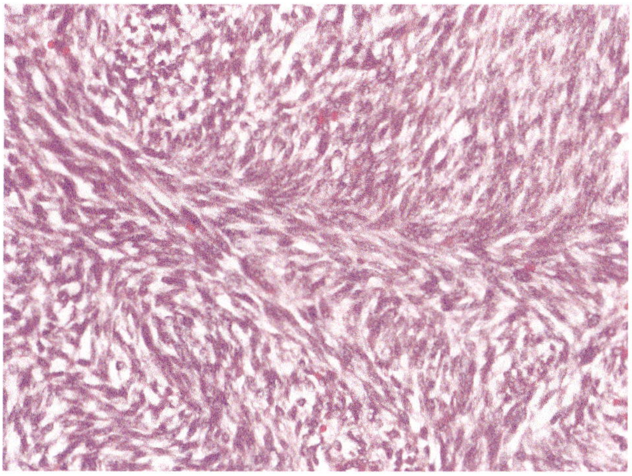

FIGURE 27.2 Higher magnification of monophasic synovial sarcoma showing uniform population of spindle cells displaying a herringbone growth pattern.

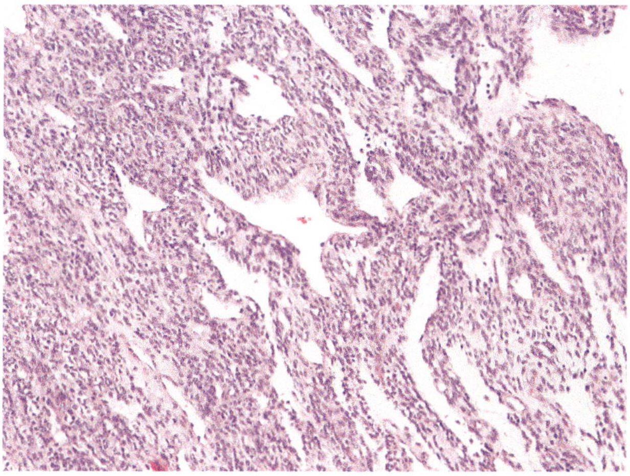

FIGURE 27.3 "Hemangiopericytic" vascular pattern in a monophasic synovial sarcoma showing numerous dilated, sharp, angulated vessels that display branching.

cytologic features and the patterns of dilated, branching vessels can be similar in both entities (Figure 27.3). Likewise, some monophasic synovial sarcomas lack the SFT-like vascular patterns or have larger, ovoid nuclei and can resemble malignant peripheral nerve sheath tumor (MPNST) more than SFT.[24]

Biphasic Synovial Sarcoma

Biphasic synovial sarcoma is characterized by an admixture of glandular structures with a compact, dense spindle cell proliferation in the stroma. A distinctive feature is that the glandular elements do not show a sharp segregation from the spindle cell elements, and the glandular structures are often flanked by strands of tightly packed atypical spindle cells. The glandular components can be quite subtle or very prominent. The presence of any glandular structures in these tumors qualifies for a diagnosis of biphasic synovial sarcoma (Figures 27.4 and 27.5). The glandular elements in biphasic synovial sarcoma can be of almost any type, including mucinous, tall columnar, simple cuboidal, with papillary excrescences, with cribriforming pattern, and with solid cords of tumor cells. Some cases can show squamous metaplasia (Figure 27.6) or areas of necrosis in the glandular component.[24]

Poorly Differentiated Synovial Sarcoma

Poorly differentiated synovial sarcoma can arise from either monophasic or biphasic synovial sarcoma; however, a precursor lesion is not always present. It is characterized by round cell differentiation that

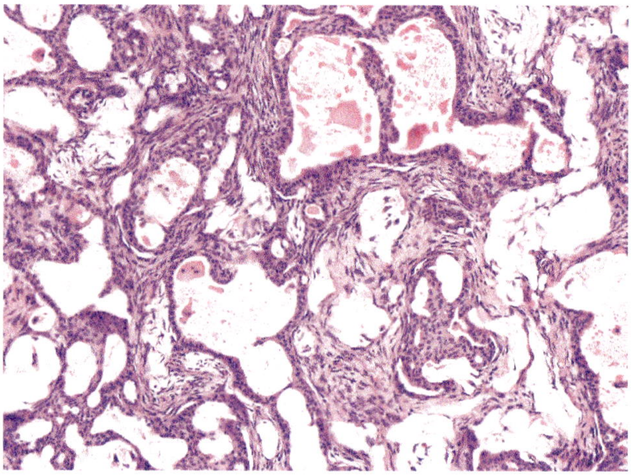

FIGURE 27.4 Biphasic synovial sarcoma shows numerous irregular glands simulating a metastatic adenocarcinoma.

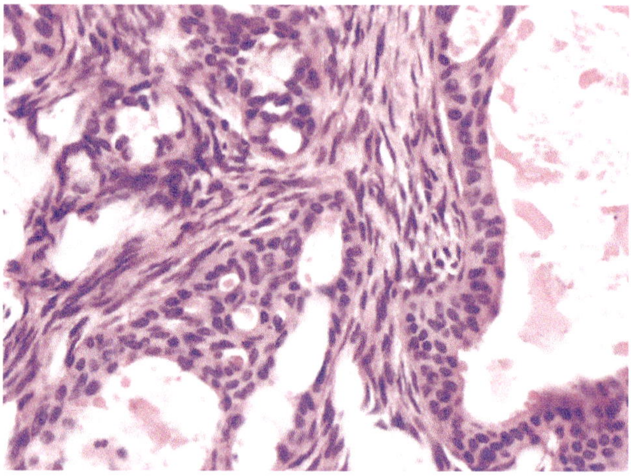

FIGURE 27.5 Higher magnification of biphasic synovial sarcoma shows glandular structures surrounded by a monotonous spindle cell stromal proliferation, corresponding to the spindle cell component of the lesion.

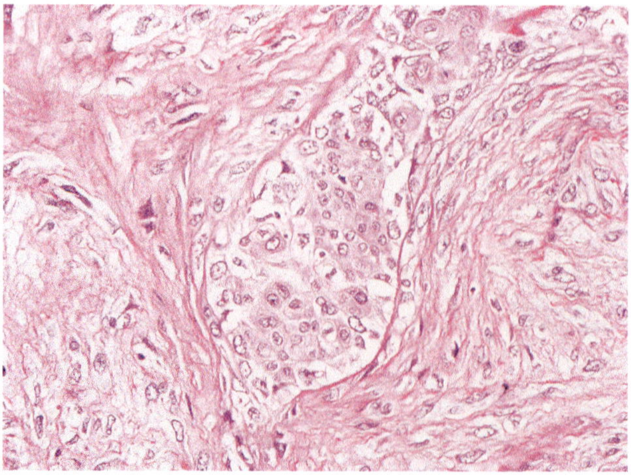

FIGURE 27.6 High-power magnification of biphasic synovial sarcoma in which the epithelial components show squamous differentiation with well-demarcated cell borders and intercellular bridges.

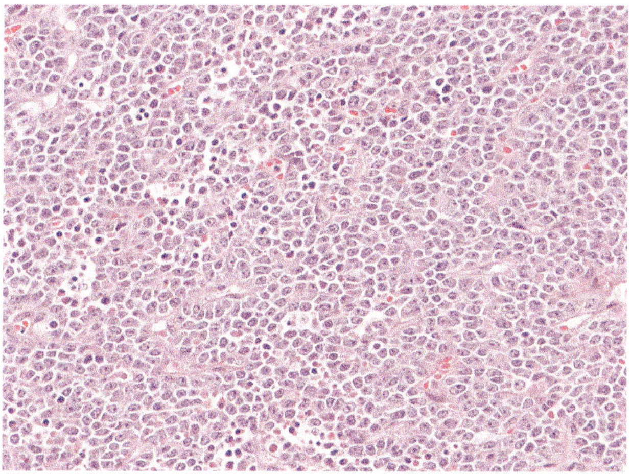

FIGURE 27.7 Poorly differentiated synovial sarcoma simulating a small round blue cell tumor with sheets of round to polygonal atypical cells with prominent nucleoli. High mitotic activity can be seen in the background.

can resemble those seen in lymphomas, Ewing sarcoma and embryonal rhabdomyosarcoma (Figure 27.7). Rhabdoid features, areas of necrosis, and a relatively higher rate of mitosis can be seen. The SFT-like vascular pattern is also often observed in poorly differentiated synovial sarcoma.[26]

Immunohistochemistry

Immunohistochemistry has a limited role in the pathologic diagnosis of synovial sarcoma. Synovial sarcomas express both low- and high-molecular-weight cytokeratins (Figures 27.8 and 27.9). Cytokeratin expression is generally focal, and it can be confined to rare cells on the section. Immunostaining can be useful for revealing occult glandular differentiation in an otherwise monophasic appearing tumor. Epithelial membrane antigen (EMA) may be positive in some cytokeratin-negative monophasic and poorly differentiated synovial sarcomas.[24] Other markers that stain synovial sarcoma include TLE1,[27] BCL-2 (Figure 27.10), vimentin, epithelial membrane antigen, and calponin. Synovial sarcoma is generally negative for CD34.

Molecular Features

A nearly invariant feature of synovial sarcoma is the reciprocal translocation between the *SS18* gene on chromosome 18 (18q11.2) and one of the three *SSX* genes (*SSX1*, *SSX2*, and rarely *SSX4*) that are

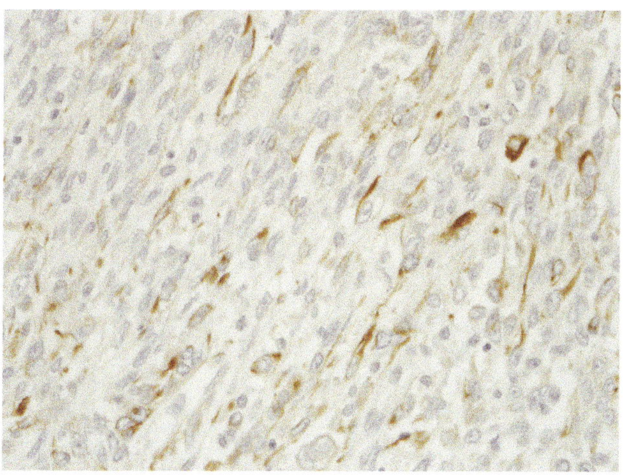

FIGURE 27.8 Characteristic staining pattern of cytokeratin (AE1/AE3) in monophasic synovial sarcoma. The staining pattern is focal and patchy, with just a few scattered positive spindle cells.

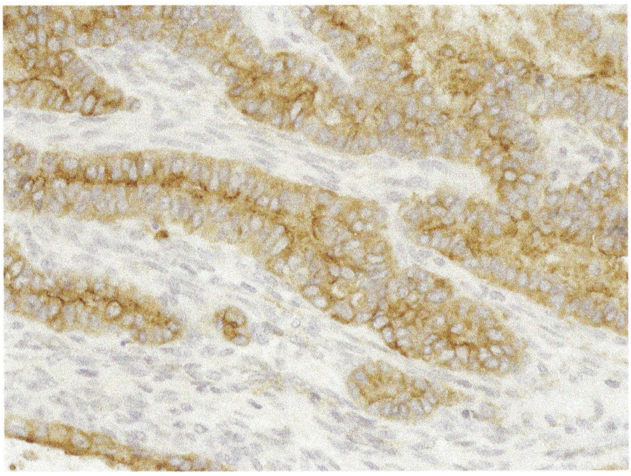

FIGURE 27.9 Immunohistochemical staining for cytokeratin (AE1/AE3) in biphasic synovial sarcoma shows strong positive staining of the glandular elements and a monotonous spindle cell proliferation in the background.

clustered on chromosome X (Xp11.2).[28,29] This translocation is unique to synovial sarcoma and is typically the only cytogenetic abnormality. It is detected in all morphologic subtypes and not observed in other human malignancies. This balanced translocation is believed to be the initiating molecular event leading to malignant transformation and development of synovial sarcoma. The translocation results in a fusion gene that codes for a chimeric protein composed of amino acids 1 to 379 of SS18 fused to the C-terminal 78 amino acids of SSX.[30–32] Detection of this fusion event is pathognomonic for synovial sarcoma. The numerous reports in the literature correlating the specific *SSX* gene involved in the translocation and the histologic subtype of synovial sarcoma are inconsistent.[33,34]

Molecular Testing for Synovial Sarcoma

Reverse transcriptase PCR has been demonstrated to be a highly effective and specific method for identifying the *SS18–SSX* fusion and is amenable to formalin-fixed, paraffin-embedded tissue.[29,35] However, the success of reverse transcriptase PCR for the detection of the *SS18–SSX* translocation is highly dependent upon both knowledge of the target sequence of the primers and the quality of RNA isolated from the tumor.

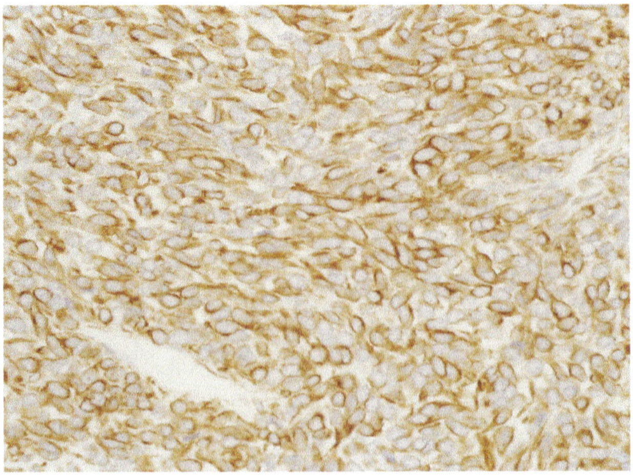

FIGURE 27.10 Strong and diffuse cytoplasmic positivity for BCL-2 in the majority of the tumor cells is also characteristic of monophasic synovial sarcoma.

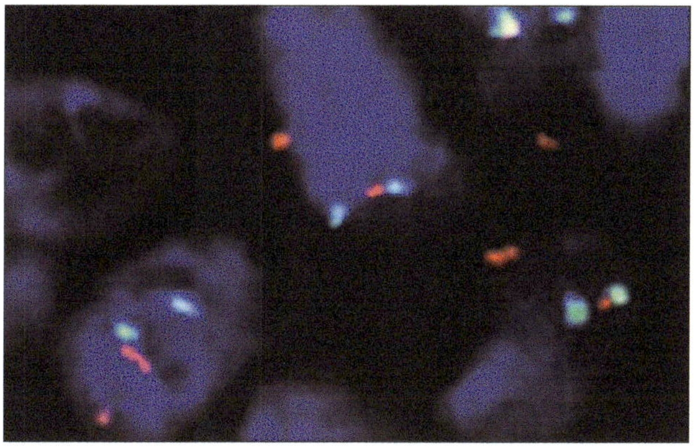

FIGURE 27.11 FISH assay demonstrating SYT translocation in synovial sarcoma using a dual color break-apart probe set with a 151-kb green probe and a 148-kb red probe flanking SYT at 18q11.2. Separate red and green signals indicate a chromosomal break at 18q11.2.
FISH, fluorescence in situ hybridization.

Fluorescence in situ hybridization (FISH)-based assays are an alternative approach to detect *SS18–SSX* translocations. These assays work well with archival or formalin-fixed, paraffin-embedded tissues in which the majority of tumor cells have interphase nuclei, and break-apart FISH probes are commonly used to detect disruption of the *SS18* gene (Figure 27.11).[36–38] In some instances, an atypical pattern consisting of loss of one of the probe signals is observed, and this should be interpreted as a peculiar unbalanced rearrangement of the *SS18* gene, and subsequent *SS18–SSX* fusion testing should be considered.[39,40] The highest analytical sensitivity and specificity (96% and 100%, respectively) have been reported by utilizing a combination of reverse transcriptase PCR and FISH.[33]

Immunohistochemistry for SYT and SSX1 proteins has been examined as an analytical method to distinguish synovial sarcoma from other soft tissue lesions. This approach is relatively sensitive— in one report, 41 of 47 cases of synovial sarcoma demonstrated strong nuclear expression of SS18.[41] However, 19 of 99 non-synovial sarcoma cases included in the study also demonstrated variable nuclear and cytoplasmic staining with SS18, and these cases included malignant peripheral nerve sheath tumor, solitary fibrous tumor, and Ewing sarcoma, all of which are in the differential diagnosis of synovial sarcoma. Therefore, immunohistochemistry for the detection of synovial sarcoma has limited application for routine testing due to low specificity.

Anchored multiplex PCR (AMP) is a novel technique for detecting gene fusion events using next-generation sequencing technology.[42] This targeted RNA sequencing strategy utilizes AMP to detect oncogenic fusion transcripts without prior knowledge of fusion partners, making this approach an attractive option to reverse transcriptase PCR, in which precise knowledge of the coding sequence for each fusion partner is required. Furthermore, the assay supports multiplex analysis of multiple fusion events and detects both common and novel fusion genes.[43] Concordance with FISH and reverse transcriptase PCR has been reported as high as 90% with advantages of this approach including superior performance and the identification of novel fusion partners.[44]

Differential Diagnosis

The main differential diagnoses include MPNST, SFT, small blue round cell tumors, and fibrosarcoma. MPNST can so closely resemble monophasic synovial sarcoma that the two entities may be indistinguishable by light microscope. The absence of CD34 tends to support the diagnosis of monophasic synovial sarcoma, whereas a clinical history of neurofibromatosis favors MPNST. Classical examples of SFT will sometimes lack alternating hypocellular and hypercellular regions ("marbling" seen in MPNST), and express CD34. In equivocal cases, immunostaining for STAT6 will show positivity in SFT and will be negative in MPNST. In addition, MPNSTs frequently demonstrate loss of H3K27me3 while synovial sarcoma and solitary fibrous tumor retain expression making immunohistochemistry for H3K27me3 useful for differentiating MPNST from synovial sarcoma.[45] Small blue round cell tumors can mimic poorly differentiated synovial sarcoma, but translocation analysis can now be used to distinguish synovial sarcoma from tumors such as Ewing sarcoma, desmoplastic small round blue cell tumor, and atypical Ewing sarcoma family tumors. Finally, fibrosarcoma, which is slowly disappearing as a diagnostic entity, is a diagnosis of exclusion to be reserved for cases in which histologic, molecular, and immunohistochemical analysis is uninformative.

MOLECULAR PATHOGENESIS OF SYNOVIAL SARCOMA

BAF Complex

Chromatin regulation is a key process that controls the appropriate timing and levels of gene expression. This complex and highly ordered epigenetic process is achieved by modulating genomic architecture through histone modification, DNA methylation, and adenosine triphosphate (ATP)-dependent chromatin remodeling, thereby altering the accessibility of transcription factors to their cognate DNA binding sites.

The BRG1/BRM associated factor (BAF) complex, which stands for Brg/Brm-associated complexes and is alternatively known as SWI/SNF complex, is one of the best characterized chromatin remodeling complexes. The BAF complex is a large, multiprotein, ATP-dependent chromatin remodeling complex and contributes to gene activation through nucleosome remodeling. The BAF complex assembles in a combinatorial manner involving 15 subunits coded by a set of gene families. Combinatorial assembly is tissue specific and plays an important role in determining cell fate.[46–48] For example, using experimental techniques to force the formation of neural-specific BAF complexes converts fibroblasts to neurons.[49]

Mutations in the BAF complex are identified in 20% of all human cancers.[50] Malignant rhabdoid tumors (MRTs) demonstrate biallelic inactivation of the *BAF47* subunit, coded by the *SMARCB1/INI1/SNF* gene, in nearly all cases.[50] *BAF47* functions as a tumor suppressor gene and reintroduction of *BAF47* into MRT cells stops cellular proliferation.[51] Other examples include *ARID1A*[52] and *PBAF*[53] mutations, which are present in the majority of ovarian clear cell and renal clear cell carcinomas, respectively. The identification of specific BAF subunit mutations in specific malignancies suggests that the different combinatorial assembly of BAF complexes underlies the tissue-specific tumor phenotype.[46] This is supported by the specialized role of BAF complexes in neural development and other cellular processes.

SSX–SS18 Fusion Protein

The SS18–SSX fusion protein effectively competes with the wild-type SS18 protein for incorporation and assembly into the BAF complex, and consequently, wild-type SS18 is displaced. Biochemical experiments suggest that SS18 and SS18–SSX do not compete for direct binding but rather the two proteins likely compete for assembly into complexes. In synovial sarcoma, the SS18–SSX outcompetes wild-type SS18 during assembly due to increased concentrations of the fusion protein.[46]

SS18–SSX-modified BAF also evicts the *BAF47* tumor suppressor from BAF complex, where it is inactivated by proteasomal degradation, indicating that *BAF47* is not required for proliferation of synovial sarcoma. SS18–SSX mediated disruption of the BAF complex is determined by two regions of the SSX protein: the C-terminal eight amino acids and two polar amino acids at positions 43 and 44. These two amino acids are conserved in SSX1, SSX2, and SSX4, but not in SSX3. In experimental models, SS18–SSX3 fusion proteins, which lack these two amino acids, can incorporate into BAF, but are deficient in eliciting *BAF47* displacement, thus underscoring their role in BAF disruption.[46] This is noteworthy from a therapeutic standpoint in that such a small region leads to complex disruption and may represent a potential target for the development of pharmaceutical inhibitors.

The SS18–SSX-modified BAF complex demonstrates global genomic relocalization encompassing both the gain and loss of BAF target sites.[23] The dual gain and loss of genomic sites of the SS18–SSX-modified BAF complex is a unique feature of synovial sarcoma. In contrast, *BAF47*-deficient tumors (for example, malignant rhabdoid tumors) demonstrate near exclusive loss of BAF complex occupancy on chromatin due to decreased BAF affinity.[54]

The key mechanism driving proliferation in synovial sarcoma is the gain of function activity and subsequent genome wide targeting of SS18–SSX-modified BAF complexes from enhancers, where wild-type BAF complexes normally localize, to polycomb repressive complex 2 (PRC2)-occupied domains resulting in the opposition of PRC2-mediated repression.[23] This in turn leads to activation of bivalent genes, activation of the synovial sarcoma gene expression signature, and initiation of cellular pathways that drive proliferation. Furthermore, SS18–SSX-modified BAF opposition results in reduced PRC2-mediated methylation of H3 K27 and activation of bivalent genes including *SOX2*. *SOX2*, which is normally targeted for repression by PRC2, is universally expressed in synovial sarcoma secondary to SS18–SSX modified BAF and is essential for proliferation.

The gene expression profile of synovial sarcoma is transcriptionally distinct from other cancers with BAF complex perturbations.[23] Synovial sarcoma specific genes include *TLE1*, regulators of neural development, regulators of myogenesis (e.g., *PAX3* and *PAX7*), and putative oncogenes (*SOX2* and *MYC*). Transcription of these genes correlates with the respective proteins as determined by immunohistochemistry. Furthermore, *MYC* expression is mutually exclusive with *PAX7* and *SOX2*. Expression of *PAX7* and *SOX2* is observed more frequently in primary synovial sarcoma, whereas *MYC* expression is more often observed in metastatic synovial sarcoma. Thus, SS18–SSX globally alters BAF-controlled gene regulation through a retargeting mechanism leading to inappropriate gene activation that drives synovial sarcoma proliferation and growth.[55]

Potential Therapeutic Implications

Activation of bivalent genes by SS18–SSX-modified BAF is positively modulated by underlying H3K4me3 levels. This suggests reduction of H3K4me3 methylation via inhibition of MLL2/COMPASS as a potential therapeutic strategy to achieve abrogation of SS18–SSX-modified BAF-mediated gene activation.[23] Furthermore, as *BAF47* is evicted in SS18–SSX-modified BAF complexes and cellular levels are reduced to varying degrees, it is uncertain that selective inhibition of EZH2 (i.e., tazemetostat), which is indicated for *BAF47*-deficient solid tumors (e.g., malignant rhabdoid tumors), will demonstrate significant benefit for treatment of synovial sarcoma since its mechanism of sensitivity is based on INI1 depletion and EZH2 dependency.

Synovial sarcoma is dependent upon a noncanonical BAF complex (ncBAF) for maintaining proliferation, implicating subunits of the ncBAF complex as a potential therapeutic target.[56] Biochemical studies demonstrate that synovial sarcoma is dependent upon the ncBAF subunit BRD9, and synovial sarcoma proliferation is highly sensitive to perturbations of BRD9. This is significant in light of the development of selective BRD9 inhibitors.[57–59]

PROGNOSIS

General

Synovial sarcoma may behave aggressively, with reported 5-year survival rate of patients presenting with localized disease ranging from 60% to 70%.[3,60,61] For patients with localized synovial sarcoma, larger tumor size, high grade, invasion of local structures such as bones or neurovascular structures, and axial primary tumor locations (as opposed to extremity tumors) are associated with increased likelihood of distant metastases and worse survival.[62–64] The American Joint Committee on Cancer (AJCC) staging system incorporates factors such as tumor size and the presence or absence of regional lymph node or distant metastases to estimate prognosis.

Lymph Node Involvement

Historically, synovial sarcoma has been associated with elevated risk of regional lymph node metastases, with published rates greater than 13%,[65] and has been grouped with other sarcoma subtypes, such as clear cell sarcoma, angiosarcoma, rhabdomyosarcoma, and epithelioid sarcoma as requiring particular attention to regional nodes. More recent analyses, including large data sets from SEER and the National Cancer Database (NCDB) as well as several large institutional databases, have found rates of regional lymph node involvement among synovial sarcoma patients ranging from 3.3% to 5.1%, similar to the overall rate for soft tissue sarcoma.[66–70] Sentinel lymph node biopsy (SLNB) was evaluated in a prospective study of patients with localized soft tissue sarcoma subtypes with presumed high risk, but no clinical evidence, of lymph node involvement. Four of 68 patients with synovial sarcoma (5.9%) were identified as having lymph node metastases (three positive sentinel lymph nodes, one false negative). The investigators proposed that SLNB would not be relevant for patients with localized synovial sarcoma.

Prognostic Tools

Prognostic tools have been developed to help clinicians estimate sarcoma patient outcomes. A nomogram, developed at Memorial Sloan Kettering, uses patient and postoperative tumor characteristics (including histologic type) to estimate risk of sarcoma-related mortality.[71] More recently, updated nomograms that estimate the risk of distant recurrence or death for patients with soft tissue sarcoma treated with curative intent have been developed and are the basis for Sarculator, a smart phone application that can be used as a prognostic tool.[72]

THERAPEUTIC APPROACH: LOCALIZED DISEASE

Surgery

Surgery is the mainstay of treatment for all soft tissue sarcomas, including synovial sarcomas. Amputation is rarely necessary and limb-sparing resection is possible for the majority of patients.[73] Resection should be performed by a fellowship-trained oncologic surgeon to ensure complete resection and minimize postoperative morbidity. Every attempt should be made to achieve a negative-margin resection to decrease the probability of local recurrence at the primary site. The goal of surgery should be an R0 resection with no ink on tumor. Acceptable local recurrence rates have been demonstrated in oncologically excised tumors with close margins of less than 1 mm.[74,75] Careful dissection should take place through normal tissue planes without contaminating the resection bed by contacting the tumor. In the case of an open biopsy, the biopsy site should be resected. Nerves or vessels that are adjacent to synovial sarcomas do not need to be excised if the adventitia and perineurium are removed and there is no involvement of the underlying neurovascular structure. Surgical clips may be placed in the resection cavity to guide postoperative radiation, if warranted.[17]

Depending on the clinical scenario, radiation therapy may be performed in conjunction with surgery, either preoperatively or postoperatively, to decrease the risk of local recurrence. The utilization of radiation therapy should be strongly considered if close surgical margins are anticipated.

In the clinical setting of metastatic disease, surgery may be considered based on performance status, disease burden, response to systemic therapy, and progression-free interval. Patients with oligometastatic disease or pulmonary-only disease may benefit from surgical management of symptomatic or bulky disease.[76,77]

Radiation Therapy

External beam radiation therapy may be used in the preoperative or postoperative setting in synovial sarcomas. Although historically radiotherapy was delivered postoperatively, the several advantages of preoperative radiation include smaller field size, decreased dose and number of treatments, facilitation of surgical resection, and decreased fibrosis. One disadvantage, however, is the increased risk of postoperative wound complications.[78]

Radiation should be considered in tumors that are greater than 5 cm, high grade, or low-grade sarcomas that abut neurovascular structures. Additionally, radiation should be considered when a closer surgical margin will allow for a meaningful decrease in morbidity for the patient[17] or when the risk of positive margins might result in tumor seeding, such as thoracic lesions, from which pleural seeding might occur.

Brachytherapy delivers radiation through multiple catheters and may be considered; however, external beam is routinely used. Brachytherapy may be of particular benefit in the setting of local recurrence in a previously radiated field.

Chemotherapy

Although the use of chemotherapy in the adjuvant and neoadjuvant treatment of soft tissue sarcoma has been associated with both recurrence-free survival and overall survival, it has not been universally accepted by all sarcoma centers. Clinical trials have been difficult to interpret because of heterogeneous patient populations, variable treatment regimens, and small study sizes. A meta-analysis of data from studies of adjuvant anthracycline-based chemotherapy, published in 1997, found improved recurrence-free, but not overall, survival associated with chemotherapy.[79] An updated meta-analysis reported statistically significant recurrence-free and overall survival benefit associated with adjuvant chemotherapy in the treatment of patients with localized, resectable soft tissue sarcoma. Benefit was most pronounced in patients treated with anthracycline and ifosfamide combination therapy, with reduction in risk of death with a hazard ratio of 0.56 ($p = .01$).[80] Use of adjuvant chemotherapy has not been universally accepted because several older studies showed no significant benefit associated with adjuvant chemotherapy in the setting of localized, resected soft tissue sarcoma.[81,82]

Prospective, randomized trials that have shown perioperative anthracycline–ifosfamide chemotherapy to be beneficial share several features—patients have high risk soft tissue sarcoma (>5 cm, high-grade tumors), treatment is limited to histologic subtypes of sarcoma known to be chemotherapy responsive (including synovial sarcoma), and ifosfamide was given at adequate doses (for example ≥9 g/m^2 per cycle).[83,84] It is clear that there is a dose–response relationship with ifosfamide.[85]

The European Society for Medical Oncology (ESMO) sarcoma guidelines state that adjuvant chemotherapy be considered as an option with individual patients at high risk for poor outcomes.[86] The

National Comprehensive Cancer Network (NCCN) soft tissue sarcoma guidelines also suggest that neoadjuvant or adjuvant anthracycline-based chemotherapy be considered according to individual patient factors for stage II and III soft tissue sarcoma of the extremities and trunk.[87]

Additional data support the importance of anthracycline–ifosfamide chemotherapy, specifically in the treatment of localized synovial sarcoma. Several retrospective studies reported significantly better disease-specific survival for patients treated with ifosfamide-containing chemotherapy, compared to those who received no chemotherapy.[88,89] Another study compared standard neoadjuvant epirubicin–ifosfamide chemotherapy to histotype-tailored chemotherapy, which was high-dose ifosfamide (14 g/m^2 continuous infusion over 14 days, every 28 days) in the synovial sarcoma cohort. Standard therapy was associated with significantly better disease-free survival.[84]

FOLLOW-UP

Follow-up for primary synovial sarcomas should involve a more rigorous schedule for several years after surgery, including interval history, physical exam, and baseline postoperative imaging of the primary site, with MRI or contrast-enhanced CT scan as an alternative with subsequent imaging based on the risk of recurrence and accessibility of the primary site to physical exam, and chest imaging every 3 to 6 months for the first 2 to 3 years, then every 6 months until year 5, and yearly thereafter. Owing to the propensity to develop late recurrence, follow-up is recommended for at least 10 years.[17,90,91] The frequency of follow-up may be modified based on tumor location, patient function, tumor grade, and symptoms and clinical exam findings.

METASTATIC RECURRENCE

Synovial sarcoma has a propensity for metastatic spread. In several retrospective series, 40% to 45% of patients with localized synovial sarcoma have metastatic disease at 5 years.[3,60,92] Median time to metastatic recurrence is less than 3 years, but metastases may also develop late, 10 years or more from initial diagnosis.[3,60,92,93] Metastases are found in the lungs in at least 80% of cases, and much less commonly in regional lymph nodes and other sites, such as soft tissue, bone, and pleura.[3,94] Metastatic synovial sarcoma is generally considered incurable, but there are some patients with limited extent of metastatic disease who may achieve long-term survival.[93]

THERAPEUTIC APPROACH: METASTATIC DISEASE

Systemic therapy, with several cytotoxic chemotherapies or the multikinase inhibitor pazopanib, is commonly used in the treatment of metastatic synovial sarcoma. Radiation therapy, ablative therapies such as cryoablation, and surgery may be used in certain situations for disease or symptom control. Immunotherapeutic approaches are being studied and show significant promise.

Chemotherapy

Synovial sarcoma is considered a chemotherapy responsive sarcoma. In a review of first-line chemotherapy trials for advanced soft tissue sarcoma, it was noted that, compared to other sarcoma subtypes, synovial sarcoma patients experienced better objective response rates (28% vs. 19%), longer progression-free survival (PFS; 6.3 vs. 3.7 months), and longer overall survival (15 vs. 11.7 months).[95]

Anthracyclines, such as doxorubicin and epirubicin, are standard first-line treatment alone or in combination for advanced soft tissue sarcomas. Doxorubicin acts on cancer cells by inhibiting topoisomerase-II-mediated repair of DNA.[96] As a single agent, at doses of 70 to 80 mg/m^2 per cycle, doxorubicin achieves response rates of 14% to 20%.[97–99] In a retrospective review of advanced synovial sarcoma patients treated at a sarcoma center, the response rate to single-agent doxorubicin was 25%.[100]

Olaratumab, a monoclonal antibody to platelet-derived growth factor alpha (PDGFRα), was granted Food and Drug Administration (FDA) approval in 2016, in combination with doxorubicin, for treatment of incurable soft tissue sarcoma. Approval was based on a randomized Phase II study that showed significant improvement in overall survival compared to single-agent doxorubicin (26.5 vs. 14.7 months).[101] Unfortunately, the randomized Phase III study comparing doxorubicin to doxorubicin plus olaratumab found no benefit for the combination in response rates, PFS, and overall survival.

Ifosfamide, an alkylating agent, at doses less than 10 g/m^2 per cycle, is an active single agent treatment for advanced soft tissue sarcoma, with response rates ranging between 10% and 25% in several studies,[85,102,103] and clear difference in response rates depending on dose, with doses of 5 g/m^2 and 9 g/m^2 per cycle defining the lower and upper ends of that range of response rates.[85] For treatment of advanced sarcoma in general, it is used more frequently in combination with doxorubicin than as a single agent.[104] Ifosfamide has particularly good antitumor activity in synovial sarcoma.[95,105] In one retrospective review, among patients with advanced soft tissue sarcoma who had been previously treated with ifosfamide, there was treatment response noted on rechallenge with ifosfamide. Nearly half (14 of 29) of synovial sarcoma patients achieved partial response or stable disease.[106] High-dose ifosfamide (HDI), 12 to 14 g/m^2 per cycle, given as continuous infusion, has activity in advanced sarcoma as well, but is associated with significant toxicity including high rates of neutropenia fever.[107,108] One study of HDI in first- or second-line treatment of advanced soft tissue sarcoma included 22 synovial sarcoma patients, eight of whom had objective responses.[108]

The combination of ifosfamide with anthracycline chemotherapy, for advanced soft tissue sarcoma in general, results in higher response rates and longer PFS, showed a trend toward an improvement in overall survival (1 year overall survival 60% vs. 51%, $p = .07$).[99] Toxicity, including myelosuppression, is more pronounced with combination therapy. For these reasons, combination therapy is an option for synovial sarcoma patients with metastatic disease, particularly if a patient is symptomatic or has a large tumor burden. When doxorubicin/ifosfamide chemotherapy is assessed specifically in patients with synovial sarcoma, response rates are particularly impressive, with 88% of the synovial sarcoma subset of patients responding to combination therapy in one clinical trial,[98] and 59% responding in another retrospective report.[100]

Pazopanib is an oral tyrosine kinase inhibitor with activity against vascular endothelial growth factor (VEGF) and platelet-derived growth factor (PDGF), which was FDA-approved in April 2012 for treatment of patients with metastatic nonadipocytic soft tissue sarcoma. Approval was based on the pazopanib for metastatic soft tissue sarcoma (PALETTE) trial, in which patients who had progressed on standard therapy were randomized to pazopanib 800 mg daily or placebo. Median PFS was significantly better in the pazopanib arm, 4.6 months versus 1.6 months.[109] PFS in the synovial sarcoma subset was similar to that for the study population as a whole.

While pazopanib is the only tyrosine kinase inhibitor FDA approved for treatment of metastatic soft tissue sarcoma, regorafenib, and sunitinib have demonstrated activity against synovial sarcoma as well.[110,111] One example of this was a study of off-label use of targeted therapies by the French Sarcoma Group that included 15 patients with synovial sarcoma; eight of these patients were treated with sunitinib, and four had partial responses.[112]

Trabectedin was approved in 2007 by the European Medicines Agency and European Commission for treatment of advanced soft tissue sarcoma after failure of anthracycline and ifosfamide, and it was FDA approved in 2015 for advanced liposarcoma and leiomyosarcoma after failing anthracycline. FDA approval was based on a clinical trial that compared trabectedin to dacarbazine 1.5 mg/m^2 as a 24-hour infusion every 3 weeks to dacarbazine. Median PFS was significantly longer in the trabectedin arm of the study, 4.2 months versus 1.5 months.[113] A retrospective analysis of outcomes in patients with translocation-related sarcomas, treated in several Phase II trabectedin trials, included 45 synovial sarcoma patients. The synovial sarcoma patients had median PFS of 3 months.[114] Multicenter retrospective review of synovial sarcoma patients treated with trabectedin included 61 patients, and found 15% objective response rate, median PFS 3 months, with 23% of patients without progression at 6 months.[115]

Gemcitabine-based therapy and various other cytotoxic chemotherapy agents are also used in the treatment of metastatic soft tissue sarcoma.[116,117] There is insufficient data to report specific outcomes for synovial sarcoma patients.

Tazemetostat, an EZH2 inhibitor, was studied in malignant rhabdoid tumors and sarcoma types with reduction or loss of INI1. There was limited activity in synovial sarcoma, with five of 33 patients achieving stable disease for 16 weeks or more.[118]

Immunotherapy

Immune checkpoint inhibitors of PD-1 (programmed cell death protein 1) and CTLA-4 (cytotoxic T-lymphocyte-associated protein 4) have been studied as treatment for soft tissue sarcoma patients. Two clinical trials, one with single-agent pembrolizumab and the other with nivolumab or a combination of nivolumab and ipilimumab, included 12 synovial sarcoma patients.[119,120] One of these patients, treated with pembrolizumab, had brief tumor response.[120] It is noted that, compared to undifferentiated pleomorphic sarcoma and dedifferentiated liposarcoma, synovial sarcoma expresses fewer inflammatory genes, has less PD-L1 (PD-1 ligand) staining, and lower T-cell fraction and T-cell clonality, suggesting synovial sarcoma is less likely to respond to these therapies.

NY-ESO-1 is a cancer testis antigen expressed by various tumors, but with very limited expression in normal tissue, and it has been studied as a target for immunotherapy. Synovial sarcoma expresses NY-ESO-1 in 80% of cases.[121] LV305 is a lentiviral vector NY-ESO-1 vaccine that targets dendritic cells, which then induce, or prime, an NY-ESO-1-specific T-cell response. CMB305, a prime-boost immunotherapy regimen, consisting of LV305 priming followed by repeated dosing with G305 (recombinant NY-ESO-1 protein combined with a TLR-4 agonist), has been studied in patients with NY-ESO-1 expressing solid tumors. This vaccine therapy was well tolerated, and 53% of the synovial sarcoma patients in the study had a best response of stable disease, with a 1-year survival rate of 86%.[122] Another approach under investigation is genetic modification of autologous T cells so that the T-cell receptors recognize NY-ESO-1. This strategy is restricted to specific HLA type, HLA-A*02:01 or in another study HLA-A2*02:06.[123,124] Objective responses among synovial sarcoma cohorts were noted in at least 50% of patients.

Multidisciplinary Management of Metastatic Disease

Pulmonary Metastectomy

For patients with oligometastatic sarcoma, NCCN guidelines recommend consideration of metastectomy or use of other modalities, such as stereotactic body radiation therapy (SBRT) or ablation, in addition to management of the primary tumor and systemic therapy, as indicated.[87] Lungs are a common site of sarcoma metastasis, and there are a number of reports of outcomes following pulmonary metastectomy. Median overall survival following pulmonary metastectomy ranges from 33 to 45 months,[125,126] and 5-year survival rates range from 25% in a systematic review of the literature including all subtypes of soft tissue sarcoma to 58% in a single institution series of synovial sarcoma patients.[127,128] Longer time from primary tumor treatment (>1 year), solitary metastasis, and complete resection of pulmonary metastases are factors associated with better survival after pulmonary metastectomy.

Radiation Therapy

SBRT may be an alternative when surgical excision of lung metastases is not feasible. Several series have been published, with varying radiation dosing regimens and follow-up periods, demonstrating lesion control rates of 82% to 96%.[129–132] As there has not been randomized, prospective study of pulmonary metastectomy or SBRT as therapy for soft tissue sarcoma metastatic lesions, the true impact on survival is unclear.

SUMMARY

Synovial sarcoma can present in patients of any age, but it tends to occur in younger patients. Correct diagnosis is important, and molecular diagnostic tools play an important role in making a diagnosis of synovial sarcoma. Synovial sarcoma is an aggressive disease, with propensity for metastatic spread. At the same time, it is considered a chemotherapy-sensitive type of soft tissue sarcoma. In the setting of high-risk, localized disease, multimodality therapy, including chemotherapy and radiation therapy, should be considered along with complete excision by an orthopedic oncologist or surgical oncologist with sarcoma expertise. Treatment options for metastatic soft tissue sarcoma, including synovial sarcoma, are increasing, including exciting immunotherapy advances.

CASE STUDY

A 31-year-old woman presented with a 3-month history of cough, dyspnea on exertion, and one episode of hemoptysis. This was initially thought to represent upper respiratory tract infection, but persistence of symptoms prompted a chest radiograph, which showed a mass-like density in the right lower hemithorax. CT scan confirmed a large, pleural-based mass in the posterior right chest, along with two 5-mm left lower lobe nodules. CT-guided core-needle biopsy showed atypical spindle cells, and other areas of epithelioid tumor cells in nests and glands, with >5 mitoses per high power field, and immunohistochemical stains positive for TLE1, and FISH positive for *SS18* gene rearrangement, consistent with a diagnosis of biphasic synovial sarcoma.

She was treated with preoperative radiation therapy to the right lung mass, to a total dose of 50 Gy. This was followed by radical resection, including the right lower lobe, partial diaphragm, and chest wall, with negative margins. Unfortunately, postoperative chest CT scan showed the left lower lobe lung nodules to be enlarging. Biopsy of one of the lung nodules was positive for metastatic synovial sarcoma.

Over the next 5 months, she was treated with six cycles of doxorubicin and ifosfamide, with partial response of visible tumors. Following chemotherapy, wedge resection of a portion of the left lung was done to resect residual disease. CT scan 4 months later showed new nodules in both lungs. She was treated with pazopanib, with stable disease for 5 months. At the time of disease progression, she was treated with two cycles of doxorubicin/olaratumab, with partial response. She then enrolled in a clinical trial at a major cancer center, and was treated with genetically engineered NY-ESO-1-specific T cells, after cyclophosphamide and fludarabine conditioning chemotherapy. She had a partial response to the T cells, lasting 5 months.

Since then, she experienced continued progression of the metastatic disease in both lungs. Over the course of 7 months, she was treated with ifosfamide, though treatment was complicated by pancytopenia and several hospital admissions for neutropenic fever. She has recently initiated treatment with trabectedin, and treatment is ongoing.

REFERENCES

1. Herzog CE. Overview of sarcomas in the adolescent and young adult population. *J Pediatr Hematol Oncol*. 2005;27(4):215–218. doi:10.1097/01.mph.0000161762.53175.e4
2. Mastrangelo G, Coindre JM, Ducimetière F, et al. Incidence of soft tissue sarcoma and beyond: a population-based prospective study in 3 European regions. *Cancer*. 2012;118(21):5339–5348. doi:10.1002/cncr.27555
3. Ferrari A, Gronchi A, Casanova M, et al. Synovial sarcoma: a retrospective analysis of 271 patients of all ages treated at a single institution. *Cancer*. 2004;101(3):627–634. doi:10.1002/cncr.20386
4. Kerouanton A, Jimenez I, Cellier C, et al. Synovial sarcoma in children and adolescents. *J Pediatr Hematol Oncol*. 2014;36(4):257–262. doi:10.1097/MPH.0000000000000154
5. Palmerini E, Staals EL, Alberghini M, et al. Synovial sarcoma: retrospective analysis of 250 patients treated at a single institution. *Cancer*. 2009;115(13):2988–2998. doi:10.1002/cncr.24370
6. Naing KW, Monjazeb AM, Li CS, et al. Perioperative radiotherapy is associated with improved survival among patients with synovial sarcoma: a SEER analysis. *J Surg Oncol*. 2015;111(2):158–164. doi:10.1002/jso.23780
7. Harb WJ, Luna MA, Patel SR, et al. Survival in patients with synovial sarcoma of the head and neck: association with tumor location, size, and extension. *Head Neck*. 2007;29(8):731–740. doi:10.1002/hed.20564
8. Essary LR, Vargas SO, Fletcher CDM. Primary pleuropulmonary synovial sarcoma: reappraisal of a recently described anatomic subset. *Cancer*. 2002;94(2):459–469. doi:10.1002/cncr.10188
9. Varma T, Adegboyega P. Primary cardiac synovial sarcoma. *Arch Pathol Lab Med*. 2012;136(4):454–458. doi:10.5858/arpa.2011-0008-RS
10. Sinniah RP, Roche E, Cameron D. GI synovial sarcomas. *Clin Transl Gastroenterol*. 2012;3:e11. doi:10.1038/ctg.2012.6
11. Zhang Q, Wang H, Ren L, et al. Primary synovial sarcoma of the prostate metastatic to the liver and lung: a case report. *World J Surg Oncol*. 2014;12:194. doi:10.1186/1477-7819-12-194
12. Cohen IJ, Issakov J, Avigad S, et al. Synovial sarcoma of bone delineated by spectral karyotyping. *Lancet*. 1997;350(9092):1679–1680. doi:10.1016/s0140-6736(05)64278-x
13. Hiraga H, Nojima T, Isu K, et al. Histological and molecular evidence of synovial sarcoma of bone. A case report. *J Bone Joint Surg Am*. 1999;81(4):558–563. doi:10.2106/00004623-199904000-00014
14. Ashamalla M, Guirguis A, Mokhtar BE, Ashamalla H. Clinical presentation and patterns of care in SCARE soft tissue sarcoma. *Int J Radiat Oncol Biol Phys*. 2017;99(2):E749. doi:10.1016/j.ijrobp.2017.06.2403
15. Soudack M, Nachtigal A, Vladovski E, et al. Sonographically guided percutaneous needle biopsy of soft tissue masses with histopathologic correlation. *J Ultrasound Med*. 2006;25(10):1271–1277; quiz 1278–1279. doi:10.7863/jum.2006.25.10.1271
16. Tsukushi S, Nishida Y, Yamada Y, et al. CT-guided needle biopsy for musculoskeletal lesions. *Arch Orthop Trauma Surg*. 2010;130(5):699–703. doi:10.1007/s00402-009-1030-6

17. Heslin MJ, Lewis JJ, Woodruff JM, Brennan MF. Core needle biopsy for diagnosis of extremity soft tissue sarcoma. *Ann Surg Oncol*. 1997;4(5):425–431. doi:10.1007/bf02305557
18. Renne SL, Iwenofu OH. Pathology of retroperitoneal sarcomas: a brief review. *J Surg Oncol*. 2018;117(1):12–24. doi:10.1002/jso.24928
19. Choi H, Varma DG, Fornage BD, et al. Soft-tissue sarcoma: MR imaging vs sonography for detection of local recurrence after surgery. *AJR Am J Roentgenol*. 1991;157(2):353–358. doi:10.2214/ajr.157.2.1853821
20. von Mehren M, Randall RL, Benjamin RS, et al. Soft tissue sarcoma, Version 2.2018, NCCN Clinical Practice Guidelines in Oncology. *J Natl Compr Canc Netw*. 2018;16(5):536–563. doi:10.6004/jnccn.2018.0025
21. Chang KJ, Lim I, Park JY, et al. The role of (18)F-FDG PET/CT as a prognostic factor in patients with synovial sarcoma. *Nucl Med Mol Imaging*. 2015;49(1):33–41. doi:10.1007/s13139-014-0301-5
22. Siddiqi MA, Kim HS, Jede F, Han I. Association of core needle biopsy tract resection with local recurrence in extremity soft tissue sarcoma. *Skeletal Radiol*. 2017;46(4):507–512. doi:10.1007/s00256-017-2579-8
23. McBride MJ, Pulice JL, Beird HC, et al. The SS18-SSX fusion oncoprotein hijacks BAF complex targeting and function to drive synovial sarcoma. *Cancer Cell*. 2018;33(6):1128.e7–1141.e7. doi:10.1016/j.ccell.2018.05.002
24. *Fletcher C, Bridge JA, Hogendoorn P, Mertens F, eds. WHO Classification of Tumours of Soft Tissue and Bone*. 4th ed, Vol. 5. Lyon, France: International Agency for Research on Cancer; 2013.
25. Bianchi G, Sambri A, Righi A, et al. Histology and grading are important prognostic factors in synovial sarcoma. *Eur J Surg Oncol*. 2017;43(9):1733–1739. doi:10.1016/j.ejso.2017.05.020
26. van de Rijn M, Barr FG, Xiong QB, et al. Poorly differentiated synovial sarcoma: an analysis of clinical, pathologic, and molecular genetic features. *Am J Surg Pathol*. 1999;23(1):106–112. doi:10.1097/00000478-199901000-00012
27. Valente AL, Tull J, Zhang S. Specificity of TLE1 expression in unclassified high-grade sarcomas for the diagnosis of synovial sarcoma. *Appl Immunohistochem Mol Morphol*. 2013;21(5):408–413. doi:10.1097/PAI.0b013e318279f9ee
28. Crew AJ, Clark J, Fisher C, et al. Fusion of SYT to two genes, SSX1 and SSX2, encoding proteins with homology to the Kruppel-associated box in human synovial sarcoma. *EMBO J*. 1995;14(10):2333–2340. doi:10.1002/j.1460-2075.1995.tb07228.x
29. Fligman I, Lonardo F, Jhanwar SC, et al. Molecular diagnosis of synovial sarcoma and characterization of a variant SYT-SSX2 fusion transcript. *Am J Pathol*. 1995;147(6):1592–1599. https://www.ncbi.nlm.nih.gov/pubmed/7495284
30. Clark J, Rocques PJ, Crew AJ, et al. Identification of novel genes, SYT and SSX, involved in the t(X;18)(p11.2;q11.2) translocation found in human synovial sarcoma. *Nat Genet*. 1994;7(4):502–508. doi:10.1038/ng0894-502
31. de Leeuw B, Balemans M, Olde WD, Geurts van Kessel A. Identification of two alternative fusion genes, SYT-SSX1 and SYT-SSX2, in t(X;18)(p11.2;q11.2)-positive synovial sarcomas. *Hum Mol Genet*. 1995;4(6):1097–1099. doi:10.1093/hmg/4.6.1097
32. Skytting B, Nilsson G, Brodin B, et al. A novel fusion gene, SYT-SSX4, in synovial sarcoma. *J Natl Cancer Inst*. 1999;91(11):974–975. doi:10.1093/jnci/91.11.974
33. Amary MFC, Berisha F, Bernardi FDC, et al. Detection of SS18-SSX fusion transcripts in formalin-fixed paraffin-embedded neoplasms: analysis of conventional RT-PCR, qRT-PCR and dual color FISH as diagnostic tools for synovial sarcoma. *Mod Pathol*. 2007;20(4):482–496. doi:10.1038/modpathol.3800761
34. Shipley J, Crew J, Birdsall S, et al. Interphase fluorescence in situ hybridization and reverse transcription polymerase chain reaction as a diagnostic aid for synovial sarcoma. *Am J Pathol*. 1996;148(2):559–567. https://www.ncbi.nlm.nih.gov/pubmed/8579118
35. Lasota J, Jasinski M, Debiec-Rychter M, et al. Detection of the SYT-SSX fusion transcripts in formaldehyde-fixed, paraffin-embedded tissue: a reverse transcription polymerase chain reaction amplification assay useful in the diagnosis of synovial sarcoma. *Mod Pathol*. 1998;11(7):626–633. https://www.ncbi.nlm.nih.gov/pubmed/9688183
36. Terry J, Barry TS, Horsman DE, et al. Fluorescence in situ hybridization for the detection of t(X;18)(p11.2;q11.2) in a synovial sarcoma tissue microarray using a breakapart-style probe. *Diagn Mol Pathol*. 2005;14(2):77–82. doi:10.1097/01.pas.0000155021.80213.c9
37. Motoi T, Kumagai A, Tsuji K, et al. Diagnostic utility of dual-color break-apart chromogenic in situ hybridization for the detection of rearranged SS18 in formalin-fixed, paraffin-embedded synovial sarcoma. *Hum Pathol*. 2010;41(10):1397–1404. doi:10.1016/j.humpath.2010.02.009
38. Kato K, Tanaka M, Toyoda Y, et al. A novel fluorescence in situ hybridization assay for synovial sarcoma. *Pathol Res Pract*. 2013;209(5):309–313. doi:10.1016/j.prp.2013.02.013
39. Papp G, Mihály D, Sápi Z. Unusual signal patterns of break-apart FISH Probes used in the diagnosis of soft tissue sarcomas. *Pathol Oncol Res*. 2017;23(4):863–871. doi:10.1007/s12253-017-0200-z
40. Jiang D, Peng R, Yan X, et al. Synovial sarcoma showing loss of a green signal in SS18 fluorescence in situ hybridization: a clinicopathological and molecular study of 12 cases. *Virchows Arch*. 2017;471(6):799–807. doi:10.1007/s00428-017-2211-2
41. He R, Patel RM, Alkan S, et al. Immunostaining for SYT protein discriminates synovial sarcoma from other soft tissue tumors: analysis of 146 cases. *Mod Pathol*. 2007;20(5):522–528. doi:10.1038/modpathol.3800766
42. Zheng Z, Liebers M, Zhelyazkova B, et al. Anchored multiplex PCR for targeted next-generation sequencing. *Nat Med*. 2014;20(12):1479–1484. doi:10.1038/nm.3729

43. Zhu G, Benayed R, Ho C, et al. Diagnosis of known sarcoma fusions and novel fusion partners by targeted RNA sequencing with identification of a recurrent ACTB-FOSB fusion in pseudomyogenic hemangioendothelioma. *Mod Pathol*. 2019;32(5):609–620. doi:10.1038/s41379-018-0175-7
44. Lam SW, Cleton-Jansen AM, Cleven AHG, et al. Molecular analysis of gene fusions in bone and soft tissue tumors by anchored multiplex PCR-based targeted next-generation sequencing. *J Mol Diagn*. 2018;20(5):653–663. doi:10.1016/j.jmoldx.2018.05.007
45. Schaefer IM, Fletcher CDM, Hornick JL. Loss of H3K27 trimethylation distinguishes malignant peripheral nerve sheath tumors from histologic mimics. *Mod Pathol*. 2016;29(1):4–13. doi:10.1038/modpathol.2015.134
46. Kadoch C, Crabtree GR. Reversible disruption of mSWI/SNF (BAF) complexes by the SS18-SSX oncogenic fusion in synovial sarcoma. *Cell*. 2013;153(1):71–85. doi:10.1016/j.cell.2013.02.036
47. Ho L, Crabtree GR. Chromatin remodelling during development. *Nature*. 2010;463(7280):474–484. doi:10.1038/nature08911
48. Tea JS, Luo L. The chromatin remodeling factor Bap55 functions through the TIP60 complex to regulate olfactory projection neuron dendrite targeting. *Neural Dev*. 2011;6:5. doi:10.1186/1749-8104-6-5
49. Yoo AS, Sun AX, Li L, et al. MicroRNA-mediated conversion of human fibroblasts to neurons. *Nature*. 2011;476(7359):228–231. doi:10.1038/nature10323
50. Dawson MA, Kouzarides T. Cancer epigenetics: from mechanism to therapy. *Cell*. 2012;150(1):12–27. doi:10.1016/j.cell.2012.06.013
51. Kia SK, Gorski MM, Giannakopoulos S, Verrijzer CP. SWI/SNF mediates polycomb eviction and epigenetic reprogramming of the INK4b-ARF-INK4a locus. *Mol Cell Biol*. 2008;28(10):3457–3464. doi:10.1128/MCB.02019-07
52. Jones S, Wang TL, Shih IM, et al. Frequent mutations of chromatin remodeling gene ARID1A in ovarian clear cell carcinoma. *Science*. 2010;330(6001):228–231. doi:10.1126/science.1196333
53. Varela I, Tarpey P, Raine K, et al. Exome sequencing identifies frequent mutation of the SWI/SNF complex gene PBRM1 in renal carcinoma. *Nature*. 2011;469(7331):539–542. doi:10.1038/nature09639
54. Nakayama RT, Pulice JL, Valencia AM, et al. SMARCB1 is required for widespread BAF complex-mediated activation of enhancers and bivalent promoters. *Nat Genet*. 2017;49(11):1613–1623. doi:10.1038/ng.3958
55. Morgan MA, Shilatifard A. Epigenetic conFUSION: SS18-SSX fusion rewires BAF complex to activate bivalent genes in synovial sarcoma. *Cancer Cell*. 2018;33(6):951–953. doi:10.1016/j.ccell.2018.05.011
56. Michel BC, D'Avino AR, Cassel SH, et al. A non-canonical SWI/SNF complex is a synthetic lethal target in cancers driven by BAF complex perturbation. *Nat Cell Biol*. 2018;20(12):1410–1420. doi:10.1038/s41556-018-0221-1
57. Hohmann AF, Martin LJ, Minder JL, et al. Sensitivity and engineered resistance of myeloid leukemia cells to BRD9 inhibition. *Nat Chem Biol*. 2016;12(9):672–679. doi:10.1038/nchembio.2115
58. Martin LJ, Koegl M, Bader G, et al. Structure-based design of an in vivo active selective BRD9 inhibitor. *J Med Chem*. 2016;59(10):4462–4475. doi:10.1021/acs.jmedchem.5b01865
59. Remillard D, Buckley DL, Paulk J, et al. Degradation of the BAF complex factor BRD9 by heterobifunctional ligands. *Angew Chem Int Ed Engl*. 2017;56(21):5738–5743. doi:10.1002/anie.201611281
60. Canter RJ, Qin LX, Maki RG, et al. A synovial sarcoma-specific preoperative nomogram supports a survival benefit to ifosfamide-based chemotherapy and improves risk stratification for patients. *Clin Cancer Res*. 2008;14(24):8191–8197. doi:10.1158/1078-0432.CCR-08-0843
61. Vlenterie M, Ho VKY, Kaal SEJ, et al. Age as an independent prognostic factor for survival of localised synovial sarcoma patients. *Br J Cancer*. 2015;113(11):1602–1606. doi:10.1038/bjc.2015.375
62. Brecht IB, Ferrari A, Int-Veen C, et al. Grossly-resected synovial sarcoma treated by the German and Italian Pediatric Soft Tissue Sarcoma Cooperative Groups: discussion on the role of adjuvant therapies. *Pediatr Blood Cancer*. 2006;46(1):11–17. doi:10.1002/pbc.20502
63. Lewis JJ, Antonescu CR, Leung DH, et al. Synovial sarcoma: a multivariate analysis of prognostic factors in 112 patients with primary localized tumors of the extremity. *J Clin Oncol*. 2000;18(10):2087–2094. doi:10.1200/JCO.2000.18.10.2087
64. ten Heuvel SE, Hoekstra HJ, Bastiaannet E, Suurmeijer AJH. The classic prognostic factors tumor stage, tumor size, and tumor grade are the strongest predictors of outcome in synovial sarcoma: no role for SSX fusion type or ezrin expression. *Appl Immunohistochem Mol Morphol*. 2009;17(3):189–195. doi:10.1097/PAI.0b013e31818a6f5c
65. Mazeron JJ, Suit HD. Lymph nodes as sites of metastases from sarcomas of soft tissue. *Cancer*. 1987;60(8):1800–1808. doi:10.1002/1097-0142(19871015)60:8<1800::aid-cncr2820600822>3.0.co;2-n
66. Keung EZ, Chiang YJ, Voss RK, et al. Defining the incidence and clinical significance of lymph node metastasis in soft tissue sarcoma. *Eur J Surg Oncol*. 2018;44(1):170–177. doi:10.1016/j.ejso.2017.11.014
67. Johannesmeyer D, Smith V, Cole DJ, et al. The impact of lymph node disease in extremity soft-tissue sarcomas: a population-based analysis. *Am J Surg*. 2013;206(3):289–295. doi:10.1016/j.amjsurg.2012.10.043
68. Riad S, Griffin AM, Liberman B, et al. Lymph node metastasis in soft tissue sarcoma in an extremity. *Clin Orthop Relat Res*. 2004;426:129–134. doi:10.1097/01.blo.0000141660.05125.46
69. Behranwala KA, A'Hern R, Omar AM, Thomas JM. Prognosis of lymph node metastasis in soft tissue sarcoma. *Ann Surg Oncol*. 2004;11(7):714–719. doi:10.1245/ASO.2004.04.027
70. Jacobs AJ, Morris CD, Levin AS. Synovial sarcoma is not associated with a higher risk of lymph node metastasis compared with other soft tissue sarcomas. *Clin Orthop Relat Res*. 2018;476(3):589–598. doi:10.1007/s11999.0000000000000057

71. Kattan MW, Leung DHY, Brennan MF. Postoperative nomogram for 12-year sarcoma-specific death. *J Clin Oncol*. 2002;20(3):791–796. doi:10.1200/JCO.2002.20.3.791
72. Callegaro D, Miceli R, Bonvalot S, et al. Development and external validation of two nomograms to predict overall survival and occurrence of distant metastases in adults after surgical resection of localised soft-tissue sarcomas of the extremities: a retrospective analysis. *Lancet Oncol*. 2016;17(5):671–680. doi:10.1016/S1470-2045(16)00010-3
73. Eilber FC, Dry SM. Diagnosis and management of synovial sarcoma. *J Surg Oncol*. 2008;97(4):314–320. doi:10.1002/jso.20974
74. Ahmad R, Jacobson A, Hornicek F, et al. The width of the surgical margin does not influence outcomes in extremity and truncal soft tissue sarcoma treated with radiotherapy. *Oncologist*. 2016;21(10):1269–1276. doi:10.1634/theoncologist.2015-0534
75. King DM, Hackbarth DA, Kirkpatrick A. Extremity soft tissue sarcoma resections: how wide do you need to be? *Clin Orthop Relat Res*. 2012;470(3):692–699. doi:10.1007/s11999-011-2167-5
76. Bedi M, King DM, Charlson J, et al. Multimodality management of metastatic patients with soft tissue sarcomas may prolong survival. *Am J Clin Oncol*. 2014;37(3):272–277. doi:10.1097/COC.0b013e318277d7e5
77. Gadd MA, Casper ES, Woodruff JM, et al. Development and treatment of pulmonary metastases in adult patients with extremity soft tissue sarcoma. *Ann Surg*. 1993;218(6):705–712. doi:10.1097/00000658-199312000-00002
78. O'Sullivan B, Davis AM, Turcotte R, et al. Preoperative versus postoperative radiotherapy in soft-tissue sarcoma of the limbs: a randomised trial. *Lancet*. 2002;359(9325):2235–2241. doi:10.1016/S0140-6736(02)09292-9
79. Sarcoma Meta-analysis Collaboration. Adjuvant chemotherapy for localised resectable soft-tissue sarcoma of adults: meta-analysis of individual data. *Lancet*. 1997;350(9092):1647–1654. doi:10.1016/S0140-6736(97)08165-8
80. Pervaiz N, Colterjohn N, Farrokhyar F, et al. A systematic meta-analysis of randomized controlled trials of adjuvant chemotherapy for localized resectable soft-tissue sarcoma. *Cancer*. 2008;113(3):573–581. doi:10.1002/cncr.23592
81. Le CA, Ouali M, Leahy MG, et al. Doxorubicin-based adjuvant chemotherapy in soft tissue sarcoma: pooled analysis of two STBSG-EORTC phase III clinical trials. *Ann Oncol*. 2014;25(12):2425–2432. doi:10.1093/annonc/mdu460
82. Woll PJ, Reichardt P, Le CA, et al. Adjuvant chemotherapy with doxorubicin, ifosfamide, and lenograstim for resected soft-tissue sarcoma (EORTC 62931): a multicentre randomised controlled trial. *Lancet Oncol*. 2012;13(10):1045–1054. doi:10.1016/S1470-2045(12)70346-7
83. Frustaci S, Gherlinzoni F, De Paoli A, et al. Adjuvant chemotherapy for adult soft tissue sarcomas of the extremities and girdles: results of the Italian randomized cooperative trial. *J Clin Oncol*. 2001;19(5):1238–1247. doi:10.1200/JCO.2001.19.5.1238
84. Gronchi A, Ferrari S, Quagliuolo V, et al. Histotype-tailored neoadjuvant chemotherapy versus standard chemotherapy in patients with high-risk soft-tissue sarcomas (ISG-STS 1001): an international, open-label, randomised, controlled, phase 3, multicentre trial. *Lancet Oncol*. 2017;18(6):812–822. doi:10.1016/S1470-2045(17)30334-0
85. van Oosterom AT, Mouridsen HT, Nielsen OS, et al. Results of randomised studies of the EORTC Soft Tissue and Bone Sarcoma Group (STBSG) with two different ifosfamide regimens in first- and second-line chemotherapy in advanced soft tissue sarcoma patients. *Eur J Cancer*. 2002;38(18):2397–2406. doi:10.1016/s0959-8049(02)00491-4
86. Casali PG, Abecassis N, Aro HT, et al. Soft tissue and visceral sarcomas: ESMO-EURACAN Clinical Practice Guidelines for diagnosis, treatment and follow-up. *Ann Oncol*. 2018;29(suppl 4):iv51–iv67. doi:10.1093/annonc/mdy096
87. von Mehren M, Randall RL, Benjamin RS, et al. Soft Tissue Sarcoma, Version 2.2018, NCCN Clinical Practice Guidelines in Oncology. *J Natl Compr Canc Netw*. 2018;16(5):536–563. doi:10.6004/jnccn.2018.0025
88. Chen Y, Yang Y, Wang C, Shi Y. Adjuvant chemotherapy decreases and postpones distant metastasis in extremity stage IIB/III synovial sarcoma patients. *J Surg Oncol*. 2012;106(2):162–168. doi:10.1002/jso.23061
89. Eilber FC, Brennan MF, Eilber FR, et al. Chemotherapy is associated with improved survival in adult patients with primary extremity synovial sarcoma. *Ann Surg*. 2007;246(1):105–113. doi:10.1097/01.sla.0000262787.88639.2b
90. Rutkowski P, Lugowska I. Follow-up in soft tissue sarcomas. *Memo*. 2014;7(2):92–96. doi:10.1007/s12254-014-0146-8
91. Krieg AH, Hefti F, Speth BM, et al. Synovial sarcomas usually metastasize after >5 years: a multicenter retrospective analysis with minimum follow-up of 10 years for survivors. *Ann Oncol*. 2011;22(2):458–467. doi:10.1093/annonc/mdq394
92. Guadagnolo BA, Zagars GK, Ballo MT, et al. Long-term outcomes for synovial sarcoma treated with conservation surgery and radiotherapy. *Int J Radiat Oncol Biol Phys*. 2007;69(4):1173–1180. doi:10.1016/j.ijrobp.2007.04.056
93. Ferrari A, De Salvo GL, Dall'Igna P, et al. Salvage rates and prognostic factors after relapse in children and adolescents with initially localised synovial sarcoma. *Eur J Cancer*. 2012;48(18):3448–3455. doi:10.1016/j.ejca.2012.06.017
94. Salah S, Yaser S, Salem A, et al. Factors influencing survival in metastatic synovial sarcoma: importance of patterns of metastases and the first-line chemotherapy regimen. *Med Oncol*. 2013;30(3):639. doi:10.1007/s12032-013-0639-z
95. Vlenterie M, Litière S, Rizzo E, et al. Outcome of chemotherapy in advanced synovial sarcoma patients: review of 15 clinical trials from the European Organisation for Research and Treatment of Cancer Soft Tissue and Bone Sarcoma Group; setting a new landmark for studies in this entity. *Eur J Cancer*. 2016;58:62–72. doi:10.1016/j.ejca.2016.02.002

96. Thorn CF, Oshiro C, Marsh S, et al. Doxorubicin pathways: pharmacodynamics and adverse effects. *Pharmacogenet Genomics*. 2011;21(7):440–446. doi:10.1097/FPC.0b013e32833ffb56
97. Borden EC, Amato DA, Rosenbaum C, et al. Randomized comparison of three adriamycin regimens for metastatic soft tissue sarcomas. *J Clin Oncol*. 1987;5(6):840–850. doi:10.1200/JCO.1987.5.6.840
98. Edmonson JH, Ryan LM, Blum RH, et al. Randomized comparison of doxorubicin alone versus ifosfamide plus doxorubicin or mitomycin, doxorubicin, and cisplatin against advanced soft tissue sarcomas. *J Clin Oncol*. 1993;11(7):1269–1275. doi:10.1200/JCO.1993.11.7.1269
99. Judson I, Verweij J, Gelderblom H, et al. Doxorubicin alone versus intensified doxorubicin plus ifosfamide for first-line treatment of advanced or metastatic soft-tissue sarcoma: a randomised controlled phase 3 trial. *Lancet Oncol*. 2014;15(4):415–423. doi:10.1016/S1470-2045(14)70063-4
100. Spurrell EL, Fisher C, Thomas JM, Judson IR. Prognostic factors in advanced synovial sarcoma: an analysis of 104 patients treated at the Royal Marsden Hospital. *Ann Oncol*. 2005;16(3):437–444. doi:10.1093/annonc/mdi082
101. Tap WD, Jones RL, Van Tine BA, et al. Olaratumab and doxorubicin versus doxorubicin alone for treatment of soft-tissue sarcoma: an open-label phase 1b and randomised phase 2 trial. *Lancet*. 2016;388(10043):488–497. doi:10.1016/s0140-6736(16)30587-6
102. Bramwell VH, Mouridsen HT, Santoro A, et al. Cyclophosphamide versus ifosfamide: a randomized phase II trial in adult soft-tissue sarcomas. The European Organization for Research and Treatment of Cancer [EORTC], Soft Tissue and Bone Sarcoma Group. *Cancer Chemother Pharmacol*. 1993;31(suppl 2):S180–S184. doi:10.1007/bf00647440
103. Antman KH, Ryan L, Elias A, et al. Response to ifosfamide and mesna. *J Clin Oncol*. 1989;7(9):1369–1369. doi:10.1200/jco.1989.7.9.1369
104. Nagar SP, Mytelka DS, Candrilli SD, et al. Treatment patterns and survival among adult patients with advanced soft tissue sarcoma: a retrospective medical record review in the United Kingdom, Spain, Germany, and France. *Sarcoma*. 2018;2018:5467057. doi:10.1155/2018/5467057
105. Sleijfer S, Ouali M, van Glabbeke M, et al. Prognostic and predictive factors for outcome to first-line ifosfamide-containing chemotherapy for adult patients with advanced soft tissue sarcomas: an exploratory, retrospective analysis on large series from the European Organization for Research and Treatment of Cancer-Soft Tissue and Bone Sarcoma Group (EORTC-STBSG). *Eur J Cancer*. 2010;46(1):72–83. doi:10.1016/j.ejca.2009.09.022
106. Noujaim J, Constantinidou A, Messiou C, et al. Successful ifosfamide rechallenge in soft-tissue sarcoma. *Am J Clin Oncol*. 2018;41(2):147–151. doi:10.1097/COC.0000000000000243
107. Lee SH, Chang MH, Baek KK, et al. High-dose ifosfamide as second- or third-line chemotherapy in refractory bone and soft tissue sarcoma patients. *Oncology*. 2011;80(3–4):257–261. doi:10.1159/000328795
108. Nielsen OS, Judson I, van Hoesel Q, et al. Effect of high-dose ifosfamide in advanced soft tissue sarcomas. A multicentre phase II study of the EORTC Soft Tissue and Bone Sarcoma Group. *Eur J Cancer*. 2000;36(1):61–67. doi:10.1016/s0959-8049(99)00240-3
109. van der Graaf WTA, Blay JY, Chawla SP, et al. Pazopanib for metastatic soft-tissue sarcoma (PALETTE): a randomised, double-blind, placebo-controlled phase 3 trial. *Lancet*. 2012;379(9829):1879–1886. doi:10.1016/s0140-6736(12)60651-5
110. George S, Merriam P, Maki RG, et al. Multicenter phase II trial of sunitinib in the treatment of nongastrointestinal stromal tumor sarcomas. *J Clin Oncol*. 2009;27(19):3154–3160. doi:10.1200/JCO.2008.20.9890
111. Mir O, Brodowicz T, Italiano A, et al. Safety and efficacy of regorafenib in patients with advanced soft tissue sarcoma (REGOSARC): a randomised, double-blind, placebo-controlled, phase 2 trial. *Lancet Oncol*. 2016;17(12):1732–1742. doi:10.1016/S1470-2045(16)30507-1
112. Eberst L, Cropet C, Le CA, et al. The off-label use of targeted therapies in sarcomas: the OUTC'S program. *BMC Cancer*. 2014;14:870. doi:10.1186/1471-2407-14-870
113. Demetri GD, von Mehren M, Jones R, et al. Efficacy and safety of trabectedin or dacarbazine for metastatic liposarcoma or leiomyosarcoma after failure of conventional chemotherapy: results of a phase III randomized multicenter clinical trial. *J Clin Oncol*. 2016;34(8):786–793. doi:10.1200/JCO.2015.62.4734
114. Le CA, Cresta S, Maki RG, et al. A retrospective analysis of antitumour activity with trabectedin in translocation-related sarcomas. *Eur J Cancer*. 2012;48(16):3036–3044. doi:10.1016/j.ejca.2012.05.012
115. Sanfilippo R, Dileo P, Blay JY, et al. Trabectedin in advanced synovial sarcomas: a multicenter retrospective study from four European institutions and the Italian Rare Cancer Network. *Anticancer Drugs*. 2015;26(6):678–681. doi:10.1097/CAD.0000000000000228
116. Villalobos VM, Byfield SD, Ghate SR, Adejoro O. A retrospective cohort study of treatment patterns among patients with metastatic soft tissue sarcoma in the US. *Clin Sarcoma Res*. 2017;7:18. doi:10.1186/s13569-017-0084-4
117. Leahy M, del Muro XG, Reichardt P, et al. Chemotherapy treatment patterns and clinical outcomes in patients with metastatic soft tissue sarcoma. The SArcoma treatment and Burden of Illness in North America and Europe (SABINE) study. *Ann Oncol*. 2012;23(10):2763–2770. doi:10.1093/annonc/mds070
118. Schoffski P, Agulnik M, Stacchiotti S, et al. Phase 2 multicenter study of the EZH2 inhibitor tazemetostat in adults with synovial sarcoma (NCT02601950). *J Clin Oncol*. 2017;35(15_suppl):11057–11057. doi:10.1200/jco.2017.35.15_suppl.11057

119. D'Angelo SP, Mahoney MR, Van Tine BA, et al. Nivolumab with or without ipilimumab treatment for metastatic sarcoma (Alliance A091401): two open-label, non-comparative, randomised, phase 2 trials. *Lancet Oncol.* 2018;19(3):416–426. doi:10.1016/S1470-2045(18)30006-8
120. Tawbi HA, Burgess M, Bolejack V, et al. Pembrolizumab in advanced soft-tissue sarcoma and bone sarcoma (SARC028): a multicentre, two-cohort, single-arm, open-label, phase 2 trial. *Lancet Oncol.* 2017;18(11):1493–1501. doi:10.1016/S1470-2045(17)30624-1
121. Jungbluth AA, Chen YT, Stockert E, et al. Immunohistochemical analysis of NY-ESO-1 antigen expression in normal and malignant human tissues. *Int J Cancer.* 2001;92(6):856–860. doi:10.1002/ijc.1282
122. Somaiah N, Chawla SP, Block MS, et al. Immune response, safety, and survival impact from CMB305 in NY-ESO-1+ recurrent soft tissue sarcomas (STS). *J Clin Oncol.* 2017;35(15_suppl):11006–11006. doi:10.1200/jco.2017.35.15_suppl.11006
123. Robbins PF, Kassim SH, Tran TLN, et al. A pilot trial using lymphocytes genetically engineered with an NY-ESO-1-reactive T-cell receptor: long-term follow-up and correlates with response. *Clin Cancer Res.* 2015;21(5):1019–1027. doi:10.1158/1078-0432.CCR-14-2708
124. D'Angelo SP, Melchiori L, Merchant MS, et al. Antitumor activity associated with prolonged persistence of adoptively transferred NY-ESO-1 T cells in synovial sarcoma. *Cancer Discov.* 2018;8(8):944–957. doi:10.1158/2159-8290.CD-17-1417
125. Chudgar NP, Brennan MF, Munhoz RR, et al. Pulmonary metastasectomy with therapeutic intent for soft-tissue sarcoma. *J Thorac Cardiovasc Surg.* 2017;154(1):319.e1–330.e1. doi:10.1016/j.jtcvs.2017.02.061
126. Schur S, Hoetzenecker K, Lamm W, et al. Pulmonary metastasectomy for soft tissue sarcoma—report from a dual institution experience at the Medical University of Vienna. *Eur J Cancer.* 2014;50(13):2289–2297. doi:10.1016/j.ejca.2014.05.009
127. Treasure T, Fiorentino F, Scarci M, et al. Pulmonary metastasectomy for sarcoma: a systematic review of reported outcomes in the context of Thames Cancer Registry data. *BMJ Open.* 2012;2(5):e001736. doi:10.1136/bmjopen-2012-001736
128. Lee K, Kang MC, Lee HW, et al. Pulmonary metastasectomy in adult patients with synovial sarcoma: a single-center experience. *Korean J Thorac Cardiovasc Surg.* 2016;49(6):451–455. doi:10.5090/kjtcs.2016.49.6.451
129. Dhakal S, Corbin KS, Milano MT, et al. Stereotactic body radiotherapy for pulmonary metastases from soft-tissue sarcomas: excellent local lesion control and improved patient survival. *Int J Radiat Oncol Biol Phys.* 2012;82(2):940–945. doi:10.1016/j.ijrobp.2010.11.052
130. Frakulli R, Salvi F, Balestrini D, et al. Stereotactic radiotherapy in the treatment of lung metastases from bone and soft-tissue sarcomas. *Anticancer Res.* 2015;35(10):5581–5586. https://www.ncbi.nlm.nih.gov/pubmed/26408729
131. Lindsay AD, Haupt EE, Chan CM, et al. Treatment of sarcoma lung metastases with stereotactic body radiotherapy. *Sarcoma.* 2018;2018:1–6. doi:10.1155/2018/9132359
132. Navarria P, Ascolese AM, Cozzi L, et al. Stereotactic body radiation therapy for lung metastases from soft tissue sarcoma. *Eur J Cancer.* 2015;51(5):668–674. doi:10.1016/j.ejca.2015.01.061

III

Other Treatment Approaches

28

Immunotherapy for Sarcoma

Catherine M. Albert and Seth M. Pollack

INTRODUCTION

Sarcomas are mesenchymal malignancies with over 50 distinct subtypes; hence, it is no surprise that this diverse group of diseases interacts with the immune system in many different ways. However, it is only over the past few years that the community of sarcoma physicians and researchers has started to appreciate how the incredible diversity of sarcoma tumors may shape their responses to immunotherapy.[1] Over 100 years ago, William Coley first administered streptococcal infection with therapeutic intent that successfully resulted in the spontaneous cancer regression observed in a patient with advanced sarcoma. In the 1980s, Rosenberg and colleagues at the National Cancer Institute ran pioneering trials using high doses of interleukin 2 (IL-2), observing durable disease response in a minority of melanoma and renal cell carcinoma (RCC) patients.[2] The potential benefits of cellular therapies were demonstrated through the "graft vs. malignancy" effect seen following allogeneic transplantation and through the observation that tumor infiltrating lymphocytes (TIL) expanded ex vivo could induce durable tumor regression in patients with advanced and refractory melanoma.[3,4]

Today, the field of immunotherapy is exploding. Monoclonal antibodies targeting immune checkpoints and cell surface proteins that downregulate T-cell activation have demonstrated incredible efficacy across a range of cancer types, in most cases with an excellent toxicity profile.[5–7] T cells with engineered antigen specificity have transformed the treatment of lymphoid malignancies[8] and are under investigation in many solid tumors.[8] Fulfilling the long-discussed promise of immunotherapy for metastatic sarcoma, we are finally starting to observe results that may incorporate immunotherapy into the standard of care for certain sarcoma subtypes. Analysis of the specific sarcoma subtypes and interactions with the tumor microenvironment have proved crucial for this evolution. However, much work remains to move these gains to the vast majority of sarcoma subtypes and to discover the optimal regimens to use them.[9]

NOVEL COMBINATIONS OF CHECKPOINT INHIBITORS

More work is needed to characterize the response pattern of sarcoma patients using programmed death protein-1 (PD-1) and programmed death ligand-1 (PD-L1) inhibitors, but we starting to see patterns emerge. The first effort to characterize the response of soft tissue sarcoma (STS) and bone sarcoma patients to PD-1 inhibition was the SARC028 study. This single-arm, Phase II study tested the PD-1 inhibitor, pembrolizumab, in patients with refractory disease.[10] The study included 40 patients with bone sarcoma and 40 with STS. Responses were mostly limited to patients with undifferentiated pleomorphic sarcoma (UPS) and dedifferentiated liposarcoma (DD LPS) along with one short-lived partial response within the synovial sarcoma (SS) cohort. No responses were seen in leiomyosarcoma (LMS) patients on the SARC028 study and this was a bit surprising as LMS often has both PD-L1 expression and T-cell infiltration. This finding was supported in a separate study of nivolimab in advanced uterine LMS, where again little activity was observed.[11] Only one patient of 22 with osteosarcoma (OST) and none of the Ewing sarcoma patients responded, but one of five patients with chondrosarcoma responded. Interestingly, in one responding LMS patient, a phosphatase and tensin homolog (*PTEN*) mutation may have induced treatment resistance.[12] Expansion cohorts were performed for UPS and DD LPS, which yielded promising results, recently reported by the American Society of Clinical Oncology (ASCO).[13] In one of the biggest success stories for checkpoint inhibitors in sarcoma, the combination of pembrolizumab and axitinib has induced impressive and often durable responses in alveolar soft part sarcoma, including in refractory patients.[14] PD-1 inhibitors are being tested in other clinical settings, including neoadjuvant, in the multicenter SARC032 study (NCT03092323).

Cytotoxic T-lymphocyte associated protein-4 (CTLA-4) inhibition combined with anti-PD-1 therapy improves survival for melanoma patients, albeit with more toxicity.[15] A study of CTLA-4 inhibition in SS patients showed no value for this treatment in this subtype as a single agent.[16] A study combining nivolimab plus a reduced dose of ipilimumab (1 mg/kg) showed impressive clinical activity with the combination.[17] Because CTLA4 and PD-1/PD-L1 modulate specific and distinct mechanisms of T-cell immunity, combined checkpoint inhibition has been pursued with even more favorable results.[18–20] The Alliance A091401 trial treated patients with the PD-1 inhibitor nivolumab alone or in combination with ipilumumab to adults with advanced STS.[21] Patients were randomized to monotherapy or the combined regimen with a total of 96 patients enrolled to the study. Responses were observed in 5% patients on the nivolumab arm and 16% on the nivolumab + ipilumumab arm, suggesting the possibility of benefit to the combination. Responses were observed in patients with UPS, LPS, angiosarcoma, LMS, and myxofibroid sarcoma. Combinations of PD-1 and CTLA-4 are being tested in ongoing studies for gastrointestinal stromal tumor (GIST) at University of California at Los Angeles (UCLA; NCT02880020) and all sarcomas at MD Anderson Cancer Center (NCT02815995).

While these initial studies are encouraging, novel combinations will be critical for using these results to make the benefits more durable and applicable to more subtypes. Doxorubicin may achieve tumor degradation and antigen presentation with a relatively low level of lymphodepletion and a recent presentation suggested encouraging signs of activity.[22] Gemcitabine may have a similar impact by modulating vasculature in addition to direct cytotoxicity (NCT03123276). A recent presentation at European Society of Medical Oncology (ESMO) suggested that sunitinib in combination with nivolimab may be effective in refractory patients (NCT03277924). Unfortunately, not all immunotherapy combinations have been successful. The combination of low-dose cyclophosphamide and pembrolizumab had great rationale as metronomic cyclophosphamide can both help treat sarcomas as well as eliminate Tregs, but unfortunately little activity was seen in the combination.[23] Novel agents targeting receptors, such as B7-H3, OX40, GITR, IDO, and ICOS have not all panned out as hoped for in other cancers but may still be effective in the right combination regimens when applied to certain sarcoma subtypes.[24–27]

CELLULAR THERAPIES

The field of cellular therapy for cancer outside transplantation began with the use of tumor-infiltrating lymphocyte (TIL) for melanoma and other tumors with some success. While the plethora of other immunotherapeutic options for melanoma has reduced interest in TIL for melanoma, the use of TIL in sarcoma is having a bit of a resurgence. Historically, we have seen studies of TIL isolation and expansion with excellent in vitro activity in the setting of multiple bone tumors.[28] This work has complemented work in preclinical OST models with TIL phenotypically similar to those seen in OST tumors. More recent work suggests that state-of-the-art technique and truly fresh tumor specimen can lead to excellent rates of expansion.[29,30] Now clinical trials are ongoing using TIL in the context of intensive lymphodepletion and IL-2 (NCT04052334).

While these approaches remain under investigation with resurgent enthusiasm, T-cell therapy targeting the cancer testis antigens (CT antigens) MAGE-A4 and NY-ESO-1 are continuing to generate excitement. CT antigens are a family of highly immunogenic proteins expressed on a protein level in many cancers and but not in normal adult tissues apart from the testis and the trophoblast.[31] In some tumor types, CT antigen expression may confer worse prognosis.[32,33] Many cancer types express NY-ESO-1 and MAGE family antigens in a minority of cases and in a heterogeneous pattern. However, SS and myxoid round cell liposarcoma (MRCL) are unique as they both consistently and homogeneously express these immunotherapeutic targets. Over 80% of SS tumors express NY-ESO-1 by immunohistochemistry (IHC),[34] generally with a homogeneous pattern.[34] MRCL tumors almost always express NY-ESO-1 with homogeneous expression in a majority of cases.[35] Endogenous cytotoxic T lymphocytes (CTLs) have been successfully produced from SS and MRCL patients following ex vivo expansion and selection in the presence of whole autologous tumor cells or tumor antigen-pulsed dendritic cells (DCs),[36] but gene transfer allows for the production of T cells with uniform and consistently high-affinity TCRs. Cellular therapy targeting multiple CT antigens (NY-ESO-1, MAGE family and PRAME) using this method is being tested at Baylor University (NCT02239861).

Because TCRs recognize cancer-specific peptides, which can be intracellular, they must be recognized in the context of major histocompatibility complexes (MHC), which means they must be matched to patients with specific HLA types. HLA-A0201 is among the most common HLA types, expressed by 20% to 40% of the Caucasian population. Multiple investigators conducted clinical trials engineering T cells to target the 157–165 CD8 T-cell epitope of NY-ESO-1, which is presented by HLA-A*02:01.[37] Objective responses were observed in a majority of patients following cellular therapy targeting NY-ESO-1, demonstrating that NY-ESO-1 is an excellent target for these tumor types.[38,39] In a pilot study testing a high affinity, NY-ESO-1-specific T-cell receptor (TCR), responses were seen in the majority of patients.[38,39] More recent studies have only improved on those original results and also underscored the importance of lymphodepletion as part of the conditioning for these patients.[40] Much work remains to be done to improve on these results as the responses patients have are rarely durable. UCLA has been investigating combinations with dendritic cell vaccination[41] and CTLA-4 inhibition. CT antigen targets other than NY-ESO-1 may make this more successful; MAGE-A4 remains an extremely promising target, and high response rates were reported in early trials.[42]

More recently, the dramatic successes of T cells engineered to express chimeric antigen receptors (CARs) targeting lymphoid malignancies have generated a desire to apply these approaches to solid tumors and sarcoma in particular.[43] It is important to recognize that CAR T cells have a number of important differences from TCR-engineered T cells. These receptors recognize their target with the scFv portion of an antibody bound to a costimulatory domain (CD28 or 41BB) and a CD3ζ chain of the TCR so they can recognize cell surface, membrane bound proteins in a way that is HLA-independent. Identification of CAR targets is challenging, but there are some exciting emerging possibilities. CAR T-cells targeting Her-2 were used for patients with OST and epithelioid sarcoma (ES) resulting in tumor necrosis,[44] and novel approaches may further enhance these responses.[45] B7-H3, along with possibly G2D, may be a particularly exciting target,[46] and it is currently in clinical trials ongoing now (NCT00902044, NCT02107963, NCT01953900).

MANIPULATING THE SARCOMA IMMUNE MICROENVIRONMENT

A plethora of studies have analyzed PD-L1, PD-1, and other immune-related biomarkers in sarcoma tumors. One of the earliest of these reports examined 105 sarcoma tumors, including specimens from a diverse group of subtypes.[47] PD-1 expressing TIL and PD-L1 expression on tumor cells was observed in 65% and 58% of cases. Both PD-1 and PD-L1 expression were associated with both higher tumor grade and advanced stage, and were independent prognostic indicators for OST and progression-free survival (PFS). A later study of 50 STS patients with a broad mix of subtypes found lower levels of PD-1 and PD-L1 expression emphasizing that it is difficult to generate broad characterization of sarcomas because the expression of these immune markers varies so much from subtype to subtype.[17] Another study used the nanostring gene expression platform with a focus on UPS, LMS, SS, and liposarcoma subtypes, and found that UPS had high levels of genes related to antigen presentation and T-cell infiltration. SS and MRCL tumors showed significantly lower expression of such genes including low levels of the MHC/HLA that are essential for antigen recognition by T cells as well as the of genes associated with T-cell infiltration, such as the IL-7 receptor-encoding (IL-7R) gene.[48] These patterns of expression appeared to also apply to expression of PD-L1 on tumor and PD-1 on infiltrating T cells, with the levels of expression highly correlated to T-cell infiltration and expression of genes related to antigen presentation.

The very low levels of T-cell infiltration, MHC expression, and expression of PD-L1 suggest an overall "quiet" or "cold" tumor immune microenvironment in STS. However, a phase 0 trial suggested that interferon gamma may be able to transform this into a "hot" environment as evidenced by increased T-cell infiltration and MHC expression; however, this regimen also resulted in the upregulation of PD-L1 in tumors.[49] An ongoing National Cancer Institute (NCI)-sponsored Phase 2 trial of pembrolizumab in combination with interferon gamma-1b has recently been amended to include metastatic and unresectable SS and MRCL (NCT03063632).

Other investigators have sought alternative strategies for manipulating the sarcoma immune microenvironment. Macrophages are myeloid derived cells that play a crucial role in manipulating the tumor immune microenviroment and have a critical prognostic importance for LMS patients[50–52] but may also play an important role for many other types of sarcoma.[53,54] These monocyte-derived cells can shift phenotype and function on a spectrum between the inflammatory M1 phenotype, which secretes IL-12 and has high class II MHC expression, and the M2 phenotype, which plays a role in wound healing and secretes inhibitory cytokines including IL-10 and transforming growth factor beta (TGFβ).[55] Pexidartinib is tyrosine kinase inhibitor (TKI) selective for the colony-stimulating factor 1 receptor (CSF1R) kinase, recently Food and Drug Administration (FDA) approved for the treatment of tenosynovial giant cell tumor based on marked clinical activity.[56] CSF1R (also known as CD115) is a classic marker for immune inhibitory macrophages, and inhibiting this receptor could play an important role in combination immunotherapies. A Phase I study combining pexidartinib and sirolimus is recruiting patients with advanced sarcomas (NCT02584647).[57] A number of groups have attempted to target macrophages through targeting CD47.[58] Trabectedin is part of standard of care treatment for sarcoma and also has potent anti-macrophage activity,[59,60] and trials combining trabectedin and checkpoint inhibitors are also ongoing (NCT03074318, NCT03138161). Manipulation of the tumor microenvironment with other agents, including a Toll-like receptor (TLR) agonist, may induce a globally inflamed environment including conversion of tumor-associated macrophages (TAMs) from M2 to M1, and trials are ongoing to attempt to exploit this effect.[61]

OTHER PROMISING STRATEGIES

Oncoytic Viral Therapies

Oncolytic viruses are attenuated or engineered viruses that either have direct cytolytic activity in tumors with at least some tumor specificity and targeting and/or operate by attracting an inflammatory antitumor immune response into the tumor that can then fight cancer systemically.[62,63] A wide variety of viral vectors have been gaining traction with encouraging activity against a variety of tumors.[64] Talimogene laherparepvec (Tvec) is a modified herpes simplex-1 virus engineer express GM-CSF (granulocyte macrophage colony-stimulating factor) that has been FDA approved as a treatment for melanoma and works better in combination with checkpoint inhibition.[65] Because STS can be superficial and injectable at the bedside, there has been some interest in finding applications for Tvec in this space. There is some evidence it may have applicability for other solid tumors.[66] Because sarcomas are often large and difficult to resect, the University of Iowa has been exploring its use in the localized setting both alone and with checkpoint blockade (NCT02453191). Memorial Sloan Kettering Cancer Center (MSKCC) investigated the use of Tvec along with pembrolizumab in 20 patients with metastatic sarcoma who had injectable lesions and reported responses in four, suggesting that this might be an area for further investigation.[67] Combinations with other immunotherapies, chemotherapy, and radiation may further potentiate responses. Preclinical activity using other oncolytic viral therapies has been demonstrated in a variety of models and this is will undoubtedly be an active area of future research.[68–70]

Cytokine Treatments

Cytokine formulations, such as pegylated IL-2,[71] may work well in combination with checkpoint strategies. IL-15 may be a key cytokine for future studies and novel formulations and compounds could potentially make this active either as a single agent or a part of a combination.[72] Delivery remains a challenge for IL-12 therapy but multiple investigators are working to bring novel formulations to the clinic.[73]

Vaccines

The field of sarcoma, like many fields in oncology, has a frustrating history with vaccines. These treatments work by stimulating the endogenous antitumor immune response. One of the most prominent disappointments for the field was a placebo-controlled, multicenter trial that tested a trivalent peptide vaccine against multiple ganglioside antigens. Vaccinologists have long suspected that peptide-induced vaccine responses can be slow in onset, so the trial focused on patients with no evidence of disease following metastectomy in a placebo-controlled, multicenter trial.[74] Although more serologic responses were seen following vaccination, there was no significant difference in PFS between trial arms. A pilot study using peptides spanning the *SYT–SSX* fusion in SS patients resulted in one transient response.[75]

There is a long history of using vaccines to induce responses against cancer testis antigens with some success at inducing immune responses with potential evidence of clinical activity.[76] LV305 was an integration-deficient lentiviral vector that selectively targeted CD209[77–79] on DCs and was able to induce strong T-cell responses in trials targeting NY-ESO-1 in SS and MRCL patients.[80,81] Phase I/II studies of this vaccine showed impressive results with 1-year overall survival (OS) of 82%.[82] Combining this vaccine with a TLR4 agonist and protein vaccine (NCT02387125) resulted in an even deeper induction of antibody and $CD4^+$ T-cell responses[83] and may have worked even better in combination with a PD-L1 inhibitor.[84] However, weak activity and logistical issues with a complicated trial design led to an abandonment of a pivotal Phase III trial. DC were also targeted in another vaccine trial that included an NY-ESO-1 protein bound to CD205, which did appear to have immunologic activity in some sarcoma patients; however, this therapy is no longer in development.[85]

Regardless, there are a number of promising strategies that may still have activity in the optimal regimen and clinical setting. A number of different trials have attempted to use DC vaccines pulsed with autologous tumor proteins, tumor lysate, or tumor-specific peptides with varying degrees of success.[86–88] Other strategies using autologous tumor have engineered tumor cells for increased immunogenicity. DC pulsed with sarcoma tumor lysate and other tumor-specific targets are being examined in combination with gemcitabine and in other regimens (NCT01803152; NCT03034304). The Vigil trial is an ongoing study in Ewing sarcoma patients receiving second-line chemotherapy (NCT03495921). This trial uses autologous tumor that has been engineered to express GM-CSF and to inhibit production of Furin, an enzyme that activated TGFβ.[89]

SUMMARY

Immunotherapy has transformed the treatment of many cancers leading to longer lives for countless patients with improved quality of life. In sarcoma, these advances have been slower, but we are finally making progress. We have started to identify areas where anti-PD-1 therapy can be incorporated into the standard of care, and T cells engineered to recognize HLA-restricted epitopes of cancer testis antigens are likely to become used more widely. As our understanding of the tumor immune microenvironment continues to evolve, novel agents and therapeutic combinations will undoubtedly continue to lead to improved care for patients with sarcoma.

REFERENCES

1. Katz D, Palmerini E, Pollack SM. More than 50 subtypes of soft tissue sarcoma: paving the path for histology-driven treatments. *Am Soc Clin Oncol Educ Book*. 2018;38:925–938. doi:10.1200/EDBK_205423
2. Rosenberg SA, Yang JC, Topalian SL, et al. Treatment of 283 consecutive patients with metastatic melanoma or renal cell cancer using high-dose bolus interleukin 2. *JAMA*. 1994;271(12):907–913. doi:10.1001/jama.1994.03510360033032
3. Dudley ME, Yang JC, Sherry R, et al. Adoptive cell therapy for patients with metastatic melanoma: evaluation of intensive myeloablative chemoradiation preparative regimens. *J Clin Oncol*. 2008;26(32):5233–5239. doi:10.1200/JCO.2008.16.5449
4. Copelan EA. Hematopoietic stem-cell transplantation. *N Engl J Med*. 2006;354(17):1813–1826. doi:10.1056/NEJMra052638
5. Topalian SL, Sznol M, McDermott DF, et al. Survival, durable tumor remission, and long-term safety in patients with advanced melanoma receiving nivolumab. *J Clin Oncol*. 2014;32(10):1020–1030. doi:10.1200/JCO.2013.53.0105
6. Brahmer JR, Tykodi SS, Chow LQM, et al. Safety and activity of anti-PD-L1 antibody in patients with advanced cancer. *N Engl J Med*. 2012;366(26):2455–2465. doi:10.1056/NEJMoa1200694
7. Herbst RS, Baas P, Kim DW, et al. Pembrolizumab versus docetaxel for previously treated, PD-L1-positive, advanced non-small-cell lung cancer (KEYNOTE-010): a randomised controlled trial. *Lancet*. 2016;387(10027):1540–1550. doi:10.1016/S0140-6736(15)01281-7
8. Turtle CJ, Hanafi LA, Berger C, et al. CD19 CAR-T cells of defined CD4+:CD8+ composition in adult B cell ALL patients. *J Clin Invest*. 2016;126(6):2123–2138. doi:10.1172/JCI85309
9. Pollack SM, Ingham M, Spraker MB, Schwartz GK. Emerging targeted and immune-based therapies in sarcoma. *J Clin Oncol*. 2018;36(2):125–135. doi:10.1200/JCO.2017.75.1610
10. Tawbi HA, Burgess M, Bolejack V. Pembrolizumab in advanced soft-tissue sarcoma and bone sarcoma (SARC028): a multicentre, two-cohort, single-arm, open-label, phase 2 trial. *Lancet Oncol*. 2017;18:1493–1501. doi:10.1016/S1470-2045(17)30624-1
11. Ben-Ami E, Barysauskas CM, Solomon S, et al. Immunotherapy with single agent nivolumab for advanced leiomyosarcoma of the uterus: results of a phase 2 study. *Cancer*. 2017;123(17):3285–3290. doi:10.1002/cncr.30738
12. George S, Miao D, Demetri GD, et al. Loss of PTEN is associated with resistance to anti-PD-1 checkpoint blockade therapy in metastatic uterine leiomyosarcoma. *Immunity*. 2017;46(2):197–204. doi:10.1016/j.immuni.2017.02.001
13. Nghiem P, Bhatia S, Lipson EJ, et al. Durable tumor regression and overall survival in patients with advanced Merkel cell carcinoma receiving pembrolizumab as first-line therapy. *J Clin Oncol*. 2019;37(9):693–702. doi:10.1200/JCO.18.01896
14. Wilky BA, Trucco MM, Subhawong TK, et al. Axitinib plus pembrolizumab in patients with advanced sarcomas including alveolar soft-part sarcoma: a single-centre, single-arm, phase 2 trial. *Lancet Oncol*. 2019;20(6):837–848. doi:10.1016/S1470-2045(19)30153-6
15. Weber JS, Kudchadkar RR, Yu B, et al. Safety, efficacy, and biomarkers of nivolumab with vaccine in ipilimumab-refractory or -naive melanoma. *J Clin Oncol*. 2013;31(34):4311–4318. doi:10.1200/JCO.2013.51.4802

16. Maki RG, Jungbluth AA, Gnjatic S, et al. A pilot study of anti-CTLA4 antibody ipilimumab in patients with synovial sarcoma. *Sarcoma*. 2013;2013:168145. doi:10.1155/2013/168145
17. D'Angelo SP, Larkin J, Sosman JA, et al. Efficacy and safety of nivolumab alone or in combination with ipilimumab in patients with mucosal melanoma: a pooled analysis. *J Clin Oncol*. 2017;35(2):226–235. doi:10.1200/JCO.2016.67.9258
18. Hammers HJ, Plimack ER, Infante JR, et al. Phase I study of nivolumab in combination with ipilimumab in metastatic renal cell carcinoma (mRCC). *J Clin Oncol*. 2014;32:4504. doi:10.1200/jco.2014.32.15_suppl.4504
19. Wolchok JD, Kluger H, Callahan MK, et al. Nivolumab plus ipilimumab in advanced melanoma. *N Engl J Med*. 2013;369(2):122–133. doi:10.1056/NEJMoa1302369
20. Hellmann MD, Rizvi NA, Goldman JW, et al. Nivolumab plus ipilimumab as first-line treatment for advanced non-small-cell lung cancer (CheckMate 012): results of an open-label, phase 1, multicohort study. *Lancet Oncol*. 2017;18(1):31–41. doi:10.1016/S1470-2045(16)30624-6
21. D'Angelo SP, Mahoney MR, Van Tine BA, et al. Nivolumab with or without ipilimumab treatment for metastatic sarcoma (Alliance A091401): two open-label, non-comparative, randomised, phase 2 trials. *Lancet Oncol*. 2018;19(3):416–426. doi:10.1016/S1470-2045(18)30006-8
22. Pollack S, Redman MW, Wagner M, et al. A phase I/II study of pembrolizumab (Pem) and doxorubicin (Dox) in treating patients with metastatic/unresectable sarcoma. *J Clin Oncol*. 2019;37:11009. doi:10.1200/JCO.2019.37.15_suppl.11009
23. Toulmonde M, Penel N, Adam J, et al. Use of PD-1 targeting, macrophage infiltration, and IDO pathway activation in sarcomas: a phase 2 clinical trial. *JAMA Oncol*. 2018;4(1):93–97. doi:10.1001/jamaoncol.2017.1617
24. Curti BD, Kovacsovics-Bankowski M, Morris N, et al. OX40 is a potent immune-stimulating target in late-stage cancer patients. *Cancer Res*. 2013;73(24):7189–7198. doi:10.1158/0008-5472.CAN-12-4174
25. Mahne AE, Mauze S, Joyce-Shaikh B, et al. Dual roles for regulatory T-cell depletion and costimulatory signaling in agonistic GITR targeting for tumor immunotherapy. *Cancer Res*. 2017;77(5):1108–1118. doi:10.1158/0008-5472.CAN-16-0797
26. Zamarin D, Holmgaard RB, Ricca J, et al. Intratumoral modulation of the inducible co-stimulator ICOS by recombinant oncolytic virus promotes systemic anti-tumour immunity. *Nat Commun*. 2017;8:14340. doi:10.1038/ncomms14340
27. Seaman S, Zhu Z, Saha S, et al. Eradication of tumors through simultaneous ablation of CD276/B7-H3-positive tumor cells and tumor vasculature. *Cancer Cell*. 2017;31(4):501.e8–515.e8. doi:10.1016/j.ccell.2017.03.005
28. Théoleyre S, Mori K, Cherrier B, et al. Phenotypic and functional analysis of lymphocytes infiltrating osteolytic tumors: use as a possible therapeutic approach of osteosarcoma. *BMC Cancer*. 2005;5:123. doi:10.1186/1471-2407-5-123
29. Mesiano G, Leuci V, Giraudo L, et al. Adoptive immunotherapy against sarcomas. *Expert Opin Biol Ther*. 2015;15(4):517–528. doi:10.1517/14712598.2015.987121
30. Zhu H, Gu S, Yin M, et al. Analysis of infantile fibrosarcoma reveals extensive T-cell responses within tumors: Implications for immunotherapy. *Pediatr Blood Cancer*. 2018;65:e26813. doi:10.1002/pbc.26813
31. Scanlan MJ, Simpson AJ, Old LJ. The cancer/testis genes: review, standardization, and commentary. *Cancer Immun*. 2004;4:1–15. http://www.cancerimmunity.org/v4p1/031220.htm
32. Szender JB, Papanicolau-Sengos A, Eng KH, et al. NY-ESO-1 expression predicts an aggressive phenotype of ovarian cancer. *Gynecol Oncol*. 2017;145(3):420–425. doi:10.1016/j.ygyno.2017.03.509
33. Iura K, Kohashi K, Hotokebuchi Y, et al. Cancer-testis antigens PRAME and NY-ESO-1 correlate with tumour grade and poor prognosis in myxoid liposarcoma. *J Pathol Clin Res*. 2015;1(3):144–159. doi:10.1002/cjp2.16
34. Jungbluth AA, Antonescu CR, Busam KJ, et al. Monophasic and biphasic synovial sarcomas abundantly express cancer/testis antigen NY-ESO-1 but not MAGE-A1 or CT7. *Int J Cancer*. 2001;94(2):252–256. doi:10.1002/ijc.1451
35. Pollack SM, Jungbluth AA, Hoch BL, et al. NY-ESO-1 is a ubiquitous immunotherapeutic target antigen for patients with myxoid/round cell liposarcoma. *Cancer*. 2012;118(18):4564–4570. doi:10.1002/cncr.27446
36. Pollack SM, Jones RL, Farrar EA, et al. Tetramer guided, cell sorter assisted production of clinical grade autologous NY-ESO-1 specific CD8(+) T cells. *J Immunother Cancer*. 2014;2(1):36. doi:10.1186/s40425-014-0036-y
37. Robbins PF, Kassim SH, Tran TL, et al. A pilot trial using lymphocytes genetically engineered with an NY-ESO-1-reactive T cell receptor: long term follow up and correlates with response. *Clin Cancer Res*. 2015;21(5):1019–1027. doi:10.1158/1078-0432.CCR-14-2708
38. Robbins PF, Morgan RA, Feldman SA, et al. Tumor regression in patients with metastatic synovial cell sarcoma and melanoma using genetically engineered lymphocytes reactive with NY-ESO-1. *J Clin Oncol*. 2011;29(7):917–924. doi:10.1200/JCO.2010.32.2537
39. Robbins PF, Kassim SH, Tran TLN, et al. A pilot trial using lymphocytes genetically engineered with an NY-ESO-1-reactive T-cell receptor: long-term follow-up and correlates with response. *Clin Cancer Res*. 2015;21(5):1019–1027. doi:10.1158/1078-0432.CCR-14-2708
40. D'Angelo SP, Melchiori L, Merchant MS, et al. Antitumor activity associated with prolonged persistence of adoptively transferred NY-ESO-1 T cells in synovial sarcoma. *Cancer Discov*. 2018;8(8):944–957. doi:10.1158/2159-8290.CD-17-1417
41. Nowicki TS, Berent-Maoz B, Cheung-Lau G, et al. A pilot trial of the combination of transgenic NY-ESO-1-reactive adoptive cellular therapy with dendritic cell vaccination with or without ipilimumab. *Clin Cancer Res*. 2019;25(7):2096–2108. doi:10.1158/1078-0432.CCR-18-3496

42. Hong DS, Butler MO, Johnson M, et al. Initial safety assessment of MAGE-A4 SPEAR T-cells. *Ann Oncol*. 2018;29:viii412. doi:10.1093/annonc/mdy288.029
43. Brentjens RJ, Davila ML, Riviere I, et al. CD19-targeted T cells rapidly induce molecular remissions in adults with chemotherapy-refractory acute lymphoblastic leukemia. *Sci Transl Med*. 2013;5(177):177ra38. doi:10.1126/scitranslmed.3005930
44. Ahmed N, Brawley VS, Hegde M, et al. Human epidermal growth factor receptor 2 (HER2)-specific chimeric antigen receptor-modified T cells for the immunotherapy of HER2-positive sarcoma. *J Clin Oncol*. 2015;33(15):1688–1696. doi:10.1200/JCO.2014.58.0225
45. Mata M, Gerken C, Nguyen P, et al. Inducible activation of MyD88 and CD40 in CAR T cells results in controllable and potent antitumor activity in preclinical solid tumor models. *Cancer Discov*. 2017;7(11):1306–1319. doi:10.1158/2159-8290.CD-17-0263
46. Majzner RG, Theruvath JL, Nellan A, et al. CAR T cells targeting B7-H3, a pan-cancer antigen, demonstrate potent preclinical activity against pediatric solid tumors and brain tumors. *Clin Cancer Res*. 2019;25(8):2560–2574. doi:10.1158/1078-0432.CCR-18-0432
47. Bertucci F, Finetti P, Perrot D, et al. PDL1 expression is a poor-prognosis factor in soft-tissue sarcomas. *Oncoimmunology*. 2017;6:e1278100. doi:10.1080/2162402X.2016.1278100
48. Pollack SM, He Q, Yearley JH, et al. T-cell infiltration and clonality correlate with programmed cell death protein 1 and programmed death-ligand 1 expression in patients with soft tissue sarcomas. *Cancer*. 2017;123(17):3291–3304. doi:10.1002/cncr.30726
49. Ni L, Lu J. Interferon gamma in cancer immunotherapy. *Cancer Med*. 2018;7(9):4509–4516. doi:10.1002/cam4.1700
50. Lee CH, Espinosa I, Vrijaldenhoven S, et al. Prognostic significance of macrophage infiltration in leiomyosarcomas. *Clin Cancer Res*. 2008;14(5):1423–1430. doi:10.1158/1078-0432.CCR-07-1712
51. Espinosa I, Beck AH, Lee CH, et al. Coordinate expression of colony-stimulating factor-1 and colony-stimulating factor-1-related proteins is associated with poor prognosis in gynecological and nongynecological leiomyosarcoma. *Am J Pathol*. 2009;174(6):2347–2356. doi:10.2353/ajpath.2009.081037
52. Ganjoo KN, Witten D, Patel M, et al. The prognostic value of tumor-associated macrophages in leiomyosarcoma: a single institution study. *Am J Clin Oncol*. 2011;34(1):82–86. doi:10.1097/coc.0b013e3181d26d5e
53. Nabeshima A, Matsumoto Y, Fukushi J, et al. Tumour-associated macrophages correlate with poor prognosis in myxoid liposarcoma and promote cell motility and invasion via the HB-EGF-EGFR-PI3K/Akt pathways. *Br J Cancer*. 2015;112(3):547–555. doi:10.1038/bjc.2014.637
54. Fujiwara T, Fukushi JI, Yamamoto S, et al. Macrophage infiltration predicts a poor prognosis for human Ewing sarcoma. *Am J Pathol*. 2011;179(3):1157–1170. doi:10.1016/j.ajpath.2011.05.034
55. Biswas SK, Mantovani A. Macrophage plasticity and interaction with lymphocyte subsets: cancer as a paradigm. *Nat Immunol*. 2010;11(10):889–896. doi:10.1038/ni.1937
56. Tap WD, Gelderblom H, Palmerini E, et al. Pexidartinib versus placebo for advanced tenosynovial giant cell tumour (ENLIVEN): a randomised phase 3 trial. *Lancet*. 2019;394(10197):478–487. doi:10.1016/S0140-6736(19)30764-0
57. Patwardhan PP, Surriga O, Beckman MJ, et al. Sustained inhibition of receptor tyrosine kinases and macrophage depletion by PLX3397 and rapamycin as a potential new approach for the treatment of MPNSTs. *Clin Cancer Res*. 2014;20(12):3146–3158. doi:10.1158/1078-0432.CCR-13-2576
58. Liu J, Wang L, Zhao F, et al. Pre-clinical development of a humanized anti-CD47 antibody with anti-cancer therapeutic potential. *PLoS One*. 2015;10:e0137345. doi:10.1371/journal.pone.0137345
59. Germano G, Frapolli R, Simone M, et al. Antitumor and anti-inflammatory effects of trabectedin on human myxoid liposarcoma cells. *Cancer Res*. 2010;70(6):2235–2244. doi:10.1158/0008-5472.CAN-09-2335
60. Germano G, Frapolli R, Belgiovine C, et al. Role of macrophage targeting in the antitumor activity of trabectedin. *Cancer Cell*. 2013;23(2):249–262. doi:10.1016/j.ccr.2013.01.008
61. Seo YD, Zhou J, Morse K, et al. Effect of intratumoral (IT) injection of the toll-like receptor 4 (TLR4) agonist G100 on a clinical response and CD4 T-cell response locally and systemically. *J Clin Oncol*. 2018;36:71–71. doi:10.1200/JCO.2018.36.5_suppl.71
62. Fukuhara H, Ino Y, Todo T. Oncolytic virus therapy: a new era of cancer treatment at dawn. *Cancer Sci*. 2016;107(10):1373–1379. doi:10.1111/cas.13027
63. Lang FF, Conrad C, Gomez-Manzano C, et al. Phase I study of DNX-2401 (Delta-24-RGD) oncolytic adenovirus: replication and immunotherapeutic effects in recurrent malignant glioma. *J Clin Oncol*. 2018;36(14):1419–1427. doi:10.1200/JCO.2017.75.8219
64. Hardcastle J, Mills L, Malo CS, et al. Immunovirotherapy with measles virus strains in combination with anti-PD-1 antibody blockade enhances antitumor activity in glioblastoma treatment. *Neuro Oncol*. 2017;19(4):493–502. doi:10.1093/neuonc/now179
65. Chesney J, Puzanov I, Collichio F, et al. Randomized, open-label phase II study evaluating the efficacy and safety of talimogene laherparepvec in combination with ipilimumab versus ipilimumab alone in patients with advanced, unresectable melanoma. *J Clin Oncol*. 2018;36(17):1658–1667. doi:10.1200/JCO.2017.73.7379
66. Dummer R, Hoeller C, Gruter IP, Michielin O. Combining talimogene laherparepvec with immunotherapies in melanoma and other solid tumors. *Cancer Immunol Immunother*. 2017;66(6):683–695. doi:10.1007/s00262-017-1967-1

67. Kelly CM, Bowler TG, Munhoz RR, et al. A phase II study of talimogene laherparepvec (T-VEC) and pembrolizumab in patients with metastatic sarcoma. *J Clin Oncol*. 2018;36:11516–11516. doi:10.1200/JCO.2018.36.15_suppl.11516
68. Hoffmann D, Heim A, Nettelbeck DM, et al. Evaluation of twenty human adenoviral types and one infectivity-enhanced adenovirus for the therapy of soft tissue sarcoma. *Hum Gene Ther*. 2007;18(1):51–62. doi:10.1089/hum.2006.132
69. Berchtold S, Lampe J, Weiland T, et al. Innate immune defense defines susceptibility of sarcoma cells to measles vaccine virus-based oncolysis. *J Virol*. 2013;87(6):3484–3501. doi:10.1128/JVI.02106-12
70. Deyle DR, Escobar DZ, Peng KW, Babovic-Vuksanovic D. Oncolytic measles virus as a novel therapy for malignant peripheral nerve sheath tumors. *Gene*. 2015;565(1):140–145. doi:10.1016/j.gene.2015.04.001
71. Charych DH, Hoch U, Langowski JL, et al. NKTR-214, an engineered cytokine with biased IL2 receptor binding, increased tumor exposure, and marked efficacy in mouse tumor models. *Clin Cancer Res*. 2016;22(3):680–690. doi:10.1158/1078-0432.CCR-15-1631
72. Hu Q, Ye X, Qu X, et al. Discovery of a novel IL-15 based protein with improved developability and efficacy for cancer immunotherapy. *Sci Rep*. 2018;8:7675. doi:10.1038/s41598-018-25987-4
73. Zhao Q, Hu J, Mitra A, et al. Tumor-targeted IL-12 combined with tumor resection yields a survival-favorable immune profile. *J Immunother Cancer*. 2019;7:154. doi:10.1186/s40425-019-0631-z
74. Chapman PB, Morrisey D, Panageas KS, et al. Vaccination with a bivalent G_{M2} and G_{D2} ganglioside conjugate vaccine: a trial comparing doses of G_{D2}-keyhole limpet hemocyanin. *Clin Cancer Res*. 2000;6(12):4658–4662. https://clincancerres.aacrjournals.org/content/6/12/4658
75. Kawaguchi S, Tsukahara T, Ida K, et al. SYT-SSX breakpoint peptide vaccines in patients with synovial sarcoma: a study from the Japanese Musculoskeletal Oncology Group. *Cancer Sci*. 2012;103(9):1625–1630. doi:10.1111/j.1349-7006.2012.02370.x
76. Maraskovsky E, Sjölander S, Drane DP, et al. NY-ESO-1 protein formulated in ISCOMATRIX adjuvant is a potent anticancer vaccine inducing both humoral and CD8+ t-cell-mediated immunity and protection against NY-ESO-1+ tumors. *Clin Cancer Res*. 2004;10(8):2879–2890. doi:10.1158/1078-0432.ccr-03-0245
77. Yang L, Yang H, Rideout K, et al. Engineered lentivector targeting of dendritic cells for in vivo immunization. *Nat Biotechnol*. 2008;26(3):326–334. doi:10.1038/nbt1390
78. Tareen SU, Kelley-Clarke B, Nicolai CJ, et al. Design of a novel integration-deficient lentivector technology that incorporates genetic and posttranslational elements to target human dendritic cells. *Mol Ther*. 2014;22(3):575–587. doi:10.1038/mt.2013.278
79. Pollack SM, Lu H, Gnjatic S, et al. First-in-human treatment with a dendritic cell-targeting lentiviral vector-expressing NY-ESO-1, LV305, induces deep, durable response in refractory metastatic synovial sarcoma patient. *J Immunother*. 2017;40(8):302–306. doi:10.1097/CJI.0000000000000183
80. Odegard JM, Flynn PA, Campbell DJ, et al. A novel HSV-2 subunit vaccine induces GLA-dependent CD4 and CD8 T cell responses and protective immunity in mice and guinea pigs. *Vaccine*. 2016;34(1):101–109. doi:10.1016/j.vaccine.2015.10.137
81. Albershardt TC, Campbell DJ, Parsons AJ, et al. LV305, a dendritic cell-targeting integration-deficient ZVex(TM)-based lentiviral vector encoding NY-ESO-1, induces potent anti-tumor immune response. *Mol Ther Oncolytics*. 2016;3:16010. doi:10.1038/mto.2016.10
82. Pollack S, Lu H, Somaiah N, et al. Association of CMB305 or LV305-induced and baseline anti-NY-ESO-1 immunity is associated with survival in recurrent cancer patients. *J Clin Oncol*. 2017;35:3090. doi:10.1200/JCO.2017.35.15_suppl.3090
83. Wagner AJ, Banerji U, Mahipal A, et al. Phase I trial of the human double minute 2 inhibitor MK-8242 in patients with advanced solid tumors. *J Clin Oncol*. 2017;35(12):1304–1311. doi:10.1200/JCO.2016.70.7117
84. Pollack SM. The potential of the CMB305 vaccine regimen to target NY-ESO-1 and improve outcomes for synovial sarcoma and myxoid/round cell liposarcoma patients. *Expert Rev Vaccines*. 2018;17(2):107–114. doi:10.1080/14760584.2018.1419068
85. Dhodapkar MV, Sznol M, Zhao B, et al. Induction of antigen-specific immunity with a vaccine targeting NY-ESO-1 to the dendritic cell receptor DEC-205. *Sci Transl Med*. 2014;6(232):232ra51. doi:10.1126/scitranslmed.3008068
86. Goldberg JM, Fisher DE, Demetri GD, et al. Biologic activity of autologous, granulocyte-macrophage colony-stimulating factor secreting alveolar soft-part sarcoma and clear cell sarcoma vaccines. *Clin Cancer Res*. 2015;21(14):3178–3186. doi:10.1158/1078-0432.CCR-14-2932
87. Himoudi N, Wallace R, Parsley KL, et al. Lack of T-cell responses following autologous tumour lysate pulsed dendritic cell vaccination, in patients with relapsed osteosarcoma. *Clin Transl Oncol*. 2012;14(4):271–279. doi:10.1007/s12094-012-0795-1
88. Mahvi DM, Shi FS, Yang NS, et al. Immunization by particle-mediated transfer of the granulocyte-macrophage colony-stimulating factor gene into autologous tumor cells in melanoma or sarcoma patients: report of a phase I/IB study. *Hum Gene Ther*. 2002;13(14):1711–1721. doi:10.1089/104303402760293556
89. Ghisoli M, Rutledge M, Stephens PJ, et al. Case report: immune-mediated complete response in a patient with recurrent advanced Ewing sarcoma (EWS) after vigil immunotherapy. *J Pediatr Hematol Oncol*. 2017;39(4):e183–e186. doi:10.1097/MPH.0000000000000822

29

Cellular Therapy

John C. Hardaway and Steven C. Katz

INTRODUCTION

Nature often gives us hints to her profoundest secrets.[1]

—William B. Coley, Memorial-Sloan Kettering surgeon and immunotherapy pioneer

Given the increasingly prominent role of immunotherapy, clinicians must learn the intricacies of emerging cellular immunotherapies for solid tumors. For solid tumors, progress has been limited, consequent to a unique set of challenges imposed by the tumor microenvironment and the technical challenges of delivering cells into tumors. Sarcomas are certainly challenging with respect to these factors, in addition to complexity imposed by extreme biologic heterogeneity across a myriad of subtypes. These caveats result in some tumor types being more amenable to immunotherapeutic approaches than others.

This chapter begins with an overview of the history and development of cellular therapy, which notably originated in transplantation and has experienced early success in treatment of hematopoietic malignancies. Following introduction of key molecular and immunologic underpinnings, challenges currently limiting the field will be considered, in addition to the unique set of complications and adverse events that are imposed. Throughout the chapter, more recent and modest attempts at applying these therapies toward treating sarcoma will be contextually incorporated.

CELLULAR IMMUNOTHERAPY: HISTORICAL BACKGROUND AND PRINCIPLES

Historical Background

It has been more than a century since William B. Coley boldly repurposed live cultures of *Streptococcus pyogenes* and *Serratia marcescens* for the treatment of soft tissue sarcoma (STS) and bone sarcoma patients—a strategy that would later employ heat-killed strains in a process known as "mixed bacterial vaccination."[2] Despite the profound insight gleaned by Coley, only recently has immunotherapy gained broad acceptance as an integral component of multidisciplinary cancer care. Indeed, the term "Coley's toxins" was far from a term of endearment, a label applied by his many fierce critics based on the treatment's associated toxicities. Thankfully, with the establishment of several key immunologic principles, the wisdom and rationale of using cellular products to stimulate an immune response is now better understood.

While Coley's approach aimed to stimulate, or otherwise induce an anticancer immune response through vaccination, much of modern-day cell therapy focuses on isolating, expanding, or manipulating immune cell products that have tumor killing capacity. Early efforts centered around isolation of tumor reactive T cells from patients and then reinfusion following stimulation and expansion. Presently, our group and others use genetically engineered cell therapy products to engender tumor antigen recognition through T-cell receptor, antibody, or natural receptor/ligand-based systems. Previously, these approaches were limited in their feasibility and scalability, but now these products are readily manufactured.

To date, much of the success with cellular immunotherapy for cancer has been realized with leukemia and lymphoma, commonly referred to as "liquid tumors."[3] Progress with solid tumors, such as STS, has been more difficult, save some notable clinical results in melanoma patients.[4] Promising clinical programs are underway for synovial cell sarcoma, but there are no effective immunotherapies for the majority STS subtypes.[5,6] Success for solid tumors will require a more comprehensive approach to account for immunosuppressive tumor microenvironments and delivery issues.[7,8]

Clinical Adaptation and Classes of Cellular Immunotherapies

Cellular immunotherapy arose from a series of cumulative advances in genetic and molecular engineering, which synergized with parallel advances in cell and tissue culture technique. While working in the field of transplant tolerance in the 1950s, Mitchison made the seminal observation that the cellular arm of the immune system is responsible for tissue rejection.[9] When Billingham, Brent, and Medawar transferred cellular material to fetuses in utero, seeking to induce a state of "actively-acquired tolerance," they performed the first adoptive cellular transfer (ACT) and provided a delivery platform that could be exploited for a panoply of future cellular immunotherapies.[10]

Other major discoveries that contributed to the modern-day manifestation of cellular therapies included the theory of clonal selection and the technique of hybridoma formation for the generation of monoclonal antibodies.[11] The theory of clonal selection solidified the concept that the immune system is composed of distinct functional cell populations and provided irrefutable evidence of the clonality of adaptive immune cells. Meanwhile, monoclonal antibodies provided an armamentarium of specific investigative probes that facilitated the identification of novel molecules and subsequent knowledge of immune signaling pathways. While details of these discoveries are outside the scope of this text, their collective influence undoubtedly shaped the evolution of cellular immunotherapies and the availability of monoclonal antibodies enabled the development of chimeric antigen receptor T cell (CAR-T) products (see later discussion of CAR-T).

Lymphokine-Activated Killer Cells

In a key technological advance, the Gallo Laboratory of Tumor Cell Biology at the National Cancer Institute (NCI) in Bethesda, Maryland, published reliable methodology for in vitro culture of T lymphocytes isolated from human bone marrow.[12] Shortly after the identification, cloning and recombinant expression of interleukin 2 (IL-2), also known as T-cell growth factor, allowed for selection and expansion of tumor-specific lymphocytes for therapeutic purposes.[13–15] One of the first applications of ACT against cancer involved the transfer of lymphokine-activated killer (LAK) cells, which are bulk, heterogeneous, nonspecific autologous lymphocytes cultured in recombinant IL-2.[16] In a preclinical model of metastatic sarcoma, LAKs were significantly more effective at reducing the number of pulmonary micrometastases than were splenocytes or IL-2 alone.[17] A subsequent NCI clinical trial examined the therapeutic response to LAK cells with supplemental IL-2 infusions against a variety of human cancers, including melanoma, renal cell carcinoma, and four sarcoma subtypes—osteosarcoma, neurofibrosarcoma, synovial cell sarcoma, and undifferentiated pleomorphic sarcoma—with objective clinical responses observed in 11 of 25 patients, though none with sarcoma responded. The therapeutic utility of LAK cells was short-lived, however, as a subsequent study in a larger cohort of 181 melanoma and renal cell carcinoma patients compared LAK + IL-2 with IL-2 alone, with no significant benefit seen in patients who received LAK cells.[18]

Tumor-Infiltrating Lymphocytes

Given that LAK therapy involved ACT of nonspecific lymphocytes without defined tumor reactivity, the next iteration of cellular therapies focused on isolation and expansion of tumor-infiltrating lymphocytes (TILs) from surgically resected tumor specimens. Contemporary TIL manufacturing generally involves tumor excision, culturing of tumor fragments supplemented with IL-2, and screening cells for tumor recognition prior to expansion.[19] Production of TILs requires a resectable tumor specimen and the presence of infiltrating lymphocytes that can be selected on the basis of their avidity for a tumor-associated antigen (TAA).[20] TIL can alternatively be expanded in bulk using anti-CD3/CD28, without the use of TAA, which offers a conceptual advantage over genetically engineered strategies that require a designated TAA. Further, since TILs occur naturally and have matured through the process of thymic selection, there is no concern with off-target tissue damage, which is a concern with other forms of cellular therapy.[21] Frequency of TILs does vary by tumor type, as evidenced by Balch et al, who prepared single-cell suspensions from 120 human tumor specimens and quantified the percentage of TILs among tumor cells.[22] Renal cell carcinoma had more TILs (65%) than tumor cells (35%), while melanoma had 30% to 35% TILs, and sarcoma had 36% TILs.[22]

The Rosenberg group from the NCI Surgery Branch were among the first to publish the effectiveness of TIL-based ACT in a mouse model of metastatic sarcoma that uses intravenously injected MCA-105 cells.[23] In this model, TILs cleared pulmonary micrometastases and were 50 to 100 times more potent on a cell-by-cell basis as compared to LAK cells, but were unable to eradicate larger, more established metastases. To promote in vivo expansion of TILs, preconditioning treatment with cyclophosphamide was incorporated to lymphodeplete the host prior to ACT, which resulted in curing 50% of mice with advanced sarcoma pulmonary metastases with a median survival time (MST) of 84 days, as compared to 0% cure and MST of 21 days among untreated mice.

Based on these preclinical findings, an NCI-sponsored clinical trial was similarly designed and conducted to examine therapeutic efficacy of TILs in patients with metastatic melanoma who were preconditioned with cyclophophamide.[24] Eleven out of 20 subjects demonstrated an objective response with greater than 50% reduction in tumor burden, and one patient had a complete response (CR), though the durability of response was variable (range 2–13 months). This study also highlighted the difficulty using TILs in the clinical setting, as there were 17 additional enrolled patients who were intended for TIL ACT, but did not receive treatment owing to disease progression during treatment preparation. While the duration of TIL expansion ranged from 24 to 56 days among the 20 patients who received TIL, the inability or delay in culturing TIL for the remaining patients underscores the need for efficient cellular manufacturing processes. This remains an ongoing challenge in the field and has implications for more advanced technologies including autologous CAR-T cell platforms. A shift toward allogeneic, "off the shelf," products has been advocated by some groups as a possible solution to progression during the production period.

In summary, the genesis and early development of TIL ACT was primarily conducted at the NCI over the past three decades. Multiple Phase 1 and 2 trials were conducted to treat metastatic melanoma, in which objective remission rates of 49% to 72%, that is, complete and partial responses, were observed. Two separate publications provide an overview of the TIL experience at the NCI, spanning the periods from 1989 to 1993 and from 2002 to 2007.[20,25] Improvements in the ability to culture TIL from tumor specimens are noted, with 60% of tumor specimens yielding TIL in the 1989 to 1993 cohort as compared to 94% from 2002 to 2007. Interestingly, extranodal tumor specimens had greater cytolytic activity in the older data set, while TILs were more easily cultured from lymph node specimens in the recent data set. TILs isolated from metastatic melanoma tumor deposits in gastrointestinal tissue were less likely to yield functional therapeutic TILs, whereas pulmonary and lymph node metastases were generally more successful. These series suggest that greater functional heterogeneity exists among TILs with respect to their tissue of origin and that further methodologic refinements may exist to improve their therapeutic utility.

Preconditioning Lymphodepletion Regimens

The majority of cell-based therapy protocols involve a preconditioning regimen intended to eliminate suppressive immune cells and create a cytokine milieu that will expand and stimulate adoptively transferred cells. Endogenous T regulatory (Treg) cells were thought to significantly influence local cytokine concentrations in the tumor microenvironment (TME) by acting as "IL-2 sinks" or by inhibiting adoptively transferred TILs through direct cell-cell contact mechanisms. Preclinical models had demonstrated a correlation between the extent of pre-ACT lymphodepletion and clinical response.[26] Thus, to improve the objective response rate in humans and to further mitigate the contributions by endogenous Treg cells, investigators incorporated total-body irradiation (TBI) and cytotoxic agents to preconditioning regimens. Compared to a 49% response rate seen with cyclophosphamide and fludarabine preconditioning, addition of TBI, at a dose of 2 or 12 Gy, increased response rates to 52% and 72%, respectively, in metastatic melanoma patients.[27] Aggressive preconditioning regimens have been associated with increased serum concentrations of IL-7 and IL-15, which are integral to lymphocyte homeostasis and also promote engraftment. Unfortunately, preconditioning regimens may also increase the likelihood of uncontrolled cell therapy activity, which may lead to severe cytokine release syndrome (CRS) and neurotoxic manifestations, both of which will be addressed below. We have adopted a multidose regional infusion strategy to avoid such complications and provide a more controllable cell therapy clinical treatment platform (NCT01373047, NCT02416466, NCT02850536, NCT03682744).[28,29] However, the need for preconditioning will likely vary with the nature of the cell therapy product, disease burden, and clinical indication.

Characteristics of Effective TIL

Seeking to identify histopathologic correlates of effective TILs, the number of TILs in resected colorectal and ovarian tumors were examined with respect to clinical outcomes, where patients with a higher frequency of T helper type 1 (Th1) TILs demonstrated a survival advantage.[30] Th1 cells are activated and differentiated $CD4^+$ T helper cells, which characteristically secrete cytokines, such as interferon-γ (IFN-γ) and IL-2 to promote cell-mediated antitumor responses. Additional phenotypic characteristics of TILs, such as telomere length and expression of the costimulatory molecule, CD28, correlate with objective clinical responses and TIL persistence/engraftment following TIL ACT.[31] Defining an ideal TIL phenotype for broad application in solid tumors will be challenging, given the vast biologic heterogeneity among patients, and even further among each patient's varied metastatic tumor deposits.

TIL Approaches in Sarcoma

The application of TIL ACT for the treatment of sarcoma has been limited, partly because of the difficulty posed by the existence of more than 50 histologic subtypes with a broad range of biologic features.[32,33] In one sample of 249 STSs containing at least eight histologic subtypes, only 15% of patients had high-frequency CD8+ TILs.[34] Yet, in another study of more common STS subtypes, such as well-differentiated liposarcoma, a substantial number of CD3, CD4, and CD8 lymphocytes were observed.[35] To potentially improve lymphocyte frequency within sarcoma specimens prior to TIL production, a Phase 2 trial for patients with advanced/metastatic STS opened in October 2018 and is designed to evaluate the safety and efficacy of an oncolytic peptide injection (LTX-315), which is hypothesized to induce T-cell infiltration prior to tumor resection (NCT03725605). The study is projected to complete enrollment in February 2023.

TIL Summary

TIL-based ACT has shown objective response rates of approximately 40% in patients with metastatic melanoma, even among those who have failed checkpoint inhibitor therapy.[36] However, widespread adoption of this approach has been impeded by the technical difficulties in generating TILs from all patients, the amount of time required to expand TILs, and the toxicities associated with harsh preconditioning regimens. As will be discussed in the next section, T-cell receptor (TCR) or chimeric antigen receptor (CAR) engineered strategies offer alternative cellular therapies for patients whose tumors are not suitable for TIL isolation and production. Furthermore, advanced cell therapy products have shown more promise for sarcoma patients as compared to TIL therapy.

Chimeric Antigen Receptor T Cells (CAR-T)

Introduction

Over the past decade, the introduction of CAR-T has led to meaningful improvements in outcomes for patients, largely for those with hematopoietic malignancies. These "liquid tumors" are readily treated by systemic infusion of CAR-T, but treatment of solid tumors, such as skeletal and soft tissue sarcomas, is hampered by delivery and trafficking challenges inherent to an organized tumor mass. Barriers to delivering CAR-T to solid tumors include aberrant vasculature, migration through dense stroma, and an elevated interstitial fluid pressure (IFP). Furthermore, systemic CAR-T infusions are associated with severe CRS, among other toxicities including on-target/off-tumor effects. Herein, the cellular and molecular principles behind CAR-T immunotherapy, the current limitations of CAR-T treatment for solid tumors, and recent progress in clinical trials using CAR-T to treat sarcoma will be reviewed.

Evolution of CAR Therapy

Reliable production of highly specific cellular therapeutics has become possible because of advances in genetic engineering of autologous T cells. In 1987, the first immunoglobulin T-cell receptor (IgTCR) fusion proteins were created by Kuwana et al.[37] In contrast to TILs, these novel CARs allow production of antigen-specific T cells without isolation from patient tumor samples. Advancement in understanding the TCR signaling apparatus, whereby the TCR CD3 complex was identified as the conduit to T-cell activation, prompted development of the first-generation CAR, where CD3-ζ replaced the α and β TCR chains of the IgTCR (Figure 29.1). Further advances led to the inclusion of costimulatory molecules such as CD28 and 4–1BB in second-generation CAR to enhance activation and persistence in vivo.

CAR platforms have the advantage of enabling products to exploit a major histocompatibility complex (MHC)-independent means of antigen-specific activation, thereby enabling its use in any patient with tumors that express the relevant antigen. Other investigators transduced autologous T cells with high-affinity, tumor-specific TCRs, which are MHC-dependent and require HLA haplotype matching between the TCR clone and the patient to avoid the issue of graft–host histocompatibility. One significant advantage of TCR and TIL approaches is that intracellular antigens, presented by MHC, can be targeted. CAR-T, on the other hand, are capable of binding only to tumor antigens expressed on the cell surface.

CAR Construct Design and Delivery

CAR constructs are composed of an ectodomain, a transmembrane domain, and an endodomain (Figure 29.1). The ectodomain typically consists of an antigen-binding, single chain variable fragment

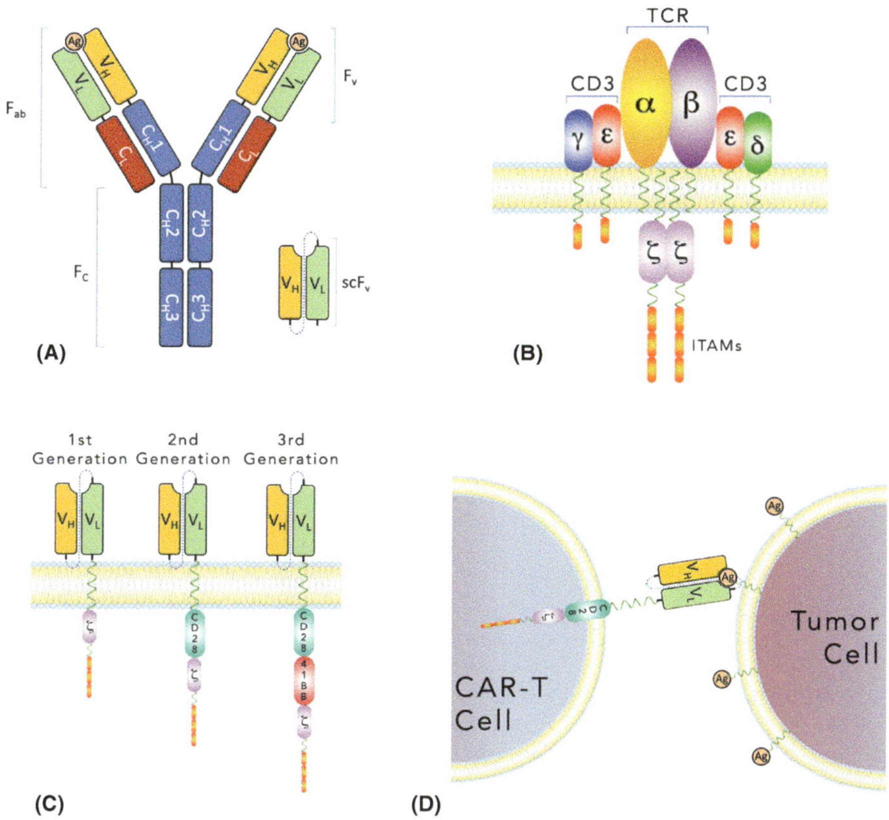

FIGURE 29.1 Evolution of chimeric antigen receptors (CARs). (A) Native immunoglobulin structure consisting of 2 heavy (H) chains and 2 light (L) chains, each with variable (VH, VL) and constant (CH, CL) regions. Antigen (Ag) binding site occurs in the variable fragment (Fv) region. Single-chain Fv (scFv) regions are engineered for use in CAR. (B) Native antibody T-cell receptor (TCRs) with associated CD3 subunits propagate intracellular signals through immunoreceptor tyrosine-based activation motifs. (C) First-generation CARs (left) are typically made of scFv and CD3z, joined by a transmembrane linker. Second-generation CARs (middle) are similar to first-generation CARs but have an additional intracellular costimulatory domain (e.g., CD28 or 4–1BB). Third-generation CARs (right) have >1 costimulatory domain. (D) CAR T cells (CAR-T) engage targeted cell surface Ag, resulting in cytokine secretion and tumor cell lysis.

Source: Reprinted with permission from Hardaway JC, Prince E, Arepally A, Katz SC. Regional infusion of chimeric antigen receptor T cells to overcome barriers for solid tumor immunotherapy. *J Vasc Interv Radiol*. 2018;29:1019. doi:10.1016/j.jvir.2018.03.001.

(scFv) derived from the light and heavy chains of an immunoglobulin, as well as a peptide linker and a hinge domain. The endodomain contains the CD3-ζ chain to propagate the signal, as well as a costimulatory domain(s). CAR constructs are generally introduced to activated lymphocytes using a lentiviral or retroviral vector, which randomly integrates in the host genome and may cause deleterious effects. Consequently, newer CAR strategies have employed knock-in approaches with gene-editing technologies such as CRISPR-Cas9 to achieve a more controlled, targeted insertion of the CAR transgene.[38]

Currently, the two FDA-approved CAR-T cell products utilize a second-generation design. More recently, third-generation CAR constructs containing multiple costimulatory domains have emerged, but have not shown clear superiority over first- or second-generation CARs. Fourth-generation CARs that incorporate additional transgenes have also emerged. This class is diverse and covers inducible on/off promoters to regulate CAR expression, suicide genes to eliminate CAR-T in settings of severe immune-mediated toxicities, cytokines, decoy checkpoint receptors, or other immune-modulatory molecules to combat the hostile tumor microenvironment.

CAR-T Successes and Challenges

Hematopoietic Malignancy

The most successful CAR-T therapy to date is CTL019, which targets the B-cell surface antigen CD19. CTL019 was initially approved for treatment of relapsed acute lymphoblastic leukemia (ALL).

Remarkably, CTL019 achieved complete remission in 90% of patients with refractory ALL, which was sustained in 67% at 6 months.[3] Negative effects of CAR-T therapy included CRS, with symptoms ranging from a mild flu-like illness to hypotension, increased vascular permeability, and multiorgan system failure. Neurotoxicity was also seen in the CTL019 trial, occurring mostly as a self-limited encephalopathy but causing seizure activity in some patients.

CAR-T Trafficking and Delivery Barriers in Solid Tumors

Systemic administration of CAR-T for solid malignancy suffers from an inability to discretely traffic to the tumor bed, which may result in "on target, off tumor" toxicity. This ineffective delivery can result in dose-limiting toxicities, as was the case in Phase 1 trial patients with metastatic colorectal adenocarcinoma, who developed severe colitis upon systemic infusion of CAR-T directed against carcinoembryonic antigen (CEA).[39] More devastating consequences occurred in a patient with colorectal metastases to the lung and liver who developed massive CRS after systemic infusion of CAR-T directed against ERBB2 (human epidermal growth factor receptor 2/neu).[40] The patient developed respiratory distress, cardiac arrest within 12 hours of infusion, and ultimately died 5 days later. Postmortem analysis revealed low-level ERBB2 expression on lung epithelia, which was thought to have engaged CAR-T and caused massive cytokine release.

Two important factors that determine the efficiency of CAR-T delivery into solid tumors include the pressure gradient and distribution of infused cells based on normal blood flow patterns. Pressures within solid tumors can be substantial and can reach up to 130 mmHg, due to disorganized neovasculature with highly permeable capillaries and high levels of extracellular matrix proteins, such as hyaluronan.[41,42] As a result, pressures are generally highest at the tumor center with lower levels toward the periphery. Effective intratumoral delivery of any cellular therapy via systemic infusion therefore occurs as a function of the pressure gradient, or the differential between intratumoral and mean arterial pressure. Thus, tumors with elevated pressures impede delivery of CAR-T when standard devices and methods are used. As such, we have combined our regional infusion strategies with high-pressure delivery devices to optimize CAR-T penetration into solid tumors (see "Regional Delivery of CAR-T").[43]

From a molecular perspective, many receptor–ligand interactions influence CAR-T navigation into tumor tissue. Our conceptual understanding of T cell homing mechanisms has accumulated from homeostatic and infectious disease studies, whereas manipulation of lymphocyte homing mechanisms is a common immunoevasive strategy employed by tumors.[44] More recently, coexpression of the CCR2 chemokine receptor in mesothelin-directed CAR-T was able to increase infiltration by 12.5-fold into mesotheliomas.[45] In the sarcoma context, infantile fibrosarcoma (IFS) tumor cells have been shown to express high levels of CXCL10 and CXCL16 chemokines, yet no sarcoma-directed ACT has yet incorporated the use of additional homing mechanisms to increase their efficacy.[46] Presumptively, we will see an increasing number of fourth-generation CAR-T that leverage inherent lymphocyte homing machinery to increase therapeutic delivery of CAR-T.

Immunosuppressive Tumor Microenvironment

Even if CAR-T are adequately delivered to, or effectively trafficked to, a solid tumor, their effect is limited by the tumor microenvironment (TME), which exploits preexisting counterregulatory mechanisms that exist to prevent immune-mediated damage to normal host tissue. The TME is thus immunosuppressed, bathed with inhibitory cytokines secreted by a diverse constituency of myeloid derived suppressor cells (MDSC), Tregs, and tumor-associated macrophages (TAMs). Tregs and MDSCs also express cell surface programmed death ligand-1 (PD-L1) and CD80/86, which directly inhibit CAR-T, TAM, and cytotoxic T lymphocytes (CTLs) through programmed death-1 (PD-1) and cytotoxic T lymphocyte-associated antigen 4 (CTLA-4) receptors.

In an osteosarcoma xenograft model using disialoganglioside (GD2)-directed CAR-T, tumor cells were eradicated in vitro, but were ineffective when delivered in vivo due to expansion of murine MDSC.[47] However, when mice were treated with all-trans retinoic acid (ATRA), a clinically approved drug that differentiates immature myeloid cells to a nonsuppressive phenotype, GD2-CAR-T regained antitumor effect against osteosarcoma xenografts. Studies from our laboratory have implicated a similar role of hepatic MDSCs as potent mediators of CAR-T suppression in a model of colorectal liver metastasis.[7,8]

Many studies have identified prognostic correlates of the TME, such as the presence of TILs and improved survival seen among patients with Ewing sarcoma, gastrointestinal stromal tumor (GIST), cutaneous angiosarcoma, and for mixed subtypes, such as leiomyosarcoma, synovial sarcoma, liposarcoma, and undifferentiated pleomorphic sarcoma (UPS).[48,49] In another TME analysis of 163 STS specimens—predominantly UPS, synovial sarcoma, fibrosarcoma, and liposarcoma subtypes—PD-L1 expression and Treg infiltration were associated with tumors that were high grade in patients of advanced age (>65 years old), implicating a potential immunoevasive synergism between PD-L1 expression and Tregs.[50] As such, strategies that disrupt PD-L1 and/or deplete Tregs may prove as useful adjuncts in overcoming the immunosuppressive TME in context of cellular therapies.

TAMs are also significant contributors to the sarcoma TME, but do not always behave according to classical M1 and M2 subtypes. That is, M1 macrophages are regarded as proinflammatory, secrete both tumor necrosis factor α (TNFα) and IL-12, and directly mediate tumor lysis, whereas M2 macrophages secrete IL-10 and proangiogenic factors to quell inflammation and favor tumor growth. Based on these functional designations, M2-polarized TAMs are characteristically found in the vast majority of human and murine tumors, but not among GISTs, which are M1-polarized at baseline. When mice with spontaneous GIST were treated with imatinib, TAM transitioned to M2, followed by a return to an M1 phenotype among imatinib-resistant tumors. While the unique oncogenes that drive GIST pathophysiology likely influence the behavior of GIST TAM, these observations underscore the likelihood of unique and complex interrelationships between TME constituents and therapeutic interventions.[51] As data regarding the sarcoma TME accumulate, it is apparent that the heterogeneous behavior of the sarcoma TME mirrors the diversity of sarcoma subtypes.

Regional Delivery of CAR-T

Regional infusion of cellular immunotherapies for treatment of hepatic and pancreatic malignancies has been performed using dendritic cells, macrophages, or LAK cells via portal vein injection or hepatic artery infusion (HAI).[52] Radiolabeled lymphocytes infused via HAI persist in the liver for up to 120 hours, with only 20% escaping to systemic circulation. Side effects of these therapies are self-limited in nature, with fever and chills most commonly observed. Safety of HAI for delivery of anti-CEA CAR-T (Sorrento/TNK Therapeutics, San Diego, CA) for adenocarcinoma liver metastases was demonstrated in our Phase 1 Hepatic Immunotherapy for Metastases (HITM) trial (NCT01373047), in which the maximum dose was reached without observation of any grade 4 or 5 adverse events.[53] Reduced serum tumor marker levels, increased serum interferon-γ, and increased fibrosis/necrosis in posttreatment biopsy specimens were observed. The safety profile of the HITM trial protocol contrasts with the dose-limiting severe colitis that was observed with systemic delivery of anti-CEA CAR-T.

We have expanded the HITM method in subsequent Phase 1 trials: HITM-SIR (NCT02416466), which utilized adjunctive yttrium-90 resin microspheres (SIR-TeX Medical, Sydney, Australia) sequentially delivered in delayed fashion after CAR-T and HITM-SURE (NCT02850536), which incorporated the use of a pressure-enabled drug delivery (PEDD) catheter (TriSalus Life Sciences, Westminster, CO) to increase CAR-T delivery.[43,54] In the HITM-SURE trial, two of five treated patients demonstrated a complete metabolic response by PET, with one patient remaining alive after 20 months. Recently, we opened a first-in-human, dose-escalation Phase 1 trial with intraperitoneal CAR-T (IPC) infusion for peritoneal metastases or malignant ascites (NCT03682744). As cellular immunotherapies emerge and are refined for the treatment of sarcoma, regional delivery strategies may prove useful to overcome the physical barriers that impede effective delivery. Several abdominal sarcoma subtypes, including GIST and leiomyosarcoma, may metastasize to the liver or recur as disseminated peritoneal sarcomatosis, thereby potentially benefiting from the HITM and IPC methods.[55,56]

CHALLENGES RELATED TO SARCOMA BIOLOGIC HETEROGENEITY

Sarcomas display myriad anatomic, biologic. and patient-related heterogeneity. This diversity demands a complementary armamentarium. Thus, a diverse array of cellular targets will likely need to be elucidated, with additional therapeutic considerations made for their respective TMEs, anatomic restraints, and age-associated influences. Current data sets have been curated from similarly heterogeneous populations or specimens and are inadequate toward these goals. For example, a study seeking to examine factors relevant to local recurrence of sarcoma among a population of patients largely composed of leiomyosarcoma has failed to acknowledge the biologic tendency of leiomyosarcoma to recur distantly.[57] Investigators who are developing autologous cellular therapies for pediatric sarcomas are working with a functionally different leukocyte donor population than would be expected from a geriatric donor, based on observations that geriatric CAR-T are functionally impaired with respect to proliferation, signaling activation, and perforin/granzyme B mediated cytotoxicity.[58] Combining the intricacies and complexities of cellular immunotherapy with the multifaceted heterogeneity of sarcoma, the corresponding investigative approaches must be cogently designed to account for unique biologic features of specific sarcoma subtypes.

Target Antigens in Sarcoma

Before delving into relevant trials in which engineered TCR and CAR-T were used to treat sarcomas, a discussion of suitable target antigens is warranted. The family of cancer testis antigens (CTAs) have garnered attention as target antigens for sarcoma, as well as other malignancies. Expression of CTA is restricted to germline tissues, placental trophoblasts, and a variety of malignancies.[59] Further, germline cells do not express MHC molecules, which renders them immunologically privileged and thus "invisible" to TCR-based approaches, which rely on MHC recognition. Thus, any cellular therapy directed against these CTAs would preferentially attack cancerous cells. Expression of several HLA*02.01 restricted CTA family members NY-ESO-1, LAGE-1, PRAME, MAGE-A3, MAGE-A4, MAGE-A9, and SSX-2 were reported across multiple sarcoma subtypes.[60] Though there were fewer than 10 tumor specimens examined for each subtype, characteristic expression patterns were observed for synovial cell sarcoma, liposarcoma, and leiomyosarcoma, as seen in Table 29.1. The majority of synovial cell sarcomas express NY-ESO-1, particularly the monophasic histologic type; however they typically do not express MAGE-A1 or CT7.[61] Myxoid and nonmyxoid liposarcoma were found to be positive for LAGE in >70% and 60% of specimens tested, respectively.[62] Expression of MAGE-A3 was seen in 66% of uterine leiomyosarcomas, but only in 14% nonuterine leiomyosarcomas.[63] Lastly, treatment with 5-aza-2-deoxycitabine (5-Aza-dC) was shown to induce expression of NY-ESO-1, LAGE-1s, and PRAME among chondrosarcoma cell lines and tumors that previously had no or low-level expression of these CTAs.[64] GD2 was shown to be highly expressed (>60% of tumor cells) among 83% of pediatric osteosarcomas and 13% of pediatric rhabdomyosarcomas, with 20% of pediatric Ewing sarcomas having low-level expression.[47] Additional osteosarcoma targets include ERBB2 and IL-11 receptor α (IL-11Rα), both of which are expressed on the cell membrane and are suitable for CAR-T therapies.[65,66]

CAR-T and TCR Trials for Sarcoma

Clinical trials of cellular therapy for sarcoma patients have been challenging and have evolved over time. Table 29.2 provides an overview of completed and ongoing sarcoma clinical trials. Owing to the general difficulty in generating TILs from nonmelanoma tumor specimens, early clinical trials using cellular immunotherapy for sarcoma utilized autologous T cells isolated from peripheral blood that were engineered to express TCRs against NY-ESO-1, because NY-ESO-1 is expressed in >80% of synovial cell sarcomas. Robbins et al. from the Surgery Branch of the NCI were the first to report a series of six patients with metastatic synovial cell sarcoma, previously treated with high-dose IL-2, who received a single dose of anti-NY-ESO-1 TCR T cells and supplemental IL-2 infusion after a preconditioning regimen of cyclophosphamide and fludarabine.[6] Partial responses were observed in four of six patients, which lasted up to 18 months in one patient who received two infusions of TCR-transduced T cells, whereas one of the patients with progressive disease had only received one-third of the dose that others in the cohort received.[6] A follow-up report from the same group 3 years later included an additional 11 patients, with six partial responses (maximum duration 47+ months) and one complete response that had persisted beyond 20 months.[5] Cumulatively, 11 of 18 patients (61%) developed an objective response, and there was one treatment-related death during the course of the trial, which

TABLE 29.1 Target Antigen Expression by Sarcoma Subtype

Sarcoma Subtype	NY-ESO-1	LAGE-1	MAGE-A3	MAGE-A4	MAGE-A9	SSX-2
Gastrointestinal stromal tumor	++	+	++	+		+
Synovial sarcoma	+++	+++			+++	
Uterine leiomyosarcoma	++	++	++	+++		+++
Nonuterine leiomyosarcoma	-	+	+	+		
Angiosarcoma						
Undifferentiated pleomorphic sarcoma	+	-	+	-		
Liposarcoma	+++	++	++	+++		
Osteosarcoma	+++	+++	+++	+++		
Chondrosarcoma	+++	+++	+++	++		
Ewing sarcoma	-	-	+	+		

TABLE 29.2 Cellular Immunotherapy Clinical Trials for Sarcoma

Title/Description	Cellular Therapy	Target Antigen	Status	Trial Number	Phase	Pts	Est. Completion
NY-ESO-1-Specific T-cells in Treating Patients With Advanced NY-ESO-1-Expressing Sarcomas Receiving Palliative Radiation Therapy	TCR	NY-ESO-1	Completed	NCT02319824	1	2	
NK White Blood Cells and Interleukin in Children and Young Adults With Advanced Solid Tumors	NK	N/A	Completed	NCT01875601	1	16	
A Pilot Study of Autologous T-Cell Transplantation With Vaccine Driven Expansion of Anti-Tumor Effectors After Cytoreductive Therapy in Metastatic Pediatric Sarcomas	CTL Vaccine	EF-1, EF-2, PXFK	Completed	NCT00001566	2	42	
Autologous T Cells and Cyclophosphamide in Treating Patients With Soft Tissue Sarcoma That is Metastatic or Cannot Be Removed By Surgery	TCR	NY-ESO-1	Completed	NCT01477021	1	6	
A Phase I Trial of T Cells Expressing an Anti-GD2 Chimeric Antigen Receptor in Children and Young Adults With GD2+ Solid Tumors	CAR-T	GD2	Completed	NCT02107963	1	15	
TAA-Specific CTLS for Solid Tumors (TACTASOM)	TCR	NY-ESO-1, MAGE-A4, PRAME, Survivin, and SSX	Active, not recruiting	NCT02239861	1	16	
NY-ESO-1-specific T Cell Receptor (TCR) T Cell in Sarcoma	TCR	NY-ESO-1	Recruiting	NCT03462316	1	20	2020
LTX-315 and Adoptive T-cell Therapy in Advanced Soft Tissue Sarcoma	TIL LTX-315	Not defined	Recruiting	NCT03725605	2	10	2023
To Evaluate the Efficacy of NY-ESO-1-specific T Cell Receptor (TCR) Affinity Enhancing Specific T Cell in Solid Tumors	TCR	NY-ESO-1	Recruiting	NCT03159585	1	20	2019
A Pilot Study of Genetically Engineered NY-ESO-1 Specific NY-ESO-1(c259) in HLA-A2+ Patients With Synovial Sarcoma	TCR	NY-ESO-1(c259)	Recruiting	NCT01343043	1	10	2020
Study of TBI-1301 (NY-ESO-1 T Cell Receptor Gene Transduced Autologous T Lymphocytes) in Patients With Synovial Sarcoma	TCR	NY-ESO-1	Recruiting	NCT03250325	1/2	8	2020
MAGE-A4(c1032) T for Multi-Tumor	TCR	MAGE-A4	Recruiting	NCT03132922	1	42	2020

(continued)

TABLE 29.2 Cellular Immunotherapy Clinical Trials for Sarcoma (*continued*)

Title/Description	Cellular Therapy	Target Antigen	Status	Trial Number	Phase	Pts	Est. Completion
Her2 Chimeric Antigen Receptor Expressing T Cells in Advanced Sarcoma	CAR-T	HER2	Recruiting	NCT00902044	1	36	2031
A Pilot Study of NY-ESO-1(c259) T Cells in Subjects With Advanced Myxoid/ Round Cell Liposarcoma	TCR	NY-ESO-1	Recruiting	NCT02992743	2	10	2020
iC9-GD2-CAR-VZV-CTLs/ Refractory or Metastatic GD2-positive Sarcoma and Neuroblastoma	CAR-T	GD2 (14g2a mAb)	Recruiting	NCT01953900	1	26	2036
Safety and Efficacy Evaluation of 4th Generation Safety-engineered CAR T Cells Targeting Sarcomas	CAR-T	Sarcoma surface antigens'	Recruiting	NCT03356782	1/2	20	2020
T Cell Receptor-transduced T Cells Targeting NY-ESO-1 for Treatment of Patients With NY-ESO-1- Expressing Malignancies	TCR	NY-ESO-1	Recruiting	NCT02457650	1	36	2019
Combination of Cryosurgery and NK Immunotherapy for Recurrent Sarcoma	NK	Not applicable	Recruiting	NCT02849366	1/2	30	2019
EGFR806 CAR T Cell Immunotherapy for Recurrent/ Refractory Solid Tumors in Children and Young Adults	CAR-T	EGFR	Recruiting	NCT03618381	1	36	2036
Study of Adoptive Immunotherapy Using Autologous CD8+ NY-ESO-1-Specific T Cells and the NY-ESO-1 Immunostimulatory Agents LV305 or CMB305 For Patients With Sarcoma	TCR LV305	NY-ESO-1	Recruiting	NCT03450122	1	18	2019
Study of TBI-1301 (NY-ESO-1 Specific TCR Gene Transduced Autologous T Lymphocytes) in Patients With Solid Tumors	TCR	NY-ESO-1	Recruiting	NCT02869217	1	15	2020
Autologous Tumor Infiltrating Lymphocytes MDA-TIL in Treating Patients With Recurrent or Refractory Ovarian Cancer, Osteosarcoma, or Pancreatic Ductal Adenocarcinoma	TIL	Not defined	Recruiting	NCT03610490	2	60	2021

CAR-T, chimeric antigen receptor T cell; CTL, cytotoxic T lymphocytes; NK, natural killer cells; TCR, T-cell receptor; TIL, tumor-infiltrating lymphocytes.

occurred as a consequence of neutropenic septic shock 3 days after ACT. The number of T cells specifically reactive to NY-ESO-1 peptide-pulsed target cells correlated with response to therapy, while the overall persistence of adoptively transferred T cells did not. An additional trial is currently underway to more broadly examine NY-ESO-1 TCR-based approaches for skeletal and STS (NCT03462316). Other CTAs, such as MAGE-A3, MAGE-A4, and MAGE-A10 are being targeted with TCR-engineered T cells for multiple sarcoma subtypes (NCT03132922, NCT03132922, NCT02989064, NCT03139370, NCT02111850, NCT02153905).[67]

As described previously, GD2 has previously been targeted in sarcoma clinical trials. A recent Phase 1 clinical trial (NCT01953900) obtained T cells from patients with advanced osteosarcoma and a history of infection/vaccination with varicella zoster virus (VZV) to examine the therapeutic efficacy and safety of GD2-redirected CAR-T cells (CARiC9-GD2-CAR-VZV-CTLs) and the role of previous VZV exposure on the in vivo expansion and persistence of the generated CAR-T cells. In a separate Phase 1 trial (NCT02107963), a third-generation CAR with an ICD9 caspase dimerization domain as a suicide switch will be used for patients with sarcoma and osteosarcoma, among other malignancies.[68]

Cellular immunotherapy for GIST is a practical consideration given that activation of $CD8^+$ TIL and apoptosis of intratumoral Treg have been implicated in the mechanism of tumor clearance by imatinib.[69] Further, patients with high-risk and/or metastatic GIST often develop resistance to imatinib or other tyrosine kinase inhibitor (TKI) therapies, which unfortunately manifests as progressive disease. For these patients, CAR-T targeting KIT (CD117) may offer an attractive therapeutic alternative, because KIT is expressed on nearly all GIST.[70] We previously reported the design and generation of a CAR construct that incorporates the natural ligand for KIT, KIT-ligand (KL), also known as stem cell factor (SCF), as its antigen-binding domain.[71] These anti-KIT CAR-T demonstrated tumor-specific activity against hKIT+ GIST cells in a subcutaneous xenograft model but have yet to be incorporated into a clinical trial. As noted earlier, regional infusion of such cell therapy products may have application for liver and peritoneal metastases for GIST and other sarcomas with similar metastatic patterns.

NATURAL KILLER CELLS

Activated and Expanded Natural Killer Cells

Activated and expanded natural killer cells (NKAE) have previously shown in vitro cytotoxicity against osteosarcoma and Ewing sarcoma.[72] To further explore these findings in vivo, a preclinical model of metastatic sarcoma demonstrated that while NKAE treatment prevented large tumor deposits from implanting, pulmonary micrometastases were still evident. CXCR4, which is upregulated in 33% to 73% of sarcomas, was targeted using an anti-CXCR4 monoclonal antibody (mAb) (MDX1338, Bristol Myers Squibb). When MDX1338 was coadministered with NKAE, no micro- or macrometastatic tumors were found.[73]

Along similar lines, Ewing sarcoma and rhabdomyosarcoma are exquisitely sensitive to killing by expanded NK cells, while NK cells also exhibit some activity against osteosarcoma cells. A Phase 1 trial (NCT02409576) seeks to use expanded activated haploidentical NK cell infusions in this context. One favorable feature of NK cell infusions is that they have been well tolerated when administered to patients with leukemia; that is, they do not induce graft versus host disease (GvHD). An alternative approach, using NK cells from non-HLA matched donors, provides the design of a trial (NCT02849366) that incorporates investigation of ALT803, a purported NK cell survival factor.

SUMMARY

The application of cellular therapies for the treatment of sarcoma is in its infancy, but is rapidly evolving in an era of technological advancement with increasing integration into multidisciplinary oncology care. Progress in sarcoma cellular therapy is hindered by the low incidence and heterogeneity inherent to this disease process, but preclinical and clinical data presented in this chapter should provide hope that sarcoma patients will soon benefit from tailored cellular therapies. Many of the hindrances to cellular immunotherapy for sarcoma reflect the limitations for solid tumors in general. Through coupling of effective tumor killing cell therapy products, effective delivery strategies, and modulation of immunosuppression in the TME, cell therapy for sarcoma will be realized.

REFERENCES

1. Coley WB. Contribution to the knowledge of sarcoma. *Ann Surg*. 1891;14:199–220. doi:10.1097/00000658-189112000-00015
2. Nauts HC, Swift WE, Coley BL. The treatment of malignant tumors by bacterial toxins as developed by the late William B. Coley, M.D., reviewed in the light of modern research. *Cancer Res*. 1946;6:205–216. https://cancerres.aacrjournals.org/content/6/4/205
3. Maude SL, Frey N, Shaw PA, et al. Chimeric antigen receptor T cells for sustained remissions in leukemia. *N Engl J Med*. 2014;371(16):1507–1517. doi:10.1056/NEJMoa1407222

4. Andersen R, Donia M, Ellebaek E, et al. Long-lasting complete responses in patients with metastatic melanoma after adoptive cell therapy with tumor-infiltrating lymphocytes and an attenuated IL2 regimen. *Clin Cancer Res*. 2016;22(15):3734–3745. doi:10.1158/1078-0432.CCR-15-1879
5. Robbins PF, Kassim SH, Tran TLN, et al. A pilot trial using lymphocytes genetically engineered with an NY-ESO-1-reactive T-cell receptor: long-term follow-up and correlates with response. *Clin Cancer Res*. 2015;21(5):1019–1027. doi:10.1158/1078-0432.CCR-14-2708
6. Robbins PF, Morgan RA, Feldman SA, et al. Tumor regression in patients with metastatic synovial cell sarcoma and melanoma using genetically engineered lymphocytes reactive with NY-ESO-1. *J Clin Oncol*. 2011;29(7):917–924. doi:10.1200/JCO.2010.32.2537
7. Thorn M, Guha P, Cunetta M, et al. Tumor-associated GM-CSF overexpression induces immunoinhibitory molecules via STAT3 in myeloid-suppressor cells infiltrating liver metastases. *Cancer Gene Ther*. 2016;23(6):188–198. doi:10.1038/cgt.2016.19
8. Burga RA, Thorn M, Point GR, et al. Liver myeloid-derived suppressor cells expand in response to liver metastases in mice and inhibit the anti-tumor efficacy of anti-CEA CAR-T. *Cancer Immunol Immunother*. 2015;64(7):817–829. doi:10.1007/s00262-015-1692-6
9. Mitchison NA. Studies on the immunological response to foreign tumor transplants in the mouse. I. The role of lymph node cells in conferring immunity by adoptive transfer. *J Exp Med*. 1955;102(2):157–177. doi:10.1084/jem.102.2.157
10. Billingham R, Brent L, Medawar P. Quantitative studies on tissue transplantation immunity. III. Actively acquired tolerance. *Philos Trans R Soc Lond B Biol Sci*. 1956;239(666):357–414. doi:10.1098/rstb.1956.0006
11. Cambrosio A, Keating P. Between fact and technique: the beginnings of hybridoma technology. *J Hist Biol*. 1992;25(2):175–230. doi:10.1007/bf00162840
12. Morgan DA, Ruscetti FW, Gallo R. Selective in vitro growth of T lymphocytes from normal human bone marrows. *Science*. 1976;193(4257):1007–1008. doi:10.1126/science.181845
13. Rosenberg SA, Grimm EA, McGrogan M, et al. Biological activity of recombinant human interleukin-2 produced in Escherichia coli. *Science*. 1984;223(4643):1412–1414. doi:10.1126/science.6367046
14. Smith KA, Lachman LB, Oppenheim JJ, Favata MF. The functional relationship of the interleukins. *J Exp Med*. 1980;151(6):1551–1556. doi:10.1084/jem.151.6.1551
15. Smith KA, Gilbride KJ, Favata MF. Lymphocyte activating factor promotes T-cell growth factor production by cloned murine lymphoma cells. *Nature*. 1980;287(5785):853–855. doi:10.1038/287853a0
16. Rosenberg SA, Lotze MT, Muul LM, et al. Observations on the systemic administration of autologous lymphokine-activated killer cells and recombinant interleukin-2 to patients with metastatic cancer. *N Engl J Med*. 1985;313(23):1485–1492. doi:10.1056/NEJM198512053132327
17. Mule JJ, Shu S, Schwarz SL, Rosenberg SA. Adoptive immunotherapy of established pulmonary metastases with LAK cells and recombinant interleukin-2. *Science*. 1984;225(4669):1487–1489. doi:10.1126/science.6332379
18. Rosenberg SA, Lotze MT, Yang JC, et al. Prospective randomized trial of high-dose interleukin-2 alone or in conjunction with lymphokine-activated killer cells for the treatment of patients with advanced cancer. *J Natl Cancer Inst*. 1993;85(8):622–632. doi:10.1093/jnci/85.8.622
19. Rosenberg SA, Restifo NP. Adoptive cell transfer as personalized immunotherapy for human cancer. *Science*. 2015;348(6230):62–68. doi:10.1126/science.aaa4967
20. Goff SL, Smith FO, Klapper JA, et al. Tumor infiltrating lymphocyte therapy for metastatic melanoma: analysis of tumors resected for TIL. *J Immunother*. 2010;33(8):840–847. doi:10.1097/CJI.0b013e3181f05b91
21. Hopewell EL, Cox C, Pilon-Thomas S, Kelley LL. Tumor-infiltrating lymphocytes: streamlining a complex manufacturing process. *Cytotherapy*. 2019;21:1–8. doi:10.1016/j.jcyt.2018.11.004
22. Balch CM, Riley LB, Bae YJ, et al. Patterns of human tumor-infiltrating lymphocytes in 120 human cancers. *Arch Surg*. 1990;125(2):200–205. doi:10.1001/archsurg.1990.01410140078012
23. Rosenberg SA, Spiess P, Lafreniere R. A new approach to the adoptive immunotherapy of cancer with tumor-infiltrating lymphocytes. *Science*. 1986;233(4770):1318–1321. doi:10.1126/science.3489291
24. Rosenberg SA, Packard BS, Aebersold PM, et al. Use of tumor-infiltrating lymphocytes and interleukin-2 in the immunotherapy of patients with metastatic melanoma. A preliminary report. *N Engl J Med*. 1988;319(25):1676–1680. doi:10.1056/NEJM198812223192527
25. Yannelli JR, Hyatt C, McConnell S, et al. Growth of tumor-infiltrating lymphocytes from human solid cancers: summary of a 5-year experience. *Int J Cancer*. 1996;65(4):413–421. doi:10.1002/(SICI)1097-0215(19960208)65:4<413::AID-IJC3>3.0.CO;2-#
26. Muranski P, Boni A, Wrzesinski C, et al. Increased intensity lymphodepletion and adoptive immunotherapy—how far can we go? *Nat Clin Pract Oncol*. 2006;3(12):668–681. doi:10.1038/ncponc0666
27. Dudley ME, Yang JC, Sherry R, et al. Adoptive cell therapy for patients with metastatic melanoma: evaluation of intensive myeloablative chemoradiation preparative regimens. *J Clin Oncol*. 2008;26(32):5233–5239. doi:10.1200/JCO.2008.16.5449
28. Katz SC, Point GR, Cunetta M, et al. Regional CAR-T cell infusions for peritoneal carcinomatosis are superior to systemic delivery. *Cancer Gene Ther*. 2016;23(5):142–148. doi:10.1038/cgt.2016.14
29. Saied A, Licata L, Burga RA, et al. Neutrophil:lymphocyte ratios and serum cytokine changes after hepatic artery chimeric antigen receptor-modified T-cell infusions for liver metastases. *Cancer Gene Ther*. 2014;21(11):457–462. doi:10.1038/cgt.2014.50

30. Zhang L, Conejo-Garcia JR, Katsaros D, et al. Intratumoral T cells, recurrence, and survival in epithelial ovarian cancer. *N Engl J Med*. 2003;348(3):203–213. doi:10.1056/NEJMoa020177
31. Zhou J, Shen X, Huang J, et al. Telomere length of transferred lymphocytes correlates with in vivo persistence and tumor regression in melanoma patients receiving cell transfer therapy. *J Immunol*. 2005;175(10):7046–7052. doi:10.4049/jimmunol.175.10.7046
32. Théoleyre S, Mori K, Cherrier B, et al. Phenotypic and functional analysis of lymphocytes infiltrating osteolytic tumors: use as a possible therapeutic approach of osteosarcoma. *BMC Cancer*. 2005;5:123. doi:10.1186/1471-2407-5-123
33. Rivoltini L, Arienti F, Orazi A, et al. Phenotypic and functional analysis of lymphocytes infiltrating paediatric tumours, with a characterization of the tumour phenotype. *Cancer Immunol Immunother*. 1992;34(4):241–251. doi:10.1007/bf01741792
34. Sorbye SW, Kilvaer T, Valkov A, et al. Prognostic impact of lymphocytes in soft tissue sarcomas. *PLoS ONE*. 2011;6(1):e14611. doi:10.1371/journal.pone.0014611
35. Tseng WW, Malu S, Zhang M, et al. Analysis of the intratumoral adaptive immune response in well differentiated and dedifferentiated retroperitoneal liposarcoma. *Sarcoma*. 2015;2015(8):547460–547469. doi:10.1155/2015/547460
36. Yee C. Adoptive T cell therapy: points to consider. *Curr Opin Immunol*. 2018;51:197–203. doi:10.1016/j.coi.2018.04.007
37. Kuwana Y, Asakura Y, Utsunomiya N, et al. Expression of chimeric receptor composed of immunoglobulin-derived V regions and T-cell receptor-derived C regions. *Biochem Biophys Res Commun*. 1987;149(3):960–968. doi:10.1016/0006-291x(87)90502-x
38. Eyquem J, Mansilla-Soto J, Giavridis T, et al. Targeting a CAR to the TRAC locus with CRISPR/Cas9 enhances tumour rejection. *Nature*. 2017;543(7643):113–117. doi:10.1038/nature21405
39. Parkhurst MR, Yang JC, Langan RC, et al. T cells targeting carcinoembryonic antigen can mediate regression of metastatic colorectal cancer but induce severe transient colitis. *Mol Ther*. 2011;19(3):620–626. doi:10.1038/mt.2010.272
40. Morgan RA, Yang JC, Kitano M, et al. Case report of a serious adverse event following the administration of T cells transduced with chimeric antigen receptor recognizing Erbb2. *Mol Ther*. 2009;18(4):843–851. doi:10.1038/mt.2010.24
41. Jain RK. Delivery of molecular and cellular medicine to solid tumors. *Adv Drug Deliv Rev*. 2001;46(1–3):149–168. doi:10.1016/s0169-409x(00)00131-9
42. Provenzano PP, Cuevas C, Chang AE, et al. Enzymatic targeting of the stroma ablates physical barriers to treatment of pancreatic ductal adenocarcinoma. *Cancer Cell*. 2012;21(3):418–429. doi:10.1016/j.ccr.2012.01.007
43. Katz SC, Guha P, Hardaway JC, et al. HITM-SURE: Phase Ib CAR-T hepatic artery infusion trial for stage IV adenocarcinoma using pressure-enabled drug delivery technology. Presented at: Society for Immunotherapy and Cancer Annual Meeting; November 7–11, 2018; Washington, DC.
44. Sackstein R, Schatton T, Barthel SR. T-lymphocyte homing: an underappreciated yet critical hurdle for successful cancer immunotherapy. 2017;97(6):669–697. doi:10.1038/labinvest.2017.25
45. Moon EK, Carpenito C, Sun J, et al. Expression of a functional CCR2 receptor enhances tumor localization and tumor eradication by retargeted human T cells expressing a mesothelin-specific chimeric antibody receptor. *Clin Cancer Res*. 2011;17(14):4719–4730. doi:10.1158/1078-0432.CCR-11-0351
46. Zhu H, Gu S, Yin M, et al. Analysis of infantile fibrosarcoma reveals extensive T-cell responses within tumors: Implications for immunotherapy. *Pediatr Blood Cancer*. 2018;65(2). doi:10.1002/pbc.26813
47. Long AH, Highfill SL, Cui Y, et al. Reduction of MDSCs with all-trans retinoic acid improves CAR therapy efficacy for sarcomas. *Cancer Immunol Res*. 2016;4(10):869–880. doi:10.1158/2326-6066.CIR-15-0230
48. Berghuis D, Santos SJ, Baelde HJ, et al. Pro-inflammatory chemokine-chemokine receptor interactions within the Ewing sarcoma microenvironment determine CD8(+) T-lymphocyte infiltration and affect tumour progression. *J Pathol*. 2011;223(3):347–357. doi:10.1002/path.2819
49. Lee A, Huang P, DeMatteo RP, Pollack SM. Immunotherapy for soft tissue sarcoma: tomorrow is only a day away. *Am Soc Clin Oncol Educ Book*. 2016;35(36):281–290. doi:10.1200/EDBK_157439
50. Que Y, Xiao W, Guan Y-X, et al. PD-L1 expression is associated with FOXP3+ regulatory T-cell infiltration of soft tissue sarcoma and poor patient prognosis. *J Cancer*. 2017;8(11):2018–2025. doi:10.7150/jca.18683
51. Cavnar MJ, Zeng S, Kim TS, et al. KIT oncogene inhibition drives intratumoral macrophage M2 polarization. *J Exp Med*. 2013;210(13):2873–2886. doi:10.1084/jem.20130875
52. Hardaway JC, Prince E, Arepally A, Katz SC. Regional infusion of chimeric antigen receptor T cells to overcome barriers for solid tumor immunotherapy. *J Vasc Interv Radiol*. 2018;29(7):1017.e1–1021.e1. doi:10.1016/j.jvir.2018.03.001
53. Katz SC, Burga RA, McCormack E, et al. Phase I hepatic immunotherapy for metastases study of intra-arterial chimeric antigen receptor-modified T-cell therapy for CEA+ liver metastases. *Clin Cancer Res*. 2015;21(14):3149–3159. doi:10.1158/1078-0432.CCR-14-1421
54. Katz SC, Prince E, Cunetta M, et al. HITM-SIR: Phase Ib trial of CAR-T hepatic artery infusions and selective internal radiation therapy for liver metastases [abstract]. Presented at: *American Association for Cancer Research Annual Meeting*; April 2017; Washington, DC.
55. Bilimoria MM, Holtz DJ, Mirza NQ, et al. Tumor volume as a prognostic factor for sarcomatosis. *Cancer*. 2002;94(9):2441–2446. doi:10.1002/cncr.10504

56. Ng EH, Pollock RE, Munsell MF, et al. Prognostic factors influencing survival in gastrointestinal leiomyosarcomas. Implications for surgical management and staging. *Ann Surg*. 1992;215(1):68–77. doi:10.1097/00000658-199201000-00010
57. Katz SC. Tailoring surgical therapy for extremity soft tissue sarcoma. *Ann Surg Oncol*. 2016;24(1):13–14. doi:10.1245/s10434-016-5468-9
58. Guha P, Cunetta M, Somasundar P, et al. Frontline science: functionally impaired geriatric CAR-T cells rescued by increased α5β1 integrin expression. *J Leukoc Biol*. 2017;102(2):201–208. doi:10.1189/jlb.5HI0716-322RR
59. Figueroa JA, Reidy A, Mirandola L, et al. Chimeric antigen receptor engineering: a right step in the evolution of adoptive cellular immunotherapy. *Int Rev Immunol*. 2015;34(2):154–187. doi:10.3109/08830185.2015.1018419
60. Pollack SM, Loggers ET, Rodler ET, et al. Immune-based therapies for sarcoma. *Sarcoma*. 2011;2011:438940. doi:10.1155/2011/438940
61. Jungbluth AA, Antonescu CR, Busam KJ, et al. Monophasic and biphasic synovial sarcomas abundantly express cancer/testis antigen NY-ESO-1 but not MAGE-A1 or CT7. *Int J Cancer*. 2001;94(2):252–256. doi:10.1002/ijc.1451
62. Skubitz KM, Pambuccian S, Manivel JC, Skubitz APN. Identification of heterogeneity among soft tissue sarcomas by gene expression profiles from different tumors. *J Transl Med*. 2008;6:23. doi:10.1186/1479-5876-6-23
63. Ayyoub M, Taub RN, Keohan M-L, et al. The frequent expression of cancer/testis antigens provides opportunities for immunotherapeutic targeting of sarcoma. *Cancer Immun*. 2004;4:7. https://cancerimmunolres.aacrjournals.org/content/canimmarch/4/1/7
64. Pollack SM, Li Y, Blaisdell MJ, et al. NYESO-1/LAGE-1s and PRAME are targets for antigen specific T cells in chondrosarcoma following treatment with 5-Aza-2-deoxycitabine. *PLoS ONE*. 2012;7(2):e32165. doi:10.1371/journal.pone.0032165
65. Ahmed N, Salsman VS, Yvon E, et al. Immunotherapy for osteosarcoma: genetic modification of T cells overcomes low levels of tumor antigen expression. *Mol Ther*. 2009;17(10):1779–1787. doi:10.1038/mt.2009.133
66. Huang G, Yu L, Cooper LJ, et al. Genetically modified T cells targeting interleukin-11 receptor α-chain kill human osteosarcoma cells and induce the regression of established osteosarcoma lung metastases. *Cancer Res*. 2012;72(1):271–281. doi:10.1158/0008-5472.CAN-11-2778
67. Pollack SM, Ingham M, Spraker MB, Schwartz GK. Emerging targeted and immune-based therapies in sarcoma. *J Clin Oncol*. 2018;36(2):125–135. doi:10.1200/JCO.2017.75.1610
68. Han S, Latchoumanin O, Wu G, et al. Recent clinical trials utilizing chimeric antigen receptor T cells therapies against solid tumors. *Cancer Lett*. 2017;390:188–200. doi:10.1016/j.canlet.2016.12.037
69. Balachandran VP, Cavnar MJ, Zeng S, et al. Imatinib potentiates antitumor T cell responses in gastrointestinal stromal tumor through the inhibition of Ido. *Nat Med*. 2011;17(9):1094–1100. doi:10.1038/nm.2438
70. Katz SC, DeMatteo RP. Gastrointestinal stromal tumors and leiomyosarcomas. *J Surg Oncol*. 2008;97(4):350–359. doi:10.1002/jso.20970
71. Katz SC, Burga RA, Naheed S, et al. Anti-KIT designer T cells for the treatment of gastrointestinal stromal tumor. *J Transl Med*. 2013;11(1):46. doi:10.1186/1479-5876-11-46
72. Cho D, Shook DR, Shimasaki N, et al. Cytotoxicity of activated natural killer cells against pediatric solid tumors. *Clin Cancer Res*. 2010;16(15):3901–3909. doi:10.1158/1078-0432.CCR-10-0735
73. Vela M. Anti CXCR4 antibody combined with activated and expanded natural killer cells for sarcoma immunotherapy. *J Clin Oncol*. 2018;36(suppl):11541

30

Interventional Radiology

Shree Venkat, Kyle Maughan, Jagteshwar Sandhu, and Prasoon Mohan

INTRODUCTION

Multidisciplinary management at high-volume sarcoma centers lead to improved short and long-term outcomes in these patients when compared to treatment at low-volume centers.[1,2] Multidisciplinary management involves experienced teams consisting of oncologists, surgeons, radiation oncologists, pathologists, and interventional radiologists with the goal of treatment being long-term survival while minimizing morbidity and maximizing function. This chapter presents the role of the interventional radiologist in the multidisciplinary team for the management of these patients.

IMAGE GUIDANCE

The use and advances in image guidance are essential in the diagnosis and treatment of these patients. These advances in imaging guidance, percutaneous ablation techniques, and embolotherapy have led interventional radiologists to play a large role in the multidisciplinary management of these patients. Image-guided core-needle percutaneous biopsy is one of the most common techniques and is routinely performed for the diagnosis of the initial tumor.[3,4] Here we discuss the different types of imaging guidance used by interventional radiologists in the management of these patients.

Ultrasound

Ultrasound (US) technology has been used to image the body for over 50 years.[5] Benefits of this technology is that it is portable, without radiation exposure, and inexpensive. For image guidance during a procedure, the needle or probe adjustments can be seen in real time rather than requiring intermittent scans. The US pulse (frequency range of 2–15 MHz) is sent from a transducer and echoes are generated by the interaction with structures in the tissue medium. Imaging is difficult for deeper structures, patients with larger body habitus, and through tissues with high acoustic impedance increases, for example, bone. Color Doppler evaluation can help in identifying vessels and avoiding such structures.

Magnetic Resonance Imaging

As with US, MRI does not use radiation to obtain information. The soft tissue delineation of MRI is exquisite. This technology combines the external magnetic field provided by a magnet with the localized magnetic field provided by gradient and shim coils with the application of radiofrequency (RF) pulse from the RF coils.[6] Adjusting the pulse sequences can provide unique information regarding differentiation of pathologic disorders or evaluating treatment response. Given their complexity, scans often take longer than US or CT evaluation, and are more expensive.

Computed Tomography

CT involves the use of ionizing radiation with the use of x-rays through the patient, creating a three-dimensional (3-D) image data set. CT is best used when high spatial resolution is needed and for rapid imaging of a patient. If malignancy cannot be excluded on plain film in bone sarcomas, MRI should be used to characterize the lesions over CT. MRI is also preferred in the initial diagnosis of soft tissue sarcomas (STS), but CT can be used to characterize calcified lesions along with retroperitoneal tumors. In the workup of STS, a chest-spiral CT is mandatory for staging purposes.[3,4] Interventional radiologists use CT to guide many procedures. In the diagnosis and treatment of sarcomas, complex biopsies are often done under CT guidance. Percutaneous radiofrequency ablation (RFA), microwave ablation (MWA), and cryoablation are also performed with CT guidance.

Positron-Emitting Tomography/Computed Tomography

The basis of PET imaging is infusing the patient with proton-rich radioactive nucleotides that emit positrons via B+ decay, which is composed of a positron and a neutrino. This decay leads to a more stable nucleus. The positron travels a very short distance before colliding with an electron in an annihilation event, which produces two photons of equal energy. These photons are detected by the scanner. The F-18 isotope gets incorporated into a glucose analog called ^{18}F-deoxyglucose, which is given to the patient prior to scanning. This molecule gets taken up by highly metabolic tissue, which will often be abnormal oncologic tissue. In sarcoma PET/CT has been studied in diagnosis, grading, staging, biopsy guidance, therapeutic monitoring, and prognostication. However, the cost effectiveness of performing PET/CT versus the standard of care in these areas has not been studied. Interventional radiologists have used PET/CT guidance in biopsies and ablations in these patients. For biopsies, the PET/CT will show the most metabolically active portion of the tumor. In ablations, interventional radiologists can monitor the tumor response to the ablation and areas of necrosis using PET/CT. Future studies in cost effectiveness when compared to the standard CT guidance for complex biopsies and ablations need to be performed before advocating PET/CT guidance as first line.[7]

Fluoroscopy

Fluoroscopy is an imaging technique that uses x-rays, ionizing radiation, to create real-time moving images of a patient. Interventional radiologists use fluoroscopy to guide many different types of procedures in the treatment of these patients. Intra-arterial embolotherapy is guided by fluoroscopy as well as the placement of lines, catheters, and ports.

CENTRAL VENOUS ACCESS

Obtaining central venous access via placement of a central venous catheter (CVC) is becoming one of the most common procedures done by an interventional radiologist. It is particularly prevalent among oncology patients, as central venous access is required for both diagnostic and therapeutic interventions. Trained interventional radiologists, with the assistance of image guidance, can routinely insert long-term venous access devices, a procedure that has shown to be safe, cost-effective, and efficacious. By using real-time imaging (fluoroscopy and/or sonography) CVCs are placed with their tip in the right atrium or at the cavo-atrial junction. While it is possible to place CVCs without image guidance, radiologically guided percutaneous insertion has higher technical success rates, shorter procedure times, lower cost, and fewer complications, making it the preferred approach to gain central access.[8]

Types of Devices

Peripherally inserted central catheters (PICCs), tunneled central catheter, and implanted ports are the most common devices used for central venous access. Benefits and indications for each type are discussed next. Most devices are made of silicone or polyurethane, which have been associated with fewer infections when compared to previously used materials.[8] Catheters can have one, two, or three lumens, allowing for multiple therapies to be administered simultaneously. Terminal end holes or side valves are designed to allow fluid injection and blood aspiration, while preventing blood or air from entering the catheter when it is not in use.

Peripherally Inserted Central Catheter

PICCs are nontunneled central catheters that are inserted through a vein in the arm. They are generally used in patients who require less than 3 months of central venous access for antibiotic administration or peripheral nutrition. PICCs can be used in the outpatient or inpatient setting among patients requiring long-term continuous or intermittent infusions. PICC placement is less invasive than placement of other CVCs, but they have a higher rate of infection and malfunction (fourfold increase when compared to ports); thus, risks and benefits must be considered before PICC placement.[8]

Tunneled Catheters

Tunneled catheters are recommended in patients requiring more than 1 month of central access. They can be used for chemotherapy administration, dialysis, plasmapheresis, or total parenteral nutrition. The catheter travels through an 8- to 15-cm subcutaneous tract, usually 5 to 10 mm beneath the surface of the skin, before entering the venous system.[9] The proximal end of the catheter contains a cuff, which induces an inflammatory reaction within the subcutaneous tissue. Three to 4 weeks after placement, the inflammatory reaction leads to fibrosis and catheter fixation. This inhibits migration of organisms down the catheter, thus reducing the incidence of catheter-related infections. Some chemotherapies, particularly trabectedin for STS, have shown to have a local sterile inflammation along the catheter trajectory.[10] Placing the tunnel deeper in the subcutaneous tissue has been shown to be the best way to prevent this complication.[10] When central venous access is no longer required, infusion of local anesthetic and blunt instrument dissection are necessary to pull the cuff free.

Ports

Ports consist of a tunneled catheter that terminates in a subcutaneous, self-sealing reservoir. The reservoir has a silicon window that can be accessed through the skin with a noncoring needle. The reservoir is normally placed in the subcutaneous tissue of the chest (preferred) or arm (usually near the antecubital fossa). Ports are generally indicated in patients who require >3 months of intermittent central venous access, and are often used for chemotherapy, chronic transfusion, or chronic blood tests.[9] Ports have the lowest rate of infection when compared to tunneled catheters and PICCs.[11]

Indications

The indications for central venous access are numerous and are notably prevalent in oncology patients who often require venous access for the duration of their disease. Therapeutic indications for central venous access include administration of chemotherapy, total parenteral nutrition, blood products, intravenous medications, fluids, plasmapheresis, and/or hemodialysis. Diagnostic indications include establishing diagnosis/prognosis, monitoring response to treatment, and/or repeated blood sampling.[11] Central venous access is recommended for boluses of vesicant drugs and is essential for continuous infusions of those agents.[8] Guidelines exist to aid in deciding which type of device to use and are summarized in Table 30.1. Devices with multiple lumens are indicated in patients who receive multiple simultaneous therapies or require peripheral nutrition in addition to chemotherapy. Although many factors are considered when choosing a device, patient involvement in the decision has been shown to result in greater patient satisfaction, fewer delays in therapy related to loss of vascular access, fewer device complications, shorter hospital stays, fewer ED visits, and decreased costs.[8] Thus, it is important to remember that patients should always be involved in decision-making.

Contraindications

Owing to the safety of the procedure and the benefits it offers to patients, absolute contraindications to central venous access are rare. Relative contraindications include coagulopathy, thrombocytopenia, and sepsis. It is preferred that a patient with bacteremia or sepsis be afebrile for 48 hours prior to the procedure, though it can still be done in emergent situations. International normalized ratio (INR) <2 and platelet count <25,000 are considered contraindications, but infusion of platelets or fresh frozen plasma can be used to circumvent this issue in emergent cases.[12] Additionally, studies show that experienced physicians can safely perform CVC placement in the presence of abnormal coagulation parameters.[13] Cannulation is generally avoided in sites with anatomic distortion or vascular injury, but a different site of entry can generally be selected in order to gain central access.

Patient Workup and Preparation

In most patients, the right internal jugular vein is the preferred access site because of its large size and proximity to the skin. It also provides a short, straight route to the superior vena cava and right atrium. Patients receiving a PICC are generally accessed via the basilic vein for similar reasons: it is closer to the

TABLE 30.1 Guidelines for Central Venous Access Device Selection

Device	Length of Use	Common indications
PICC	<3 months	Antibiotics, TPN
Tunneled catheter	>1 month	Chemotherapy, TPN, dialysis, plasmapheresis
Implantable port	>3 months	Chemotherapy, chronic transfusion, chronic blood tests

PICC, peripherally inserted central catheter; TPN, total parenteral nutrition.
Source: Reproduced with permission from Valji K. Vascular access placement and foreign body retrieval. In: Valji K, ed. *The Practice of Interventional Radiology.* Philadelphia, PA: Elsevier; 2012:559–580.

surface and larger than surrounding veins, thus resulting in decreased vasospasm and fewer complications.[8] These sites should be examined in all patients to rule out any anatomic variations or deformity.[9] Coagulation parameters should be checked and corrected before the procedure. With the exception of PICCs, placement of a CVC requires the same aseptic environment found in the operating room.

Follow-Up

Postprocedure imaging to confirm successful placement may include fluoroscopy, a chest radiograph, or contrast injection through the catheter.[14] Standard of practice is to position the catheter tip in the upper to mid-right atrium with the patient supine, allowing for migration of the tip when the patient switches from the supine to standing position.[12] Technical success is defined as catheter introduction into the desired location, with adequate catheter function. Catheter function is defined as withdrawal of blood and infusion of saline without significant resistance. Nursing staff should be well trained in venous access care and able to recognize device failures and identify and treat potential complications.[14]

Complications and Troubleshooting

Complications are rare, with success rates >96%. Complications can be classified as early (<24 hours after placement) and late (>30 days after placement).[14] Selected complication rates when using image guidance can be seen in Table 30.2. Some of the more common and serious complications are discussed individually.

Infection

Chemotherapy and radiotherapy can cause significant neutropenia, and over 60% of catheter-related sepsis (CRS) occurs during periods of neutropenia. Oncology patients with central venous catheters are therefore at an increased risk of catheter-related bloodstream infection (CRBSI.) CRBSI is defined as at least two blood cultures positive with the same organism, obtained from two different sites at two separate times, in association with evidence of colonization of the catheter with the same organism. This differs from central line–associated bloodstream infection (CLABSI), which is defined as recovery of a pathogen from a blood culture (single if not related to the skin or two or more cultures for an organism commonly present on the skin) in a patient who had a central line at the time of infection or within 48 hours developing an infection.[15] The most common symptoms associated with infection are fever or chills followed by erythema/induration at the insertion site.[15]

Measures can be taken to reduce the incidence of CRBSI. Insertion should occur with appropriate hand hygiene, maximum sterile barrier precautions, and proper skin preparation. Dressings at CVC sites should be changed weekly until the insertion site has healed, and then dressings should no longer be used. Site selection can also decrease infections, with internal jugular placement showing lower

TABLE 30.2 Central Venous Access Complication Rates

Complication	Rate (%)
Tunneled catheter and port placement	
Pneumothorax	1–3
Hematoma	1–3
Perforation	0.5–1
Air embolism	1
Thrombosis	4
Procedure-induced sepsis	1–3
PICC placement	
Pneumothorax	0
Hematoma	1
Phlebitis	4
Thrombosis	3
Procedure-induced sepsis	1

PICC, peripherally inserted central catheter.

Source: Data from Dariushnia SR, Wallace MJ, Siddiqi NH, et al. Quality improvement guidelines for central venous access. *J Vasc Interv Radiol*. 2010;21(7):976–981. doi:10.1016/j.jvir.2010.03.006.

rates of infection compared to femoral. Devices impregnated with a combination of minocycline and rifampin have been shown to reduce infection rates, and current evidence suggests that such catheters are cost effective for high-risk patients compared with standard CVCs. Use of prophylactic antibiotics before central venous access is controversial, and there are no current recommendations for their use. Catheters should be removed promptly when no longer needed.

Management centers around the isolated organism and its antibiotic sensitivities. Antibiotics should be administered, and then a decision to remove the catheter or to keep it in place must be made. Patients with limited access may benefit from keeping the catheter in place, even in the setting of infection. The catheter should be removed if the patient has unexplained sepsis, erythema, or purulence at the catheter insertion site, or CRBSI associated with supportive thrombophlebitis, endocarditis, or osteomyelitis. Likewise, it should be removed if the organism isolated from blood cultures is *Staphylococcus aureus*.[8,16]

Thrombosis

Thrombotic complications are relatively common and are generally marked by catheter malfunction or symptoms of deep vein thrombosis (DVT). The buildup of fibrin around the catheter can cause a partial or complete occlusion of the lumen. Thrombosis occurs as intraluminal thrombosis, fibrin sheaths, and mural thrombosis. Complications include pulmonary embolism, DVT recurrence, and postphlebitic syndrome.

Prevention can be accomplished by selecting the proper device and access point, and ensuring proper tip placement. Silicone and polyurethane are now the most common materials used because of their decreased risk of thrombosis. A greater vessel length increases the risk of thrombosis; therefore, the shortest possible route should be selected. Device placement against the wall of the right atrium has been shown to increase risk of thrombosis; therefore, the correct anatomic placement is crucial. Image guidance reduces endothelial damage and decreases the risk of catheter-associated thrombosis. Catheters should be flushed routinely with saline or unfractionated heparin. Tissue plasminogen activator (tPA) can be used weekly as a locking solution. There is inadequate evidence to support the use of routine heparin or warfarin for prevention of thrombosis.

Management of partial thrombotic occlusion includes unfractionated heparin 5,000 to 25,000 units over 6 to 24 hours. Complete occlusion requires one to two doses of urokinase or recombinant tPA. Fibrin sheaths can be treated with a catheter exchange, angioplasty balloon, or fibrin sheath stripping, all of which are reserved for instances when pharmacologic therapy fails to reestablish patency.

Patients with catheter-related DVT should be placed on anticoagulation for a minimum of 3 months. Catheters affected by thrombosis should be removed whenever possible. Some studies show utility in thrombolysis. Catheter-directed thrombolysis has been shown to be safer than systemic thrombolysis, and can be considered in patients with extensive thrombosis.[8]

Catheter Malfunction

Catheter malfunction manifests as increased resistance on infusion or the inability to aspirate blood. Patients may also complain of pain during injection. Such patients should be evaluated promptly for evidence of device malfunction. Troubleshooting consists of physical exam, chest radiograph, or injection of contrast to assess device position and integrity. The most common cause is fibrin deposition and venous thrombosis, as mentioned previously. Other causes include catheter malposition, kinking, and catheter fracture.[9] Occlusion can also be due to precipitation of drugs with low or high pH or lipid-rich parenteral infusions. Such occlusions can be treated with sodium bicarbonate, hydrochloric acid, or ethanol, respectively. These agents should fill the catheter for up to 20 minutes.[8] Nonfunctioning catheters with no signs of infection can usually be replaced over a guidewire through the original tunnel.

BIOPSY

Biopsy of suspected sarcoma is the diagnostic standard and is necessary prior to the development and application of treatment strategies.[17] In an age when personalized oncology and targeted therapies provide the best outcomes, determining relevant cellular and molecular signatures of tissue via a histologic sample is critical. Different approaches exist, including open biopsy, fine-needle aspiration, and percutaneous core-needle biopsy. Image-guided percutaneous biopsy has been shown to be safe, effective, and considerably less invasive than open biopsy. Positive and negative predictive values, sensitivity, and specificity of tissue samples obtained via image-guided percutaneous biopsy have been reported to be similar to those found in open incisional biopsies.[18,19] Biopsies of suspected sarcomas are technically challenging, high-risk procedures. They should only be done at institutions with specialty sarcoma centers made up of an interdisciplinary team.

Indications

Percutaneous biopsy of bone or soft tissue is performed whenever histologic confirmation is required for definitive diagnosis and/or treatment. Soft tissue tumors are often heterogeneous and it can be difficult to determine if they are benign or malignant from imaging alone. Benign soft tissue masses are 100 times more common than malignant sarcomas, and it can therefore be challenging to determine which soft tissue masses require further workup, evaluation, and biopsy. Published criteria for referral to sarcoma center for potential biopsy of a soft tissue lesion include any lesion that is >5 cm, painful, rapidly increasing in size, deep to the muscle fascia, or recurrent after previous excision.[20] Other common indications are to assist in staging or to determine if a mass is secondary to metastasis or primary sarcoma when PET/CT is equivocal.[21]

Contraindications

There are no absolute contraindications; however, there are a handful of relative contraindications in which risk versus benefit should be carefully considered. Biopsy is not indicated in a patient if the results will not change management or if surgery is indicated irrespective of the outcome of the biopsy.[22] Biopsy may be contraindicated in patients that exhibit uncorrectable coagulation abnormalities. Severely compromised cardiopulmonary function or hemodynamic instability could potentially incur too much risk to safely complete the procedure.[23] Lesions that are located in a position where there is no safe percutaneous approach should be avoided. Additionally, caution should be taken when performing an image-guided percutaneous biopsy in a patient who is unable or unwilling to limit movement during the procedure. If repeat core-needle biopsy is unable to obtain adequate tissue for diagnosis, an incisional biopsy may need to be performed.[21]

Approach

Patients should undergo INR and activated partial thromboplastin time (aPTT) (if receiving heparin) prior to the procedure. If INR is less than 1.5 it should be corrected. It is recommended that platelets be transfused if platelet count is less than 50,000. Low-molecular-weight heparin (LMWH) (1 day) and clopidogrel (5 days) should be withheld before the procedure. There is no need to withhold aspirin.[13]

Generally, the shortest path to the lesion is considered when planning the imaging approach. Choice of imaging modality for biopsy is based on lesion characteristics and operator preference. The most common modalities are fluoroscopy, sonography, and CT, each having its own advantages and disadvantages. Fluoroscopy is commonly used for biopsy of lung and pleural masses and is useful for its ability to give real-time images. Disadvantages include increased radiation exposure and inability to visualize adjacent structures. Ultrasound is used for biopsy of intra-abdominal lesions, masses in the retroperitoneum, and other peripheral lesions. Advantages include the lack of radiation, real-time imaging, and multiplanar imaging. Disadvantages include impaired visualization of deep lesions and obscuration by overlying structures. CT is reserved for biopsy of smaller or deeper lesions not well visualized by sonography or fluoroscopy. Advantages include high-quality images and the ability to clearly visualize all surrounding structures. Disadvantages include increased radiation, lack of real-time feedback, and patient movement after capturing the CT image. CT fluoroscopy can be used to obtain near real-time imaging when necessary.

Single-needle and two-needle techniques can be used in obtaining the biopsy. In the single-needle technique, a needle is advanced into position and imaging is obtained. If the needle is not positioned in the desired location, it is left in place to guide the placement of a second needle. Each biopsy then requires a new needle to be placed in the lesion, allowing for sampling of different regions of the mass. In the two-needle technique, the initial needle is inserted into the desired location within the mass and is used as the landmark for subsequent needles. With the coaxial method, a large needle is inserted just superficial to the mass. The biopsy is then performed with longer, smaller-gauge needles, allowing for a single puncture of viscera or pleura.[22]

A multidisciplinary team should be assembled to treat all patients with sarcoma. Interventional radiologists should work closely with the medical and radiation oncologists and pathologists to

TABLE 30.3 Percutaneous Needle Biopsy Complication Rates

Complication	Rate (%)
Bleeding requiring intervention	0.1–8.3
Tract seeding	0.3–4.0
Pneumothorax	0.5
Pneumothorax in transthoracic percutaneous needle biopsy	12–45

Source: Data from Gupta S, Wallace MJ, Cardella JF, et al. Quality improvement guidelines for percutaneous needle biopsy. *J Vasc Interv Radiol.* 2010;21(7):969–975. doi:10.1016/j.jvir.2010.01.011.

determine the best treatment and biopsy approach for the patient. Additionally, they should be in close communication with the surgeon to determine the best route for biopsy in the event that the biopsy tract needs to be resected (see Table 30.3).

Multiple passes may be needed owing to the heterogeneity of many sarcomas. After the biopsy is completed, imaging can be performed to exclude potential complications. The patient should be monitored for up to 4 hours, with frequent monitoring of vital signs. The patient may be discharged home if vital signs remain stable.[22]

Complications

Complications are rare, with a rate of 1.1% in image-guided percutaneous needle biopsy (PNB) of musculoskeletal (MSK) lesions.[19] Complication rates of PNB in general are shown in Table 30.3.

Compartmental anatomic guidelines for biopsy of MSK tumors have been published and used with the hopes of decreasing complication rates. Recommendations are extensive and include avoidance of critical structures and breaching more than one anatomic compartment. However, recent studies have shown that nonadherence to these recommendations does not result in increased complications or tumor recurrence.[24]

Tract Seeding and Tumor Spillage

In theory, disruption of the tumor pseudocapsule with the biopsy needle could result in tumor cells spilling into adjacent tissue and seeding of the biopsy tract. Rates of needle tract seeding (NTS) vary for different tumors, with the incidence in hepatocellular carcinoma (HCC) as high as 3%. In such cases, pretreatment biopsy is rarely used. However, in suspected sarcomas, NTS is obscure and a diagnosis without biopsy is frequently unreliable. Correct treatment cannot be safely initiated without diagnosis; therefore, biopsy is routinely performed. Studies are inconclusive, but recent reports indicate that there is no significant increased risk of NTS in soft tissue biopsies. One study showed that 13% of needle tracts had evidence of sarcoma cells, but those tracts did not have an increased incidence of tumor recurrence. Case reports of tumor recurrence along the biopsy tract seem to be decreasing, perhaps due to the widespread use of coaxial sheathed biopsy needles. However, because of existing case reports and the paucity of quality evidence regarding NTS in sarcoma, it is generally recommended that the biopsy trajectory be planned in conjunction with a team of surgeons so that the tract is resected with the tumor in order to avoid any potential complications.[25]

Pneumothorax

Pneumothoraces occur commonly in transthoracic biopsies and can also occur (although not as commonly) in nontransthoracic biopsies. Complications can be divided into major and minor complications. Chest tube placement is required if a pneumothorax becomes symptomatic or continually enlarges. Pneumothorax requiring thoracotomy tube placement is considered a minor complication if it only requires an overnight hospital stay. It is considered a major complication if hospitalization is longer than 48 hours for management of a persistent leak, or if the pneumothorax results in delay of chest tube removal for more than 3 days.

Measures can be taken to reduce the incidence of pneumothorax. Patients should be instructed not to move, talk, cough or breathe deeply during and immediately after the procedure. If possible, the pleura should only be punctured once and a coaxial technique should be used.[26] Pneumothorax rates range between 17% and 26%; however, only 1% to 14% of patients require a chest tube.[26] Risk factors include chronic obstructive pulmonary disease, depth of lesion, size of lesion, and number of pleural punctures.[26]

TRANSARTERIAL APPROACH

With the introduction of the Seldinger technique of catheterization, arterial access evolved in the 1970s and continues to do so. Access sites have evolved to less minimally invasive approaches from translumbar, to transaxillary to transfemoral and now transradial.[27,28] Angiography offers a diagnostic evaluation paired with a unique minimally invasive access to tumor vasculature that can help decrease perioperative hemorrhage, permit targeted chemotherapy delivery, or perform focused brachytherapy. These procedures can last anywhere from less than 2 hours to over 4 hours. While patients only require a combination of local anesthesia and conscious sedation, general anesthesia may be provided. Postprocedure care is centered around decreasing access site complications and supportive care. For the former, this may include lying flat for up to 6 hours if femoral access is used. This is not required with radial artery access.[28]

Contraindications

Angiographic intervention is contraindicated in a medically unstable patient with multisystem organ failure.[29] Relative contraindications include cardiac abnormalities, such as a recent myocardial infarction, serum electrolyte imbalances, severe contrast agent reactions, impaired renal status, inability to lay flat (agitation or impaired respiratory status), pregnancy, and Ehlers–Danlos syndrome.[27,29] Severe contrast reactions are marked by angioedema or bronchospasm. Dermal reactions can be managed with premedication. Impaired renal status may be addressed with prehydration or limiting the use of iodinated contrast agent by replacing it with carbon dioxide (CO_2.) Patients with Ehlers–Danlos syndrome have a high risk for arterial injury, such as arterial dissection.[29]

Complications

Puncture Site–Related Complications

Common arterial injuries caused by femoral artery catheterization include hemorrhage, postcatheterization pseudoaneurysm formation, arterial obstruction, arteriovenous fistula, and limb amputation.[27,30] Incidence rates are reported between 0.05% and 14%.[30] Risk factors include obesity, use of anticoagulation, use of large-caliber sheaths in access (greater than 7F [French]), puncture above the inguinal ligament, brief manual compression, hypertension, calcified atherosclerotic arteries, and history of hemodialysis, to name a few.[30] Pseudoaneurysm formation presents with pain, swelling, and dramatic bruising around the puncture site after recent arterial puncture. Diagnosis is made with US, which would reveal a mass with to-and-fro flow pattern on color Doppler mode.[30] While spontaneous thrombosis has been seen in pseuodoaneurysms less than 3 cm in size, management by US-guided compression, US-guided thrombin injection, coil embolization, stent placement, or surgical repair is recommended, given risk of rupture.[30]

Contrast-Induced Nephropathy

Contrast-induced nephropathy (CIN) is defined as a 0.5 mg/dL or 25% to 50% increase in serum creatinine or a 25% or greater decrease in estimated glomerular filtration rate (eGFR). This change can be seen as early as 24 hours or up 7 days after contrast administration.[29,31] Risk is low if renal function is normal.[29] If the patient has a eGFR <30 indicating stage 4 or 5 chronic kidney disease, incidence has been reported as high as 40%.[29] Other risk factors include dehydration, diabetes mellitus, congestive heart failure, and the use of angiotensin-converting enzyme inhibitors.[29,31] Prevention with hydration with 0.9% saline prior to the procedure has been effective.[32] Behavior modification of the operator has also been shown to help, examples of which include diluting contrast agent or using alternative agents, such as CO_2.[31]

Postembolization Syndrome

Postembolization syndrome (PES) presents as fatigue, nausea, vomiting, abdominal pain, and/or fever.[29,33] Incidence ranges between 60% and 90% with chemoembolization, and is also seen in bland embolization of the liver.[29] Possible causes include a systemic inflammatory response caused by the ischemia or necrosis of hepatocytes. The incidence can be reduced with the administration of dexamethasone.[33] The remainder of care is supportive with antiemetics, pain control, and hydration, and can lead to prolonged hospitalization.[33–35] With radioembolization, the symptoms are milder; therefore, it is classified as postradioembolization syndrome (PRS), which includes fatigue, nausea, anorexia, fever, abdominal discomfort, and cachexia.[29,34,35] Incidence ranges between 20% and 55% and can be minimized with postprocedure course of steroids and antiemetics.[34]

Radiation Safety

Intra-arterial procedures require fluoroscopic guidance; therefore delivering significant doses of radiation to the patient and the operator.[29,36] Tissue reactions are deterministic in that there is a threshold dose below which no injury is seen (2 Gy). Cancer risks from unrepaired or incorrectly repaired DNA are stochastic, indicating a linear, no threshold model. In other words, as exposure increases, so does risk. Given that sarcoma patients are often young, the risk of induction of cancers, such as leukemia or thyroid, skin, breast, or brain cancer, is greater.[29,37] Strategies to decrease dose include decreasing procedure time, effective shielding, using personal protective equipment, and improved equipment, which allows low dose rates without compromising on imaging quality.[29,36,38]

Indications

Liver Metastases

Locoregional therapy that has been used to manage primary liver cancer and metastatic disease, particularly colorectal cancer, includes transcatheter arterial embolization (TAE), transcatheter arterial chemoembolization (TACE), and transcatheter arterial radioembolization (TARE.) This has led to transarterial approach to treat sarcoma metastases in the liver, particularly the mesenchymal tumor, gastrointestinal stromal tumor (GIST.)[39] Incidence of liver metastases is 55% to 72% of the time with GIST and control of metastases is a determinant of survival.[40,41]

Special considerations when evaluating intra-arterial liver metastases include performance status and liver function.[40] It is preferred that liver function is Child-Pugh class A or B, as nontarget embolization or treatment can potentiate liver failure.[40] Radioembolization requires a closer attention to bilirubin levels; they should be less than 2 mg/dL given risk of radiation-induced liver disease (RILD.)[34,35] RILD results from radiation exposure to normal liver parenchyma and rates are reported between 0% and 4%.[34] Centers use a bilirubin of less than 3 mg/dL as a cutoff for TAE or TACE.[40,41] This technique exploits the dual supply to the liver; therefore, the portal vein is preferred to be used for patients with hepatopedal flow.[41]

Risk of liver injury may be mitigated by decreasing the amount of liver parenchyma exposed, which can be performed by favoring a subselective technique over a lobar or segmental approach. In this approach, the liver lesions are targeted through their third and fourth order arterial branches with a microcatheter, decreasing exposure of embolic to uninvolved segments. A sequential lobar approach could be used if there are diffuse metastases with interventions spaced out between 2 and 4 weeks, targeting the lobe with the most extensive involvement first.[41]

Procedure time is determined by anatomy and approach; for example, subselective embolization requires more time. TAE and TACE can be repeated in regular intervals, with imaging follow-up obtained 1 month after the procedure.[41,42] TARE requires a mapping angiogram to evaluate tumor supply, embolize branches to bowel, and evaluate lung shunt function.[43] Lung shunts greater than 20% can limit ability to give a dose that is effective at treating the tumor, without damaging lung parenchyma.[34,43] Treatment is then delivered at most centers 10 to 14 days after mapping procedure.[43,44] Imaging follow-up is performed 3 months after delivery of the radioembolic therapy as radiation changes can be mistaken for progression.[43,44]

With TAE and TACE, different embolics include gelfoam reabsorbable sponges to particles, such as polyvinyl alcohol (PVA) or trisacyl microspheres. There are two types of radioembolic devices with yttrium embedded in glass spheres or on resin microspheres. With chemoembolization, different agents include cisplatin, mytomycin C, doxorubicin, and vinblastine. Some series mix GIST with leiomyosarcoma (LMS). An example of bland embolization for GIST and LMS in shown in Figures 30.1 and 30.2, respectively.

Patients with GIST tend to do better than those with LMS.[45] The addition of a targeted agent, such as imatinib, improved overall survival (OS).[41] There is evidence to support embolization in patients with GIST who are imatinib resistant; however, patient performance status drives survival benefit.[40,42,46] There is also evidence to support embolization in LMS resistant to chemotherapy.[47,48] Extrahepatic disease, poor imaging response, and progression after embolization were associated with poor OS.[41] Initial data with TARE are promising; one multicenter study between four institutions with the majority of patients with LMS (GIST excluded) showed an OS of 30 months treated with resin and glass microspheres, depending on institution protocol.[49] A summary of these studies is included in Table 30.4.

Given that patients often have had prior surgery, attention to prior biliary interventions is needed.[40,52] This can result in an increased risk of infection or biloma formation, for example, in the series by Maluccio. Two patients developed abscess requiring intervention and one bactermia.[34,45,52] One patient in the series also developed a duodenal stricture from nontarget embolization, requiring

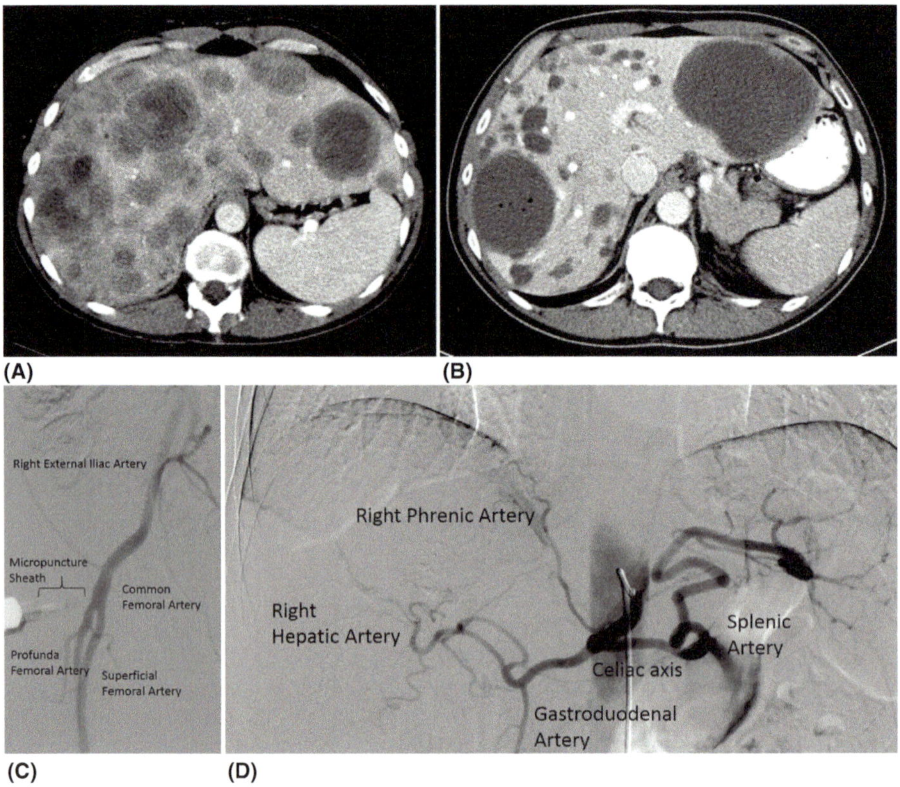

FIGURE 30.1 A 40-year-old man diagnosed with GIST after a small bowel tumor was seen during workup for abdominal pain. His original tumor was an over 9 cm mass. He was maintained on imatinib until 4 years later when he was found to have progression of liver lesions. The dose of imatinib was increased; he underwent bland embolization. His liver function was preserved (Child-Pugh class A) and his performance status was excellent (ECOG grade 0). Bland embolization was performed and showed dramatic response likely related to the adjustment of the imatanib dosing and embolization. Over the next 5 years, he underwent eight different bland embolizations to control the liver lesions. He was given different targeted agents including sunitinib, regorafanib, pazopanib, and ponatinib. Just before succumbing to the disease in the liver, omentum, and mesentery, his liver function deteriorated with elevation of his total bilirubin to 1.8 mg/dL. (A) Contrast-enhanced axial image showed multiple bilateral hypoattenuating lesions. (B) After embolization, lesions have decreased in number and enhancement. (C) Angiogram showing common femoral artery access over the midfemoral head away from the bifurcation. (D) Angiogram showing conventional anatomy of the celiac axis.

ECOG, Eastern Cooperative Oncology Group; GIST, gastrointestinal stromal tumor.

surgical bypass.[45] In the TARE series with 39 patients by Miller et al, one patient with a hepatojejeunostomy developed a liver abscess.[49] The other grade 3 adverse events included one gastroduodenal ulcer and one patient developed radiation pneumonitis.[49] In a second series of TARE with 11 patients, one developed a gastric ulcer.[51] A strategy to mitigate risks when a patient with an incompetent ampulla of Vater is to begin preprocedure antibiotics days prior to the procedure and follow an extended course of postprocedure antibiotics.[34,52]

Intra-Arterial Therapy Prior to Limb Salvage Surgery

A combined strategy of preoperative chemotherapy followed by limb salvage surgery and adjuvant therapy gives hope to balance quality of life without jeopardizing OS. The preoperative chemotherapy may be given via continuous intravenous infusion (CI) or intra-arterial (IA) route, or a combination of the approaches. The IA approach has been favored over cisplatin infusion to lower the rate of complication such as hearing loss, although hematologic toxicities have been found to be comparable.[53,54] Despite promising necrosis results from initial evaluations, improvement in local recurrence rates has not been noted.[54–58] In a pair of randomized control trials comparing IA to CI cisplatin along with a three-drug regimen (high-dose methotrexate [MTX] and doxorubicin) initially, histologic outcomes were significantly improved with IA route, but when a fourth drug was added to the regimen (ifosfomide), there was no difference.[54] There is evidence to suggest that if electing to perform IA cisplatin

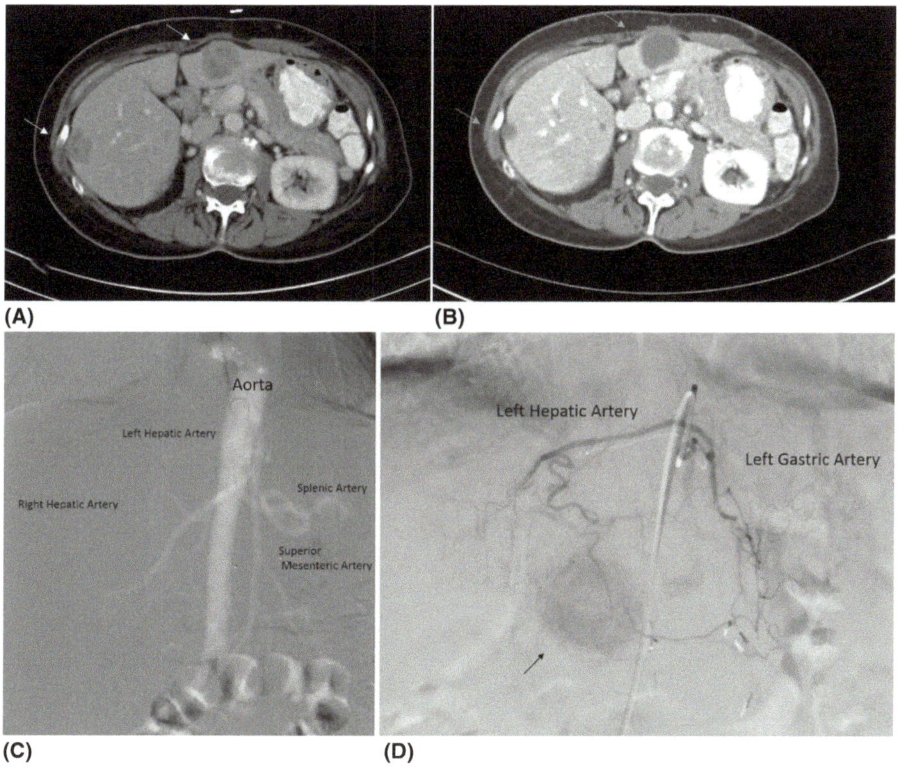

FIGURE 30.2 A 71-year-old woman originally diagnosed 15 years previously with retroperitoneal leiomyosarcoma. Metastases to the thigh, shoulder, small bowel, and lung have been managed with radiation and resection. Prior chemotherapy regimens included doxorubicin and darbazine, gemcitabine/taxotere, trabectedin, erbulin, and keytruda. While on immunotherapy, progression of liver lesions was noted. After multidisciplinary discussion, the patient was referred for bland embolization to control liver metastases. Liver function was preserved (Child-Pugh class A) and performance status was excellent (ECOG grade 0). Bilateral subselective bland embolization was performed with 100–300 µm Embospheres® (Merit Medical, Jordan, UT). (A) Precontrast axial CT in the portal venous phase of imaging shows enhancement in dominant segment III mass and small segment V mass (white arrows). (B) Postcontrast axial CT shows hypoattenuation without any residual enhancement in both lesions (gray arrows). (C) CO_2 aortogram through a 4F flush catheter was performed to evaluate vascular anatomy. (D) Subselective angiogram through 2.9F microcatheter advanced coaxially through a 5F reverse curve catheter revealed an anatomic variant, in which the left hepatic and left gastric arteries share a common origin also known as a gastrohepatic trunk. Tumor blush is seen in the dominant segment III lesion (black arrow). The procedure was complicated by nausea. She was discharged on the same day.

ECOG, Eastern Cooperative Oncology Group.

infusion, more cycles will improve necrosis; for example, in one study, when four cycles were given greater than 90%, necrosis was achieved two-thirds of the time.[57,59] IA MTX did not show as favorable a response as IA cisplatin.[56] Another approach is to also embolize the tumor to decrease blood loss during surgery. Adjuvant chemotherapy regimens either mirrored the neoadjuvant regiments if necrosis was favorable, or salvage option was offered. This may include doxorubicin, MTX, or ifosfamide.[53,55–57,59–63] In cases of positive surgical margins, radiation therapy can be offered.[57] An example of IA cisplatin infusion is shown in Figure 30.3.

The procedure involves femoral artery access. For a lower extremity tumor, the contralateral groin is generally used.[53,63,64] The accessed is maintained with a vascular sheath on the order of a 5F or 6F. The sheath is connected to a heparinized saline drip to maintain patency.[53,54] Through this, the contralateral artery is accessed with a diagnostic catheter (4F–5F). If infusion is planned, a multi-side hole infusion catheter is favored over an end-hole diagnostic catheter, which could sub-select a small branch. The catheter is secured and infusion is performed either in the procedure room or in the comfort of the patient room. If embolic agent is to be delivered, this is done through a microcatheter (on the order of 1.8F–2.9 F) to allow sub-selection of tumor branches and limit nontarget embolization. On removal of the catheter(s) and sheath, hemostasis may be achieved with manual pressure or a vascular closure device. Vascular closure devices are associated with a reduced time to hemostasis.[65]

TABLE 30.4 Hepatic Embolization Response Rates

Study	Etiology	*N*	Chemotherapy	Embolic Method	1-Year OS (%)	3-Year OS (%)	Median OS (Months)
Maluccio et al.[45]	GIST	16	None	PVA or trisacyl microspheres			36
	LMS	7					18
	Liposarcoma	1			-	-	-
	Total	24			62	29	24
Maglivit et al.[47]	LMS	14	Cisplatin followed by vinblastine	PVA	-	-	12
Rajan et al.[50]	GIST	11	Cisplatin, doxorubicin, mitomycin C	Lipiodol and PVA	67	40	13
	Total	16					
Kobayashi et al.[41]	GIST	110	Cisplatin, or cisplatin followed by vinblastine	Gelfoam and/ or PVA	62	21	17.2
Kobayashi et al.[42]	GIST (imatinib resistant)	14			45.8	45.8	9.7
Cao et al.[40,46]	GIST (imatinib resistant)		Doxorubicin	Lipiodol and gelfoam	-	-	17
Cao et al.[40]	GIST	45	None	Trisacyl microspheres	-	-	18.5
		26	Doxorubicin	Lipiodol and gelfoam			15.4
Miller et al.[49]	LMS	20	None	Resin and glass microspheres	-	-	30
	Total	39					
Rathmann et al.[51]	GIST (imatinib resistant)	11	None	Resin microspheres	-	-	29.8

GIST, gastrointestinal stromal tumor; LMS, leiomyosarcoma; OS, overall survival; PVA, polyvinyl alcohol.

Response Rates

Limb salvage surgery rates ranged between 83% and 92% after IA chemoinfusion.[54,57,64,66] Event-free survival rates ranged between 55% and 84%[54,62,64] OS rates ranged between 78% and 92%.[62,64,66] Local recurrence rates ranges from 0% to 6%.[54,64,66] Despite positive results in a few studies, the role of IA cisplatin infusion in the treatment of osteosarcoma is unclear.[58]

Angiography and Tumor Response

High-grade sarcomas can be identified by their dramatic tumor neovascularity on angiography. The few series where this is mentioned showed significant reduction in arterial perfusion.[53,57] The change of this vascularity with treatment has been shown to predict response.[53,64,66]

Complications

Complication rates are not uniformly reported with some as high as 2.5%.[53] In one series, 1/40 patients experienced major hearing loss.[57] One series evaluated ototoxicity with audiogram in 21 patients and noted 18 grade 2 or less toxicities and one patient required a hearing aid.[64] Myocutaneous inflammation and skin toxicities range between 0% and 10%, with reports of one patient requiring skin graft; however, limb-salvage surgery was not compromised.[64,66] The benefit of the angiographic intervention should be weighed with the morbidity of added procedures.[58]

PERCUTANEOUS TUMOR ABLATION

Tumor ablation is a technique to directly apply thermal or chemical therapy to a lesion to destroy or eradicate tumor cells. As the interventional radiologist is involved in obtaining the biopsy to diagnose

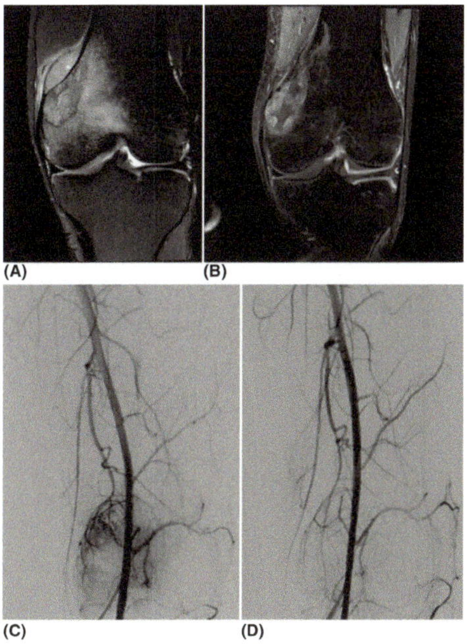

FIGURE 30.3 A 22-year-old man who was experiencing knee pain was found to have a high-grade osteosarcoma of the distal left femur. He underwent four cycles of IA cisplatin with IV doxorubicin (Adriamycin). This was followed by resection and long femur arthroplasty. The pathology revealed 92% necrosis. For adjuvant chemotherapy, he had four cycles of doxorubicin and ifosfamide. Surgery was complicated by postoperative infection that was resolved after IV antibiotics. He was lost to follow-up, transferring to a different institution after 2 years. No local recurrence or metastases were identified. (A) A proton-density (PD) fat saturation (FAT SAT) coronal image shows a 7-cm avid cortically based mass in the distal medial femoral metaphysis, eroding the cortex, resulting in aggressive periosteal reaction, subperiosteal edema, with an extraosseous soft tissue component. (B) After completing four cycles of IA cisplatin with IV doxorubicin, the mass shows less enhancement, edema, and soft tissue component. (C) Initial angiogram showed dramatic vascularity to the mass in the medial femoral metaphysis. (D) Angiogram performed before final IA cisplatin infusion shows dramatic decrease in vascularity to the mass.

IA, intra-arterial; IV, intravenous.

different sarcomas, newer technology using the same approach to accompany the biopsy can offer treatment and palliation, especially in oligometastatic disease.[67] The image-guided approach offers decreased risks of morbidity and mortality, increased precision, and repeatability.[68] Modalities that have been employed include but are not limited to radiofrequency ablation (RFA), microwave ablation (MWA), cryoablation (Cryo), irreversible electroporation (IRE), percutaneous ethanol injection (PEI), percutaneous acetic acid injection, and high-intensity focused ultrasound (HIFU).[68]

Modalities

Radiofrequency Ablation

RFA employs alternative current directly into tumor tissue, which returns through grounding pads on the skin. Friction is generated as the current causes tissue ions to oscillate, resulting in coagulative necrosis. Charring, desiccation, and water vapor can increase impedance and can limit that amount of current and heat delivered.[69] Heat conduction is dependent on tissue characteristics and is affected by adjacent perfusion and ventilation.[70] Temperatures in the range of 50°C to 55°C result in irreversible cellular damage, and those between 60°C and 100°C can result in immediate coagulation; however, when temperatures exceed 100°C, carbonization occurs. Carbonization or gas formation insulates the probe as well as slows the ability to form an effective RF field.[71] In order to overcome these limitations, internal cooling, saline infusion, multi tyne, or multiple probe (oscillating between probes) systems have been developed.[69,71] Ablation zones are limited by probe size and configuration. The risk of skin burns increases as current increases.[69]

Microwave Ablation

MWA allows placement of a microwave antenna into a tumor.[68] This antenna delivers radiation with frequencies between 900 and 2450 MHz that agitates water molecules by flipping the electrical charge on the order of 2 to 5 billion times a second.[71] This agitation produces friction and heat, and resultant cell death via coagulation necrosis.[68,71] Changing the power setting and length (time) of treatment allows different ablation zones to be created. The connection from the generator is a coaxial cable, which can be bulky, given the extent of insulation required. Grounding pads are not required, given the electromagnetic waves; therefore, there is no risk of grounding pad burns. The electromagnetic waves are also less susceptible to tissue characteristics that cause impedance, resulting in faster treatment times, bigger ablation zones, and less susceptibility to heat sink.[68,69]

Cryoablation

Cryoablation causes cell death in several different ways. First, intracellular ice crystals form, damaging the cell membrane and organelles.[69] Second, extracellular ice crystals induce cell dehydration by changing the osmolality.[69] Third, there is microvascular damage.[71] Finally, apoptosis is induced; however, this mechanism is not well understood.[69] To achieve this, freeze and thaw cycles are alternated, which results in longer ablation times on the order of 30 minutes.[69,72] There is an increase in hyperemia to the ablation zone, which allows breakdown products to move rapidly to the systemic circulation and can induce cryoshock.

Two common cryogens are argon and liquid nitrogen; however, their properties require different delivery systems. The heat exchange is caused by the expansion of argon gas to a liquid, along the probe tip, also known as the Joule–Thompson effect.[71] This heat transfer is passive and is dependent on the probe surface area. The liquid nitrogen system boils or phase shifts to a gas, thus extracting heat from surrounding structures.[71] While lower temperatures can be achieved, this approach is limited by the Leidenfrost phenomenon, in which the gas accumulates around the treatment zone, slowing the delivery of the liquid nitrogen to the tissue. Ideal temperatures are between −40 to 50°C, which are achieved just adjacent to the probe.[71] In both systems, to achieve larger ablation zones, more probes are often required as the lethal ice centers around the probes.[69]

Unique to cryoablation is the ability to visualize the ice ball leading edge with CT or MRI guidance. When treating in close proximity to critical structures such as nerves, bowel, and vessels the ice ball not only can be monitored but can be combined with protective techniques, such as hydrodissection, CO_2 dissection, and temperature monitoring.

Irreversible Electroporation

Electroporation is the process of applying high-electric-field pulses to create pores in the cell membrane.[73,74] Given the correct voltage (magnitude of the pulse) and duration (time), these pores can be so large that the damage is irreversible.[73,74] Reversible formation of these pores has aided in penetration of anticancer agents into cells and gene therapy.[73] In 2011, Thomson et al. showed that irreversible electroporation (IRE) was safe and effective in treating tumor in humans as long as ECG-gating was employed.[75] The mechanism of cell death is not known, but a combination of apoptosis and necrosis has been noted.[74]

Benefits of the therapy are that it is nonthermal when used as recommended.[74,76] This allows for ablation adjacent to critical structures that are often susceptible to or adversely affect thermal techniques, such as vessels and bile ducts.[77,78] The technique of creating an adequate ablation zone, however, involves placement of multiple electrodes approximately 1 mm in diameter (probes) in a parallel configuration space between 1 and 2.2 cm apart.[75,79] The treatment between pairs is on the order of 70 to 90 pulses (70 µs at 1,000–3,000 V) until a change in amperes is seen to correlate to an adequate drop in resistance.[73,75] The active electrode exposure can be adjusted.[75] When treating larger lesions, it follows that the complete treatment time can be long as shown in one series to have effective IRE delivery time on average 43 minutes and procedure time 190 minutes.[73] Elevated liver function tests are transient, not dissimilar to RFA.[80,81] In the liver, it has been shown that the hypoattenuating postablation zones decrease in size on follow-up dramatically, suggesting repair due to intact skeletal matrix, unlike thermal ablations, for which treatment zones persist, especially RFA.[80]

High-Intensity Focused Ultrasound

HIFU is a noninvasive approach to thermal ablation by focusing the ultrasound beam to raise tissue temperature and induce coagulation necrosis.[72,82] The advantage MR-HIFU has over US-guided HIFU is greater lesion characterization, real-time temperature monitoring, and posttreatment tissue evaluation.[83] The safety and efficacy have been established in the treatment of symptomatic uterine fibroids and painful bony lesions.[84–87] Currently, MR-HIFU is primarily indicated for secondary palliation.[86] Real-time guidance with ultrasound or MRI shows ablation zone and early studies have shown promise; however, there are limitations with respiratory gating, time of treatment, and barriers to adequate beam delivery.[71,88]

Additional Ablation Strategies

Other strategies include chemical ablation, cementoplasty, and laser photocoagulation. Chemical agents include but are not limited to ethanol, 50% acetic acid, steroids, sclerosants, and chemotherapeutic agents. This involves direct injection of the agent, but is dependent on diffusion through the tumor. Ablation volumes are unpredictable, but the treatment may be performed with small needles and repeated as needed.[71,72]

Percutaneous injection of polymethylmethacrylate (PMMA) or cementoplasty has been shown to offer pain relief and strengthen bone against compressive forces. Image guidance of CT or fluoroscopy aids to avoid intravasation or cement leakage. Cementoplasty has been effective in palliation of osteolytic bone metastases as a single therapy and along with ablation.[71,72]

Laser photocoagulation (Nd: YAG laser) uses the energy from infrared light to heat and ablate tumors. The applicators are small. They produce small ablation zones therefore are used for small tumors.[72]

Margins

Patient selection is not just dependent on patient performance status but also on lesion size and location. Heat-based thermal techniques are limited when lesions are adjacent to critical structures, such as vessels and nerves.[69,72,89] The ability to visualize ice ball in cryoablation can be used to control proximity of ablation to nerves.[72,89] IRE probes can abut vessels with minimal damage.[77] However, to achieve adequate treatment, anticipated ablation zones should provide adequate margins at least on the order of 5 mm.[90] This is difficult to achieve for lesions over 3 cm in size.[90]

Indications

Bone and Soft Tissue Tumors

While radiation therapy and surgery remain the main approach to painful skeletal metastases, it is reported that up to 30% of patients do not receive pain relief.[70] Ablation can provide an alternative in these cases. In a study performed by Goetz et al., 43 patients with painful bone metastases were treated by image guided RFA, including three patients with sarcoma; 95% of patients reported a clinically significant decrease in pain.[70] This was followed by a decreased opioid requirement as well after 8 weeks of the intervention.[70] Callstrom et al. showed in a prospective multicenter trial that cryoablation is also a durable method to ameliorate pain from bone metastases.[91] A combination of cryoablation and cementoplasty can help with pain control and improve mobility.[92,93]

Sarcoma specific data are limited and often combined in series with treatment of bone metastases.[94,95] Li et al. reported on a pair of studies to perform joint-sparing cryoablation (12 patients) and MWA (11 patients) of juxta-articular osteosarcoma.[96,97] Functional outcomes were good in both series, and only one patient had recurrence in the soft tissue.[96,97] Three patients in the cryoablation study developed pulmonary metastases.[97] Saumet et al. reported on seven patients with local recurrence or bone metastases from osteosarcoma, where the three patients who underwent curative RFA maintained complete remission beyond 45 months.[98] Several studies report improvement in pain relief of primary malignant bone tumors with HIFU.[85,99,100] In one series of 80 patients, complete necrosis was achieved in 86% of tumors, but 40 experienced complications, of which 14 patients required surgical intervention.[100] These include third-degree skin burn, bone fractures, epiphysiolysis, and secondary infections.[100] In the other two series, complication rates were dramatically lower; however, complete ablation was only achieved in 7% and 46% of patients.[85,99]

Chondroblastoma

Ablation can be used as an alternative to surgical curettage for chondroblastoma. Owing to the common location in the epiphysis and apophysis, surgical intervention can result in limb shortening and early osteoarthritis.[72,101–103] Reports of this approach are small.[101,102] Xie et al. reviewed 25 patients who underwent RFA for lesions that were on average 2 cm, with 88% of patients reporting complete relief of symptoms.[103] Rate of local recurrence was 12%, which is not dissimilar to those reported in surgery.[72,103] Rybak et al. reported on a series of 17 patients, of which 100% reported immediate pain relief, and of those who were not lost to follow-up, 93% did not require further pain medications.[104] Recurrence rate was 6%, resulting in the single adverse event of delayed articular collapse.[104] Hospital stays were very short, often one night.[72]

Desmoids

Several studies have shown safe and effective ablation of extra-abdominal desmoid tumors, which tend to be very locally aggressive.[94,105–107] Havez et al. treated 13 patients and had a disease-free survival

(DFS) rate of 82%, with local recurrence in two patients (12%) after 2 years.[106] Kujak et al. reported on five patients; two patients with less than 5-cm lesions showed resolution and complete pain response.[105] For the two lesions over 9 cm, size reduction was minimal and pain reduction returned to baseline.[105] Schmitz et al. treated 18 patients with 26 tumors, and showed volume reduction in 95.7% of lesions and complete response in 39%.[107] Progressive disease was seen in 4.3% of patients.[107] Muscular injury, though a concern, is often negligible when treating soft tissue tumors. Bing et al. described myositis that was seen in over 87% of patients and was only symptomatic in two of 21 patients.[108] A case example is shown in Figure 30.4.

Complications

Concerns are proximity to critical structures and technical issues regarding the devices and when performing ablation in bone risk of fracture. For example, in the study performed by Goetz et al., one patient had transient bowel and bladder incontinence when targeting the upper sacrum, one patient had a skin burn from grounding pad, and one patient had a fracture of the acetabulum 6 weeks after RFA that required surgical arthroplasty.[70] Neural injury rates when treating bone and soft tissue tumors range between 0% and 25%.[89] Though rare, injury to the artery of Adamkiewicz or the great anterior segmental radiculomedullary artery, which through the anterior spinal artery supplies the anterior two-thirds of the spinal cord, can result in paraplegia.[89] Littrup et al. reported on 220 cyroablation procedures for oligometastatic soft tissue tumors and showed a complication rate of only 2.3%.[109]

Avoiding Complications

After identifying the structure at risk, different techniques can be employed to mitigate risks without compromising efficacy. Two main problems are visibility and proximity. In the case of neural structures, MR guidance provides unique visibility that CT guidance cannot.[89] Contrast agent or CO_2 injection can help outline nerves.[89]

Optimizing the distance away from critical structures can be done by careful selection of approach, for example, transpedicular access to the vertebral body rather than parapedicular. Displacement techniques vary between the use of liquid, gas, or balloons. With hydrodissection of artificial ascites, nonionic solutions are preferred in the setting of RFA to prevent inadvertent energy conduction to adjacent structures.[89] CO_2 is preferred over room air not only because it is a better insulator, but to prevent risks such as air embolism and pneumocephalus.[89] Maintaining a safe skin temperature can eliminate the risk of skin injury. For example, when performing cryoablation, warm the skin with gauze soaked in warm water or fill a sterile glove with warm water and apply it to the area in question.[89] An example is shown in Figure 30.4.

When critical structures, such as the nerves, cannot be avoided, monitoring can be performed to avoid reaching critical temperatures. Neural injury occurs when temperatures reach below 10°C and above 44°C.[89] Thermocouples can be placed in the epidural space or between the nerve and the impending ablation zone to give real-time feedback of risk. Monitoring of somatosensory or motor evoked potentials can be evaluated during ablation to detect injury, but at times this may already be irreversible.[89]

Liver

Image-guided ablation has been shown to be safe and effective in treating primary and oligometastatic disease in the liver.[110] Approaches are mixed between percutaneous, laparoscopic, and open surgery in order of increasing invasiveness. The goal of ablation is to provide local control requiring at minimum 5 mm margins in a full 360 degrees around the tumor; however, 1-cm margins are better at reducing local progression.[90,110]

RFA, MWA, cryoablation, and IRE have been shown to be effective with different benefits of each treatment. In general, RFA has a high rate of local control in tumor less than 3 cm and is well supported in the literature.[71,110] However, it is susceptible to heat sink, requires grounding pads, has longer ablation times, and may cause thermal injury to adjacent structures. MWA is a new technology with less wealth of evidence, but can ablate lesions greater than 3 cm effectively.[71,110] While MWA is less susceptible to heat sink, there is a greater risk of thermal injury than RFA.[69,110] Cryoablation provides the ability to perform large ablations and the ice ball is visible. However, there is a higher risk of bleeding and cryoshock.[110,111] IRE allows treatment very close to critical structures without any impact of heat sink.[77,78] However, treatment times are longer, requiring neuromuscular blockage (anesthesia) and cardiac gating.[75]

Data specific to ablation of sarcoma metastases in the liver are limited a few series. Littrup et al. and Thomson et al. showed safety of efficacy of liver ablation metastatic sarcoma to the liver for

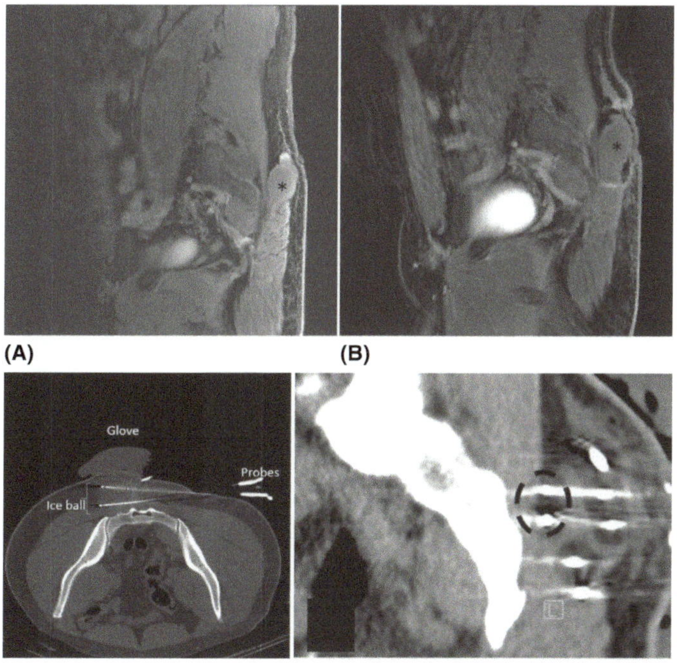

FIGURE 30.4 A 42-year-old man with a biopsy-proven desmoid on his right lower back causing pressure and discomfort when he exercises and limits his ability to perform all the aspects of his work. This did not respond to celecoxib. He is referred for cryoablation to palliate and control the lesion, which measured approximately 3.5 x 4.8 x 5.0 cm at the time of treatment. Procedure was performed under general anesthesia. Seven probes were positioned around the lesion. To limit skin injury, the subcutaneous fat was infiltrated with saline. During the freezing, a sterile glove filled with warm saline was placed on the skin as well. The patient tolerated the procedure well and was discharged the next day. There was minimal postprocedure numbness over the right gluteal region. Over the next 6 months, he noted decreased pressure. He was able to resume his original exercise routine and return to full duty at work. (A) Sagittal image of a contrast-enhanced MRI showing homogeneous enhancement of the mass extending above the right gluteus muscle (asterisk). (B) Sagittal image of a contrast-enhanced MRI obtained 6 months after ablation, showing decreased enhancement and rim denoting margin of ablation zone (asterisk). (C) A pair of probes covering the mid aspect of the mass after initial 10-minute freeze cycle. (D) Saggital reformatted image showing small ice balls around each probe (dotted circle) after initial 5 minutes into first freeze cycle.

cryoablation and IRE, respectively.[75,111] RFA in the treatment of GIST liver metastases combined with tyrosine kinase inhibitor therapy (TKI) has been shown to be feasible and safe.[112,113] In a unique study performed by Hakimé et al., three cohorts were compared one with RFA after TKI therapy was discontinue with 2-year PFS rate of 29%, a second where curative RFA was performed and TKI therapy was maintained with a 2-year PFS rate of 75%, and a third where RFA was performed only on those lesions progressing under TKI therapy with a 2-year PFS rate of 20%.[112] This suggests that ablation should be approached with curative intent and that TKI therapy should be maintained for improved results.[112] In a study by Jones et al., similar 2-year OS of 77% was achieved with the combination of RFA and imatinib.[113] Both series were small with 17 and 13 patients, respectively.[112,113] Jones et al. studied another 12 patients with a mixture of leiomyosarcoma, chondrosarcoma, and fibrosarcoma metastases to the liver who did not respond as well with a 2-year OS rate of 40%.[113,114] Gravel et al. studied a series of thermal ablation (RFA, MWA, and cryoablation) of leiomyosarcoma metastases to the liver and found 1, 3, and 5-year OS rates of 96%, 62%, and 28%, respectively.[114] Thomson et al. showed that IRE was safe and effective to control epitheloid hepatic hemandioendothelioma (HEHE) within their large initial series and followed this with a report suggesting it may be efficacious to add antibiotics.[75,79] A case example is presented in Figure 30.5.

Major complication rates reported after percutaneous image-guided thermal ablation are low, ranging between 2% and 5%.[115] A review of 1000 RFA treatments revealed tumor seeding (1.5%), liver abscess formation (0.7%), hemorrhage requiring transfusion (0.4%), pleural effusion requiring thoracentesis (0.4%), hepatic infarction (0.2%), bronchobiliary fistula (0.2%), pneumothorax requiring intervention (0.1%), hemothorax requiring drainage (0.1%), bile peritonitis (0.1%), bowel injury

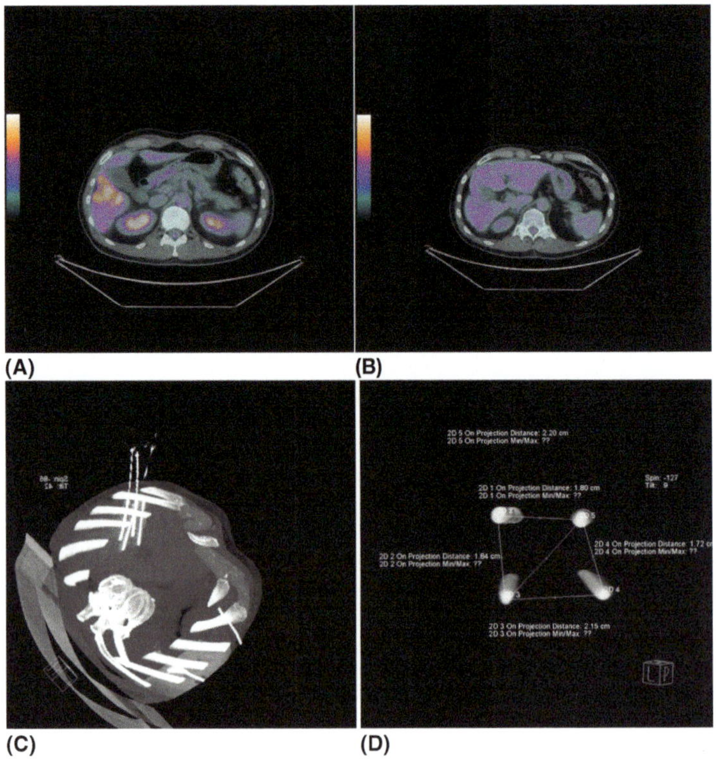

FIGURE 30.5 A 50-year-old man was found to have multiple liver lesions that on biopsy proved to be hepatic epithelioid hemangioendothelioma (HEHE). He was referred for IRE for local control. Owing to pain on the right side, the fluorodeoxyglucose (FDG) avid segment VI lesion was targeted. The lesion measured 5.2 x 3.4 x 4.5 cm. Because of its size, four treatments were performed dividing the lesion into cranial and caudal components. Probes were exposed to 2.5 cm. A mixture of four, five, and three probe arrays were used to cover the area. Immediate pain procedure was managed with patient-controlled anesthesia pump. This resolved and the patient continues to state that initial pain has not returned. At 3-month follow-up, PET/CT shows resolution of the segment VI lesion, but progression in segment VII. He later underwent an IRE of segment VII lesion. This showed partial response and appears stable on follow-up imaging. (A) Axial fused PET/CT image showing FDG avid lesion in segment VI adjacent to the gallbladder. (B) Axial fused PET/CT image from 3-month follow-up scan, which showed no residual activity. (C) Volume rendering technique shows the spacing and approach in the intercostal spaces of a four-probe IRE array. (D) Maximum intensity projection of the probe tips en face to measure distances between the pairs to allow for treatment.

IRE, irreversible electroporation.

(0.3%), biloma (0.7%), portal vein thrombosis (0.4%), hemobilia (0.3%), and skin burns (0.3%.)[116] Postablation syndrome as marked by malaise, nausea, vomiting, fever, and body aches, which is usually self-limiting, was reported in up to 18% of thermal and 15% of IRE treatments.[117] Infection and abscess formation are more frequently in patients with a bilioenteric anastomosis or prior biliary manipulation with rates as 50% to 100%, but can be decreased dramatically with extended prophylactic antibiotic therapy.[115] With cryoablation in the large series reported by Littrup et al., death from cryoshock was reported in 1.2% of the cohort.[111] Decrease in platelets and hemoglobin was seen in 5.2% of cases, but was dramatically less when controlled for initial platelet counts and tumors greater than 4 cm.[111] In the same series, reactive pleural effusion that required intervention was seen in 1.2% of the patients.[111] One patient had a bowel injury.[111]

Lung Metastases

Ablation of lung metastasis has been shown to be safe and effective with RFA, cryoablation, and MWA.[118–121] As shown in a prospective Phase II trial performed by Ricke et al., IRE was not effective in the treatment of lung metastases, with high local recurrence rates likely related to the interference of the air.[122] Determinants of success include size and location of tumors. Generally, ablation has been successful with tumors as large as 3.5 cm, with planned ablation achieving at least 5 mm margin.[120,121,123] Multiple tumors can be treated in one setting; however, bilateral treatment is not recommended.[118,123] Preferred location is in the outer two-thirds of the lung to decrease bleeding risk and bronchopulmonary fistula risk.[124]

Centers vary between performing the ablations under general anesthesia versus moderate conscious sedation.[121,124]

In theory, MWA should be more effective than RFA as ventilated lung has a high electrical resistivity.[120] However, meta-analysis has shown improved median OS of 34.8 months over 18.7 months with RFA over MWA for pulmonary metastasis.[121] MWA technology does continue to evolve, as does operator experience.[68] Cryoablation can create larger ablation zones, offers pain control benefits, and is often preferred when tumors are pleural based.[118]

In a unique study, seven centers reported on their experience with pulmonary tumor RFA complications for a combined 493 procedures.[124] While pneumothoraxes occurred in up to 30% of interventions, less than 10% required drainage.[124] Mortality rate was approximately 0.4%.[124] Of the pleural effusions that developed, only 10% needed drainage.[124] This mirrors the meta-analysis performed by Yuan et al., in which pneumothoraces were reported in ~34% of cases, of which only ~12% required intervention.[121] In this analysis, the rate of pleural effusions were less ~5% to 10%, of which only 0.6% required drainage.[121] Bronchopleural fistula is very rarely reported on the order of 0.5% and can be treated by pleurodesis, bronchoscopic, or surgical repair.[120,125] The effect of ablation on pulmonary function is generally self-limiting, unless severe pleuritis is induced or large parenchymal volumes are ablated, but is still shown to be less than surgery and stereotactic body radiation therapy (SBRT).[67,119,120,126] NTS is rarely reported to be 0.3% per RFA treatment in a cohort of 374 patients with 1,024 tumor treated.[67,127]

Ablation of lung metastases from sarcomas has been reported within larger cohorts as safe and effective.[118,119,121] Those that are specific to sarcoma show negative prognostic factors including noncurative ablation and extrapulmonary metastasis.[123,128] For example, in one study to treat lung metastases from musculoskeletal sarcomas, 1- and 3-year survival rates after RFA were 58% and 29% for all patients and 89% and 59% when complete tumor ablation was performed.[128] For those patients who underwent incomplete ablation, 1 and 3-year survival rates were 30% and 0%.[128] Another study of RFA of lung metastases from sarcoma reported 1- and 3-year survival rates of 80% and 47% for all patients, and 100% and 63% for curative ablation.[123] Overall, lung ablation is safe and can offer local control of pulmonary metastases.

SUMMARY

Sarcoma management requires participation by the interventional radiology team to provide adequate biopsies and appropriate venous access to allow for chemotherapy delivery. Moving beyond these established roles offers unique opportunities for local control and treatment. Percutaneous image-guided ablation of liver, lung, soft tissue, and bone metastases from sarcoma is safe. Data regarding primary lesions are limited. Palliation of pain, particularly of bone lesions, is well established. The ability to target lesions selectively through the intraarterial route can augment local control, especially when tumors are resistant to systemic agents. As the technology available to interventional radiologists and the techniques continue to advance, further investigation is required to establish their role in current sarcoma treatment algorithms.

REFERENCES

1. Bagaria SP, Chang YH, Gray RJ, et al. Improving long-term outcomes for patients with extra-abdominal soft tissue sarcoma regionalization to high-volume centers, improved compliance with guidelines or both? *Sarcoma*. 2018;2018:8141056. doi:10.1155/2018/8141056
2. Hoekstra HJ, Haas RLM, Verhoef C, et al. Adherence to guidelines for adult (Non-GIST) soft tissue sarcoma in the Netherlands: a plea for dedicated sarcoma centers. *Ann Surg Oncol*. 2017;24(11):3279–3288. doi:10.1245/s10434-017-6003-3
3. Casali PG, Bielack S, Abecassis N, et al. Bone sarcomas: ESMO-PaedCan-EURACAN Clinical Practice Guidelines for diagnosis, treatment and follow-up. *Ann Oncol*. 2018;29(Suppl 4):iv79–iv95. doi:10.1093/annonc/mdy310
4. ESMO/European Sarcoma Network Working Group. Soft tissue and visceral sarcomas: ESMO Clinical Practice Guidelines for diagnosis, treatment and follow-up. *Ann Oncol*. 2014;25(suppl 3):iii102–iii12. doi:10.1093/annonc/mdu254
5. Hangiandreou NJ. AAPM/RSNA physics tutorial for residents. Topics in US: B-mode US: basic concepts and new technology. *Radiographics*. 2003;23(4):1019–1033. doi:10.1148/rg.234035034
6. Jacobs MA, Ibrahim TS, Ouwerkerk R. AAPM/RSNA physics tutorials for residents: MR imaging: brief overview and emerging applications. *Radiographics*. 2007;27(4):1213–1229. doi:10.1148/rg.274065115

7. Becher S, Oskouei S. PET imaging in sarcoma. *Orthop Clin North Am*. 2015;46(3):409–415, xi. doi:10.1016/jocl.2015.03.001
8. Shaw CM, Shah S, Kapoor BS, et al. ACR appropriateness criteria radiologic management of central venous access. *J Am Coll Radiol*. 2017;14(11S):S506–S529. doi:10.1016/j.jacr.2017.08.053
9. Kaufman JA. Upper extremity, neck, and central thoracic veins. In: Kaufman J, Lee MJ, eds. *Vascular and Interventional Radiology: The Requisites*. 2nd ed. Philadelphia, PA: Elsevier; 2014:136–158.
10. Verboom MC, Ouwerkerk J, Steeghs N, et al. Central venous access related adverse events after trabectedin infusions in soft tissue sarcoma patients; experience and management in a nationwide multi-center study. *Clin Sarcoma Res*. 2017;7:2. doi:10.1186/s13569-017-0066-6
11. Dariushnia SR, Wallace MJ, Siddiqi NH, et al. Quality improvement guidelines for central venous access. *J Vasc Interv Radiol*. 2010;21(7):976–981. doi:10.1016/j.jvir.2010.03.006
12. Valji K. Vascular access placement and foreign body retrieval. In: Valji K, ed. *The Practice of Interventional Radiology*. Philadelphia, PA: Elsevier; 2012:559–580.
13. Patel IJ, Davidson JC, Nikolic B, et al. Consensus guidelines for periprocedural management of coagulation status and hemostasis risk in percutaneous image-guided interventions. *J Vasc Interv Radiol*. 2012;23(6):727–736. doi:10.1016/j.jvir.2012.02.012
14. Silberzweig JE, Sacks D, Khorsandi AS, et al. Reporting standards for central venous access. *J Vasc Interv Radiol*. 2003;14(9 Pt 2):S443–S452. doi:10.1097/01.rvi.0000094617.61428.bc
15. Haddadin Y, Regunath H. Central line associated blood stream infections (CLABSI). In: *StatPearls*. Treasure Island, FL: StatPearls Publishing; 2020. https://www.ncbi.nlm.nih.gov/books/NBK430891
16. Miller DL, O'Grady NP, Society of Interventional Radiology. Guidelines for the prevention of intravascular catheter-related infections: recommendations relevant to interventional radiology for venous catheter placement and maintenance. *J Vasc Interv Radiol*. 2012;23(8):997–1007. doi:10.1016/j.jvir.2012.04.023
17. Trieu J, Sinnathamby M, Di Bella C, et al. Biopsy and the diagnostic evaluation of musculoskeletal tumours: critical but often missed in the 21st century. *ANZ J Surg*. 2016;86(3):133–138. doi:10.1111/ans.13251
18. Welker JA, Henshaw RM, Jelinek J, et al. The percutaneous needle biopsy is safe and recommended in the diagnosis of musculoskeletal masses. *Cancer*. 2000;89(12):2677–2686. doi:10.1002/1097-0142(20001215)89:12<2677::aid-cncr22>3.0.co;2-l
19. Traina F, Errani C, Toscano A, et al. Current concepts in the biopsy of musculoskeletal tumors. *J Bone Joint Surg Am*. 2015;97(1):e7. doi:10.2106/JBJS.N.00661
20. Sinha S, Peach AH. Diagnosis and management of soft tissue sarcoma. *BMJ*. 2010;341:c7170. doi:10.1136/bmj.c7170
21. Irani FG, Buy X, Gangi A. Musculoskeletal intervention. In: Kaufman J, Lee MJ, eds. *Vascular and Inverventional Radiology: The Requisites*. 2nd ed. Philadelphia, PA: Elsevier; 2014:527–546
22. Aryafar H, Kinney TB. Percutaneous biopsy. In: Valji K, ed. *The Practice of Interventional Radiology*. Philadelphia, PA: Elsevier; 2012:84–105.
23. Gupta S, Wallace MJ, Cardella JF, et al. Quality improvement guidelines for percutaneous needle biopsy. *J Vasc Interv Radiol*. 2010;21(7):969–975. doi:10.1016/j.jvir.2010.01.011
24. UyBico SJ, Motamedi K, Omura MC, et al. Relevance of compartmental anatomic guidelines for biopsy of musculoskeletal tumors: retrospective review of 363 biopsies over a 6-year period. *J Vasc Interv Radiol*. 2012;23(4):511–518, 518.e1–2. doi:10.1016/j.jvir.2012.01.058
25. Berger-Richardson D, Swallow CJ. Needle tract seeding after percutaneous biopsy of sarcoma: risk/benefit considerations. *Cancer*. 2017;123(4):560–567. doi:10.1002/cncr.30370
26. Wu CC, Maher MM, Shepard JA. Complications of CT-guided percutaneous needle biopsy of the chest: prevention and management. *AJR Am J Roentgenol*. 2011;196(6):W678–W682. doi:10.2214/AJR.10.4659
27. Hessel SJ, Adams DF, Abrams HL. Complications of angiography. *Radiology*. 1981;138(2):273–281. doi:10.1148/radiology.138.2.7455105
28. Iezzi R, Pompili M, Posa A, et al. Transradial versus transfemoral access for hepatic chemoembolization: intrapatient prospective single-center study. *J Vasc Interv Radiol*. 2017;28(9):1234–1239. doi:10.1016/j.jvir.2017.06.022
29. Kandarpa K, Machan L, Durham J. *Handbook of interventional radiologic procedures*. 5th ed. New York, NY: Wolters Kluwer; 2016.
30. Morgan R, Belli AM. Current treatment methods for postcatheterization pseudoaneurysms. *J Vasc Interv Radiol*. 2003;14(6):697–710. doi:10.1097/01.RVI.0000071089.76348.6A
31. Singh R, Zughaib M. Timeout for contrast: using physician behavior modification to reduce contrast in the catheterization laboratory. *Cardiol Res Pract*. 2019;2019:9238124. doi:10.1155/2019/9238124
32. Brar SS, Aharonian V, Mansukhani P, et al. Haemodynamic-guided fluid administration for the prevention of contrast-induced acute kidney injury: the POSEIDON randomised controlled trial. *Lancet*. 2014;383(9931):1814–1823. doi:10.1016/S0140-6736(14)60689-9
33. Yang H, Seon J, Sung PO, et al. Dexamethasone prophylaxis to alleviate postembolization syndrome after transarterial chemoembolization for hepatocellular carcinoma: a randomized, double-blinded, placebo-controlled study. *J Vasc Interv Radiol*. 2017;28(11):1503.e2–1511.e2. doi:10.1016/j.jvir.2017.07.021
34. Riaz A, Lewandowski RJ, Kulik LM, et al. Complications following radioembolization with yttrium-90 microspheres: a comprehensive literature review. *J Vasc Interv Radiol*. 2009;20(9):1121–1130; quiz 1131. doi:10.1016/j.jvir.2009.05.030

35. Salem R, Gilbertsen M, Butt Z, et al. Increased quality of life among hepatocellular carcinoma patients treated with radioembolization, compared with chemoembolization. *Clin Gastroenterol Hepatol*. 2013;11(10):1358.e1–1365.e1. doi:10.1016/j.cgh.2013.04.028
36. Balter S. Reducing unnecessary radiation in fluoroscopically guided interventional procedures: vigilance and feedback are needed. *Radiology*. 2019;290(3):750–751. doi:10.1148/radiol.2019182738
37. Laurent O, Ancelet S, Richardson DB, et al. Potential impacts of radon, terrestrial gamma and cosmic rays on childhood leukemia in France: a quantitative risk assessment. *Radiat Environ Biophys*. 2013;52(2):195–209. doi:10.1007/s00411-013-0464-y
38. Steele JR, Jones AK, Ninan EP. Quality initiatives: establishing an interventional radiology patient radiation safety program. *Radiographics*. 2012;32(1):277–287. doi:10.1148/rg.321115002
39. Pierce DB, Johnson GE, Monroe E, et al. Safety and Efficacy Outcomes of Embolization in Hepatic Sarcomas. *AJR Am J Roentgenol*. 2018;210(1):175–182. doi:10.2214/AJR.16.17573
40. Cao G, Zhu X, Li J, et al. A comparative study between Embosphere(®) and conventional transcatheter arterial chemoembolization for treatment of unresectable liver metastasis from GIST. *Chin J Cancer Res*. 2014;26(1):124–131. doi:10.3978/j.issn.1000-9604.2014.02.11
41. Kobayashi K, Gupta S, Trent JC, et al. Hepatic artery chemoembolization for 110 gastrointestinal stromal tumors: response, survival, and prognostic factors. *Cancer*. 2006;107(12):2833–2841. doi:10.1002/cncr.22336
42. Kobayashi K, Szklaruk J, Trent JC, et al. Hepatic arterial embolization and chemoembolization for imatinib-resistant gastrointestinal stromal tumors. *Am J Clin Oncol*. 2009;32(6):574–581. doi:10.1097/COC.0b013e31819cca35
43. Murthy R, Nunez R, Szklaruk J, et al. Yttrium-90 microsphere therapy for hepatic malignancy: devices, indications, technical considerations, and potential complications. *Radiographics*. 2005;25 Suppl 1:S41-55. doi:10.1148/rg.25si055515
44. Atassi B, Bangash AK, Bahrani A, et al. Multimodality imaging following 90Y radioembolization: a comprehensive review and pictorial essay. *Radiographics*. 2008;28(1):81–99. doi:10.1148/rg.281065721
45. Maluccio MA, Covey AM, Schubert J, et al. Treatment of metastatic sarcoma to the liver with bland embolization. *Cancer*. 2006;107(7):1617–1623. doi:10.1002/cncr.22191
46. Cao G, Li J, Shen L, Zhu X. Transcatheter arterial chemoembolization for gastrointestinal stromal tumors with liver metastases. *World J Gastroenterol*. 2012;18(42):6134–6140. doi:10.3748/wjg.v18.i42.6134
47. Mavligit GM, Zukwiski AA, Ellis LM, et al. Gastrointestinal leiomyosarcoma metastatic to the liver. Durable tumor regression by hepatic chemoembolization infusion with cisplatin and vinblastine. *Cancer*. 1995;75(8):2083–2088. doi:10.1002/1097-0142(19950415)75:::aid-cncr2820750809>3.0.co;2-h
48. Mavligit GM, Zukiwski AA, Salem PA, et al. Regression of hepatic metastases from gastrointestinal leiomyosarcoma after hepatic arterial chemoembolization. *Cancer*. 1991;68(2):321–323. doi:10.1002/1097-0142(19910715)68:::aid-cncr2820680219>3.0.co;2-b
49. Miller MD, Sze DY, Padia SA, et al. Response and Overall Survival for Yttrium-90 Radioembolization of Hepatic Sarcoma: A Multicenter Retrospective Study. *J Vasc Interv Radiol*. 2018;29(6):867–873. doi:10.1016/j.jvir.2018.01.775
50. Rajan DK, Soulen MC, Clark TW, et al. Sarcomas metastatic to the liver: response and survival after cisplatin, doxorubicin, mitomycin-C, Ethiodol, and polyvinyl alcohol chemoembolization. *J Vasc Interv Radiol*. 2001;12(2):187–193. doi:10.1016/s1051-0443(07)61824-7
51. Rathmann N, Diehl SJ, Dinter D, et al. Radioembolization in patients with progressive gastrointestinal stromal tumor liver metastases undergoing treatment with tyrosine kinase inhibitors. *J Vasc Interv Radiol*. 2015;26(2):231–238. doi:10.1016/j.jvir.2014.09.020
52. Khan W, Sullivan KL, McCann JW, et al. Moxifloxacin prophylaxis for chemoembolization or embolization in patients with previous biliary interventions: a pilot study. *AJR Am J Roentgenol*. 2011;197(2):W343-5. doi:10.2214/AJR.10.6019
53. Cullen JW, Jamroz BA, Stevens SL, et al. The value of serial arteriography in osteosarcoma: delivery of chemotherapy, determination of therapy duration, and prediction of necrosis. *J Vasc Interv Radiol*. 2005;16(8):1107–1119. doi:10.1097/01.RVI.0000167856.31329.F8
54. Bacci G, Ferrari S, Tienghi A, et al. A comparison of methods of loco-regional chemotherapy combined with systemic chemotherapy as neo-adjuvant treatment of osteosarcoma of the extremity. *Eur J Surg Oncol*. 2001;27(1):98–104. doi:10.1053/ejso.2000.1056
55. Winkler K, Bielack SS, Delling G, et al. Treatment of osteosarcoma: experience of the Cooperative Osteosarcoma Study Group (COSS). Cancer Treat Res. 1993;62:269–277. doi:10.1007/978-1-4615-3518-8_32
56. Jaffe N, Robertson R, Ayala A, et al. Comparison of intra-arterial cis-diamminedichloroplatinum II with high-dose methotrexate and citrovorum factor rescue in the treatment of primary osteosarcoma. J Clin Oncol. 1985;3(8):1101–1104. doi:10.1200/JCO.1985.3.8.1101
57. Kempf RA, Irwin LE, Menendez L, et al. Limb salvage surgery for bone and soft tissue sarcoma. A phase II pathologic study of preoperative intraarterial cisplatin. *Cancer*. 1991;68(4):738–743. doi:10.1002/1097-0142(19910815)68:::aid-cncr2820680413>3.0.co;2-j
58. Rao BN, Rodriguez-Galindo C. Intra-arterial cisplatin in osteosarcoma: same question, different answer. Ann Surg Oncol. 2003;10(5):481–483. doi:10.1245/aso.2003.04.903
59. Jaffe N, Raymond AK, Ayala A, et al. Effect of cumulative courses of intraarterial cis-diamminedichloroplatin-II on the primary tumor in osteosarcoma. *Cancer*. 1989;63(1):63–67. doi:10.1002/1097-0142(19890101)63:::aid-cncr2820630110>3.0.co;2-o

60. Bacci G, Ferrari S, Longhi A, et al.; Italian Sarcoma Group/Scandinavian Sarcoma Group. High dose ifosfamide in combination with high dose methotrexate, adriamycin and cisplatin in the neoadjuvant treatment of extremity osteosarcoma: preliminary results of an Italian Sarcoma Group/Scandinavian Sarcoma Group pilot study. *J Chemother*. 2002;14(2):198–206. doi:10.1179/joc.2002.14.2.198
61. Harrison DJ, Geller DS, Gill JD, et al. Current and future therapeutic approaches for osteosarcoma. *Expert Rev Anticancer Ther*. 2018;18(1):39–50. doi:10.1080/14737140.2018.1413939
62. Rha SY, Chung HC, Gong SJ, et al. Combined pre-operative chemotherapy with intra-arterial cisplatin and continuous intravenous adriamycin for high grade osteosarcoma. Oncol Rep. 1999;6(3):631–637. doi:10.3892/or.6.3.631
63. Zhang H-J, Yang J-J, Lu J-P, et al. Use of intra-arterial chemotherapy and embolization before limb salvage surgery for osteosarcoma of the lower extremity. *Cardiovasc Intervent Radiol*. 2009;32(4):672–678. doi:10.1007/s00270-009-9546-2
64. Wilkins RM, Cullen JW, Odom L, et al. Superior survival in treatment of primary nonmetastatic pediatric osteosarcoma of the extremity. Ann Surg Oncol. 2003;10(5):498–507. doi:10.1245/aso.2003.03.061
65. Robertson L, Andras A, Colgan F, Jackson R. Vascular closure devices for femoral arterial puncture site haemostasis. *Cochrane Database Syst Rev*. 2016;3:CD009541. doi:10.1002/14651858.CD009541.pub2
66. Hugate RR, Wilkins RM, Kelly CM, et al. Intraarterial chemotherapy for extremity osteosarcoma and MFH in adults. Clin Orthop Relat Res. 2008;466(6):1292–1301. doi:10.1007/s11999-008-0252-1
67. de Baere T, Tselikas L, Gravel G, et al. Interventional radiology: role in the treatment of sarcomas. *Eur J Cancer*. 2018;94:148–155. doi:10.1016/j.ejca.2018.02.017
68. Simon CJ, Dupuy DE, Mayo-Smith WW. Microwave ablation: principles and applications. *Radiographics*. 2005;25(suppl 1):S69–S83. doi:10.1148/rg.25si055501
69. Hinshaw JL, Lubner MG, Ziemlewicz TJ, et al. Percutaneous tumor ablation tools: microwave, radiofrequency, or cryoablation—what should you use and why? *Radiographics*. 2014;34(5):1344–1362. doi:10.1148/rg.345140054
70. Goetz MP, Callstrom MR, Charboneau JW, et al. Percutaneous image-guided radiofrequency ablation of painful metastases involving bone: a multicenter study. *J Clin Oncol*. 2004;22(2):300–306. doi:10.1200/JCO.2004.03.097
71. Mueller PR, Adam A, eds. *Interventional Oncology: A Practical Guide for the Interventional Radiologist*. New York, NY: Springer Publishing; 2012.
72. Foster RC, Stavas JM. Bone and soft tissue ablation. *Semin Intervent Radiol*. 2014;31(2):167–179. doi:10.1055/s-0034-1373791
73. Dunki-Jacobs EM, Philips P, Martin RC 2nd. Evaluation of resistance as a measure of successful tumor ablation during irreversible electroporation of the pancreas. *J Am Coll Surg*. 2014;218(2):179–187. doi:10.1016/j.jamcollsurg.2013.10.013
74. Golberg A, Yarmush ML. Nonthermal irreversible electroporation: fundamentals, applications, and challenges. *IEEE Trans Biomed Eng*. 2013;60(3):707–714. doi:10.1109/TBME.2013.2238672
75. Thomson KR, Cheung W, Ellis SJ, et al. Investigation of the safety of irreversible electroporation in humans. *J Vasc Interv Radiol*. 2011;22(5):611–621. doi:10.1016/j.jvir.2010.12.014
76. Faroja M, Ahmed M, Appelbaum L, et al. Irreversible electroporation ablation: is all the damage nonthermal? *Radiology*. 2013;266(2):462–470. doi:10.1148/radiol.12120609
77. Narayanan G, Bhatia S, Echenique A, et al. Vessel patency post irreversible electroporation. *Cardiovasc Intervent Radiol*. 2014;37(6):1523–1529. doi:10.1007/s00270-014-0988-9
78. Silk MT, Wimmer T, Lee KS, et al. Percutaneous ablation of peribiliary tumors with irreversible electroporation. *J Vasc Interv Radiol*. 2014;25(1):112–118. doi:10.1016/j.jvir.2013.10.012
79. Neal RE 2nd, Kavnoudias H, Cheung W, et al. Hepatic epithelioid hemangioendothelioma treated with irreversible electroporation and antibiotics. *J Clin Oncol*. 2013;31(27):e422–e426. doi:10.1200/JCO.2012.44.9736
80. Scheck J, Bruners P, Schindler D, et al. Comparison of chronologic change in the size and contrast-enhancement of ablation zones on CT images after irreversible electroporation and radiofrequency ablation. *Korean J Radiol*. 2018;19(4):560–567. doi:10.3348/kjr.2018.19.4.560
81. Froud T, Venkat SR, Barbery KJ, et al. Liver function tests following irreversible electroporation of liver tumors: experience in 174 procedures. *Tech Vasc Interv Radiol*. 2015;18(3):140–146. doi:10.1053/j.tvir.2015.06.004
82. Rodrigues DB, Stauffer PR, Vrba D, Hurwitz MD. Focused ultrasound for treatment of bone tumours. *Int J Hyperthermia*. 2015;31(3):260–271. doi:10.3109/02656736.2015.1006690
83. Geiger D, Napoli A, Conchiglia A, et al. MR-guided focused ultrasound (MRgFUS) ablation for the treatment of nonspinal osteoid osteoma: a prospective multicenter evaluation. *J Bone Joint Surg Am*. 2014;96(9):743–751. doi:10.2106/JBJS.M.00903
84. Huisman M, Lam MK, Bartels LW, et al. Feasibility of volumetric MRI-guided high intensity focused ultrasound (MR-HIFU) for painful bone metastases. *J Ther Ultrasound*. 2014;2:16. doi:10.1186/2050-5736-2-16
85. Yu W, Tang L, Lin F, et al. High-intensity focused ultrasound: noninvasive treatment for local unresectable recurrence of osteosarcoma. *Surg Oncol*. 2015;24(1):9–15. doi:10.1016/j.suronc.2014.10.001
86. Hurwitz MD, Ghanouni P, Kanaev SV, et al. Magnetic resonance-guided focused ultrasound for patients with painful bone metastases: phase III trial results. *J Natl Cancer Inst*. 2014;106(5). doi:10.1093/jnci/dju082
87. Pron G. Magnetic resonance-guided high-intensity focused ultrasound (MRgHIFU) treatment of symptomatic uterine fibroids: an evidence-based analysis. *Ont Health Technol Assess Ser*. 2015;15(4):1–86. https://www.ncbi.nlm.nih.gov/pmc/articles/PMC4558769

88. Shim J, Staruch RM, Koral K, et al. Pediatric sarcomas are targetable by MR-guided high intensity focused ultrasound (MR-HIFU): anatomical distribution and radiological characteristics. *Pediatr Blood Cancer*. 2016;63(10):1753–1760. doi:10.1002/pbc.26079
89. Kurup AN, Schmit GD, Morris JM, et al. Avoiding complications in bone and soft tissue ablation. *Cardiovasc Intervent Radiol*. 2017;40(2):166–176. doi:10.1007/s00270-016-1487-y
90. Sotirchos VS, Petrovic LM, Gönen M, et al. Colorectal cancer liver metastases: biopsy of the ablation zone and margins can be used to predict oncologic outcome. *Radiology*. 2016;280(3):949–959. doi:10.1148/radiol.2016151005
91. Callstrom MR, Dupuy DE, Solomon SB, et al. Percutaneous image-guided cryoablation of painful metastases involving bone: multicenter trial. *Cancer*. 2013;119(5):1033–1041. doi:10.1002/cncr.27793
92. Coupal TM, Pennycooke K, Mallinson PI, et al. The hopeless case? palliative cryoablation and cementoplasty procedures for palliation of large pelvic bone metastases. *Pain Physician*. 2017;20(7):E1053–E1061. https://www.painphysicianjournal.com/current/pdf?article=NDcxMg%3D%3D&journal=108
93. Deschamps F, de Baere T. Cementoplasty of bone metastases. *Diagn Interv Imaging*. 2012;93(9):685–689. doi:10.1016/j.diii.2012.06.009
94. Thompson SM, Schmitz JJ, Schmit GD, et al. Image-guided thermal ablative therapies in the treatment of sarcoma. *Curr Treat Options Oncol*. 2017;18(4):25. doi:10.1007/s11864-017-0465-1
95. Deschamps F, Farouil G, Ternes N, et al. Thermal ablation techniques: a curative treatment of bone metastases in selected patients? *Eur Radiol*. 2014;24(8):1971–1980. doi:10.1007/s00330-014-3202-1
96. Li J, Guo Z, Wang Z, et al. Does microwave ablation of the tumor edge allow for joint-sparing surgery in patients with osteosarcoma of the proximal tibia? *Clin Orthop Relat Res*. 2015;473(10):3204–3211. doi:10.1007/s11999-015-4447-y
97. Li J, Guo Z, Yang Q, et al. Adjuvant argon-based cryoablation for joint-preserving tumor resection in patients with juxta-articular osteosarcoma around the knee. *Cryobiology*. 2015;71(2):236–243. doi:10.1016/j.cryobiol.2015.07.005
98. Saumet L, Deschamps F, Marec-Berard P, et al. Radiofrequency ablation of metastases from osteosarcoma in patients under 25 years: the SCFE experience. *Pediatr Hematol Oncol*. 2015;32(1):41–49. doi:10.3109/08880018.2014.926469
99. Li C, Zhang W, Fan W, et al. Noninvasive treatment of malignant bone tumors using high-intensity focused ultrasound. *Cancer*. 2010;116(16):3934–3942. doi:10.1002/cncr.25192
100. Chen W, Zhu H, Zhang L, et al. Primary bone malignancy: effective treatment with high-intensity focused ultrasound ablation. *Radiology*. 2010;255(3):967–978. doi:10.1148/radiol.10090374
101. Christie-Large M, Evans N, Davies AM, James SLJ. Radiofrequency ablation of chondroblastoma: procedure technique, clinical and MR imaging follow up of four cases. *Skeletal Radiol*. 2008;37(11):1011–1017. doi:10.1007/s00256-008-0526-4
102. Lalam RK, Cribb GL, Tins BJ, et al. Image guided radiofrequency thermo-ablation therapy of chondroblastomas: should it replace surgery? *Skeletal Radiol*. 2014;43(4):513–522. doi:10.1007/s00256-014-1820-y
103. Xie C, Jeys L, James SLJ. Radiofrequency ablation of chondroblastoma: long-term clinical and imaging outcomes. *Eur Radiol*. 2015;25(4):1127–1134. doi:10.1007/s00330-014-3506-1
104. Rybak LD, Rosenthal DI, Wittig JC. Chondroblastoma: radiofrequency ablation—alternative to surgical resection in selected cases. *Radiology*. 2009;251(2):599–604. doi:10.1148/radiol.2512080500
105. Kujak JL, Liu PT, Johnson GB, Callstrom MR. Early experience with percutaneous cryoablation of extra-abdominal desmoid tumors. *Skeletal Radiol*. 2010;39(2):175–182. doi:10.1007/s00256-009-0801-z
106. Havez M, Lippa N, Al-Ammari S, et al. Percutaneous image-guided cryoablation in inoperable extra-abdominal desmoid tumors: a study of tolerability and efficacy. *Cardiovasc Intervent Radiol*. 2014;37(6):1500–1506. doi:10.1007/s00270-013-0830-9
107. Schmitz JJ, Schmit GD, Atwell TD, et al. Percutaneous cryoablation of extraabdominal desmoid tumors: a 10-year experience. *AJR Am J Roentgenol*. 2016;207(1):190–195. doi:10.2214/AJR.15.14391
108. Bing F, Garnon J, Tsoumakidou G, et al. Imaging-guided percutaneous cryotherapy of bone and soft-tissue tumors: what is the impact on the muscles around the ablation site? *AJR Am J Roentgenol*. 2014;202(6):1361–1365. doi:10.2214/AJR.13.11430
109. Littrup PJ, Bang HJ, Currier BP, et al. Soft-tissue cryoablation in diffuse locations: feasibility and intermediate term outcomes. *J Vasc Interv Radiol*. 2013;24(12):1817–1825. doi:10.1016/j.jvir.2013.06.025
110. Lencioni R, de Baere T, Martin RC, et al. Image-guided ablation of malignant liver tumors: recommendations for clinical validation of novel thermal and non-thermal technologies—a western perspective. *Liver Cancer*. 2015;4(4):208–214. doi:10.1159/000367747
111. Littrup PJ, Aoun HD, Adam B, et al. Percutaneous cryoablation of hepatic tumors: long-term experience of a large U.S. series. *Abdom Radiol (NY)*. 2016;41(4):767–780. doi:10.1007/s00261-016-0687-x
112. Hakimé A, Le Cesne A, Deschamps F, et al. A role for adjuvant RFA in managing hepatic metastases from gastrointestinal stromal tumors (GIST) after treatment with targeted systemic therapy using kinase inhibitors. *Cardiovasc Intervent Radiol*. 2014;37(1):132–139. doi:10.1007/s00270-013-0615-1
113. Jones RL, McCall J, Adam A, et al. Radiofrequency ablation is a feasible therapeutic option in the multi modality management of sarcoma. *Eur J Surg Oncol*. 2010;36(5):477–482. doi:10.1016/j.ejso.2009.12.005
114. Gravel G, Yevich S, Tselikas L, et al. Percutaneous thermal ablation: a new treatment line in the multidisciplinary management of metastatic leiomyosarcoma? *Eur J Surg Oncol*. 2017;43(1):181–187. doi:10.1016/j.ejso.2016.06.391

115. Welch BT, Schmitz JJ, Atwell TD, et al. Evaluation of infectious complications following percutaneous liver ablation in patients with bilioenteric anastomoses. *Abdom Radiol (NY)*. 2017;42(5):1579–1582. doi:10.1007/s00261-017-1051-5
116. Akahane M, Koga H, Kato N, et al. Complications of percutaneous radiofrequency ablation for hepato-cellular carcinoma: imaging spectrum and management. *Radiographics*. 2005;25(suppl 1):S57–S68. doi:10.1148/rg.25si055505
117. Verloh N, Jensch I, Lürken L, et al. Similar complication rates for irreversible electroporation and thermal ablation in patients with hepatocellular tumors. *Radiol Oncol*. 2019;53(1):116–122. doi:10.2478/raon-2019-0011
118. de Baere T, Tselikas L, Woodrum D, et al. Evaluating cryoablation of metastatic lung tumors in patients—safety and efficacy: the ECLIPSE trial—interim analysis at 1 year. *J Thorac Oncol*. 2015;10(10):1468–1474. doi:10.1097/JTO.0000000000000632
119. Lencioni R, Crocetti L, Cioni R, et al. Response to radiofrequency ablation of pulmonary tumours: a prospective, intention-to-treat, multicentre clinical trial (the RAPTURE study). *Lancet Oncol*. 2008;9(7):621–628. doi:10.1016/S1470-2045(08)70155-4
120. Vogl TJ, Nour-Eldin A, Albrecht MH, et al. Thermal ablation of lung tumors: focus on microwave ablation. *Rofo*. 2017;189(9):828–843. doi:10.1055/s-0043-109010
121. Yuan Z, Wang Y, Zhang J, et al. A meta-analysis of clinical outcomes after radiofrequency ablation and microwave ablation for lung cancer and pulmonary metastases. *J Am Coll Radiol*. 2019;16(3):302–314. doi:10.1016/j.jacr.2018.10.012
122. Ricke J, Jürgens JHW, Deschamps F, et al. Irreversible electroporation (IRE) fails to demonstrate efficacy in a prospective multicenter phase II trial on lung malignancies: the ALICE trial. *Cardiovasc Intervent Radiol*. 2015;38(2):401–408. doi:10.1007/s00270-014-1049-0
123. Sato T, Iguchi T, Hiraki T, et al. Radiofrequency ablation of pulmonary metastases from sarcoma: single-center retrospective evaluation of 46 patients. *Jpn J Radiol*. 2017;35(2):61–67. doi:10.1007/s11604-016-0601-z
124. Steinke K, Sewell PE, Dupuy D, et al. Pulmonary radiofrequency ablation—an international study survey. *Anticancer Res*. 2004;24(1):339–343. http://ar.iiarjournals.org/content/24/1/339.full.pdf+html
125. Zheng A, Wang X, Yang X, et al. Major complications after lung microwave ablation: a single-center experience on 204 sessions. *Ann Thorac Surg*. 2014;98(1):243–248. doi:10.1016/j.athoracsur.2014.03.008
126. Tada A, Hiraki T, Iguchi T, et al. Influence of radiofrequency ablation of lung cancer on pulmonary function. *Cardiovasc Intervent Radiol*. 2012;35(4):860–867. doi:10.1007/s00270-011-0221-z
127. Hiraki T, Mimura H, Gobara H, et al. Two cases of needle-tract seeding after percutaneous radiofrequency ablation for lung cancer. *J Vasc Interv Radiol*. 2009;20(3):415–418. doi:10.1016/j.jvir.2008.12.411
128. Nakamura T, Matsumine A, Yamakado K, et al. Lung radiofrequency ablation in patients with pulmonary metastases from musculoskeletal sarcomas [corrected]. *Cancer*. 2009;115(16):3774–3781. doi:10.1002/cncr.24420

Index